Clinical Manual

for the Oncology Advanced Practice Nurse

Edited by
Dawn Camp-Sorrell, RN, MSN, FNP, AOCN®
Rebecca A. Hawkins, RN, MSN, ANP, AOCN®

Oncology Nursing Press, Inc.
A subsidiary of the Oncology Nursing Society
Pittsburgh, PA

Oncology Nursing Press, Inc.
Publisher: Leonard Mafrica, MBA, CAE
Director of Commercial Publications: Barbara Sigler, RN, MNEd
Staff Editor: Lisa M. George, BA
Copy Editor: Krista, Ramsey, BA
Creative Services Assistant: Dany Sjoen, Chad Chronick

Clinical Manual for the Oncology Advanced Practice Nurse

Library of Congress Card Catalog Number: 00-106771

ISBN 1-890504-19-X

Publisher's Note
This book is published by the Oncology Nursing Press, Inc. (ONP). ONP neither represents nor guarantees that the practices described herein will, if followed, ensure safe and effective patient care. The recommendations contained in this manual reflect ONP's judgment regarding the state of general knowledge and practice in the field as of the date of publication. The recommendations may not be appropriate for use in all circumstances. Those who use this book should make their own determinations regarding specific safe and appropriate patient-care practices, taking into account the personnel, equipment, and practices available at the hospital or other facility at which they are located. The editors and publisher cannot be held responsible for any liability incurred as a consequence from the use or application of any of the contents of these guidelines. Figures and tables are used as examples only. They are not meant to be all-inclusive, nor do they represent endorsement of any particular institution by the Oncology Nursing Society (ONS). Mention of specific products and opinions related to those products do not indicate or imply endorsement by ONS or ONP.

ONS and ONP publications are originally published in English. Permission has been granted by the ONS Board of Directors for foreign translation. (Individual tables and figures that are reprinted or adapted require additional permission from the original source.) However, because translations from English may not always be accurate and precise, ONS and ONP disclaim any responsibility for inaccurate translations. Readers relying on precise information should check the original English version.

Printed in the United States of America

Oncology Nursing Press, Inc.
A subsidiary of the Oncology Nursing Society

To our patients, who have taught us about the cancer experience, developed our hunger for knowledge, and made us strive to be better nurses.

We would also like to acknowledge the love and support of our family and friends who never let us lose the vision of this accomplishment.

DCS
RAH

Contributors

Co-Editors

Dawn Camp-Sorrell, RN, MSN, FNP, AOCN®
Oncology Nurse Practitioner
Central Alabama Hematology-Oncology Associates
Alabaster, Alabama
Chapter 1. Hiccups
Chapter 56. Hepatomegaly
Chapter 157. Phlebitis

Rebecca A. Hawkins, RN, MSN, ANP, AOCN®
Oncology Nurse Practitioner
St. Mary Regional Cancer Center
Pendleton, Oregon
Chapter 52. Constipation
Chapter 150. Hypothyroidism

Terri S. Armstrong, RN, MS, NP, CS
Neuro-Oncology Nurse Practitioner
Department of Neurosurgery
Emory Healthcare
The Emory Clinic, Inc.
Atlanta, Georgia
Chapter 134. Brain Metastasis
Chapter 136. Meningitis
Chapter 137. Neurotoxicity

Susan Baird-Powell, RN, MSN, CRNP
Panama City Beach, Florida
Chapter 143. Diabetes Mellitus, Types 1 and 2
Chapter 147. Hyponatremia/Hypernatremia
Chapter 149. Hyperthyroidism

Deborah McCaffrey Boyle, RN, MSN, AOCN®, FAAN
Oncology Clinical Nurse Specialist
Inova Fairfax Cancer Center
Falls Church, Virginia
Chapter 76. Hematuria
Chapter 80. Urinary Incontinence

Chapter 126. Confusion/Delirium
Chapter 131. Peripheral Neuropathy

George Bryant, ND, APN
Instructor
Myeloma and Transplantation Research Center
Arkansas Cancer Research Center
Little Rock, Arkansas
Introduction
Chapter 50. Abdominal Pain
Chapter 68. Hemorrhoids

Diane G. Cope, PhD, ARNP-CS, AOCN®
Nurse Practitioner
Florida Cancer Specialists
Fort Myers, Florida
Chapter 10. Rhinosinusitis
Chapter 42. Dyslipidemia
Chapter 66. Gastroesophageal Reflux Disease
Chapter 91. Lower Urinary Tract Infection—Cystitis
Chapter 93. Pyelonephritis
Chapter 110. Lymphedema

Aurelie C. Cormier, RN, MS, AOCN®
Clinical Nurse
Ambulatory Gyn Oncology
Brigham and Women's Hospital
Boston, Massachusetts
    Chapter 74. Amenorrhea
    Chapter 151. Menopausal Symptoms and
      Menopause

Susan A. Ezzone, MS, RN, CNP
Nurse Practitioner
Blood and Marrow Stem Cell Transplant
Arthur G. James Cancer Hospital and Rich-
    ard J. Solove Research Institute
Ohio State University Medical Center
Columbus, Ohio
    Chapter 27. Capillary Leak Syndrome
    Chapter 32. Pulmonary Edema
    Chapter 94. Syndrome of Inappropriate
      Antidiuretic Hormone
    Chapter 119. Disseminated Intravascular
      Coagulation
    Chapter 140. Fever
    Chaper 158. Total Parental Nutrition
      Ordering and Monitoring

Janet S. Fulton, PhD, RN
Associate Professor
Wright State University
Dayton, Ohio
    Chapter 16. Cellulitis
    Chapter 17. Decubitus Ulcer
    Chapter 18. Atopic Dermatitis
    Chapter 19. Contact Dermatitis
    Chapter 21. Skin Metastasis

Nancy C. Grandt, RN, CNP, MS, AOCN®
Nurse Practitioner
HealthEast Care System
St. Joseph's Hospital
St. Paul, Minnesota
    Chapter 34. Tuberculosis
    Chapter 69. Hepatitis
    Chapter 138. Spinal Cord Compression

Jeanne Held-Warmkessel, MSN, RN, CS,
    AOCN®
Clinical Nurse Specialist
Fox Chase Cancer Center
Philadelphia, Pennsylvania
    Chapter 53. Diarrhea
    Chapter 55. Hematemesis
    Chapter 58. Melena
    Chapter 60. Rectal Bleeding
    Chapter 63. Bowel Obstruction and Ileus
    Chapter 73. Peptic Ulcer Disease

Sandra C. Henke, RN, MS, ANP
Advanced Practice Nurse
Thoracic & Cardiovascular Surgery
University of Texas M.D. Anderson Cancer Cen-
    ter
Houston, Texas
    Chapter 24. Hemoptysis
    Chapter 28. Chronic Obstructive Pulmo-
      nary Disease
    Chapter 29. Pleural Effusion
    Chapter 31. Pneumothorax
    Chapter 33. Pulmonary Embolism

Cindy Jo Horrell, MS, CRNP, AOCN®
Oncology Nurse Practitioner
Clinical Associates
The Regional Cancer Center
Erie, Pennsylvania
    Chapter 36. Angina
    Chapter 57. Jaundice
    Chapter 64. Cirrhosis
    Chapter 70. Hepatotoxicity
    Chapter 72. Pancreatitis

Jennifer S. Jockel, RN, BSN, OCN®
Clinical Nurse III
Memorial Sloan Kettering Cancer Center
New York, New York
    Chapter 82. Vaginal Stenosis

Lisa Keel, RN, MSN, CNS
Clinical Nurse Specialist
Cardiology Care Unit
Johns Hopkins Hospital
Baltimore, Maryland
    Chapter 47. Myocardial Infarction

Martha E. Langhorne, MSN, RN, FNP
Oncology Advanced Practice Nurse
United Health Services Hospitals
UHS Cancer Care Center
Johnson City, New York

Joanne Lester, MSN, RNC, OCN® CNP
Nurse Practitioner
Division of Surgical Oncology
Arthur G. James Cancer Hospital and Richard J. Solove Research Institute
Ohio State University Medical Center
Columbus, Ohio

Mary Pat Lynch, CRNP, MSN, AOCN®
Oncology Nurse Practitioner
Clinical Faculty
Oncology Advanced Practice Nurse Program
University of Pennsylvania School of Nursing
Philadelphia, Pennsylvania

Karen E. Maher, ANP, MS, AOCN®
Nurse Practitioner
Radiation Oncology
Radiation Oncologists, PC

Legacy Portland Hospitals
Portland, Oregon

Madonna K. McDermott, RN, MS, ANP,
    OCN®
Adult Nurse Practitioner
United Pain Center
St. Paul, Minnesota

Debra J. Mercy, MS, CRNP, AOCN®
Adult Oncology Nurse Practitioner
Saint Alphonsus Cancer Treatment Center
Boise, Idaho

Amy Crawford Minchin, RN, MSN, ANCC
Clinical Research Coordinator
Pittsburgh Cancer Institute
Pittsburgh, Pennsylvania

Jay M. Mirtallo, MS, RPh, BCNSP
Specialty Practice Pharmacist
Nutrition/Surgery
Department of Pharmacy
Ohio State University Medical Center
Columbus, Ohio

Giselle J. Moore-Higgs, ARNP, MSN
Nurse Practitioner and Clinic Coordinator
Department of Radiation Oncology

University of Florida College of Medicine
Gainesville, Florida

Kathleen Murphy-Ende, RN, PhD, CFNP
Oncology Nurse Practitioner and Research
   Associate
School of Nursing
University of Wisconsin Hospital and Clinics
Madison, Wisconsin

Lillian M. Nail, PhD, RN, FAAN
Professor and Peery Presidential Endowed
   Chair
College of Nursing
University of Utah
Salt Lake City, Utah

Ann O'Mara, PhD, MPh, RN, AOCN®
Cancer Prevention Fellow
National Cancer Institute
Potomac, Maryland

Julie D. Painter, RNC, MSN, OCN®
Clinical Nurse Specialist
Adult Nurse Practitioner
Community Hospital of Indianapolis
Indianapolis, Indiana

Mary P. Pazdur, RN, MSN, AOCN®
Nurse Practitioner
Warren Grant Magnuson Clinical Center
National Institutes of Health
Bethesda, Maryland

Margaret Q. Rosenzweig, CRNP-C, MSN,
   AOCN®
Doctoral Candidate and Teaching Fellow
University of Pittsburgh School of Nursing
Pittsburgh, Pennsylvania

Kimberly A. Rumsey, RN, MSN
Family Practice Nurse Practitioner
Kimberly Schroeder, PADO
Tomball, Texas

Barbara St. Marie, RN, MA, CNP, ANP, GNP
Nurse Practitioner
Pain Management Center
Fairview/University Medical Center
Minneapolis, Minnesota

Gail Egan Sansivero, MS, ANP, AOCN®
Nurse Practitioner
The Institute for Vascular Health and Disease
Albany Medical College
Albany, New York

Chapter 4. Sore Throat (Pharyngitis)
Chapter 51. Ascites
Chapter 54. Heartburn/Indigestion/
    Dyspepsia
Chapter 61. Splenomegaly
Chapter 65. Dysphagia

Gena Schottmuller, RN, BA, CIC
System Director, Infection Control
HealthEast Care System
St. Joseph's Hospital
St. Paul, Minnesota
    Chapter 34. Tuberculosis

Brenda K. Shelton, RN, MS, CCRN, AOCN®
Critical Care Clinical Nurse Specialist
The Johns Hopkins Oncology Center
Baltimore, Maryland
    Chapter 37. Palpitations
    Chapter 43. Dysrhythmias
    Chapter 44. Endocarditis
    Chapter 47. Myocardial Infarction
    Chapter 48. Pericarditis/Pericardial
        Effusion/Tamponade

Wendy J. Smith, RN, MSN, ACNP, AOCN®
Acute Care Nurse Practitioner
North MS Hematology/Oncology Associates,
    Ltd.
Tupelo, Mississippi
    Chapter 144. Hypocalcemia/Hypercalcemia
    Chapter 145. Hypokalemia/Hyperkalemia
    Chapter 146. Hypomagnesemia/Hyper-
        magnesemia
    Chapter 147. Hyponatremia/
        Hypernatremia
    Chapter 148. Hypophosphatemia/
        Hyperphosphatemia

Laura M. Stempkowski, RN, MS, CUNP,
    AOCN®
Nurse Practitioner

GU Oncology
Dartmouth-Hitchcock Medical Center
Lebanon, New Hampshire
    Chapter 84. Adrenal Metastasis
    Chapter 141. Flu-Like Syndrome

Kristine Turner Story, RN, MSN, ARNP
Adult Nurse Practitioner
Physicians Clinic
Internal Medicine Midwest
Omaha, Nebraska
    Chapter 5. Tinnitus
    Chapter 7. Conjunctivitis
    Chapter 41. Deep Vein Thrombosis
    Chapter 67. Gastritis
    Chapter 71. Irritable Bowel Syndrome

Roberta A. Strohl, RN, BSN, MN, AOCN®
Clinical Nurse Specialist, Radiation Oncol-
    ogy
University of Maryland
Baltimore, Maryland
    Chapter 11. Stomatitis/Xerostomia
    Chapter 78. Penile Discharge
    Chapter 81. Vaginal Discharge
    Chapter 88. Hemorrhagic Cystitis
    Chapter 92. Prostatitis: Lower Urinary
        Tract Symptoms
    Chapter 103. Bone Metastasis
    Chapter 135. Headache

Mary Ann Winokur, CRNP, MSN
Nurse Practitioner
Department of Cardiovascular Medicine
University of Alabama at Birmingham
Birmingham, Alabama
    Chapter 38. Peripheral Edema
    Chapter 40. Congestive Heart Failure
    Chapter 45. Hypertension
    Chapter 46. Hypotension
    Chapter 49. Peripheral Vascular Disease

Reviewers

Emil (Bud) Bardana, MD
Professor of Medicine
Division of Allergy and Clinical Immunology
Oregon Health Sciences University
Portland, Oregon

Donna L. Berry, RN, PhD, AOCN®
Research Assistant Professor
Biobehavioral Nursing and Health Systems
University of Washington
Seattle, Washington

Deborah L. Bolton, RN, OCN®, MN, CNS-FNP
Clinical Nurse Specialist, Hematology/Oncology
UCLA Medical Center
Los Angeles, California

Jeannine M. Brant, RN, MS, AOCN®
Oncology Clinical Nurse Specialist and Pain Consultant
Saint Vincent Hospital and Health Center
Billings, Montana

Cynthia Chernecky, RN, PhD, CNS, AOCN®
Associate Professor
Department of Adult Health
School of Nursing
Medical College of Georgia
Augusta, Georgia
Visiting Scholar
School of Nursing
University of California Los Angeles
Los Angeles, California

Alan Fleischer, MD
Department of Dermatology
Wake Forest University Baptist Medical Center
Winston-Salem, North Carolina

Mark R. Gilbert, MD
Associate Professor
Chief, Division of Neuro-Oncology
Emory University
Atlanta, Georgia

Eric B. Goosenberg, MD
Gastroenterologist, Director of Endoscopy
Fox Chase Cancer Center
Philadelphia, Pennsylvania

Judith A. Headley, RN, PhD, AOCN®
Assistant Professor, Division of Oncology
School of Nursing
University of Texas Health Science Center–Houston
Houston, Texas

Catherine Hogan, MN, RN, CS, AOCN®
Clinical Assistant Professor of Medicine
UNC Medical Center
Chapel Hill, North Carolina

Ryan Iwamoto, ARNP, MN, AOCN®
Cancerfacts.com
Seattle, Washington

Jonas T. Johnson, MD, FACS
Vice Chairman, Department of Otolaryngology
Director, Otolaryngology Residency Training Program
University of Pittsburgh School of Medicine
Pittsburgh, Pennsylvania

Anita Yeomans Kinney, PhD, APRN
Assistant Professor
College of Nursing
University of Utah
Salt Lake City, Utah

Patricia A. Kormanik, MS, C-ANP, OCN®
Certified Adult Nurse Practitioner
University of California San Diego Cancer
    Center
La Jolla, California

Elizabeth Lowenthal, DO
Central Alabama Hematology/Oncology As-
    sociates
Baptist Health Center
Alabaster, Alabama

Terri Maxwell, RN, MSN, AOCN®
Executive Director
Center for Palliative Care
Thomas Jefferson University
Philadelphia, Pennsylvania

Richard A. Menin, MD
Director, Gastrointestinal Cancer Program
Albert Einstein Medical Center
Philadelphia, Pennsylvania

Kenneth S. O'Rourke, MD
Assistant Professor
Department of Medicine
Wake Forest University School of Medicine
Winston-Salem, North Carolina

Maureen E. O'Rourke, RN, PhD
Assistant Professor, Nursing
University of North Carolina
Greensboro, North Carolina
Adjunct Assistant Professor of Medicine
Wake Forest University School of Medicine
Winston-Salem, North Carolina

Anthony J. Pinevich, MD
Chairman, Department of Physician Assistant
Duquesne University
Pittsburgh, Pennsylvania

Vincent G. Powell, RN
Panama City Beach, Florida

Julie Rose, MD
Medical Director
St. Mary Regional Cancer Center
Walla Walla, Washington

Susan F. Rudy, MSN, CRNP, CORLN
Research Nurse Practitioner
National Institute on Deafness and Other
    Communication Disorders
Bethesda, Maryland

Deborah Rust, RN, MSN, CRNP, AOCN®
Program Coordinator, Oncology Nurse Prac-
    titioner Program
University of Pittsburgh School of Nursing
Nurse Practitioner
University of Pittsburgh Cancer Institute
Pittsburgh, Pennsylvania

Gary E. Shelton, RN, MSN, AOCN®
Research Clinical Nurse Specialist
Herbert Irving Comprehensive Cancer Center
New York Presbyterian Hospital
New York, New York

Patricia Spencer-Cisek, MS, RN, CS, ANP,
    AOCN®
Clinical Director, Oncology Services
Glens Falls Hospital
Glens Falls, New York

Malcolm Townsley, MD, PhD
Chief of Staff, St. Anthony's Hospital
Pendleton Internal Medicine Specialists
Pendleton, Oregon

Table of Contents

Preface

Oncology advanced practice nurses (OAPNs) are becoming more abundant in providing care to patients with cancer. OAPNs work differently than physicians by bringing a nursing perspective and nursing skills to patient encounters. Never before has the healthcare system so critically needed caregivers with these attributes. With radical cost-containment strategies, restricted access to medical services, increased patient self-care, and payment for preventive services, OAPNs bring a clear value to payors of care and to patients with cancer and their families. OAPNs can successfully provide holistic care to patients either collaboratively or independently with the inclusion of primary care. The result is total care that is cost-effective and quality-driven.

As advanced practitioners, OAPNs possess steadfast knowledge of oncology; however, a growing need exists for OAPNs to make clinical decisions regarding internal medicine. Often, OAPNs are faced with patient complaints that are not related to the cancer process or side effects of cancer treatment. However, management of routine medical problems presents unique challenges in the cancer population. A clinical manual is needed to provide the necessary knowledge for managing the care of the patient with cancer.

This clinical manual is geared toward OAPNs who provide care to the patient with cancer and manage general medical problems. The manual is divided into symptoms and medical diagnoses within each body system. The last section is devoted to relevant clinical information, such as how to write orders for total parenteral nutrition or perform special physical examinations.

Clinical Manual for the Oncology Advanced Practice Nurse is intended to be a quick reference to guide OAPNs in diagnosing and treating acute and chronic problems seen in the patient with cancer. For example, if a patient presented with the complaint of a cough, the OAPN could review the cough section, ask the appropriate history questions, determine the appropriate diagnostic tests, interpret the tests, and narrow down the medical diagnosis. If the diagnosis was determined to be pneumonia, the OAPN could review the pneumonia section and treat or make the appropriate referral.

The manual is presented in an easy-to-read outline format containing comprehensive clinical material. Each section can stand alone, which may lead to duplication of information; however, this allows the manual to accommodate OAPNs on an as-needed basis.

Dawn Camp-Sorrell, RN, MSN, FNP, AOCN®
Rebecca A. Hawkins, RN, MSN, ANP, AOCN®

Section **I.** Introduction

I.

Introduction

George Bryant, ND, APN, and
Ann O'Mara, PhD, MPh, RN, AOCN®

The Role of the Advanced Practice Nurse in Cancer Care

Advanced practice nurses play a pivotal role in assisting patients across the cancer trajectory. From the time of diagnosis through the rehabilitative phase of cancer care, the skills and knowledge of both clinical nurse specialists and nurse practitioners are essential to patients receiving high-quality, comprehensive cancer care. In particular, expert clinical judgment and leadership often have been cited as the two most important components in the delivery of expert patient care by advanced practice nurses (Chuk, 1997; Martin & Coniglio, 1996). Because patients with cancer are living longer with their disease, clinicians are faced not only with managing the cancer but also with managing the other chronic diseases that afflict the adult population (Bramble, 1995). Given these changing demographics, the role of the advanced practice nurse can only expand to meet the increasing healthcare needs of our surviving chronically ill population.

I. History taking: Obtaining a careful, detailed history is critical to making an accurate, definitive diagnosis.
   A. Eight categories are used as a guide when gathering data.
      1. Description of the patient
      2. The patient's chief complaint
      3. Other healthcare providers involved in the patient's care
      4. History of present illness
      5. Past medical history
      6. Social and occupational history
      7. Family history
      8. Review of systems
   B. Using the six variables of *what, where, when, how much, chronological course,* and *what exacerbates or lessens the symptom* will help to elicit a thorough documentation of the patient's problem.
   C. Several factors can limit history taking.
      1. The patient's mental state
      2. Unavailability of previous medical records
      3. Interplay of other coexisting chronic diseases that "may draw the attention of the clinician away from the patient's presenting complaint" (Szaflarski, 1997, p. 293).

D. Depth and breadth of obtaining the past medical, social, and family history are determined by the acuity of the patient's symptomatology and the clinician's relationship with the patient.

E. Interview: The process of posing questions to elicit information, which is, thus, subjective data

1. Open-ended questions allow the patient to verbalize complaints and past history information.

2. Direct questions: Seek specific information.

3. Leading questions: The information provided may be what the patient thinks the clinician wants to know. These types of questions should be avoided.

    a) Chief complaint: A brief statement by the patient on the reason for seeking medical advice

    b) Present problem: Each problem should be explored fully.

        (1) Where: Location, extent of limitation, occurrence

        (2) When: Onset, duration, frequency

        (3) What: Patient's perception, quality, intensity, aggravating factors, associated factors

        (4) How: Associated factors, past episodes, coping, support systems

        (5) Why: The answer is the solution to the presenting problem.

        (6) State of health immediately prior to presenting with the problem and complete description of the symptom must be obtained.

        (7) Review with the patient for accuracy.

    c) Past medical history

        (1) General health

        (2) Childhood illnesses: Chicken pox, measles, mumps, etc.

        (3) Major adult illnesses: Tuberculosis, hepatitis, diabetes mellitus, hypertension, infections, nonsurgical hospital admissions

        (4) Immunizations: Childhood, tetanus, hepatitis

        (5) Surgery: Dates, diagnosis, complications, physician name, hospital

        (6) Trauma: Disabilities, fractures

        (7) Current medications: Prescribed, home remedies, over-the-counter

        (8) Allergies: Food, medications, environmental

        (9) Transfusions: Type, complications, reason

       (10) Obstetric history: Gravidity and parity

       (11) Last examination date

    d) Family history

        (1) Any members of the family (or significant others) with the features of the patient's presenting problem

        (2) Health and cause of death for parents or siblings

        (3) History of heart disease, renal disease, cancer, diabetes, tuberculosis, allergies, blood dyscrasias

    e) Social history

        (1) Marital status, children

        (2) Cultural and religious background

        (3) Hobbies, coping strategies, stress relievers

      (4) Tobacco or alcohol use
      (5) Sexual history: Birth control method, protective devices
      (6) Home conditions: Housing, economic type
      (7) Occupation: Type, conditions, exposure to harmful substances
      (8) Insurance
   f) Review of systems
      (1) General: Fatigue, fever, night sweats, weight change, behavior change (irritability)
      (2) Diet: Likes, dislikes, restrictions, 24-hour recall
      (3) Skin, hair, nails: Birthmarks, skin disease, pigment or color change, mottling, change in mole, pruritus, rash, lesion, acne, easy bruising or petechiae, easy bleeding
      (4) Musculoskeletal: Arthritis, joint pain, stiffness, swelling, limitation of movement, gait, strength and coordination, muscle pain, cramps and weakness, back pain, posture, spinal curvature
      (5) Head and neck: Headache, head injury, dizziness, swollen or tender glands, limitation of movement, stiffness
      (6) Endocrine: Diabetes mellitus, thyroid disease, excessive hunger or thirst, frequent urination, unusual hair distribution, precocious or delayed puberty
      (7) Lungs: Croup, asthma, wheezing or noisy breathing, shortness of breath, chronic cough
      (8) Heart: Congenital heart problems, history of murmur and cyanosis, limitation of activity, dyspnea on exertion, palpitations, high blood pressure, coldness in the extremities
      (9) Breasts: Performance of breast self-exam, lumps, tenderness, swelling, redness, dimpling, retraction
    (10) Hematologic: Excessive bruising, lymph node swelling, exposure to toxic agents or radiation
    (11) Gastrointestinal: Abdominal pain, nausea and vomiting, history of ulcer, stool color and characteristics, diarrhea, constipation or stool-holding, rectal bleeding, anal itching, history of pinworms, use of laxatives
    (12) Genitourinary: Painful urination, polyuria/oliguria, narrowed stream, urine color, history of urinary tract infections; in men, penis or testicular pain, sores or lesions, discharge, hernia or hydrocele, swelling in scrotum; in women, genital itching, rash, vaginal discharge
    (13) Neurological: Numbness, tingling, altered sensation or mobility
    (14) Psychiatric/emotional status: Constellation of family and friends, recent losses (e.g., employment, spouse, friends), how person deals with stress
   g) Biographical data: Age, sex, race, marital status, ethnic origin, occupation
F. Types of history
  1. Complete: Thorough review of the patient's past and current state of health, associated factors, and hereditary factors; usually recorded at initial visit and added to with subsequent visits
  2. Inventory: Ascertainment of major points of the history until sufficient time can be given to obtain a complete history

3. Problem (focused): Basic information taken usually during an acute situation, such as life-threatening or requiring immediate attention
4. Interim: Obtaining information, to add onto the complete history, of chronicled events that have occurred since previous visit

II. Physical exam
   A. Goal: To elicit signs of the disease hypothesis considered as a result of the history
   B. Evaluate abnormalities unnoticed by the patient.
   C. Step-by-step approach from head to toe
   D. Four methods of examination (in order)
      1. Inspection
      2. Palpation
      3. Percussion
      4. Auscultation (done before palpation in the abdominal exam)
   E. System approach
      1. Skin, hair, and nails
         a) Texture
         b) Temperature
         c) Color
         d) Distribution
         e) Lesions
      2. Head
         a) Configuration
         b) Scalp tenderness, masses
      3. Eyes
         a) Visual acuity (chart)
         b) Extraocular movements (EOMs)
         c) Visual fields
         d) Conjunctivae, sclerae
         e) PERRLA: Pupils equal, round, reactive to light and accommodation
         f) Funduscopic exam: Lens, disc, and retina
      4. Ears
         a) Auditory acuity, Weber, and Rinne tests
         b) Otoscopic exam of canal and tympanic membranes
      5. Mouth
         a) Lips
         b) Tongue
         c) Teeth and gingiva
         d) Buccal mucosa
         e) Pharynx
      6. Neck and axillae
         a) Symmetry of neck and breasts
         b) Thyroid gland and carotid pulses
         c) Lymph node palpation

   d) Thyroid and trachea
   e) Jugular venous distention and neck distention
  7. Chest
   a) Symmetry
   b) Percuss lung fields and point of maximum intensity.
   c) Auscultate lungs and heart sounds.
   d) Perform breast examination.
   e) Assess for carotid bruits.
  8. Hands and upper extremities
   a) Evaluate skin, muscles, joints, and range of motion (ROM).
   b) Check pulses.
   c) Assess deep tendon reflexes (DTR).
   d) Evaluate strength.
  9. Abdomen
   a) Inspect for pulsations, hernias, or striae.
   b) Auscultate for bruits and bowel sounds.
   c) Percuss/palpate liver, spleen, and masses.
   d) Palpate lymph nodes and pulses.
  10. Legs and lower extremities
   a) Evaluate skin, muscles, joints, and ROM.
   b) Check pulses.
   c) Assess DTRs.
   d) Assess strength.
  11. Male genitalia
   a) Inspect and palpate.
   b) Perform digital exam of rectum and prostate.
  12. Female genitalia
   a) Inspect and palpate.
   b) Perform pelvic exam with Pap smear.
   c) Perform rectal exam.

III. Diagnostic tests
 A. Laboratory
 B. Radiological, such as
  1. Standard x-rays: Chest, bone film, kidney, ureters, and bladder (KUB)
  2. Computed tomography (CT) scans
  3. Magnetic resonance imaging (MRI)
 C. Specialized/invasive testing
  1. Nuclear medicine: Multiple-gated acquisition (MUGA) scan
  2. Nerve conduction studies: Peripheral neuropathy
  3. Ultrasound
  4. Barium studies
  5. Endoscopy/colonoscopy
 D. Natural progression in ordering studies: Basic to complex to invasive
 E. Review of data

1. Presenting symptoms
2. Physical exam findings and history
3. Diagnostic testing abnormalities or normal findings
4. Synthesis and definitive diagnosis
5. Treatment plan and management

IV. Analyzing and interpreting symptoms and history
   A. Collect all pertinent clinical data.
      1. History
      2. Physical exam
      3. Diagnostic tests
   B. Ask, "What could be the cause(s) producing the chief complaint?"
   C. Synthesize knowledge base.
      1. Classic textbook signs and symptoms
      2. Past clinical experience
      3. Current clinical picture
   D. Formulate potential list of differential diagnoses.

V. Differential diagnosis
   A. Problem-solving process
   B. Diagnostic plan to rule out other possible conditions
   C. Determining risk factors: Age, sex, family history, environment
   D. Intuition-based thinking
   E. Making hypothesis to possible diagnosis
   F. Confirmation testing to rule out other potential diagnoses
   G. Reinforcing assumptions
      1. Original diagnosis
      2. Exacerbations of chronic diseases may be secondary to a new problem.
      3. Laboratory and diagnostic testing validates findings.
   H. Confirmation of diagnosis
      1. Until certain, potentials must be considered.
      2. Ordering diagnostic workup for verification
      3. Review of synthesized information
      4. Making the definitive diagnosis
   I. Initiation of treatment and management

VI. Treatment and management
   A. Nonpharmacologic
      1. Alternative health methods: Acupuncture, therapeutic touch therapy, macrobiotics
      2. Diet and exercise
      3. Allied health methods: Physical and occupational therapy
   B. Pharmacologic
      1. Standard based on the classic textbook approach

      2. State-of-the-art based on new research
      3. Investigational/experimental

VII. Referral process
    A. Interdisciplinary care
    B. Knowledge of scope of practice
      1. Aware of limitations
      2. Written agreements (in certain states)
      3. Physician collaboration
        a) New diagnosis
        b) Initiation of pharmacologic treatment
        c) Patient unresponsive to first-line therapy
    C. Recurrence of initial presenting problem several months after treatment
    D. Requires additional diagnostic testing for diagnosis
      1. Radiographic study: Radiologist
      2. Cystoscopy: Urologist
      3. Cardiac catheterization: Cardiologist
    E. Specialized problem requiring a specialist in the field such as
      1. Myocardial infarction: Cardiologist
      2. Seizure or stroke: Neurologist
      3. Fractured femur: Orthopedist
      4. Breast cancer: Oncologist

VIII. Follow-up
    A. Short-term
      1. Evaluate new treatment.
      2. Make changes in therapy if needed (e.g., increase drug dosage).
      3. Determine if patient is tolerating treatment.
      4. Monitor compliance with regimen.
      5. Provide patient teaching for prevention of recurrent episodes.
      6. Establish long-term goal of therapy once patient is tolerating therapy and the desired results are being met.
    B. Long-term
      1. Provide a maintenance check-up.
      2. Reevaluate the current therapy for adjustment, if needed.
      3. Reinforce patient teaching.
      4. Continue with long-term goal to prevent further exacerbations.
      5. Maintain follow-up as needed.

References

Bramble, K. (1995). Spotlight on nurse practitioner practice. *Nurse Practitioner Forum, 6,* 180–182.

Chuk, P. (1997). Clinical nurse specialists and quality patient care. *Journal of Advanced Nursing, 26,* 501–506.

Cutler, P. (1998). *Problem solving in clinical medicine: From data to diagnosis* (3rd ed.). Baltimore: Williams & Wilkins.

Holleman, D.R., & Simel, D.L. (1997). Quantitative assessments from the clinical examination. How should clinicians integrate the numerous results? *Journal of General Internal Medicine, 12,* 165–171.

Martin, B., & Coniglio, J.U. (1996). The acute care nurse practitioner in collaborative practice. *AACN Clinical Issues, 7,* 309–314.

Peters, R.M. (1995). The role of intuitive thinking in the diagnostic process. *Archives of Family Medicine, 4,* 939–941.

Szaflarski, N.L. (1997). Diagnostic reasoning in acute and critical care. *AACN Clinical Issues, 8,* 291–302.

Section II.

Head and Neck

Symptoms

Medical Diagnosis

Chapter

1.

Hiccups

Dawn Camp-Sorrell, RN, MSN, FNP, AOCN®

I. Definition: Phenomenon characterized by repetitive, sharp inspiratory sounds associated with spasm of the glottis and diaphragm
   A. Bout: Episode persisting as long as 48 hours
   B. Persistent: Episode persisting longer than 48 hours but less than one month
   C. Intractable: Episode lasting longer than one month

II. Pathophysiology
   A. Synchronous clonic spasm of the intercostal muscles and diaphragm causes sudden inspiration followed by prompt closure of the glottis, causing the hiccup sound and inhibiting respirations.
   B. Hiccups are a reflex arc in the upper segments of the cervical (C) spinal cord (between C-3 and C-5) and travel an afferent pathway over vagal sympathetic and sensory fibers of the phrenic nerve.
      1. Afferent pathway of hiccup reflex encompasses the phrenic and vagus nerves and the sympathetic chain arising from thoracic (T) segments T-6 to T-12.
      2. Primary efferent reflex branch is the phrenic nerve; however, the glottis and accessory muscles of the respiratory nerves have been suggested as the efferent pathway.

III. Clinical features: Hiccups are a transient, innocuous symptom; can become exhausting and disabling (e.g., respiratory insufficiency) if they persist; and are classified as psychogenic, organic, and idiopathic. Persistent and intractable hiccups occur more frequently in men and they serve no known physiologic function.
   A. Etiology: Benign bouts are self-limited and caused by
      1. Gastric distention
      2. Alcohol intake
      3. Tobacco
      4. Sudden excitement
      5. Sudden change in gastrointestinal temperature (i.e., from drinking a hot or cold beverage)
      6. Carbonated beverage intake.
   B. History
      1. History of cancer and cancer treatment

      2. Current medications: Prescribed and over-the-counter
      3. History of presenting symptom(s): Precipitating factors, onset, location, and duration
      4. Changes in activities of daily living
      5. Past medical history: Recent abdominal, thoracic, or neurologic surgery; emotional problems
      6. Social history of alcohol intake

  C. Signs and symptoms of intractable hiccups
      1. Dyspnea
      2. Anorexia
      3. Weight loss
      4. Fatigue and exhaustion
      5. Insomnia
      6. Heartburn (from severe gastric reflux)
      7. Depression

  D. Physical exam
      1. Head, eyes, ears, nose, and throat (HEENT): Examine for evidence of trauma.
        a) Mucous membranes: Assess for dehydration.
        b) Assess for mucal rigidity, thyromegaly, and cervical adenopathy.
      2. Integument exam: Observe for wound dehiscence as a secondary problem from hiccups.
      3. Pulmonary exam
        a) Conduct percussion for evidence of reduced diaphragmatic excursion.
        b) Auscultate for abnormal sounds indicating infiltrate, effusion, or pleuritis.
      4. Abdominal exam: Examine for distention or organomegaly.
      5. Neurologic exam: Assess for mental changes indicating stroke, brain metastasis, dehydration, or trauma.

IV. Diagnostic tests
  A. Laboratory: Not indicated
  B. Radiology
      1. Chest x-ray: To rule out pulmonary, mediastinal, or cardiac abnormalities capable of irritating phrenic nerve, vagal nerve, or diaphragm
      2. CT scan of the abdomen: To evaluate for abnormalities of the subdiaphragmatic region
      3. CT scan or MRI of head: To evaluate for lesions or bleeds

V. Differential diagnosis
  A. Structural defect
      1. Pericarditis (see Chapter 48)
      2. Malignancy
      3. Subdiaphragmatic abscess
      4. Hiatal hernia
      5. Myocardial infarction (see Chapter 47)
      6. Peritonitis
      7. Pancreatitis (see Chapter 72)

      8. Biliary tract disease
      9. Feeding tube
  B. Metabolic disturbances
      1. Uremia
      2. Diabetes mellitus (see Chapter 143)
      3. Alcoholism
      4. Goiter (see Chapters 149 and 150)
  C. Central nervous system disorders
      1. Infection (see Chapter 140)
      2. Multiple sclerosis
  D. Thorax-related
      1. Ulcer
      2. Abscess
      3. Aneurysm
      4. Pleuritis
      5. Pneumonia (see Chapter 30)
  E. Drug-induced
      1. Corticosteriods (e.g., dexamethasone, methylprednisolone)
      2. Benzodiazepines (e.g., midazolam, chlordiazepoxide)
      3. Anesthesia
  F. Psychogenic disease
      1. Hysteria
      2. Anorexia nervosa
      3. Anxiety (see Chapter 152)

VI. Treatment: Overall goal is to relieve the patient of this symptom.
  A. Nonpharmacologic measures
      1. Hold breath.
      2. Breathe into a paper bag.
      3. Swallow a teaspoonful of granulated sugar.
      4. Stimulate the gag reflex.
      5. Lift uvula with a spoon.
      6. Gargle with or sip ice water.
      7. Bite a lemon wedge.
      8. Inhale a noxious irritant (e.g., ammonia).
      9. Interrupt vagal stimulation by Valsalva maneuver, carotid massage, supraorbital pressure, irritation of tympanic membrane, or digital rectal massage.
    10. Disrupt phrenic nerve transmission.
       a) Rhythmically tap over fifth cervical vertebra.
       b) Apply ice to skin over phrenic nerve.
       c) Apply electric stimulation over phrenic nerve.
    11. Counterirritation of the diaphragm.
       a) Pull knees to chest.
       b) Lean forward to compress chest.
       c) Apply pressure at points of diaphragmatic insertion.

12. Induce vomiting if cause is gastric distention.
13. Hypnosis
14. Acupuncture

B. Pharmacologic measures: To interrupt afferent and efferent pathways
   1. Antipsychotics
      a) Chlorpromazine: 25–50 mg po initially with maintenance therapy of 25 mg qid
      b) Haloperidol: 2–5 mg IM initially with maintenance of 1–4 mg po tid
   2. Anticonvulsants
      a) Valproic acid: 250 mg po per day in divided doses for two weeks; no long-term use because of potential hepatotoxicity
      b) Phenytoin: Initially 200 mg IV followed by maintenance dose of 300 mg po qd
   3. Miscellaneous
      a) Metoclopramide: 10 mg po tid after large-dose IV (2 mg/kg)
      b) Baclofen: 10 mg po qid
C. Surgical infiltration of the phrenic nerve: When other measures have not been successful
   1. Injection of long-acting anesthetic or alcohol
   2. Crushing or cutting the phrenic nerve

VII. Follow-up: Depends on etiology and occurrence of hiccups
   A. For persistent and intractable hiccups, see patient daily until interventions have been successful and maintenance dose is managed.
   B. If patient is taking anticonvulsant or antipsychotic drugs, monitor serum levels every two weeks or monthly, as well as liver function tests if indicated.
   C. Hospitalization may be warranted if patient has persistent or intractable hiccups to aggressively manage symptom.

VIII. Referrals
   A. Surgeon: If invasive procedure is necessary
   B. Anesthesiologist: For phrenic nerve block

References

Cersosimo, R.J., & Brophy, M.T. (1998). Hiccups with high dose dexamethasone administration. *Cancer, 82,* 412–416.

Johnson, R.R., & Kriel, R.L. (1996). Baclofen for chronic hiccups. *Pediatric Neurology, 15*(1), 66–67.

Okuda, Y., Kitajima, T., & Asai, T. (1998). Use of a nerve stimulator for phrenic nerve block in treatment of hiccups. *Anesthesiology, 88,* 525–526.

Petroianu, G., Hein, G., Petroianu, A., Bergler, W., & Rufer, R. (1997). Idiopathic chronic hiccup: Combination therapy with cisapride, omeprazole, and baclofen. *Clinical Therapeutics, 19,* 1031–1038.

Rousseau, P. (1995). Hiccups. *Southern Medical Journal, 88*(2), 175–181.

Thompson, D.F., & Landry, J.P. (1997). Drug-induced hiccups. *Annals of Pharmacotherapy, 31,* 367–369.

Chapter

2.

Hoarseness/Dysphonia

Joanne Lester, MSN, RNC, OCN®, CNP

I. Definition: Terms that describe voice changes

II. Physiology/Pathophysiology
   A. Normal physiology
      1. Vocal quality is determined by multiple factors.
         a) Distance between vocal cords
         b) Tenseness of vocal cords
         c) Rapidity of vibration
         d) Innervation controlling these areas
      2. Vocal cord position
         a) While breathing, the vocal cords remain apart, and air passes through the opening without making sound.
         b) When a person is speaking or singing, the vocal cords come together and vibrate to create sound.
   B. Pathophysiology: Hoarseness results when the cord structure and function are altered, preventing normal apposition.

III. Clinical features
   A. Etiology
      1. Breathy voice sounds are caused by air escaping during vocalization as a result of paresis or paralysis.
      2. Raspy or harsh voice sounds are a result of thickened or irregular vocal cords from inflammation, infection, edema, abuse, nodules, polyps, papilloma, or tumor.
      3. High, shaky voice sounds result from decreased respiratory force (i.e., phonasthenia) from neurologic impairment.
      4. Laryngitis has a chemical, traumatic, or inflammatory cause.
      5. Excessive use of voice, strain, shouting
   B. History
      1. History of cancer and cancer treatment
      2. Current medications: Prescribed and over-the-counter
      3. History of presenting symptom(s): Precipitating factors, onset, location, and duration
      4. Changes in activities of daily living

     5. Occupational history: Exposure to dust, fire, smoke, or irritant fumes
     6. Social history of alcohol and tobacco use
     7. History of recent upper respiratory tract infection, sore throat, fever, chills, thyroid disorder, myalgia (self or family member)
     8. Past medical history: Neck mass, neck or thoracic surgery, intubation, lung tumor, thyroid disorder, trauma

C. Signs and symptoms
     1. Quality of voice (e.g., completely lost, raspy, breathy, coarse, strident)
       a) Changes in volume, quality, flexibility, or pitch
       b) Continuous or intermittent; sudden onset, progressive, or chronic
     2. Nasal or pharyngeal drainage or congestion
     3. Shortness of breath
     4. Neck swelling
     5. Hemoptysis
     6. Difficulty swallowing
     7. Indigestion
     8. Sore throat

D. Physical exam: Patients experiencing hoarseness for greater than two weeks must be referred for a laryngoscopy.
     1. HEENT exam
       a) Inspection of nose, paranasal sinuses, nasopharynx, and ears: Look for abnormal anatomy, excess tissue, abnormal growths, mechanical obstruction/foreign objects, or inflammation/infection.
       b) Palpation of thyroid, head and neck lymph nodes, oral cavity: Look for abnormal anatomy, excess tissue, abnormal growths, lymphadenopathy, or inflammation/infection.
       c) Indirect laryngoscopy: Essential for patients with a history of hoarseness for greater than two weeks; visualizes the hypopharynx and larynx to detect obstruction, inflammation/infection, incomplete closure of vocal cords, abnormal anatomy, excess tissue, or abnormal growths
     2. Pulmonary exam: Assess for obstruction/absence of lung sounds or adventitious sounds.
     3. Focused neurologic exam: Examine head, face, and neck regions for abnormal response to expected normal neurologic exam, focusing on cranial nerves I–XII (see Appendix 5).

IV. Diagnostic tests
A. Laboratory
     1. Thyroid function studies (thyroid-stimulating hormone [TSH], serum T_4): If enlarged thyroid, to rule out thyroid disease
     2. Biopsy: Required for all suspicious lesions
B. Radiology
     1. Chest x-ray (PA and lateral): For suspected malignancy or nerve or chest involvement
     2. CT scan of head and neck or chest: For suspected malignancy

    3. MRI of head and neck: If CT scan results inconclusive
  C. Other: Direct laryngoscopy by skilled clinician to visualize larynx and vocal cords

V. Differential diagnosis
  A. Neoplastic and dysplastic
    1. Vocal cord cancer
    2. Supraglottic cancer with muscle invasion
    3. Leukoplakia
    4. Central nervous system (CNS) tumor affecting cranial nerve X
  B. Infectious
    1. Viral laryngitis
    2. Bacterial tracheitis or laryngitis
    3. Croup
    4. Papillomatosis
  C. Traumatic
    1. Vocal cord nodules
    2. Vocal cord polyp
    3. Smoke irritation
    4. Gastroesophageal reflux (see Chapter 66)
    5. External laryngeal trauma
    6. Senile atrophy
  D. Neurologic
    1. Tumor compression (e.g., glomus, thyroid, pulmonary, esophageal)
    2. Trauma to nerves
    3. Neural tumors
    4. Neuromuscular disease (e.g., Parkinsonism, tremor of cords, spasmodic dysphonia)
    5. Dystonia
    6. Cerebral vascular accident
  E. Functional
    1. Hysterical aphonia (i.e., absence of voice from psychiatric hysteria)
    2. Ventricular dysphonia
    3. Hyperkinetic dysphonia
    4. Vocal abuse (i.e., overuse or exaggerated use, such as screaming)
  F. Endocrine
    1. Hypothyroidism (see Chapter 150)
    2. Adrenal insufficiency
    3. Acromegaly
    4. Hormones (e.g., birth control pills, menopause)
    5. Menopause (see Chapter 151)

VI. Treatment
  A. Treatment for simple hoarseness depends on the resolution of etiologic factor(s), as well as localized, symptomatic relief.
    1. Treat underlying infectious process with antibiotics.

2. In trauma, eliminate causative factors (e.g., smoking, exposure to chemical toxins, overuse or abuse of vocal cords).
3. Patients must drink plenty of fluids, rest the voice for 24–72 hours, and use a humidifier, especially at night.
4. In severe laryngitis, inhaled or systemic corticosteroids may effectively assist rapid resolution.

B. When gastroesophageal reflux is identified as the causative factor, employ aggressive therapy to reduce the acid production and resulting acid splash (see Chapter 66).

VII. Follow-up
A. Short-term follow-up should occur within 48 hours of initial contact to verify partial or complete resolution of symptoms.
B. Long-term follow-up depends on the etiology and causative factors, as well as persistence of symptoms.

VIII. Referral
A. No referral: Patients who improve significantly or spontaneously resolve within 48 hours (without evidence of underlying disease) and patients with symptoms related to a previously diagnosed chronic illness (e.g., terminal malignancies) may possibly be managed without a physician referral.
B. Family/general practice physician: Refer patients who do not improve or resolve after 48 hours.
C. Otolaryngologist: Refer patients who have hoarseness for longer than two weeks for a complete exam, including a laryngoscopy for removal of mass, nodules, or polyps.
D. Acute or more complex etiologies must be diagnosed and managed by an otolaryngologist or pulmonologist. Hospitalization may be required, especially in cases with concurrent dyspnea.
E. Speech pathologist: Referral may be helpful to retrain the voice through vocal therapy.

References

Dettelbach, M., Eibling, D.E., & Johnson, J.T. (1994). Hoarseness: From viral laryngitis to glottic cancer. *Postgraduate Medicine, 95*(5), 143–162.

Garrett, C.G., & Ossoff, R.H. (1995). Hoarseness: Contemporary diagnosis and management. *Comprehensive Therapy, 21,* 705–710.

Lyons, B.M. (1994). Ear, nose and throat disorders: "Doctor, my voice seems husky." *Australian Family Physician, 23,* 2111–2119.

Mitchell, I.C. (1994). An approach to ear, nose and throat assessment. *Australian Family Physician, 23,* 2087–2093.

Chapter

3. Otalgia (Ear Pain)

Debra J. Mercy, MS, CRNP, AOCN®

I. Definition: The sensation of pain in or around the ear

II. Physiology/Pathophysiology
   A. Normal physiology
      1. Nerves innervating the auricle or external auditory canal include cranial nerves V, VII, IX, and X and cervical nerves C2 and C3.
      2. These nerves also innervate the pharynx, potentially causing referred pain.
   B. Pathophysiology: These nerves may be compressed by inflammation, tumor, or infection.

III. Clinical features: Otalgia can be primary or secondary (i.e., referred). The severity of otalgia does not reflect the seriousness of the etiology.
   A. Risk factors
      1. Recent swimming
      2. Injuries to the ear
      3. Recent travel in an airplane
      4. Recent deep-sea diving
   B. Etiology: See Figure 3-1
   C. History
      1. History of cancer and cancer treatment
      2. Current medications: Prescribed and over-the-counter
      3. History of presenting symptom(s): Precipitating factors, onset, location, and duration. Associated symptoms include hearing loss, ringing in the ears, dizziness, ear drainage, itching, painful teeth, difficulty or pain with chewing or swallowing, ears popping, and voice changes.
      4. Changes in activities of daily living
      5. Past medical history of injuries to the ear
   D. Signs and symptoms: Ear pain
   E. Physical exam
      1. HEENT exam
         a) External ear and external auditory canal
            (1) Tenderness to palpation or movement of the auricle or tragus
            (2) Edema or erythema, indicating cellulitis

        (3) Purulent green or yellow discharge, indicating otitis externa

        (4) Furuncle

        (5) Foreign body

    b) Tympanic membrane

        (1) Hemorrhagic vessels or blebs, indicating bullous myringitis or herpes zoster oticus

        (2) Erythema or bulging tympanic membrane with or without yellow pus, indicating otitis media or possible neoplasm (e.g., glomus tumor)

        (3) Blue tympanic membrane (from hemorrhage), indicating old blood, often from barotrauma (i.e., from flying or diving)

        (4) Perforation

    c) Hearing

        (1) Whisper test: To ascertain hearing alteration; if positive, perform Rinne and Weber tests with a 512 Hz tuning fork

        (2) Rinne and Weber tests: To compare hearing by bone and air conduction (see Appendix 13)

    d) Oral cavity

        (1) Erythematous posterior pharynx or exudate, indicating pharyngitis or tonsillitis

        (2) Base of tongue abnormalities (e.g., neoplasm, ulceration)

        (3) Tooth painful upon palpation or percussion or signs of extreme pain, indicating abscess or infection

        (4) Swelling, tenderness, or mass in parotid gland with lack of expressible saliva or purulent exudate from Stenson's duct, indicating neoplasm, calculus, or infection

        (5) Vocal hoarseness or breathiness, indicating laryngeal pathology

  2. Neurologic exam: Assess cranial nerves (see Appendix 4)

  3. Lymph exam: Lymphadenopathy indicating infection or neoplasm

  4. Musculoskeletal exam

    a) Cervical spine pain, crepitus, indicating cervical spine lesion

    b) Temporomandibular joint pain upon palpation: Malocclusion or trismus, indicating temporomandibular joint dysfunction

IV. Diagnostic tests

  A. Laboratory: Myringotomy with culture of middle-ear fluid

  B. Radiology

    1. CT of head and neck: To look for source of pain (e.g., mastoiditis, brain abscess) and complications of otitis media

    2. Panorex: To evaluate dentition

  C. Other

    1. Audiometry: Conductive versus sensorineural hearing loss

    2. Fine-needle aspiration of neck or parotid mass

V. Differential diagnosis (see Figure 3-1)

VI. Treatment

Figure 3-1. Etiology of Otalgia

Otogenic

- External ear
  - Diffuse external otitis
  - Furunculosis
  - "Malignant" external otitis
  - Impacted cerumen
  - Perichondritis
  - Foreign bodies
  - Bullous myringitis
  - Herpes zoster oticus
  - Neoplasm
  - Otomycosis
  - Trauma
  - Keratosis obturans (i.e., cholesteatoma of ear canal)

- Middle ear or mastoid
  - Acute otitis media
  - Acute mastoiditis
  - Acute aero-otitis media (barotrauma)
  - Acute eustachian tube obstruction
  - Chronic otitis media

- Complications of otitis media and mastoiditis
  - Subperiosteal abscess
  - Petrositis
  - Extradural abscess
  - Subdural abscess
  - Brain abscess
  - Lateral sinus thrombophlebitis
  - Meningitis
  - Otitic hydroencephalus

- Neoplasm

- Trauma

- Postsurgical otalgia

Nonotogenic

- Cranial nerve V
  - Nose and sinuses
    - Infection
    - Neoplasm
    - Septal deformity
  - Nasopharynx
    - Acute infection
    - Adenoidectomy
    - Neoplasm
  - Teeth and jaws
    - Impaction of molar teeth
    - Temporomandibular arthritis
    - Malocclusion
  - Salivary glands
    - Infection
    - Calculi
  - Trigeminal neuralgia
  - Sphenopalatine neuralgia

- Cranial nerve VII
  - Geniculate neuralgia

- Cranial nerves IX and X
  - Pharynx
    - Tonsillectomy
    - Acute tonsillitis
    - Peritonsillar abscess
    - Para-, retropharyngeal abscess
    - Neoplasm
  - Larynx
    - Neoplasm
    - Ulceration
  - Tongue
    - Neoplasm
    - Ulceration
  - Esophagus
  - Elongated styloid process
  - Glossopharyngeal neuralgia
  - Tympanic neuralgia

- The cervical nerves
  - Cervical spine lesions

- Miscellaneous
  - Carotidynia
  - Postauricular lymphadenitis
  - Psychogenic otalgia

Note. From "Otalgia" (p. 109) by E. Yanagisawa in K.J. Lee (Ed.), *Differential Diagnosis in Otolaryngology,* 1978, New York: Arco Publishing Co. Copyright 1978 by K.J. Lee. Adapted with permission.

      A. Treat the cause of the otalgia, if found.

      B. Prescribe topical and/or systemic analgesics.

VII. Follow-up

      A. Close follow-up after treatment is necessary to evaluate response to therapy.

      B. If expected outcome is not met, refer patient to otolaryngology for further evaluation.

VIII. Referrals

      A. Otolaryngologist for further evaluation and treatment

      B. Dentist for treatment of dental causes

      C. Neurosurgeon: If cervical abnormality is found on radiologic exam

References

Amundson, L.H. (1990). Disorders of the external ear. *Primary Care, 17,* 213–231.

Harvey, H. (1992). Diagnosing referred otalgia: The ten Ts. *Journal of Craniomandibular Practice, 10,* 333–334.

Yanagisawa, K., & Kveton, J.F. (1992). Referred otalgia. *American Journal of Otolaryngology, 13,* 323–327.

Chapter

4.

Sore Throat (Pharyngitis)

Gail Egan Sansivero, MS, ANP, AOCN®

I. Definition: A feeling of soreness in the throat

II. Physiology/Pathophysiology
   A. Normal physiology: The pharynx consists of lymphoglandular tissue and serves as the first line of defense.
   B. Pathophysiology
      1. Throat irritation occurs from external factors (e.g., physical, chemical, or microbial origin).
      2. Both viral and bacterial infections can cause acute pharyngitis, resulting in cellular inflammation and discomfort.

III. Clinical features: Chronic pharyngitis is rarely infectious in nature.
   A. Risk factors
      1. Irritants
      2. Smoking
      3. Dehydration
      4. Allergies
      5. Immunocompromised individuals
      6. Those frequently exposed to organisms (e.g., daycare workers, teachers)
   B. Etiologies
      1. Most sore throats are caused by viruses.
      2. Approximately 20% of adult sore throats are caused by bacterial infection; streptococcal infection occurs most commonly in children ages 5–18.
      3. Other infectious causes include *Mycoplasma pneumoniae, Chlamydia trachomatis,* and *Candida albicans.*
      4. In patients with exudative pharyngitis with fever, adenopathy, and absence of upper respiratory infection (URI) symptoms, 50% will have a positive streptococcal culture.
      5. Patients receiving chemotherapy (especially 5-fluorouracil, methotrexate, cyclophosphamide, and cisplatin) or radiation therapy to the head and neck area may experience pharyngitis because of inflammation, cellular death, and open lesions.
   C. History

      1. History of cancer and cancer treatment
      2. Current medications: Prescribed and over-the-counter
      3. History of presenting symptom(s): Precipitating factors, onset, location, and duration
      4. Changes in activities of daily living
      5. Social history of tobacco or alcohol
      6. Past medical history of immune disorders or sexually transmitted disease (STD)

D. Signs and symptoms
      1. Fever, headache, malaise, chills
      2. Sore throat
      3. Nonproductive cough
      4. Anorexia

E. Physical exam
      1. Vital signs: Include temperature.
      2. HEENT exam
         a) Ears: Examine for erythema, drainage, alteration of landmarks.
         b) Oropharynx cavity: Inspect for
            (1) Enlarged tonsils
            (2) Pharyngeal erythema
            (3) Tonsillar exudate
            (4) Soft palate petechiae
            (5) Exudate
            (6) Lesions (e.g., apthous ulcers, candidiasis, herpetic lesions)
            (7) Trismus
            (8) Small vesicles on pharynx, buccal mucosa, tonsils.
      3. Integument exam: Inspect for color, exanthema, and hydration status.
      4. Lymph exam: Palpate for enlarged lymph nodes.
      5. Neck exam: Assess for nuchal rigidity.
      6. Cardiac and pulmonary exam: Auscultate for abnormal sounds indicating pulmonary infection or rheumatic fever.
      7. Abdominal exam: Examine for splenomegaly and hepatomegaly.

IV. Diagnostic tests
A. Laboratory studies
      1. Throat culture: If fever, dysphagia, and cervical adenopathy present
         a) Rapid streptococcal test has positive predictive value of 86%–92%.
         b) Throat culture specificity is 76%–99%.
         c) Neither the rapid streptococcus test nor throat culture will detect chlamydia or mycoplasma.
      2. Complete blood count (CBC) with differential: Consider and expect white blood count (WBC) increase in bacterial infection.
         a) CBC has low predictive value.
         b) May help in differentiating between viral and bacterial etiologies
      3. Culture for gonorrhea: Consider if patient practices oral-genital sex.
      4. Mononucleosis spot: Perform if Epstein-Barr infection is suspected.
B. Radiology: Usually not indicated

C. Other: Laryngoscopy for patients with persistent sore throat or hoarseness lasting more than two to three weeks or accompanied by signs/symptoms suggestive of a more serious process (e.g., weight loss, dysphagia, mass); laryngoscopy will evaluate for presence or absence of masses and vocal cord mobility.

V. Differential diagnosis
   A. Stomatitis (see Chapter 11)
   B. Epiglottitis
   C. Allergic rhinitis with postnasal drip (see Chapter 6)
   D. Rhinosinusitis (see Chapter 10)
   E. Viral infection (e.g., herpangina, mononucleosis, Coxsackie, influenza)
   F. Bacterial infection (e.g., Group A beta-hemolytic streptococcus, *Neisseria gonorrheae, Corynebacterium diphtheriae*)
       1. Peritonsillar abscess
       2. Retropharyngeal abscess
   G. Fungal infections (*Candida albicans*)
   H. Mouth breathing
   I. Trauma from thermal chemical irritants
   J. Infectious mononucleosis (Epstein-Barr virus)
   K. Thyroiditis
   L. HIV (see Chapter 156)
   M. Aphthous ulcers (i.e., canker sores): Usually numerous, small ulcerated lesions on tongue, palate, and buccal mucosa associated with viral infections (e.g., Coxsackie A, herpes simplex) or antineoplastic therapy
   N. Pemphigus: Bullae or vesical formation on skin or mucous membranes
   O. Erythema multiforme
   P. Blood dyscrasia (include leukemia and lymphoma)
   Q. Carcinoma of the tonsil, tongue, soft palate, supraglottic larynx
   R. Salivary gland tumors
   S. Carotidynia (i.e., tenderness along the course of the common carotid artery)
   T. Tortuous internal carotid artery
   U. Toxic shock syndrome
   V. Acute rheumatic fever
   W. Palatal cellulitis
   X. Vincent's angina (i.e., necrotic tonsillar ulcers)
   Y. Gingivitis (i.e., "trench mouth")
   Z. Gastroesophageal reflux disease (GERD) (see Chapter 66)

VI. Treatment: In immunosuppressed patients, empiric antibiotic therapy may be indicated prior to establishing definitive diagnosis (see Table 4-1).
   A. For viral pharyngitis, treatment is aimed at symptomatic relief.
       1. Teach patients to maintain adequate fluid intake.
       2. Patient may use acetaminophen or nonsteroidal anti-inflammatory drugs (NSAIDs) for fever, pain.
       3. Patient may use lozenges, normal saline gargles or rinses to relieve pain.

Table 4-1. Pharmacologic Therapy in Pharyngitis

Type	Drug therapy	Dose	Frequency	Side Effects	Considerations
Viral	None	—	—	—	—
Group A Beta-hemolytic streptococcus	Penicillin VK	250 mg po	qid x 10 days	Superinfection, anaphylaxis, urticaria	—
	Erythromycin	250 mg po	qid x 10 days	Superinfection, GI upset, anaphylaxis, urticaria	Alternative in patients with penicillin allergy
Gonorrhea	Ceftriaxone	250 mg IM	x 1	Local reaction, anaphylaxis	—
	Cefixime (Suprax[a])	400 mg po	x 1	Diarrhea, GI upset, rash	Use caution with patients with penicillin allergy.
Candidiasis	Nystatin suspension: 100,000 units/ml	5–15 ml po	qid x 10 days swish and swallow	Diarrhea, nausea, vomiting	Retain in mouth as long as possible.
	Clotrimazole troche (Mycelex[b])	10 mg po	tid x 10 days	Nausea, vomiting	Should be dissolved slowly
	Fluconazole	200 mg initially, 100 mg po qd	x 10 days	Nausea, rash, headache, diarrhea, hepatotoxicity	May need loading dose of 400 mg po x 1. Monitor liver function in prolonged use. Potentiates warfarin, oral hypoglycemic agents, theophylline.
Chlamydia trachomatis	Nystatin pastilles	1–2 po	x 10 days	Diarrhea, GI distress	Dissolve in mouth slowly.
Mycoplasma pneumoniae	Erythromycin	250 mg po	tid–qid x 10 days	Superinfection, anaphylaxis, GI upset, urticaria	—
	Azithromycin (Zithromax[c])	500 mg po day one, 250 mg on days 2–5	x 1	GI upset	Take on empty stomach.

[a] Lederle Laboratories, Pearl River, NY; [b] Bayer Corporation Pharmaceutical Division, West Haven, CT; [c] Pfizer Inc., New York, NY

   4. Encourage smoking cessation.
   5. Humidified air with cool mist may offer symptomatic relief.
   6. Instruct patient to seek immediate medical attention if swallowing is impaired.
   B. For streptococcus throat, antibiotics are needed to reduce suppurative complications, decrease the risk of rheumatic fever, and avoid disease transmission.
      1. Therapy is initiated in those patients with a history of rheumatic fever, with positive cultures, or with a high index of clinical suspicion.
      2. Completion of prescribed therapy is crucial, as failure rate increases when therapy is shortened.
      3. Patient should avoid school/work for at least 24 hours after therapy initiation when bacterial infection is present.
   C. Treatment for pharyngeal gonorrhea is ceftriaxone 250 mg IM x 1.
   D. Treat patients with *Chlamydia trachomatis* or *Mycoplasma pneumoniae* with standard therapy. Treatment does not necessarily shorten the course of illness.
   E. Treat patients with *Candida albicans* with nystatin swish and swallow, nystatin lozenges, or systemic antifungal agents.
   F. Patients should avoid contact with infected individuals if they are immunosuppressed or are at high risk for recurrent infection.
   G. Frequent recurrent infections may be an expression of immunodeficiency; testing for Epstein-Barr virus or HIV may be indicated.
   H. Patients with epiglottitis need constant monitoring for airway compromise. Hospitalization is needed for administration of IV antibiotics and steroids.

VII. Follow-up
   A. Short-term: Not necessary in uncomplicated cases. Instruct patient to call for re-evaluation if symptoms do not resolve in three to four days. Assume patient is noninfectious after 24 hours of antibiotic therapy.
   B. Long-term
      1. Repeat throat cultures indicated only in patients at high risk for rheumatic fever or who are symptomatic after treatment.
      2. Monitor nutritional status and weight of patients with chronic pharyngitis or acute or severe pharyngitis related to cancer therapy.

VIII. Referrals
   A. Refer patients with peritonsillar abscess for IV antibiotics and possible ear, nose, throat evaluation (otolaryngologist) and surgical intervention.
   B. Surgeon, oncologist/hematologist: Refer patients with lesions that may indicate malignancy for biopsy and management.
   C. Specialist: Refer patients with suspected immunodeficiency to appropriate physician (e.g., infectious disease, AIDS specialist).
   D. Oncologist/radiation oncologist: Consult about antineoplastic treatment plan for patients with moderate to severe pharyngitis related to cancer therapy. The patient may require dose modification or treatment interruption or delay.
   E. Dietitian: Refer patients with chronic or severe pharyngitis that affects ability to maintain adequate nutritional intake/hydration.

References

Carroll, K., & Reimer, L. (1996). Microbiology and laboratory diagnosis of upper respiratory tract infections. *Clinical Infectious Diseases, 23,* 442–448.

Hedges, J.R., & Lowe, R.A. (1987). Approach to acute pharyngitis. *Emergency Medical Clinics of North America, 5,* 335–351.

Perkins, A. (1997). An approach to diagnosing the acute sore throat. *American Family Physician, 55,* 131–138.

Perlman, P.E., & Ginn, D.R. (1990). Respiratory infections in ambulatory adults. *Postgraduate Medicine, 87,* 175–184.

Ruoff, G.E. (1996). Recurrent streptococcal pharyngitis. *Postgraduate Medicine, 99,* 211–222.

Chapter

5.

Tinnitus

Kristine Turner Story, RN, MSN, ARNP

I. Definition: The subjective perception of abnormal ear or head noises that are perceived in the absence of an external noise source

II. Pathophysiology: Tinnitus most often occurs from irreversible disease of the cochlea.

III. Clinical features: Persistent tinnitus is associated with sensory hearing loss. Patients with tinnitus complain of a constant ringing or humming sensation. Intermittent periods of mild, high-pitched tinnitus for several minutes is normal and not diagnostic of tinnitus. There is no known cause in a large percentage of patients.
    A. Etiology
        1. Causes include pathologic conditions of the external ear canal, middle ear, auditory nerve, brain stem, and cerebral cortex.
        2. Exact cause is unknown; possible causes include spontaneous otoacoustic emissions from the cochlea, spontaneous electrical activity in cranial nerve VIII, and electrophysiologic events in the brain stem and cerebral cortex.
        3. Most tinnitus is bilateral. If unilateral or asymmetrical, consider a lesion proximal to the cochlea.
    B. History
        1. History of cancer and cancer treatment
        2. Current medications: Prescribed and over-the-counter
        3. History of presenting symptom(s): Precipitating factors, onset, location, and duration
        4. Changes in activities of daily living
        5. Past medical history: Exposure to ototoxic agents/events (see Figure 5-1), renal disease, head trauma
    C. Signs and symptoms
        1. High-pitched ringing, buzzing, whining sound in the ears or the head
            a) Unilateral or bilateral
            b) Continuous or intermittent
        2. If severe and persistent, may interfere with concentration and sleep resulting in psychologic distress
    D. Physical exam: There are rare cases of objective tinnitus in which the sound perceived is also audible to examiner.

Figure 5-1. Factors Contributing to the Development of Tinnitus

Medications	Noise Trauma	Physical Trauma
Salicylates	Industrial noise	Head injury
Aminoglycosides	Weapons	Radiation therapy
Loop diuretics	Loud music	
Cisplatin		
Ifosfamide		
NSAIDs		
Oral contraceptives		
Quinine/antimalarials		

1. HEENT
    - *a)* External ear should be normal.
    - *b)* Canal and tympanic membrane should be normal.
2. Neurological exam
    - *a)* Cranial nerve assessment should be normal.
    - *b)* Hearing may be normal or decreased based on the whisper test.
    - *c)* Weber test should be negative.
    - *d)* Air conduction is greater than bone conduction on the Rinne test.

IV. Diagnostic tests
   A. Laboratory: CBC, chemistry profile, electrolytes, TSH to rule out contributing causes (see Differential diagnosis, below)
   B. Radiology: MRI or CT of head to rule out intracranial lesions
   C. Other
      1. Audiometry: Perform baseline audiometry if using ototoxic agents; serial measurements may be necessary.
      2. Test auditory brain stem evoked-response (BSER) to rule out lesion.
      3. Consider doppler studies if tinnitus is pulsatile or objective to rule out vascular causes.

V. Differential diagnosis
   A. Structural lesions
      1. Malignant or benign cochlear tumor
      2. Malignant or benign glomus tumor
      3. Acoustic neuroma
      4. Meningioma
      5. Temporomandibular joint syndrome
      6. Metastatic tumors
      7. Middle ear muscle myoclonus
   B. Metabolic derangements
      1. Diabetes mellitus (see Chapter 143)
      2. Hypothyroidism (see Chapter 150)
      3. Dyslipidemia (see Chapter 42)

      4. Renal failure (see Chapter 83)

      5. Anemia (see Chapters 111–118)

  C. Infections

      1. Otitis media (see Chapter 9)

      2. Mumps

      3. Measles

      4. Syphilis (see Chapter 95)

      5. Meningitis (see Chapter 136)

  D. Autoimmune disorders

      1. Polyarteritis nodosa

      2. Lupus erythematosus

      3. Giant-cell arteritis

  E. Vascular anomalies

      1. Arteriovenous malformation

      2. Aneurysm

  F. Cardiovascular

      1. Hypertension (see Chapter 45)

      2. Arteriosclerosis

  G. Migraine headache (see Chapter 135)

  H. Cerumen impaction

   I. Menière's disease

   J. Otosclerosis

VI. Treatment

  A. Prevention

      1. Avoid exposure to ototoxic agents (see Figure 5-1).

      2. Reduce dose of causative agents, if possible.

      3. Monitor serum peak/troughs of ototoxic medications and adjust as necessary.

      4. Avoid concomitant use of ototoxic agents.

      5. Reduce dose of ototoxic agents in patients with renal impairment.

  B. Treatment: Tinnitus is usually an irreversible condition. Treatment is aimed at decreasing awareness of the symptom and limiting its impact on quality of life.

      1. Use of hearing aids to amplify normal sounds and block high-frequency noises

      2. Use of music or other ambient sounds (e.g., waves, rain, white noise) to mask tinnitus

      3. Counseling/reassurance

      4. Habituation therapy: Goal is to train the individual to become unaware of the presence of tinnitus by changing the emotional response to the sound.

      5. Biofeedback

      6. Dietary restriction

        a) Limit caffeine.

        b) Limit sodium intake.

        c) Stop smoking.

      7. Medications that may decrease the perception of tinnitus

        a) Tricyclic antidepressants

          (1) Amitriptyline (Elavil®, AstraZeneca, Wilmington, DE): 25–50 mg po q hs

        (2) Nortriptyline (Pamelor®, Novartis Pharmaceuticals Corporation, East Hanover, NJ): 25–50 mg po q hs

        (3) Trimipramine (Surmontil®, Wyeth-Ayerst Pharmaceuticals, Philadelphia, PA): 50–100 mg po q hs

        (4) Protriptyline (Vivactil®, Merck & Co., Inc., Philadelphia, PA): 15–40 mg/day in divided doses

    b) Anticonvulsants: Carbamazepine (Tegretol®, Novartis Pharmaceutical Corporation, East Hanover, NJ) 200 mg po bid initially; may titrate up (maximum 2,000 mg)

    c) Antianxiety agents

        (1) Alprazolam (Xanax®, Pharmacia & Upjohn, Peapack, NJ): 0.25–0.5 mg po tid

        (2) Clonazepam (Klonopin®, Roche Laboratories, Nutley, NJ): 0.25 mg po bid

        (3) Diazepam (Valium®, Roche Laboratories): 2–10 mg po two to four times every day

    d) Diuretics: Furosemide (Lasix®, Aktiengesellschaft, Frankfurt, Germany) 20–40 mg po qd

    e) Antihistamines: Meclizine (Antivert®, Pfizer Inc., New York, NY) 25 mg q eight hours

VII. Follow-up

    A. Short-term: Evaluate for progression of symptoms during therapy for possible dose reduction.

    B. Long-term: Evaluate for progression at long term follow-up visits.

VIII. Referrals

    A. Audiologist: For audiometry

    B. Otolaryngologist: For conductive hearing loss

    C. Neurologist/neurosurgeon: If tumor is suspected or to assess abnormal cranial nerve

    D. Psychiatrist/psychologist: For habituation therapy

References

Greenberger, N.J., & Hinthorn, D.R. (1993). *History taking and physical examination essentials and clinical correlates.* St. Louis: Mosby.

Jastreboff, P.J., Gray, W.C., & Gold, S.L. (1996). Neurophysiological approach to tinnitus patients. *The American Journal of Otology, 17,* 236–240.

Knox, G.W., & McPherson, A. (1997). Meniere's disease: Differential diagnosis and treatment. *American Family Physician, 55,* 1185–1190.

Nadol, J.B. (1993). Hearing loss. *New England Journal of Medicine, 329,* 1092–1102.

Seidman, M.D., & Jacobson, G.P. (1996). Update on tinnitus. *Otolaryngology Clinics of North America, 29,* 455–465.

Seligman, H., Podoshin, L., Ben-David, J., Frodis, M., & Goldstein, M. (1996). Drug-induced tinnitus and other hearing disorders. *Drug Safety, 14,* 198–212.

Spoelhof, G.D. (1995). When to suspect an acoustic neuroma. *American Family Physician, 52,* 1768–1774.

6.

Allergic Rhinitis

Debra J. Mercy, MS, CRNP, AOCN®

I. Definition: An immunoglobulin E IgE-mediated form of rhinitis, which occurs in response to foreign antigens

II. Pathophysiology
   A. Initial sensitization to allergen
      1. Inhalation of allergen, elution, and diffusion occur across nasal membranes.
      2. Allergen is processed by antigen-presenting cells (i.e., macrophages and dendritic cells) and presented to T-helper cells, then B cells.
      3. B cells synthesize IgE with help of interleukin-4 (IL-4) and IL-13.
      4. Allergen-specific IgE attaches to receptors on mast cells and basophils.
   B. Early-phase response
      1. Antigen challenge is initial exposure.
      2. Allergen binds to IgE antibodies on mast cells, which causes cross linking of the molecules.
      3. This signals degranulation of the mast cell, which releases inflammatory mediators (e.g., histamine) within minutes.
      4. Increased histamine causes stimulation of blood vessels, nerves, and mucous-producing glands, resulting in sneezing, itching, rhinorrhea, and congestion.
   C. Late-phase response
      1. Response occurs hours after initial challenge.
      2. After mast cell activation, the nasal epithelium is infiltrated with eosinophils, basophils, monocytes, and T lymphocytes.
      3. Mediators released by these cells include leukotriene, kinin, and histamine.
      4. Cytokine production, including IL-3, IL-4, IL-5, IL-6, IL-8, granulocyte macrophage-colony-stimulating factor (GM-CSF), is elevated and prolonged for several hours after antigen challenge.
      5. Cytokines interact with various mediators that
         a) Direct adhesion molecule expression
         b) Produce chemoattractant
         c) Recruit inflammatory cells.
      6. Neural reflex mechanism also complicates the interaction and increases the reactions in those with perennial or seasonal allergic rhinitis.

III. Clinical features
  A. Risk factors
    1. Family history of allergies
    2. Occupational exposures
  B. Etiologies
    1. Seasonal allergens specific to geographic location (e.g., grass, pollen, ragweed, trees)
    2. Perennial allergens (e.g., dust mites, molds, animal dander, saliva, cockroach antigen)
    3. Irritants (e.g., smoke, air pollutants, perfumes, detergents, soaps, solvents) and other stimuli (e.g., emotion)
    4. Perennial allergic rhinitis: Present throughout the year
    5. Seasonal allergic rhinitis: Occurs during the same time each year
    6. Episodic allergic rhinitis: Occurs after an exposure to allergen
  C. History
    1. History of cancer and cancer treatment
    2. Current medications: Prescribed and over-the-counter
    3. History of presenting symptom(s): Precipitating factors, onset, location, and duration
    4. Changes in activities of daily living
    5. Past medical history: Eczema, dermatitis, urticaria, hives, allergies
    6. Social history of smoking or secondhand smoke exposure; occupational history, living environment
  D. Signs and symptoms
    1. Nasal congestion
    2. Watery rhinorrhea
    3. Postnasal drainage
    4. Paroxysmal sneezing
    5. Itchy nose, ears, and/or throat
    6. Watery, itchy eyes
    7. Headache over paranasal sinus areas
    8. Altered sense of smell and taste
    9. Cough
    10. Periorbital and eyelid edema
  E. Physical exam
    1. Do not rely on clinical signs for diagnosis.
    2. HEENT exam
      a) Nasal passages
        (1) Pale, boggy, and swollen turbinates
        (2) Red and swollen turbinates if early in reaction
        (3) Blue (cyanotic) mucosa
        (4) Clear bilateral nasal discharge
      b) Oral cavity
        (1) Erythematous posterior pharynx
        (2) Nasal mucous drainage in posterior pharynx
        (3) Lymphoid hyperplasia in the posterior pharynx

        c) Conjunctiva and scleral injection may be observed during eye exam.

        d) Palpation of sinuses may elicit tenderness or bogginess.

        e) Allergic "shiners" may be present, which appear as dark circles under the eyes.

        f) Allergic crease, caused by upward wiping, may be present at dorsum of nose.

IV. Diagnostic tests
- A. Laboratory
    1. Wright's stain of nasal secretions
        - *a)* Collect by blowing nose directly onto wax paper or cellophane.
        - *b)* Presence of eosinophils in clumps or greater than 10% of total WBCs indicates a probable allergic process.
    2. Immunologic testing: Reserve for those not responding to symptomatic therapy.
        - *a)* Skin testing: Must discontinue antihistamines three to five days prior to testing, depending on agent.
            - (1) Allergens are applied by intracutaneous or scratch techniques.
            - (2) Allergen is identified and degree of sensitivity evaluated.
        - *b)* Radioallergosorbent test (RAST): Draw blood sample.
            - (1) Measures the patient's level of IgE for a specific allergen
            - (2) Less sensitive and more expensive
            - (3) Limited selection of antigens available
- B. Radiology
    1. Water's view x-ray: To rule out sinusitis
    2. CT of sinuses: To rule out sinusitis

V. Differential diagnosis
- A. Infectious causes
    1. Rhinitis
        - *a)* Viral
        - *b)* Bacterial
        - *c)* Fungal
    2. Rhinosinusitis (See Chapter 10)
- B. Noninfectious, nonallergic causes
    1. Vasomotor rhinitis: Chronic idiopathic or nonallergic rhinitis
    2. Rhinitis medicamentosa
        - *a)* Topically applied
            - (1) Overuse of sympathomimetic nasal drops
            - (2) Cocaine
        - *b)* Ingested
            - (1) Sympathoplegic antihypertensives (e.g., methyldopa, clonidine)
            - (2) NSAIDs
            - (3) Oral contraceptives
        - *c)* Inhalants (e.g., ozone)
    3. Structural
        - *a)* Deviated septum
        - *b)* Nasal polyps

      4. Tumor
- *a)* Benign (e.g., inverting papilloma)
- *b)* Malignant (e.g., adenocarcinoma)

C. Metabolic: Hypothyroidism (see Chapter 150)

D. Other
1. Foreign bodies
2. Granulomatous disease (Wegener's sarcoid)
3. Vasomotor rhinitis
4. Nonallergic rhinitis with eosinophilia
5. Atrophic rhinitis
6. Cerebrospinal fluid rhinorrhea

VI. Treatment

A. Antihistamine and decongestant combination (see Appendix 6)

B. Antihistamines: Best used before allergen exposure (see Appendix 4)

C. Decongestants (see Appendix 7)

D. Topical nasal steroids (see Appendix 15)

E. Mast cell stabilizer, such as cromolyn sodium

F. Immunotherapy
1. Specific therapies are based on result of RAST testing or skin testing.
2. Weekly injection of allergen decreases sensitivity.

G. Environmental modification
1. Seasonal
- *a)* Stay indoors.
- *b)* Filter room air.
- *c)* Keep bedroom windows closed.
2. Perennial
- *a)* Eliminate dust traps in the home (e.g., rugs, feather pillows).
- *b)* Remove sources of mold spores (e.g., houseplants).
- *c)* Control dust mites.
  - (1) Use washable curtains.
  - (2) Use water-sealed vacuum cleaner.
  - (3) Encase mattress, box spring, and pillows in plastic.
  - (4) Wash sheets in hot water once per week.
  - (5) Keep humidity at 50% or lower.

VII. Follow-up

A. Short-term
1. Monitor for development of secondary sinusitis.
2. Inadequate response within two to three weeks requires altering treatment regimen or referral to otolaryngologist.

B. Long-term: Prevent seasonal allergies with premedication.

VIII. Referrals

A. Otolaryngologist

      1. If anatomic or secondary disorder is suspected
      2. To rule out or treat complications
      3. To provide other treatment options when initial treatment failed
   B. Allergist
      1. For further testing to isolate a definitive diagnosis
      2. If response to treatment is inadequate

References

Ciprandi, G., Passalacqua, G., Mincarini, M., Ricca, V., & Canonica, G.W. (1997). Continuous versus on demand treatment with cetrizine for allergic rhinitis. *Annals of Allergy, Asthma, and Immunology, 79,* 507–511.

Grosclaude, M., Mees, K., Pinelli, M.E., Lucas, M., & Van de Venne, H. (1997). Cetirizine and pseudoephedrine retard, given alone or in combination, in patients with seasonal allergic rhinitis. *Rhinology, 35,* 67–73.

Meltzer, E.O. (1997). The pharmacological basis for the treatment of perennial allergic rhinitis and non-allergic rhinitis with topical corticosteroids. *Allergy, 52*(Suppl. 36), 33–40.

Naclerio, R.M. (1997). Pathophysiology of perennial allergic rhinitis. *Allergy, 52*(Suppl. 36), 7–13.

Naclerio, R., & Solomon, W. (1997). Rhinitis and inhalant allergens. *JAMA, 278,* 1842–1848.

7. Conjunctivitis

Kristine Turner Story, RN, MSN, ARNP

I. Definition: An inflammatory condition of the conjunctiva resulting in redness and irritation of the conjunctiva
   A. When the cornea is involved, condition is referred to as keratoconjunctivitis.
   B. When eyelids are involved, condition is referred to as blepharitis.

II. Pathophysiology
   A. Infectious conjunctivitis is caused by invasion of the conjunctiva by an offending organism, most commonly bacterial or viral.
   B. Noninfectious conjunctivitis has a variety of causative factors, the more common being allergic conjunctivitis and chemical conjunctivitis.

III. Clinical features: Conjunctivitis may be acute or chronic. Conjunctivitis is highly transmissible via direct contact with contaminated fingers, towels, tissues, eye droppers, etc.
   A. Etiology
       1. Common bacterial pathogens: *Staphylococcus aureus, Streptococcus pneumoniae, Haemophilus influenzae, Moraxella catarrhalis, Pseudomonas* species, *Neisseria gonorrhoeae, Chlamydia trachomatis*, pneumococcus
       2. Common viral pathogens: Adenovirus (commonly type 3, 4, or 7), picornavirus, enterovirus, herpes simplex Type I
       3. Radiation-induced from treatment of head and neck cancers
       4. Chemotherapy-induced from
           a) Doxorubicin
           b) Cytosine arabinoside
           c) 5-fluorouracil
           d) Methotrexate
           e) Ifosfamide
           f) Nitrosourea
           g) Cyclophosphamide
       5. Biotherapy-induced from interferon
   B. History
       1. History of cancer and cancer treatment
       2. Current medications: Prescribed and over-the-counter

      3. History of presenting symptom(s): Precipitating factors, onset, location, and duration
      4. Changes in activities of daily living
      5. Past medical history: Eye trauma, eye infections, or STD
      6. History of wearing glasses or contact lenses
C. Signs and symptoms
      1. Bacterial conjunctivitis
          a) Acute onset mucopurulent drainage (green or yellow): Usually unilateral at the onset, with transmission to the unaffected eye in two to five days
          b) Foreign body sensation: Common
          c) Lid edema with matting of lashes: Especially upon awakening
          d) Itching, red, burning
          e) Corneal ulcerations or infiltration
      2. Viral conjunctivitis
          a) Marked conjunctival injection
          b) Watery or mucoid discharge
          c) Large preauricular lymph nodes
          d) Coexisting symptoms of fever and pharyngitis: Common
      3. Allergic conjunctivitis
          a) Itchy eyes, edematous lids
          b) Watery discharge
          c) Chemosis (e.g., conjunctival edema): May be severe
          d) Coexisting systemic allergic symptoms (e.g., sneezing, rhinorrhea): Common
          e) Allergic shiners
      4. Chlamydial conjunctivitis
          a) Thin, mucoid discharge
          b) Photophobia
          c) Moderate eyelid edema
      5. Conjunctivitis caused by herpes simplex
          a) Vesicle on skin of lids
          b) Coexisting fever blisters on the lips or face: Common
      6. Chemical conjunctivitis
          a) Burning, itching sensation
          b) Redness extends to lids
          c) Watery discharge or excessive dryness
D. Physical exam
      1. Vital signs: May have elevated temperature
      2. HEENT exam
          a) Pupils: Equal, round, react to light and accommodation
          b) Extra-ocular movements: Intact
          c) Fundoscopic exam usually normal, ulceration may be present
          d) Normal visual acuity or slight blurred vision
          e) Clear corneas except dendrite corneal lesions can be noted with herpes
          f) Conjunctiva: More injected around periphery with extension toward the iris
          g) Observe for drainage, edema.

      h) Posterior pharynx injected

      i) Assess nasal mucosa, which could be pale and edematous.

  3. Lymph exam: Evaluate for enlarged preauricular and neck nodes.

IV. Diagnostic tests

  A. Laboratory: Culture and sensitivity and gram stain of discharge if gonorrhea or chlamydia is suspected

  B. Radiology: Noncontributory

  C. Other: Fluorescein dye stain if history of trauma is present, if corneal abrasion is suspected, or to diagnose herpes simplex virus (will see dendritic pattern on stain)

V. Differential diagnosis (see Table 7-1)

  A. Subconjunctival hemorrhage

  B. Systemic illnesses

    1. Stevens-Johnson syndrome

    2. Lupus

    3. Sarcoidosis

    4. Ankylosing spondylitis

Table 7-1. The Inflamed Eye: Differential Diagnosis of Common Causes

Characteristics	Acute Conjunctivitis	Acute Uveitis	Acute Glaucoma	Corneal Trauma or Infection
Incidence	Extremely common	Common	Uncommon	Common
Discharge	Moderate to copious	None	None	Watery or purulent
Vision	No effect on vision	Often blurred	Markedly blurred	Usually blurred
Pain	Mild	Moderate	Severe	Moderate to severe
Conjunctival injection	Diffuse; more toward fornices	Mainly circumcorneal	Mainly circumcorneal	Mainly circumcorneal
Cornea	Clear	Usually clear	Steamy	Clarify change related to cause
Pupil size	Normal	Small	Moderately dilated and fixed	Normal
Pupillary light response	Normal	Poor	None	Normal
Intraocular pressure	Normal	Commonly low but may be elevated	Elevated	Normal
Smear	Causative organisms	No organisms	No organisms	Organisms found only in corneal ulcers due to infection

Note. From "Eye" (p. 182) by P. Riordan-Eva & D.G. Vaughan in L.M. Tierney, S.J. McPhee, & M.A. Popadakis (Eds.), *Current Medical Diagnosis and Treatment* (37th ed.), 1998, Stamford, CT: Appleton & Lange. Copyright 1998 by Appleton & Lange. Reprinted with permission.

     5. Behcet's syndrome
  C. Infectious diseases
     1. Reiter's syndrome
     2. Mumps
     3. Rubella
  D. Vitamin A deficiency
  E. Chemotherapy-induced ocular toxicities
  F. Radiation-induced ocular toxicities secondary to head and neck cancers

VI. Treatment
  A. Never patch an infected eye.
  B. Avoid prescribing topical anesthetics.
  C. Reserve the use of topical steroids; ophthalmologist should consider.
  D. Symptomatic measures
     1. Apply cool compresses bid to qid.
     2. Clean lids and eyelashes with diluted baby shampoo bid.
     3. Wash hands well and dispose of used tissues; do not share wash cloths, linens, etc.
     4. Dispose of used eye makeup.
     5. Do not wear contact lenses until infection clears; disinfect before wearing, and use new pair after infection clears.
     6. Advise patient to return to school or work after drainage has cleared.
  E. Medication based on causative agent
     1. Bacterial conjunctivitis
       a) Sulfacetamide sodium 10% solution (Sulamyd®, Schering Corporation, Kenilworth, NJ; Cetamide®, Alcon Laboratories, Inc., Fort Worth, TX; Blephamide®-10, Allergan, Inc., Irvine, CA): 1–2 eye drops (gtts) q two hours while awake for two to five days
       b) Tobramycin 0.3% ophthalmic solution (Tobrex®, Alcon Laboratories, Inc.): 1–2 gtts q four hours while awake for two to five days
       c) Gentamycin ophthalmic solution (Genoptic®, Allergan, Inc.; Garamycin®, Schering Corporation; Gentacidin®, Cooper Vision, Inc., Palo Alto, CA): 1–2 gtts q four hours while awake until clear
       d) Polymixin, bacitracin (Polysporin®, Warner-Lambert Consumer Healthcare, Morris Plains, NJ) ophthalmic ointment: Small amount q three to four hours until clear
       e) Ofloxacin 0.3% ophthalmic solution (Ocuflox®, Allergan, Inc.): 1–2 gtts q two to four hours for two days, then qid until clear
       f) Ciprofloxacin 0.3% ophthalmic solution (Ciloxan®, Alcon Laboratories, Inc.): 1–2 gtts q two hours for two days, then qid for five days
       g) Avoid preparations containing neomycin because they can cause hypersensitivity.
     2. Viral conjunctivitis: None necessary; may use antibiotics to prevent secondary bacterial infection
     3. Chlamydial conjunctivitis
       a) Tetracycline or erythromycin: 250 mg po six times a day for three to five weeks

    b) Doxycyline: 300 mg po loading dose, then 100 mg po bid for three to five weeks

    c) Treat sexual partners.

  4. Gonococcal conjunctivitis

    a) If cornea not involved, ceftriaxone (Rocephin®, Roche Laboratories, Inc., Nutley, NJ) 1 g IM one time

    b) If cornea is involved, ceftriaxone (Rocephin) 1–2 g a day IV for five days

    c) Topical agents also may be used as needed (see Bacterial Conjunctivitis, p. 44).

    d) Treat sexual partners.

  5. Allergic conjunctivitis

    a) Oral antihistamines

      (1) Diphenhydramine (Benadryl®, Warner-Lambert Consumer Healthcare): 25–50 mg po q four to six hours prn

      (2) Hydroxyzine (Atarax®, Pfizer Inc., New York, NY): 25–50 po mg q four to six hours prn

      (3) Loratadine (Claritin®, Schering Corp.): 10 mg po qd

      (4) Astemizole (Hismanal®, Janssen Pharmaceutica, Inc., Titusville, NJ): 10 mg po qd

      (5) Fexofenadine (Allegra®, Hoescht Marion Roussel, Kansas City, MO): 60 mg po bid

      (6) Cetirizine (Zyrtec®, Pfizer Inc.): 10 mg po qd

    b) Mast cell stabilizers: Lodoxamide 0.1% ophthalmic solution (Alomide®, Alcon Laboratories, Inc.): 1–2 gtts qid

    c) Ocular antihistamines/vasoconstrictors: Naphazoline/pheniramine ophthalmic solution (Naphcon A®, Alcon Laboratories, Inc.): 1-2 gtts q four to six hours prn

    d) Ocular antihistamine/mast cell stabilizer: Olopatadine 0.1% ophthalmic solution (Patanol®, Alcon Laboratories, Inc.): 1–2 gtts q six to eight hours

    e) Nonsteroidal anti-inflammatory agents

      (1) Ketorolac 0.5% ophthalmic solution (Acular®, Allergan, Inc.): 1 gtt qid

      (2) Diclofenac 0.1% ophthalmic solution (Voltaren®, Novartis Pharmaceutical Corp., East Hanover, NJ): 1 gtt qid

    f) Avoid offending agents.

  6. Herpes simplex conjunctivitis

    a) Vidarabine 3% ophthalmic ointment (Vira-A®, Parke-Davis, Morris Plains, NJ): one-half inch q three hours

    b) Trifluridine 1% ophthalmic solution (Viroptic®, Monarch Pharmaceuticals, Bristol, TN): 1 gtt q two hours

    c) Avoid steroids.

VII. Follow-up

  A. Short-term

    1. See patient in office if no improvement in 48 hours.

    2. No need to follow up on mild cases if resolved.

    3. Follow up in 7–10 days for severe cases.

B. Long-term: Unnecessary unless repeat occurrences

VIII. Referrals: Ophthalmologist: Refer for diagnosis and management for STDs, cancer treatment-induced, ulceration.

References

Hara, J.H. (1996). The red eye: Diagnosis and treatment. *American Family Physician, 54,* 2423–2430.

Jaanus, S.D. (1998). Oral and topical antihistamines: Pharmacologic properties and therapeutic potential in ocular allergic disease. *Journal of the American Optometry Association, 69*(2), 77–87.

King, E., Rexavibul, N., Yee, R., Kellaway, J., & Przepiorka, D. (1998). The use of cyclosporin A in ocular graft-versus-host disease. *Bone Marrow Transplantation, 22,* 147–151.

Morrow, G.L., & Abbott, R.L. (1998). Conjunctivitis. *American Family Physician, 57,* 735–746.

Riordan-Eva, P., & Vaughan, D.G. (1998). Eye. In L.M. Tierney, Jr., S.J. McPhee, & M.A. Popadakis (Eds.), *Current medical diagnosis and treatment* (37th ed.) (pp. 156–180). Stamford, CT: Appleton & Lange.

Ruppert, S.D. (1996). Differential diagnosis of pediatric conjunctivitis (red eye). *Nurse Practitioner, 21,* 1226.

Weinstock, F.J., & Weinstock, M.B. (1996). Common eye disorders. Six patients to refer. *Postgraduate Medicine, 99*(4), 107–117.

Weinstock, F.J., & Weinstock, M.B. (1996). Common eye disorders. Six patients to treat, pitfalls to avoid. *Postgraduate Medicine, 99*(4), 119–123.

Chapter

8.

Otitis Externa

Debra J. Mercy, MS, CRNP, AOCN®

I. Definition: Inflammation and/or infection of the auricle and external auditory canal

II. Physiology/Pathophysiology
   A. Normal physiology
      1. The external ear includes the auricle, external ear canal, and the lateral surface of the tympanic membrane.
      2. The skin of the cartilaginous canal has unique qualities.
         a) Self-debridement, shedding, and migration of cells into the canal; cells are trapped by cerumen and expelled
         b) Acidic pH (6.5–6.8): Below optimal pH for most bacteria
         c) Tightly bound, water-resistant
         d) Ample blood supply and lymphatic drainage
         e) Antibacterial properties of cerumen
      3. Aging of the ear canal
         a) Subcutaneous tissue, overlying skin: Atrophy, thinning
         b) Skin: Dry, prone to breakdown or trauma
         c) Cerumen: Concentrated; possibly hard and impacted
   B. Pathophysiology: Inflammation, edema, and erythema block the canal and compress the nerve.

III. Clinical features
   A. Risk factors
      1. Swimming
      2. Tendency to retain water in the canal (from small or tortuous canal anatomy)
      3. Hot, humid climates
      4. Trauma to the ear (commonly self-induced with cotton-tipped applicators, bobby pins, or paper clips)
      5. Radiation to the head
   B. Etiology
      1. Typical organisms
         a) *Pseudomonas epidermidis*: Resident skin flora
         b) *Pseudomonas aeruginosa*: Enters by contaminated material (e.g., water)

     c)   *Streptococcus pyogenes*

     d)   *Staphylococcus aureus*

     e)   *Streptococcus pneumoniae*

     f)   *Aspergillus niger*

     g)   *Candida albicans*

   2.   Chronic infections may indicate fungal infections.

   3.   Necrotizing otitis externa results from intractable infection beginning in the external ear in diabetic or immunocompromised patients.

     a)   Usually caused by *Pseudomonas* or *Staphylococcus epidermidis*

     b)   Associated with high mortality unless diagnosed and treated early

   4.   Radiation therapy effects on the external auditory canal

     a)   Tympanic membrane: Inflammatory changes may cause erythema or congestion; also may reflect changes within the middle ear

     b)   External auditory canal: Response to radiation is similar to response of other skin.

     c)   Occasional stenosis or necrosis of the canal: Reported in cases of radiation therapy following surgery

 C.   History

   1.   History of cancer and cancer treatment

   2.   Current medications: Prescribed and over-the-counter

   3.   History of presenting symptom(s): Precipitating factors, onset, location, and duration

   4.   Changes in activities of daily living

   5.   History of self-induced trauma

   6.   Recent change of soap, lotion, hairspray, shampoo, earrings, or medication, including the use of Neosporin® (Warner-Lambert Consumer Healthcare, Morris Plains, NJ)

 D.   Signs and symptoms

   1.   Pruritus: External auditory canal and auricle

   2.   Pain: Increased with movement of ear or swallowing

   3.   Muffled hearing: From edema within canal

   4.   Discharge

   5.   Radiation-induced: Initial dry desquamation; pruritus may develop into moist desquamation or false membrane formation.

 E.   Physical exam

   1.   HEENT: External ear exam

     a)   Skin of the auditory canal: May be edematous and erythematous; suspect deeper infection or allergic reaction to ear drops.

     b)   Debris in canal

     c)   Discharge: May range from green, indicating bacterial infection, to dark, indicating fungal infection

     d)   Pain with manipulation of auricle differentiates otitis externa from otitis media; response is best elicited by pushing on the tragus; pulling back on the helix is less sensitive.

     e)   Pain increased with pressure on the tragus

   2.   Otoscopic exam: Tympanic membrane is red; appears granular and edematous with exudate in canal.

    3. Lymph exam: Enlarged lymph nodes occasionally present

IV. Diagnostic tests
- A. Laboratory
  1. CBC and erythrocyte sedimentation rate (ESR): To rule out infection if necrotizing otitis externa is suspected
  2. Culture and sensitivity of ear discharge: If patient is immunosuppressed or does not respond to treatment
  3. Potassium hydroxide, microscopic evaluation, or microscopic culture: If fungal cause is suspected
  4. Viral cultures of ear drainage: If herpes zoster is suspected
- B. Radiology: CT scan to evaluate for cartilage and bone invasion if necrotizing otitis externa is suspected
- C. Biopsy: If melanoma or metastatic disease is suspected

V. Differential diagnosis
- A. Contact dermatitis: Caused by ear drops (see Chapter 19)
- B. Bacterial infection
- C. Otomycosis: Fungal infection of ear
- D. Furunculosis: Acute localized external otitis, abscess in hair follicles
- E. Impetigo
- F. Necrotizing otitis externa
- G. Bullous myringitis
- H. Herpes zoster (see Chapter 20)
- I. Carcinoma or melanoma
- J. Seborrheic dermatitis
- K. Perichondritis or chondritis

VI. Treatment
- A. Cleansing of ear canal
  1. Proper cleansing is necessary, especially if accumulated debris prevents solution from contacting affected area.
  2. Use gentle suction or cotton-tipped applicator.
  3. Irrigate with warm saline or diluted hydrogen peroxide solution, if necessary.
  4. Dry with gentle suction, if necessary.
- B. Medications
  1. Topical antimicrobial combined with steroid or 2% acetic acid solution three to four times a day for 10 days. Apply with cotton wick if canal is narrowed or occluded. Do not use acetic acid or alcohol preparation if tympanic membrane is perforated.
     - *a)* Cortisporin® (Monarch Pharmaceuticals, Bristol, TN) otic suspension
     - *b)* Otic Domeboro® (Bayer Corporation Pharmaceutical Division, West Haven, CT)
     - *c)* VōSol HS® (Wallace Laboratories, Cranbury, NJ)
     - *d)* Orlex™ (Alberto Bartolomel, Gurabo, PR)
     - *e)* Coly-Mycin S® (Monarch Pharmaceuticals)

   2. Use oral antibiotics if cellulitis is present (see Appendix 1).
   3. Necrotizing otitis externa requires IV antibiotics that cover pseudomonas; give for six weeks (see Appendix 1).
   4. Furuncles do not require antibiotics unless inflammation of surrounding tissue is present. Spontaneous eruption usually occurs after applying warm compresses. Incision and drainage may be required.
  C. Prevention
   1. Bathing caps and earplugs do not prevent further infection.
   2. Dry the ear canal with acetic acid solution or Burrow's solution daily or after contact with water.
   3. Avoid scratching or traumatizing the ear (i.e., using cotton-tipped applicators).

 VII. Follow-up
   A. Short-term: Three to five days if patient does not respond to therapy or if oral antibiotics are required
   B. Long-term: Necrotizing otitis externa requires frequent and prolonged follow-up.

 VIII. Referrals: Otolaryngologist if patient does not respond to treatment or if necrotizing otitis externa is suspected

References

Amundson, L.H. (1990). Disorders of the external ear. *Primary Care, 17,* 213–231.

Jahn, A.F., & Hawke, M. (1993). Infections of the external ear. In C.W. Cummings, J.M Fredrickson, L.A. Harker, C.J. Krause, & D.E. Schuller (Eds.), *Otolaryngology-Head and neck surgery* (2nd ed.) (pp. 2787–2794). St. Louis: Mosby.

Bull, T.R. (1987). *A color atlas of E.N.T. diagnosis* (2nd ed.). St. Louis: Mosby.

Marcy, S.M. (1985). Infections of the external ear. *Pediatric Infectious Disease Journal, 4,* 192–201.

Roland, P.S. (1994). Clinical ototoxicity of topical antibiotic drops. *Otolaryngology-Head and Neck Surgery, 110,* 598–602.

Rubin, J., & Yu, V.L. (1988). Malignant external otitis: Insights into pathogenesis, clinical manifestations, diagnosis and therapy. *American Journal of Medicine, 85,* 391–397.

Chapter

9. Otitis Media

Debra J. Mercy, MS, CRNP, AOCN®

I. Definition: Symptomatic inflammation or effusion in the middle ear; classified as acute or chronic

II. Physiology/Pathophysiology
   A. Normal
      1. The middle ear consists of the tympanic membrane (TM), auditory ossicles (malleus, incus, and stapes), and the eustachian tube.
      2. The middle ear is lined with mucous-secreting epithelium.
      3. The eustachian tube connects the middle ear to the nasopharynx.
         a) Eustachian tube functions include equalizing pressure on both sides of the TM.
         b) The eustachian tube normally is in a collapsed, closed position, which protects the middle ear from reflux of nasopharyngeal debris.
         c) Secretions move through the tube into the nasopharynx by way of ciliary action.
         d) Normal transmission of sound to the oval window membrane requires a patent eustachian tube.
   B. Pathophysiology
      1. Acute bacterial otitis media (OM) infection occurs when the normal eustachian tube functions are altered and a pathogen enters the middle ear.
      2. As a result of pathogen invasion, inflammation, erythema, and edema occur.

III. Clinical features: OM is more common in children than adults because their eustachian tubes are shorter and more horizontal. Acute OM usually is preceded by upper respiratory infection (URI) (e.g., viral). Chronic OM is a persistent effusion in the middle ear, which usually follows acute OM, allergic rhinitis, or URI.
   A. Risk factors
      1. Male > female
      2. Exposure to URI
      3. Smoking/secondhand smoke exposure
      4. Previous episode of acute OM
      5. Allergies
      6. Alaskan/Native American heritage
      7. Down syndrome
      8. Immunocompromised status

B. Etiology: Most common pathogens ascend from the nasopharynx
    1. *Streptococcus pneumoniae* (35%)
    2. *Haemophilus influenzae* (23%)
    3. *Moraxella catarrhalis* (14%)
    4. Other pathogens that are infrequently cultured
        a) Group A beta-hemolytic streptococcus
        b) *Staphylococcus aureus*
        c) Anaerobic bacteria (chronic infections)
        d) Viruses
C. History
    1. History of cancer and cancer treatment
    2. Current medications: Prescribed and over-the-counter
    3. History of presenting symptoms: Precipitating factors, onset, location, and duration. Associated symptoms include hearing loss, ear pain, or dizziness.
    4. Changes in activities of daily living
    5. History of recent URI
D. Signs and symptoms
    1. Otalgia (ear pain)
        a) Pulling, poking, or tugging at external ear
        b) Aggravated by swallowing, belching
    2. Otorrhea
    3. Hearing loss
    4. Vertigo
    5. Tinnitus
    6. Systemic symptoms: Fever, rhinitis, sore throat, dizziness
    7. Disturbed sleep
    8. Irritability
    9. Loss of appetite
    10. Vomiting
E. Physical exam
    1. Vital signs: Temperature may be elevated.
    2. HEENT
        a) External ear exam: Observe for drainage, elicit pain
        b) Otoscopic exam
            (1) Mobility of the TM
                (a) Bulging with no mobility, indicating pus or fluid in the middle ear
                (b) Retracted with no mobility, indicating obstruction of eustachian tube with or without fluid
                (c) Mobility with negative pressure only, indicating obstruction of eustachian tube
                (d) Excess mobility (flaccid TM), indicating healed perforation or patulous eustachian tube
            (2) Color
                (a) Amber indicates serous fluid in middle ear.
                (b) Blue or deep red indicates blood or erythema.

        (c) Chalky white indicates infection.

        (d) Redness indicates infection or scarring of the middle ear.

        (e) Dullness indicates fibrosis or effusion.

        (f) White flakes or dense white plaques indicate healed inflammation or cholesteatoma.

    (3) Other findings

        (a) Fluid line, indicating fluid behind middle ear

        (b) Dark area on TM, indicating perforation

        (c) Bullae or blisters, indicating infection

        (d) Discharge, indicating infection or perforation

        (e) Air bubbles, indicating serous fluid

IV. Diagnostic tests

    A. Laboratory: CBC and culture of ear drainage to document infection (only 45% predictive value from culture)

    B. Radiology: Not indicated

    C. Other

       1. Impedance tympanometry

         a) Measurement of resonance of ear canal to changes in air pressure

         b) Sensitive and reliable method of detecting an effusion

         c) Useful for chronic OM

       2. Acoustic reflectometry: Sonar measurement of sound reflected back from TM

       3. Tympanocentesis: With or without placement of pressure equalizing tube

         a) Usually not necessary, unless patient is immunosuppressed or develops antibiotic resistance

         b) One-third of cultures show no growth.

V. Differential diagnosis: The etiology of otorrhea can be otitis externa or OM with perforation (see Table 9-1).

Table 9-1. Otitis Media Versus Otitis Externa

Symptom/Sign	Otitis Media	Otitis Externa
Systemic signs	Fever, upper respiratory infection	None
Lymphadenopathy	None	Regional
Decreased hearing	May be present	May be present
Ear pain	With swallowing or belching	With moving jaw or auricle
Auricle motion tenderness	None	Extreme
Canal edema	None	Present
Exudate	Only with perforation	May be minimal
Tympanic membrane	Fluid line, may be perforated	Normal or inflamed, no fluid line

A. Myringitis: Red TM without exudate
B. Pharyngitis (see Chapter 4)
C. Tonsillitis
D. Temporomandibular joint (TMJ) syndrome
E. Mastoiditis
F. Foreign body
G. Dental abscess
H. Furuncle
 I. Tumor (external compression)
J. Trauma
K. Ototoxicity
  1. Radiation therapy to the ear region
  2. Chemotherapy (e.g., cisplatin)
  3. Other: Aminoglycosides, salicylate, quinidine, furosemide

VI. Treatment
   A. First-line antibiotics: Amoxicillin 250–500 mg po q eight hours for 10 days
   B. If B-lactamase-producing *Haemophilus influenzae* or *Moraxella catarrhalis* is suspected
     1. Amoxicillin-clavulanate (Augmentin®, SmithKline Beecham Pharmaceuticals, Phila-delphia, PA): 250 mg po every eight hours for 10 days up to 875 mg po q 12 hours for 10 days
     2. Cephalosporin of choice
     3. Trimethoprim with sulfa (Bactrim® DS, Roche Laboratories, Inc., Nutley, NJ): One tablet po q 12 hours for 10 days
   C. If penicillin-resistant *Streptococcus pneumoniae* is suspected
     1. Azithromycin (Zithromax®, Pfizer Inc., New York, NY): 500 mg po on day 1, then 250 mg po q day for four days
     2. Clarithromycin (Biaxin®, Abbott Laboratories, Abbott Park, IL): 250–500 mg po q 12 hours for 7–14 days
   D. Antihistamines (see Appendix 4)
     1. If associated with allergic rhinitis
     2. Not documented to improve the course of OM as they may decrease ciliary motion
   E. Decongestants (see Appendix 7)
     1. Widely used
     2. Efficacy not documented in controlled studies
   F. Treatment for chronic OM should begin if the effusion has not resolved in 12 weeks. A 14–28-day antibiotic prescription should be given.

VII. Follow-up
   A. Continue to monitor for potential severe complications.
     1. CNS infection
     2. Mastoiditis
     3. Cholesteatoma
   B. Physical exam
     1. Conduct three to four weeks after start of therapy to assess for persistent effusion.
     2. Evaluate symptomatic patients sooner.

VIII. Referrals
    A. Otolaryngologist: For patients with effusions lasting 16 weeks
    B. Audiologist: For audiogram to evaluate hearing

References

Calandra, L.M. (1998). Otitis media with effusion: Strategies and controversies. *Advance for Nurse Practitioners, 6*(2), 67–70.

Carroll, K., & Reimer, L. (1996). Microbiology and laboratory diagnosis of upper respiratory tract infections. *Clinical Infectious Diseases, 23,* 442–448.

Kligman, E.W. (1992). Treatment of otitis media. *American Family Physician, 45,* 242–250.

Rosenfeld, R.M. (1996). An evidenced-based approach to treating otitis media. *Pediatric Otolaryngology, 43,* 1165–1181.

Sigler, B.A., & Schuring, L.T. (1993). *Ear, nose, and throat disorders.* St. Louis: Mosby.

Smith, C.A. (1998). Managing otitis media; Present methods, future directions. *The American Journal for Nurse Practitioners, 2*(2), 27–31.

Thoene, D.E., & Johnson, C.E. (1991). Pharmacotherapy of otitis media. *Pharmacotherapy, 11,* 212–221.

Chapter

10. Rhinosinusitis

Diane G. Cope, PhD, ARNP-CS, AOCN®

I. Definition: Inflammation of the mucous membranes lining the sinus cavities

II. Pathophysiology/Physiology (see Figure 10-1)
   A. Bacteria or allergens invade into the sinus cavities, causing acute or chronic manifestations.
   B. Inflammation occurs with resultant edema, causing obstruction to the flow of secretions and a decrease in mucociliary action.
   C. Inflammation of the mucous membranes causes an increase in mucous production, creating an environment that facilitates bacterial growth within the sinus cavities.

III. Clinical features: Chronic sinusitis often is not associated with an infection and generally does not include fever. The maxillary and frontal sinuses are most frequently involved. Consider acute bacterial rhinosinusitis if an acute URI has not improved or is worse after 10–14 days.

Figure 10-1. Adult Sinus Structures

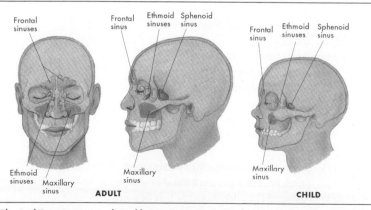

Note. From *Physical Examination and Health Assessment* (p. 387), by C. Jarvis, 1996, Philadelphia: W.B. Saunders Co. Copyright 1996 by W.B. Saunders Co. Reprinted with permission.

A. Risk factors
1. Congenital bone/cartilage/ciliary anomalies
2. Nasal polyps
3. Cystic fibrosis
4. Recent URI
5. Allergic rhinitis
6. Orofacial trauma
7. Recent dental procedures
B. Etiology: Predominant organisms are *Haemophilus influenzae*, *Streptococcus pneumoniae*, and *Straphylococcus aureus*.
C. History
1. History of cancer and cancer treatment
2. Current medications: Prescribed and over-the-counter
3. History of presenting symptom(s): Precipitating factors, onset, location, and duration. Associated symptoms include fever, headache, drainage
4. Changes in activities of daily living
5. Social history of tobacco use
6. History of recent URI or dental procedure
D. Signs and symptoms
1. Localized pain over sinuses
2. Low-grade or no fever
3. Pain
   a) In maxillary teeth
   b) Over sinuses
   c) Increases when bending over
4. Nasal obstruction
5. Cough with or without sputum production
6. Sore throat
7. Thick, purulent nasal drainage
8. Inability to expel nasal secretions
9. Headache
E. Physical exam
1. Vital signs: Low-grade or absent fever
2. HEENT exam
   a) Maxillary or frontal sinus
      (1) Tenderness to percussion
      (2) Sinus opacity on transillumination
   b) Ethmoid or sphenoid sinus
      (1) Retro-orbital pain
      (2) Mild palpebral edema
   c) Nares
      (1) Edematous, erythematous inferior turbinates
      (2) Thick or crusty purulent nasal drainage
      (3) Anosmia (i.e., decreased or loss of smell)
   d) Oral cavity/oropharynx
      (1) Purulent nasal drainage

(2) Erythematous

(3) Percuss maxillary teeth with tongue blade to assess for dental source.

   3. Pulmonary exam: Auscultate for adventitious sounds.

   4. Neurologic exam: Cranial nerves; cranial nerve I (olfactory nerve); anosmia

IV. Diagnostic tests

  A. Laboratory: Anterior nasal cultures are not accurate because of nasal contaminants.

  B. Radiology

    1. Sinus plain films: 75% specific for maxillary sinusitis; views ethmoid sinuses poorly

    2. CT scan: For definitive anatomic imaging to evaluate sinusitis

      a) Images the ethmoid sinuses

      b) 90%–100% sensitivity

      c) 60% false positives

  C. Other

    1. Flexible rhinopharyngoscopy: By otolaryngologist or allergist

    2. Sinus tap: To obtain material for culture, especially in neutropenic patients

V. Differential diagnosis

  A. Inflammatory

    1. Allergic rhinitis (see Chapter 6)

    2. Wegener's granulomatosis

    3. Sarcoidosis

  B. Non-inflammatory

    1. Idiopathic vasomotor rhinitis

    2. Drug-induced vasomotor rhinitis

    3. Hormone-induced rhinitis (e.g., from pregnancy)

  C. Mechanical

    1. Deviated septum

    2. Nasal polyps

    3. Tumor

    4. Foreign body

  D. Barotrauma: Bleeding into sinuses caused by negative pressure

  E. Other causes of headache/facial pain

    1. TMJ

    2. Migraine (see Chapter 135)

    3. Dental pathology

    4. Neuralgia

    5. CNS tumor

    6. Temporal arteritis

  F. Genetic

    1. Cystic fibrosis

    2. Ciliary dyskinesia/immobile cilia

VI. Treatment

  A. Decongestants (see Appendix 7)

    1. Pseudoephedrine HCl (Sudafed®, Warner-Lambert Consumer Healthcare, Morris Plains, NJ): 60 mg, one tablet po every six hours as needed
    2. Triprolidine HCl and pseudoephedrine HCl (Actifed®, Warner-Lambert Consumer Healthcare): One tablet every four to six hours as needed

B. Antihistamines (see Appendix 4)
    1. Diphenhydramine HCl (Benadryl®, Warner-Lambert Consumer Healthcare): 25–50 mg po every four to six hours as needed
    2. Chlorpheniramine maleate (Chlor-Trimeton®, Schering Corporation, Kenilworth, NJ): 4 mg po every four to six hours as needed
    3. Loratadine (Claritin®, Schering Corporation): 10 mg po daily
    4. Astemizole (Hismanal®, Janssen Pharmaceuticals, Belgium): 10 mg po daily
    5. Brompheniramine maleate and phenylpropanolamine HCl (Dimetapp®, A.H. Robins Co., Inc., Richmond, VA): One tablet po every four hours as needed

C. Antibiotics (see Appendix 1)
    1. Acute sinusitis
      a) Sulfamethoxazole and trimethoprim (Septra® DS, Monarch Pharmaceuticals, Bristol, TN): One tablet po every 12 hours for 10–14 days
      b) Amoxicillin (Amoxil®, SmithKline Beecham Pharmaceuticals, Philadelphia, PA): 250–500 mg po every eight hours for 10–14 days
    2. Recurrent or chronic sinusitis: Coverage for beta-lactamase, *Haemophilus influenzae* or *Moraxella catarrhalis*
      a) Amoxicillin/clavulanic acid (Augmentin®, SmithKline Beecham Pharmaceuticals): 500 mg po every eight hours or 875 mg every 12 hours for two to three weeks
      b) Cefaclor (Ceclor®, Eli Lilly & Co., Indianapolis, IN): 250 mg po every eight hours for two to three weeks
      c) Cefuroxime (Ceftin®, Glaxo Wellcome Inc., Research Triangle Park, NC): 250–500 mg po every 12 hours for two to three weeks
      d) Azithromycin (Zithromax®, Pfizer Inc., New York, NY) 500 mg po for one day, then 250 mg every day for four days
      e) Clarithromycin (Biaxin®, Abbott Laboratories, Abbott Park, IL): 500 mg po every 12 hours for two to three weeks

D. Pain
    1. Acetaminophen (Tylenol®, McNeil Consumer Healthcare, Fort Washington, PA): 325 mg, two tablets po every four to six hours as needed
    2. Ibuprofen (Advil®, American Home Products Corp., Madison, NJ; Motrin®, McNeil Consumer Healthcare; Nuprin®, The Upjohn Company, Kalamazoo, MI): 200–400 mg po every four to six hours as needed

E. Functional endoscopic sinus surgery (for chronic sinus disease)

F. Special considerations
    1. Neutropenic or immunocompromised patients
      a) Antibiotic therapy used for recurrent or chronic sinusitis
      b) Consider granulocyte-colony-stimulating factor (G-CSF) support
      c) May need to irrigate sinus for symptomatic relief
    2. Neutropenic population is at a greater risk for complications (e.g., orbital cellulitis, frontal sinus abscess, cavernous sinus thrombosis).

VII. Follow-up
    A. Short-term: Improvement in symptoms should be noted within two to three days of initiating treatment.
    B. Long-term: Chronic infections require appropriate referrals.

VIII. Referrals
    A. Otolaryngologist or allergist: For complicated sinusitis, recurrent infections, or chronic sinus disease
    B. Neurologist: If any indication of CNS involvement

References

Ahuje, G.S., & Thompson, J. (1998). What role for antibiotics in otitis media and sinusitis? *Postgraduate Medicine, 104,* 93–99, 103–104.

Bhattacharyya, T., Piccirillo, J., & Wippold, F.J. (1997). Relationship between patient-based descriptions of sinusitis and paranasal sinus computed tomographic findings. *Archives of Otolaryngology-Head and Neck Surgery, 123,* 1189–1192.

Brook, I., Yocum, P., & Frazier, E.H. (1996). Bacteriology and beta-lactamase activity in acute and chronic maxillary sinusitis. *Archives of Otolaryngology-Head and Neck Surgery, 122,* 407–413.

Fagnan, L.J. (1998). Acute sinusitis: A cost-effective approach to diagnosis and treatment. *American Family Physician, 58,* 1795–1802, 1805–1806.

Gonzales, R., Steiner, J.F., & Sande, M.A. (1997). Antibiotic prescribing for adults with colds, upper respiratory infections, and bronchitis by ambulatory care physicians. *JAMA, 278,* 901–904.

Slack, R., & Bates, G. (1998). Functional endoscopic sinus surgery. *American Family Physician, 58,* 707–718.

Slavin, R.G. (1997). Nasal polyps and sinusitis. *JAMA, 278,* 1849–1854.

Williams, J.W., Holleman, D.R., Samasa, G.P., & Simel, D.L. (1995). Randomized controlled trial of 3 vs. 10 days of trimethoprim/sulfamethoxazole for acute maxillary sinusitis. *JAMA, 273,* 1015–1021.

Williams, J.W., & Simel, D.L. (1993). Does this patient have sinusitis? Diagnosing acute sinusitis by history and physical examination. *JAMA, 270,* 1242–1246.

11. Stomatitis/Xerostomia

Roberta A. Strohl, RN, BSN, MN, AOCN®

I. Definition: Diffuse ulcerative condition of oral mucosa most commonly occurring in nonkeratinized cells
  A. Mucositis: Inflammation of the mucous membranes
  B. Xerostomia: Dryness of the mucous membranes

II. Physiology/Pathophysiology
  A. Normal: The oral cavity is composed of rapidly dividing epithelial cells.
  B. Pathophysiology
    1. Direct stomatotoxicity is the result of a decrease in oral cavity cell renewal with epithelial thinning.
    2. Ulceration of the oral cavity occurs within five to seven days of chemotherapy drug administration and within 7 to 10 days of oral cavity radiation.
      a) If there are no secondary bone marrow effects, mucositis heals in approximately 14 days after discontinuing treatment.
      b) Xerostomia or dryness of the oral cavity contributes to the development of stomatitis.
    3. Indirect stomatitis is caused by reduced myeloproliferation of bone marrow cells, resulting in neutropenic sepsis.

III. Clinical features: The mouth is the most frequently documented source of infection in immunosuppressed patients.
  A. Risk factors
    1. Chemotherapy
      a) Vincristine
      b) Vinblastine
      c) Dactinomycin
      d) Idarubicin
      e) Methotrexate
      f) 5-fluorouracil
      g) Cytarabine
      h) Etoposide
      i) Doxorubicin

      2. Radiation therapy to oral cavity

      3. Bone marrow transplantation

      4. Multimodal therapy

      5. Recent oral surgery

      6. Poor oral hygiene with gingivitis, caries, and periodontitis

  B. History

      1. History of cancer and cancer treatment

      2. Current medications: Prescribed and over-the-counter

      3. History of presenting symptom(s): Precipitating factors, onset, location, and duration

      4. Changes in activities of daily living

      5. Past medical history of HIV

      6. History of nutritional intake, current diet, weight loss, current oral hygiene practices

      7. Social history of tobacco or alcohol use

  C. Signs and symptoms

      1. Erythema

      2. Ulceration

      3. Pale mucosa

      4. Xerostomia

      5. Fever

      6. Pain

      7. Dysphagia

      8. Hoarseness

  D. Physical exam

      1. HEENT exam

          a) Remove dentures and oral prostheses to visualize oral cavity.

          b) Inspect and palpate oral cavity, noting condition of oral cavity and any lesions.

              (1) Gray-white lesions with necrotic clusters are typical appearance of stomatitis.

              (2) Raised white, curdy-looking areas indicative of *Candida albicans* are the most frequently observed fungal infection of oral cavity.

              (3) Croppy vesicular lesions with ulceration seen unilaterally and on the palate indicate herpes zoster infection.

              (4) White lacy keratotic lesions with erosive or painful bullous lesions are typical of the oral manifestations of graft-versus-host disease.

          c) Note presence, absence, and character of saliva.

          d) Assess ease of swallowing.

      2. Lymph exam: Palpate cervical and submandibular lymph nodes for enlargement.

IV. Diagnostic tests

  A. Laboratory

      1. CBC: To assess for neutropenia

      2. Culture of oral lesions: To identify organism

      3. Blood cultures: If systemic sepsis is suspected or fever is present

      4. Herpes simplex antibody status

      5. HIV status

  B. Radiology: Not indicated

V. Differential diagnosis
   A. Poor oral hygiene
   B. Kaposi's sarcoma
   C. Infection: Candida, herpes
   D. Aphthous ulcers (canker sores)
   E. Trauma to oral mucosa
   F. Oral cancers: Squamous cell carcinoma
   G. Reiter's syndrome: Triad of symptoms—conjunctivitis, urethritis, arthritis with oral, genital, or mucocutaneous lesions
   H. Behcet's syndrome: Triad of symptoms—iritis, oral lesions, and genital lesions

VI. Treatment: Prevent and minimize the oral consequences of cancer therapy.
   A. Thorough dental exam: Conduct prior to initiation of therapy. Teeth that need to be extracted should be taken out before any treatment to allow healing before therapy begins (10–14 days).
   B. Prophylactic oral hygiene
      1. Brush and floss teeth before and after meals if platelet count is > 50,000 cells/mm^3 and WBC is > 1,000 cells/mm^3.
      2. Clean teeth with a moistened 2 x 2 inch gauze sponge or soft implement if counts are low.
      3. Use fluoride mouth rinse daily for one minute.
      4. Avoid harsh chemicals or irritants (e.g., alcohol-containing mouthwashes, rough foods, alcohol, tobacco).
      5. Eat soft, nutritious foods and limit sucrose intake.
      6. Prostheses should be removed until healing occurs.
      7. Prophylactic antivirals are included in some protocols (e.g., BMT, multimodal), as herpes simplex virus infection is implicated in stomatitis.
   B. Pain management: All treatments listed can be used before meals and at bedtime.
      1. Lidocaine rinse: 5–15 cc
      2. Benadryl and Kaopectate® (The Upjohn Co., Kalamazoo, MI): Swish and spit equal proportions 5–15 cc
      3. Systemic analgesics: May be indicated (see Appendix 8a/b)
      4. Benadryl, Maalox® (Rhône-Poulenc Rorer, Collegville, PA), and viscous xylocaine: Swish and swallow 15–30 cc
   C. Xerostomia management
      1. Artificial saliva
      2. Sucrose-free lemon drops
      3. Frequent intake of fluids
      4. Pilocarpine: 5–10 mg tid is under investigation as a means of stimulating salivary flow during radiation treatment.
   D. Infection
      1. Broad spectrum antibiotic coverage with penicillin 500 mg po qid for 7–14 days for bacterial infection
      2. Candidiasis
         a) Nystatin oral suspension: Swish and swallow 200,000–400,000 units qid

          b) Ketoconazole: 200 mg po once a day for seven days

          c) Fluconazole: 200 mg po on day one, then 100 mg for three days

          d) Clotrimazole: One disc five times a day for seven days, dissolved slowly in mouth

   3. Keep oral cavity clean by rinsing with saline solution (one liter saline with one teaspoon bicarbonate of soda, swish and spit).

VII. Follow-up

    A. During the acute phase of stomatitis, inspect the oral cavity at least daily.

    B. Carefully follow patients who have had stomatitis, particularly with herpes simplex virus infection, when subsequent treatment begins, as viral reactivation is possible.

    C. Patients should report a history of stomatitis and oral cavity radiation to their dentist, as subsequent dental work may require antibiotic prophylaxis if permanent dryness or changes in the oral cavity exist.

VIII. Referrals

    A. Medical oncologist, radiation oncologist, dentist: May be involved in the patient's care

    B. Dietitian: To maintain adequate food and fluid intake

References

Alvarez, S. (1992). Infections in the compromised host. *Medical Clinics of North America, 76,* 1135–1142.

Ganley, B. (1996). Mouth care for the patient undergoing head and neck radiation therapy: A survey of radiation oncology nurses. *Oncology Nursing Forum, 23,* 1619–1623.

Madeya, M. (1996a). Oral complications from cancer therapy: Part 1. Pathophysiology and secondary complications. *Oncology Nursing Forum, 23,* 801–807.

Madeya, M. (1996b). Oral complications from cancer therapy: Part 2. Nursing implications for assessment and treatment. *Oncology Nursing Forum, 23,* 808–820.

Peterson, D.E., & Ambrosio, J.A. (1992). Diagnosis and management of acute and chronic oral complications of non-surgical cancer therapies. *Dental Clinics of North America, 36,* 945–996.

Rose, M., Shrader-Bogen, C., Korlath, G., Priem, J., & Larson, L. (1996). Identifying patient symptoms after radiotherapy using nurse-managed telephone interviews. *Oncology Nursing Forum, 23,* 99–102.

Section III. Integument

Symptoms

Medical Diagnosis

Chapter

12. Hyperpigmentation

Kathleen Murphy-Ende, RN, PhD, CFNP

I. Definition: General darkening of the skin or nails; localized or brown spots

II. Pathophysiology
   A. Causes of hyperpigmentation
      1. Increased rate of melanosome production
      2. Increased amount of melanosome transferred to keratinocytes
      3. Larger size and melanization of the melanosome, or when the pigment is deposited in anomalous sites
   B. Mechanisms that produce hyperpigmentation through the melanocyte system by stimulation of melanin formation
      1. Elevated adrenocorticotropic hormone (ACTH), which stimulates the melanocytes
      2. Direct stimulation of the melanocytes
      3. Inflammatory changes, which stimulate melanin formation
   C. Medications: Can cause hyperpigmentation by deposition of the drug or its by-product metabolite into the skin or by inducing increased melanin production by the melanocytes

III. Clinical features
   A. History
      1. History of cancer and cancer treatment
      2. Current medications: Prescribed and over-the-counter
      3. History of presenting symptom(s): Precipitating factors, onset, location, and duration
      4. Changes in activities of daily living
      5. Past medical history of skin problems, adrenal insufficiency, thyroid or liver disease
   B. Signs and symptoms
      1. Diffuse melanosis: A generalized darkening of the skin that is evenly distributed
      2. Local area of pigmentation
      3. Circumscribed
         a) Actinic keratosis: Flattened papule, dry, tan or gray
         b) Actinic or solar lentigines: Macule on the dorsum of the hand and/or wrist; often termed liver spots
         c) Chloasma or melasma: Nonuniform, hyperpigmented, flat spot seen on the forehead, cheeks, and upper lip

    d) Nevus: Slightly elevated, round, evenly pigmented
    e) Nodules: Deep, firm, raised lesion greater than 0.5 cm
    f) Ochronosis: Bluish-black or brown pigmented area of the sclerae, ears, skin, or nails
    g) Tinea pityriasis versicolor: Patchy, yellow-brown pigmented area over the trunk
  C. Physical exam
    1. Integument exam
      a) Inspect and palpate the skin and scalp, noting the color, moisture, temperature, texture, mobility, and turgor.
      b) Note location and distribution of lesions.
    2. Nails: Inspect and palpate, noting color, shape, and lesions.
    3. Oral mucosa: Inspect mucous membrane for color, moisture, and lesions.

IV. Diagnostic tests
  A. Laboratory
    1. Usually not indicated
    2. Biopsy of areas suspicious for malignancy
  B. Radiology: Usually not indicated

V. Differential diagnosis
  A. Genetic factors: Melasma is the hyperpigmentation of the face, neck, and forearms.
  B. Endocrine
    1. Addison's disease: Hyperpigmentation of creases, pressure areas, and nipples (see Chapter 149)
    2. Hypothyroidism (see Chapter 150)
    3. Pregnancy
  C. Metabolic
    1. Biliary cirrhosis (see Chapter 64)
    2. Gaucher's disease
    3. Hemosiderosis
    4. Ochronosis
  D. Nutritional
    1. Excessive carotene ingestion
    2. Folic acid deficiency (see Chapter 115)
    3. Malabsorption
    4. Pellagra (niacin deficiency)
  E. Systemic
    1. Graft-versus-host disease
    2. Hemochromatosis
    3. Hepatic insufficiency
    4. Porphyria cutanea tarda
    5. Rheumatoid arthritis (see Chapter 108)
    6. Scleroderma
  F. Malignancy-associated
    1. ACTH-producing tumors

2. Carcinoid syndrome
3. Cutaneous malignancies
4. Neurofibromatosis
5. Skin malignancy (see Chapter 21)
6. Chemotherapy-induced (e.g., bleomycin, busulfan, cyclophosphamide, dacarbazine dactinomycin, daunorubicin, doxorubicin, 5-fluorouracil, hydroxyurea, 6-mercap-topurine, mitomycin, methotrexate, thiotepa, vinblastine)
7. Radiation: Acute and late effect (see pp. 89–90)

VI. Treatment
   A. No treatment usually is necessary.
   B. Hyperpigmentation may or may not be reversible and often is permanent after the patient undergoes radiation.
   C. Reassure the patient that these changes are a side effect of the treatment and not progression of disease.
   D. Makeup for pigmented facial spots may be effective in minimizing the appearance of lesions.
      1. Bleaching preparations consisting of hydroquinone cream may lighten the lesion if the pigment is in the epidermis, but they can be irritating to the skin.
      2. Combination retinoic acid 0.1%, hydroquinone cream, and dexamethasone 0.1% in a hydrophilic ointment can be used to lighten the lesion but can be irritating to the skin.
      3. Excessive pigmented lesions can be minimized with mid-depth trichloroacetic acid or glycolic acid chemical peels or laser resurfacing.

VII. Follow-up: Periodic evaluation of the skin should be performed at consecutive visits.

VIII. Referrals: Patients with any skin lesion that is suspicious of malignancy should undergo biopsy and be referred to a dermatologist.

References

Blackmar, A. (1997). A focus on wound care: Radiation-induced skin alterations. *MEDSURG Nursing, 6*(3), 172–175.

Gallagher, J. (1995). Management of cutaneous symptoms. *Seminars in Oncology Nursing, 11,* 239–247.

Rodriguez, C., & Ash, J.C. (1996). Associated late effects. *Cancer Nursing, 19,* 455–468.

Shellow, W. (1995). Evaluation of disturbances in pigmentation. In A. Goroll, L.M. May, & A. Mulley (Eds.), *Primary care medicine: Office evaluation and management of the adult patient* (3rd ed.) (pp. 893–895). Philadelphia: Lippincott.

13. Nail Changes

Kathleen Murphy-Ende, RN, PhD, CFNP

I. Definition: Alterations in the nails or nail beds

II. Physiology/Pathophysiology
   A. Normal
      1. The nail protects the terminal phalanx and aids in perception of fine touch and the ability to perform motor skills such as to pick, lift, and scratch.
      2. The nail plate consists of keratin and is attached to and receives its nutrients from the vascular nail bed. The blood supply originates from two main arterial arches, which are branches of the digital arteries.
      3. The nail root is the living nail layer.
         a) The root lies under the proximal nail fold and extends out to form the lunula (white moon).
         b) Nail grows out from the nail root or matrix at a rate of approximately 0.1 mm daily for fingernails and 0.05 mm for toenails.
      4. Cuticles form a seal between the nail fold and the plate, protecting this space from external moisture. The side of the plate is covered by the lateral nail fold.
   B. Pathophysiology: Pigmentary changes are caused by absence of melanin or an increase, decrease, or altered distribution of melanin.

III. Clinical features: Many types of nail changes can occur in a variety of local or systemic disorders; therefore, changes must be correlated with other clinical findings.
   A. Etiology
      1. Nail changes can result from trauma, infection, dermatologic disorders, systemic disease, or medications.
      2. Similar nail changes may occur in many different conditions because the nails have a limited response capability.
   B. History
      1. History of cancer and cancer treatment
      2. Current medications: Prescribed and over-the-counter
      3. History of presenting symptom(s): Precipitating factors, onset, location, and duration
      4. Changes in activities of daily living
      5. Past medical history of recent trauma or chemical contact to the nails

C. Signs and symptoms
1. Painful or cold fingers/toes
2. Discoloration of fingers/toes
   a) Pallor
   b) Cyanosis
   c) Hyperemia
D. Physical exam: Inspect and palpate nails, noting color, shape, and lesions. Inspect tissue surrounding the nail for erythema or swelling.
1. Beau's lines: Transverse depression in the nails emerging from under the proximal nail folds growing out with the nails; usually follows one month after an acute illness
2. Brittle nails: Split or break easily
3. Clubbing: Rounded and bulbous distal phalanx; convex nail plate; angle between distal phalanx and nail bed greater than 180 degrees
4. Distortion
5. Discoloration
6. Hyperpigmentation bands: Dark brown or blue transverse lines across nail plate
7. Koilonychia (spoon nail): Concave malformation of outer surface of the nail
8. Leukonychia: White spots that grow out with the nail
9. Longitudinal nail grooves
10. Mees' lines: Transverse white lines emerging from the proximal nail folds and growing out with the nail
11. Nail atrophy or dystrophy
12. Onychauxis: Thickened nail plates
13. Onycholysis: Distal separation of the nail plate from the nail bed
14. Paronychia: Inflammation of the proximal and lateral nail folds
15. Pitting: Small pits in the nail
16. Splinter hemorrhages: Thin, longitudinal red or brown bands
17. Subungual or periungual lesions: Growth of tissue under or within the nail
18. Terry's nails: White with a distal band of reddish brown; lunulae may not be visible.
19. Yellow nail syndrome: Nails become yellow and cease to grow.

IV. Diagnostic tests: Usually not necessary
A. Laboratory
1. Complete blood count to evaluate for anemia
2. Sedimentation rate to evaluate for inflammatory process
3. Serum iron and iron-binding capacity to detect iron-deficiency anemia
4. Culture of nail or surrounding tissue for fungus or bacteria
5. Biopsy of nail or surrounding tissue if malignancy is suspected
B. Radiology: Not indicated

V. Differential diagnosis: Abnormal nail changes must be correlated with other systemic findings to derive accurate diagnosis.
A. Medication-induced: Numerous medications can cause nail changes. Examples include
1. Antimalarial: Blue-gray to yellow discoloration
2. Antibiotics

        a) Demethylchlortetracycline and doxycycline may cause painful photo-onycholysis and yellow pigmentation.

        b) Cloxacillin and cephaloridine may cause temporary nail loss.

  3. Arsenic: White lines

  4. Beta-blockers

        a) Practolol: Psoriasiform nail dystrophy, onycholysis, and subungual hyperkeratosis

        b) Propranolol: Psoriasiform eruptions with thickening, pitting, and discoloration of nails

        c) Metoprolol: Beau's lines

        d) Timolol maleate eye drops: Pigmentation

  5. Chemotherapy-induced: Most common include

        a) Bleomycin: Nail loss

        b) Cyclophosphamide: Hyperpigmentation, transverse ridging

        c) Dacarbazine and daunorubicin: Hyperpigmentation, onycholysis

        d) Doxorubicin: Hyperpigmentation of nail beds and dermal creases

        e) 5-fluorouracil: Nail loss, brittleness, cracking

        f) Hydroxyurea: Longitudinal pigmented nail bands

        g) Idarubicin: Transverse pigmented bands and hyperpigmentation

        h) Ifosfamide: Nail ridging

        i) Melphalan, mechlorethamine, methotrexate, and mitomycin: Hyperpigmentation and dark half-circles

        j) Mitoxantrone: Onycholysis

B. Infection

  1. Candidiasis: Onycholysis invading the superficial aspect of the undersurface of the nail along the distal and lateral borders, which may progress to atrophy with distal erosion of the plate

  2. Fungal: Onychia, paronychia

  3. HIV: Hyperpigmentation, transverse and longitudinal ridging, changes in the size of lunulae, and onycholysis (see Chapter 156)

  4. Paronychia: Redness, swelling, and tenderness at the lateral fold

  5. Tinea unguium: Hyperkeratosis at the lateral or distal margin of the plate progressing to fragmentation of the nail plate

C. Benign growths

  1. Warts, periungual fibroma: Fibrous tissue growing from the lateral nail fold

  2. Subungual exostosis: Firm swelling of the great toe below the nail tip, displacing the nail

  3. Pigmented nevus: Longitudinal band of pigment in nail plate caused by junctional nevus in matrix

D. Malignancy-associated

  1. Epithelioma: Chronic paronychia

  2. Melanoma

  3. Kaposi's sarcoma

  4. Squamous cell carcinoma

E. Nail changes associated with systemic disease

1. Vitamin B_{12} deficiency: Digital and nail pigmentation (see Chapter 114)
2. Digital artery insufficiency: Permanent loss of nail in a single digit
3. Diabetes mellitus (see Chapter 143)
4. Cardiovascular or pulmonary disease: Clubbing, cyanosis
5. Chronic anemia (see Chapter 112)
6. Endocarditis: Splinter hemorrhages (see Chapter 44)
7. Hyperparathyroidism: Nail dystrophy or onycholysis
8. Hypo/hyperthyroidism: Brittleness, onycholysis (see Chapters 149 and 150)
9. Hypopituitarism: Dystrophy, loss of lunula, spooning
10. Peripheral neuropathy: Nail dystrophy (see Chapter 131)
11. Raynaud's phenomenon: Longitudinal ridging, nail splitting, koilonychia, onycholysis
12. Rheumatoid arthritis: Ridging and beading (see Chapter 108)
13. Scleroderma: Partial or total loss of nail
14. Systemic lupus erythematosus: Clubbing, splinter hemorrhage, nail fold infarcts, onycholysis, pitting, ridging

F. Trauma-associated nail changes
1. Ingrown nail: Nail plate grows into the lateral nail folds; progresses to form granulation tissue and possibly infection
2. Loss, chipping, and splitting of nail: Occurs from direct blow to nail or excessive exposure to water or irritants

VI. Treatment
A. Treatment is directed at the underlying medical conditions, which may or may not result in improvement of nail condition.
B. Drug-induced changes do not require treatment and usually improve when drug is discontinued.
1. Reassure the patient that nail changes are an expected side effect and are not cancer-related.
2. Educate the patient that it takes approximately 5.5 months for fingernails to completely grow and 12–18 months for toenails to regrow.
C. Primary nail conditions
1. Candidiasis: Itraconazole 100 mg po bid for one week
2. Fungal infection
    a) Itraconazole 100 mg po qid or 400 mg po qd for one week per month for three months.
    b) Terbinafine 250 mg po qd for six weeks for fingernails and three months for toenails
3. Warts
    a) Fulguration or cryosurgery
    b) Topical solution of lactic acid 85% solution covered with flexible colloidin and waterproof tape for eight hours daily
4. Paronychia: Lance the fold and begin antibiotics appropriate for *Staphylococcus aureus*.

  a) Soak nail in warm water for 15 minutes qid and cover with a nonocclusive dressing.
  b) Chronic paronychia: Avoid excessive exposure to water and irritants.
  c) Topical corticosteroids may be helpful if inflammation is present (see Appendix 14).

5. Onycholysis: To prevent secondary bacterial infection, careful debridement, manicuring, and reduction of irritant exposure

6. Psoriasis or lichen planus: Intradermal triamcinolone acetonide suspension 2.5 mg/ml injected into the nail matrix every two to four weeks to treat inflammatory nail dystrophy as a last resort

7. Ingrown nail
  a) Pack under the free edge of the nail with a cotton wick.
  b) If the nail is growing into the tissue, clip the nail and soak the finger or toe in warm water daily.
  c) Instruct the patient on clipping toenails straight across and avoiding tight-fitting shoes.

VII. Follow-up: After initiating treatment in one to two weeks to evaluate for healing

VIII. Referrals: Nail changes that do not heal with treatment or are suggestive of malignancy should be referred to a dermatologist or podiatrist.

References

Borecky, D., Stephenson, J., Keeling, J., & Vukelja, S. (1997). Idarubicin-induced pigmentary changes of the nails. *Cutis, 59,* 203–204.

Cakir, B., Sucak, G., Haznedar, R., & Turkey, A. (1997). Longitudinal pigmented nail bands during hydroxyurea therapy. *International Journal of Dermatology, 36,* 236–237.

Creamer, J., Mortimer, P., & Powles, T. (1995). Mitoxantrone-induced onycholysis: A series of five cases. *Clinical and Experimental Dermatology, 20,* 459–461.

Lemez, P. (1995). Transverse nail ridgings induced by chemotherapy: A dose dependent phenomenon. *Acta Haematologica, 92,* 212–213.

Samman, P.D., & Fenton, D.A. (1995). *Samman's the nails in disease* (5th ed.). Boston: Butterworth-Heinemann Ltd.

Chapter

14. Pruritus

JoAnne Lester, MSN, RNC, OCN®, CNP

I. Definition: A cutaneous sensation or itch that provokes the urge to scratch or rub the skin

II. Pathophysiology
   A. Arises from sensory, unmyelinated, unspecialized free nerve endings of the skin located between cells of the epidermis, found near the dermal-epidermal junction
   B. Afferent transmission by polymodal, unmyelinated C fibers through the dorsal horn of the gray matter of the spinal cord
      1. Synapses with secondary neurons
      2. Ascending to the contralateral spinothalamic tracts
      3. Ascending to the thalamus
      4. Relayed by tertiary neurons to the level of consciousness in the cerebral cortex
   C. Unmyelinated C fibers especially concentrated in the flexor aspects of the wrists and ankles
   D. Peripheral mediators related to etiology of pruritus
      1. Histamine
      2. Neuropeptides
      3. Vasoactive peptides and proteases
      4. Arachidonic acid transformation products
      5. Platelet-activating factor
   E. Scratch response: A spinal reflex

III. Clinical features: Common complaint of the elderly
   A. Etiology
      1. May be localized or generalized, with or without skin lesions
      2. May represent an underlying disease or even a prognostic variable of an identified disease
      3. Factors modulating itching, such as psychological factors, inflammation, dry skin, vasodilatation, warmth, and cold
   B. History
      1. History of cancer and cancer treatment
      2. Current medications: Prescribed and over-the-counter
      3. History of presenting symptom(s): Precipitating factors, onset, location, and duration
      4. Changes in activities of daily living and levels of stress

     5. History of exposure to chemicals, plants, animals, topicals (e.g., soaps, creams, perfumes)

  C. Signs and symptoms

     1. Skin changes, such as scaling, rash, pustules, macules, hives/wheals, dryness, cracking, or excoriation

     2. Color changes, such as erythema or jaundice

  D. Physical exam

     1. Complete inspection of the skin is performed, including the affected area and overall skin surface, looking for scaling, dryness, xerosis, inflammation, scratch marks, breaks in skin, excoriations, lichenification, lice, scabies, stasis dermatitis, or jaundice and distribution (localized or generalized).

     2. Systemic condition requires complete physical exam to look for the following.

       a) Hepatomegaly, splenomegaly, and symptoms suggestive of liver disease

       b) Scleral icterus, indicating liver disease

       c) Lymphadenopathy, indicating infection or lymphoma

IV. Diagnostic tests: If no obvious abnormalities indicate a possible etiology, obtain in order of importance.

  A. Laboratory

     1. Complete blood count with differential to evaluate for infection or anemia

     2. Sedimentation rate to evaluate for inflammatory process

     3. Chemical profile to rule out renal or hepatic disease, hyperglycemia, hypoglycemia, effects of drugs, pancreatic disorders, endocrine disorders, dietary imbalances, cholestasis, or malignancies

     4. Thyroid function studies to rule out thyroid disorders

     5. Serum iron to rule out iron deficiency

     6. Serum protein electrophoresis, immunoelectrophoresis to rule out protein gammopathies or malignancies

     7. Antinuclear antibody (ANA), rheumatoid arthritis factor (RA) to rule out autoimmune deficiency

  B. Radiology: If laboratory studies are inconclusive, consider chest x-ray (PA and lateral) to rule out malignancies, infection, or inflammation.

  C. Other tests may be indicated: Possible skin biopsy with special stains and/or skin scrapings to determine presence of autoimmune diseases, malignancies, circulatory disorders, parasites, infections, or inflammation

V. Differential diagnosis (see Figure 14–1)

  A. Localized pruritus: Primary dermatologic condition secondary to infection or infestation

  B. Generalized pruritus: A systemic condition or psychogenic etiology

VI. Treatment

  A. Treatment for pruritus is dependent on resolution of etiologic factor(s) as well as localized, symptomatic relief. If considered to be medication-induced, stop medication.

  B. Topical applications, such as cotton clothing, heat/cold, baths, humidity, ultraviolet light, emollient soaps or lotions, antihistamine or hydrocortisone creams, or soothing

Figure 14-1. Differential Diagnosis of Pruritus

Malignancy
- Hematologic disorders
- Hodgkin's disease
- Non-Hodgkin's lymphoma
- Leukemia
- Mycosis fungoides
- Multiple myeloma
- Sarcomas
- Germ cell neoplasm
- Bowen's disease
- Invasive squamous cell carcinoma
- Visceral tumors

Hematologic
- AIDS
- Polycythemia vera
- Iron-deficiency anemia
- Paraproteinemia

Endocrine
- Hypo/Hyperthyroidism

Miscellaneous
- Radiation therapy
- Xerosis (dry skin)
- Psychosis
- Advanced age
- Multiple sclerosis
- Venous stasis
- Dermatitis—atopic/contact

Infections
- Rubella
- Varicella
- Trichinosis
- Onchocerciasis
- Psoriasis
- Herpes
- Fifth disease
- Impetigo
- Measles

Autoimmune
- Systemic lupus erythematosus
- Immunoglobulin disorders
- Graft-versus-host disease

Renal
- Chronic renal failure

Hepatic
- Cholestasis
- Obstructive biliary disease
- Primary biliary disease
- Post-hepatic obstruction

Skin diseases
- Scabies
- Mites
- Insect bites
- Eczema
- Lichen planus
- Dermitis
- Herpetiformis
- Fungal infection
- Parasitic xerosis
- Rash

Medication-Induced
- Allergic reaction
- Opioids
- Antibiotics
- Contraceptives

Note. Based on information from Seiz & Yarbro, 1999.

lotions with menthol may relieve local symptoms. Preparations such as calamine lotion can be drying and are most effective on weeping pustules.

C. Systemic antihistamines (see Appendix 4), sedatives, aspirin, or tricyclic antidepressants to relieve systemic symptoms (other drugs may be systemically taken depending on the etiology and underlying disease process).

D. Behavioral measures, such as trimmed fingernails, soft clothing, air humidification, tepid baths or showers, Aveeno® (S.C. Johnson & Son, Inc., Racine, WI) oatmeal baths, and mild, nonperfumed soaps

VII. Follow-up
A. Short-term follow-up should be done within 48 hours of initial contact to verify partial or complete resolution of symptoms. Many cases of pruritus spontaneously resolve.
B. Long-term follow-up is dependent on the etiology and causative factors.

VIII. Referrals
A. Patients who improve significantly or spontaneously resolve within 48 hours (without evidence of underlying disease) generally do not require a physician referral.
B. Patients with symptoms related to a previously diagnosed chronic illness (e.g., end-stage liver or renal disease, terminal malignancy) may possibly be managed without a physician referral.

    C. Patients who do not improve or resolve after 48 hours or show progression of symptoms require a family or general practice physician referral.

    D. Dermatology may be consulted, depending on the presentation and symptoms.

    E. Patients who present with underlying disease processes should be referred immediately to a physician.

    F. Patients with underlying psychogenic causes or distress should be referred to a psychiatrist or psychologist.

References

Blow, C. (1997). Urticaria: A rational GP approach. *The Practitioner, 241,* 80–85.

Goolsby, M.J. (1998). The elusive itch: Assessment, diagnosis and management of pruritus. *Advances for Nurse Practitioners, 6*(11), 61–65.

Kantor, G.R. (1993). Generalized pruritus: How do you manage it? *Emergency Medicine, 25,* 18–26.

Lober, C.W. (1993). Pruritus and malignancy. *Clinics in Dermatology, 11,* 125–128.

Rudikoff, D. (1998). The effect of dryness on the skin. *Clinics in Dermatology, 16,* 99–107.

Scott, C.B., & Moloney, M.F. (1996). Physical urticaria: A common misdiagnosis. *Nurse Practitioner, 21*(11), 42–56.

Seiz, A.M., & Yarbro, C.H. (1999). Pruritus. In C.H. Yarbro, M.H. Frogge, & M. Goodman (Eds.), *Cancer symptom management* (2nd ed.) (pp. 148–158). Boxton: Jones & Bartlett.

Tur, E. (1997). Physiology of the skin—Differences between women and men. *Clinics in Dermatology, 15,* 5–16.

Warner, M.R., Taylor, J.S., & Leow, Y.H. (1997). Agents causing contact urticaria. *Clinics in Dermatology, 15,* 623–635.

Chapter

15. Rash

Kathleen Murphy-Ende, RN, PhD, CFNP

I. Definition: A general term that refers to an eruption of the skin

II. Physiology/Pathophysiology
   A. Normal physiology
      1. The skin is a living organ that provides a barrier between the internal and external environment, holding fluid within and protecting the body from microorganisms and irritants.
      2. The skin helps to regulate body temperature and synthesizes vitamin D.
      3. The skin consists of three layers.
         a) Epidermis: Where melanin and keratin are formed
         b) Dermis: Contains connective tissue, sebaceous glands, and hair follicles
         c) Subcutaneous layer: Contains fat, sweat glands, and hair follicles
   B. Pathophysiology
      1. Many rashes are caused by an inflammatory response from contact with bacteria, viruses, temperature extremes, chemicals, or mechanical irritants.
      2. During the inflammatory phase, histamine and other mediators are released, causing dilation of the blood vessels and leakage of fluid.
      3. Pressure from the fluid causes release of other mediator substances, which may irritate the nerve fibers and cause pain or pruritus.

III. Clinical features
   A. Etiology: Causes include infection, allergic reaction, or systemic condition.
   B. History: Examining the rash prior to obtaining history will guide the practitioner in asking pertinent questions.
      1. History of cancer and cancer treatment
      2. Current medications: Prescribed and over-the-counter
      3. History of rashes: Precipitating factors, onset, location, and duration
      4. Changes in activities of daily living
      5. Past medical history: Exposure to people with a similar rash, diabetes mellitus, lupus, kidney disease, asthma, or skin diseases (e.g., eczema, dermatitis, psoriasis)
      6. Recent exposure to new physical or chemical agents in the home or work environment
   C. Signs and symptoms

1. Crusting
2. Elevated temperature
3. Fatigue
4. Jaundice
5. Joint swelling
6. Night sweats
7. Pain
8. Pruritus
9. Redness, warmth
10. Tingling
11. Weeping

D. Physical exam
   1. Integument: The entire skin, including the nails, scalp, palms, soles, and mucous membranes
   2. Nature of the rash: Accurate overall descriptions, including nature, distribution (localized or generalized), and associated findings
      a) Atrophy: Translucent thinning of the skin with loss of furrow
      b) Bulla: Blister greater than 0.5 cm in diameter
      c) Burrow: Slightly raised linear tunnel in the epidermis that may end in a vesicle
      d) Comedo: Black mark plugging the opening of a sebaceous gland
      e) Crust: Dried residue of serum, pus, or blood
      f) Cyst: Lesion with internal wall that contains blood or fluid
      g) Erosion: Loss of epidermis after the rupture of a vesicle or because of an abrasion; the surface is moist but does not bleed.
      h) Excoriation: Scratches
      i) Fissure: Linear loss of skin
      j) Lichenification: Thickening of the epidermis with increased skin furrow
      k) Maceration: Softening and loss of top layer of epidermis
      l) Malar rash: Erythema on face
      m) Macule: Flat lesion with color change only
      n) Nodule: Raised, solid lesion greater than 1 cm in diameter
      o) Papule: Raised, solid lesion less than 1 cm in diameter
      p) Patch: Circumscribed, flat, nonpalpable change in skin color
      q) Plaque: Flat, elevated lesion greater than 0.5 cm in diameter
      r) Pustule: Elevated lesion filled with purulent material
      s) Scale: Thin flake of exfoliated epidermis
      t) Telangiectasia: Dilation of superficial blood vessels
      u) Ulcer: Loss of skin and underlying tissue
      v) Vesicle: Blister filled with serous fluid up to 0.5 cm in diameter
      w) Weeping: Eruption of serum from the lesion
      x) Wheal: Irregular, transient superficial area of localized skin edema
   3. Distribution of the rash over the body, such as extremities, thorax, skin folds, face, or scalp
   4. Pattern of rash: Generalized versus localized
      a) Central distribution

       b) Clustered
       c) Fernlike pattern
       d) Grouped
       e) Herald patch
       f) Linear
       g) Multiple or single
       h) Symmetrical
   5. Associated findings
       a) Erythema
       b) Pigmentation

IV. Diagnostic tests: Usually not necessary for the diagnosis of most rashes; selection must be guided by the history and physical exam.
  A. Laboratory
    1. Skin biopsy: Any skin lesion suspected of being malignant
    2. Complete blood count: Increased eosinophils in allergic reactions, anemia associated with chronic diseases
    3. Wound culture to identify bacterial or fungal source
    4. Potassium hydroxide solution on skin scrapings: Positive hyphae and spores with fungal infections, such as tinea pedis
    5. Scratch test: Urticarial eruption or linear wheals a few minutes after scratching the skin with a tongue depressor; associated with dermographism, indicating an allergic reaction
  B. Radiology: Not indicated

V. Differential diagnosis
  A. Autoimmune
    1. Cutaneous lupus: Discoid or other lesions without systemic illness
    2. Erythema nodosum: Tender, erythematous, nodular 5–20 mm lesions in the extensor surface of the distal lower extremities
    3. Dermatomyositis: Inflammatory skin changes associated with proximal skeletal muscle inflammation and weakness
    4. Systemic lupus erythematosus: Butterfly rash and photodermatitis with systemic disease
    5. Thrombocytopenic purpura: Large red or purple ecchymotic lesions (see Chapter 120)
  B. Allergic
    1. Atopic dermatitis (see Chapter 18)
    2. Angioneurotic edema: Transient wheals or hives of the deep tissues and may include mucous membranes and tongue swelling
    3. Contact dermatitis (see Chapter 19)
    4. Drug allergies
       a) Abrupt onset of a widespread, symmetric erythematous rash; may include constitutional symptoms
       b) May appear similar to an inflammatory condition, such as eczema or dermatitis
       c) Appearance may vary (e.g., maculopapular, urticaria, fixed hyperpigmentation, vesicles, bullae, acneiform)

    5. Urticaria: Transient wheals or hives of the superficial tissue

C. Dermatologic
    1. Actinic keratosis: Lesions on the face, neck, dorsal hands, and forearms that are dry, scaly, and rough in texture and approximately 5 mm or less in diameter
    2. Pityriasis rosea: Oval papulosquamous patch on trunk or proximal upper extremity followed by a generalized macular eruption of small oval plaques on the trunk and proximal extremities, aligning with the skin line and forming a Christmas tree formation
    3. Psoriasis: Erythematous, scaling, hyperproliferative papulosquamous eruption; well-defined plaques with adherent, silver to white scale; commonly on the extensor surface of the knees and elbows, scalp, sacrum
    4. Rosacea: Chronic facial acneiform lesions, papules, pustules, and occasional nodules
    5. Seborrheic dermatitis: Scaling macules, papules, and plaques; yellow and thick or white and dry; may crust, fissure, and weep; usually found on the face, scalp, or folds of the skin
    6. Xerosis: Dry skin

D. Infection
    1. Acne: Comedos, papules, pustules, and nodules
    2. Candidiasis: Erythematous base, scaly or denuded, beefy red; may or may not have satellite lesions; commonly found in moist areas such as skin folds
    3. Cellulitis (see Chapter 16)
    4. Chicken pox: Multiple vesicles starting on the trunk and extending peripherally
    5. Erythema multiforme: Symmetrical multiple wheals and papules
    6. Erythema marginatum: Erythematous, rapidly spreading, flat, pale centers with raised red margins seen in streptococcal infections
    7. Fifth disease (erythema infectiosum): Erythematous, papular rash on the trunk, face, and back with central clearing
    8. Fungal infection (e.g., tinea capitis, tinea cruris, tinea pedis, tinea versicolor): Scaly lesion, nodular pustules, sharply demarcated, moist
    9. Herpes labialis or genitalis (see Chapter 89)
   10. Herpes zoster (see Chapter 20)
   11. Impetigo: Papules, vesicles, and pustules on face and neck with serum-colored crusting
   12. Measles: Maculopapular rash starting on the face and hairline, which descends and becomes confluent, may have desquamation
   13. Rubella: Maculopapular rash beginning at the face and neck and spreading to the trunk; extremities may have slight desquamation
   14. Scabies: Burrow rash on the finger webs, flexor surfaces of wrist, penis, nipples, buttocks, axillae, and toes; forms crusty, excoriated papules

E. Malignancy-associated (see Appendix 12)
    1. Abdominal/gastrointestinal malignancy: Acanthosis nigricans or freckling and hyperpigmentation in the axillary folds and elsewhere
    2. ACTH-producing tumors: Hyperpigmentation
    3. Basal cell or squamous cell carcinoma
    4. Carcinoid: Episodic general erythema and cyanosis
    5. Colon cancer: Dermatomyositis and acanthosis nigricans

      6. Cutaneous T cell lymphoma: Initial scaling, erythematous macular eruption, then well-demarcated erythematous macules progressing to plaques and to diffuse, intense erythema overlying white scales
      7. Kaposi's sarcoma: Red-purple or dark plaques or nodules
      8. Leukemia: Erythematous subcutaneous nodules
      9. Melanoma: Nevus with irregular border, irregular distribution of pigment
     10. Neurofibroma: Raised nodules

F. Physical agents
      1. Chemical irritants
      2. Overdrying or overwashing of the skin
      3. Radiation-induced (see Acute Radiation Therapy Skin Changes on page 89)
      4. Photodermatitis: Sunburn

G. Systemic
      1. Cirrhosis: Spider angioma
      2. Cushing's syndrome: Acne, flushed face, purple striae
      3. Diabetes mellitus (see Chapter 143)
      4. Renal disease: Excoriation, uremic frost (see Chapter 83)
      5. Obstructive biliary disease: Jaundice, excoriation
      6. Iron-deficiency anemia (see Chapter 116)
      7. Polycythemia vera (see Chapter 122)

VI. Treatment: Directed at providing symptomatic relief and eliminating causative factors (see Table 15-1)

VII. Follow-up: Close follow-up is necessary to evaluate the effectiveness of treatment and for symptom management.

VIII. Referrals: Consultation with a dermatologist may be necessary in establishing a diagnosis or if the rash does not heal with treatment.

Table 15-1. General Principles of Treatment for Rash

Treatment	Base	Comments
Aqueous solutions	Water is the solvent.	Drying if alcohol in the solution
Creams	Solid emulsions	Moisturizing if in oil emulsion; neutral if in oil-free or ester emulsion
Emollients	Base preparation of oil	Very moisturizing
Gels	Semisolid oil-based	Deposits film on skin; neutral to drying
Lotions	Liquid emulsions; powder suspended in oil or water	Neutral to drying
Ointments	Fat base	Very moisturizing
Powders	Agent in fine particles	Drying

References

Blackmar, A. (1997). A focus on wound care: Radiation-induced skin alterations. *MEDSURG Nursing, 6*(3),172–175.

Gallagher, J. (1995). Management of cutaneous symptoms. *Seminars in Oncology Nursing, 11,* 239–246.

Kurzrock, R., & Cohen, P. (1995). Cutaneous paraneoplastic syndromes in solid tumors. *American Journal of Medicine, 99,* 662–671.

Reifsnider, E. (1997). Common adult infectious skin conditions. *Nurse Practitioner, 22*(11), 17–33.

Rothe, M.J., & Grant-Keels, J.M. (1996). Atopic dermatitis: An update. *Journal of the American Academy of Dermatology, 35*(1), 1–13.

Acute Radiation Therapy Skin Changes

Tissue Response	Onset	Duration	Clinical Response	Suggested Therapy
Erythema (transient)	Within hours to days of first treatment	Resolves after several days but will occur with further treatment	Faint, often unnoticed redness	Topical application of lotions, creams, or ointments without alcohol, menthol, or other chemical irritants; 1% hydrocortisone ointment bid to tid (see Appendix 14)
Erythema (proper)	Following two to three weeks of standard fractionated radiation therapy	Resolves within 20–30 days following last treatment	Redness that outlines treatment field; intensifies as treatment continues; skin may be warm with edema	Topical application of lotions, creams, or ointments without alcohol, menthol, or other chemical irritants; 1% hydrocortisone ointment bid to tid (see Appendix 14)
Pruritus	When radiation exposure exceeds 20–28 Gy	—	Itching	See Chapter 14
Hyperpigmentation	Following two to three weeks of standard fractionated radiation therapy	Usually resolves three months to one year following completion of treatment but may be chronic	Tanned appearance	None
Dry desquamation	Following three to four weeks of standard fractionated radiation therapy	Resolves in one to two weeks after completion of treatment	Dryness, flaking, and peeling often accompanied by itching	Same as for erythema, including applying cornstarch
Moist desquamation	Following 40 Gy or with trauma or excess friction	Recovery usually two to four weeks after completion of treatment	Painful, brilliant erythema, sloughing skin, exposed dermis, and serous exudate oozing from the surface	Apply dressings (hydrogel, hydrocolloid, polyurethane film) (see Chapter 17). Cleanse with one-third strength hydrogen peroxide, normal saline, or a wound cleanser.

(Continued on next page)

Acute Radiation Therapy Skin Changes (Continued)

Radiation-Related Factors
- Total dose and total time
- Daily fraction size
- Type of radiation (photon versus electron)
- Use of tissue equivalent material (bolus)
- Size of treatment field

Patient-Related Factors
- Anatomic location of treatment field(s)
- Characteristics of skin in treatment field(s)
- Proximity of tumor to skin surface
- Concomitant chemotherapy
- Comorbid conditions
- Nutritional status

Acute Skin Changes
- May occur within two to three weeks of starting treatment (approx. 20–30 Gy)
- Usually repairable
- Types
  - Erythema/epilation
  - Dry desquamation
  - Moist desquamation

Chronic Skin Changes
- May occur months to years after completion of treatment
- May be permanent
- Types
  - Tissue necrosis or ulceration
  - Fibrosis
  - Edema
  - Hyperpigmentation

Suggested Management of Skin Care

There is no consensus on the optimum skincare regimen during radiation therapy because of the paucity of scientific data to support most interventions.

Goals of Skin Care:
- To enhance patient comfort
- To promote healing
- To prevent infection with skin breakdown

General Guidelines:
- Gentle care of skin in treatment field (i.e., no scrubbing, avoid extreme hot/cold, trauma)
- Topical emollient creams/lotions as per individual practice protocol
- Sun protection with sun-block products (SPF ≥ 15)
- Moist wound healing principles for management of moist desquamation

Archambieu, J.O., & Pezner, R. (1995). Pathophysiology of irradiated skin and breast. *International Journal of Radiation Oncology, Biology, Physics, 31,* 1171–1185.

Dunne-Daly, C.F. (1995). Skin and wound care in radiation oncology. *Cancer Nursing, 18,* 144–162.

Maher, K. (in press). Radiation therapy: Toxicity and management. In C.H. Yarbro, M.H. Frogge, & M. Goodman (Eds.), *Cancer nursing: Principles and practice* (5th ed.). Boston: Jones and Bartlett.

Sitton, E. (1997). Managing side effects of skin changes and fatigue. In K.H. Dow, J.D. Bucholtz, R. Iwamoto, V.K. Fieler, & L.J. Hilderley (Eds.), *Nursing care in radiation oncology* (2nd ed.) (pp. 79–100). Philadelphia: Saunders.

Note. Developed by Rebecca A. Hawkins, RN, MSN, ANP, AOCN®, and Karen E. Maher, ANP, MS, AOCN®

16. Cellulitis

Janet S. Fulton, PhD, RN

I. Definition: An acute, deep, spreading infection of the dermal and subcutaneous tissues

II. Pathophysiology
   A. An opportunistic organism enters the dermis through a cut, abrasion, or preexisting dermatologic disorder, such as an open ulcer, or it may be seeded by the hematogenous route from another source of infection in the body, such as a surgical wound.
      1. Tissue edema predisposes an individual to bacterial proliferation.
         a) Staphylococci produce disease through their ability to multiply and produce a host of extracellular enzymes, including alpha and beta hemolysin, leukocidin, coagulase, hyaluronidase, and lipases.
         b) Anaerobic bacteria can produce these extracellular enzymes and act synergistically with aerobic bacteria.
      2. The number of organisms present in the affected area usually is low. The intensity of the inflammatory response does not seem to correlate with the density of organisms.
      3. Damage to local lymphatics during an acute episode can result in residual lymphedema and predispose the patient to recurrent infections.
   B. Opportunistic organisms also may multiply in conditions of reduced lymphatic drainage or reduced capillary perfusion.

III. Clinical features
   A. Risk factors
      1. Diabetes mellitus
      2. Alcoholism
      3. Compromised immune system
      4. Impaired skin integrity
      5. Lymphedema
      6. Exposure to opportunistic organisms by skin contaminations (e.g., animals)
      7. Cellulitis of the central face increases the risk of extension to the cavernous sinus.
   B. Etiology
      1. Usually caused by Group A beta-hemolytic streptococci or *Staphylococcus aureus*
      2. Occasionally caused by other aerobic and anaerobic bacteria as well as deep fungi, such as *Cryptococcus neoformans*, particularly in patients who are immunosuppressed

3. Enteric aerobic and anaerobic bacteria can cause cellulitis of the perineum.
4. Mucosal surface injuries predispose one to anaerobic organisms, such as traumatic or extravasation wounds.
5. Infection spreads along the fascial planes once the connective tissue is involved.
6. Variants of cellulitis
   a) Erysipelas: Caused by group A streptococci; a superficial type of cellulitis involving lymphatics; margins of the lesion are raised, sharply demarcated from adjacent normal skin, and often painful. The surface has more of an "orange peel" appearance. Common sites include the face, lower legs, and areas of preexisting lymphedema.
   b) Erysipeloid: Cellulitis on the hand, especially fingers, after handling saltwater fish, shellfish, meat, hides, or poultry; caused by *Erysipelothrix rhusiopathiae;* systemic symptoms usually are not present.
   c) Ecthyma gangrenosum: Caused by *Pseudomonas aeruginosa*; usually located in the lower extremities; the limb rapidly becomes ulcerated, leading to necrosis.
   d) Cryptococcal cellulitis: Presents as red, hot, tender, edematous plaque, usually on an extremity, rarely involving multiple noncontiguous sites; patients are almost exclusively immunocompromised.
   e) Infectious gangrene (gangrenous cellulitis): A rapidly progressive cellulitis associated with extensive necrosis of subcutaneous tissue and overlying skin; usually caused by Clostridium species; prognosis is guarded.
7. Local fibrosis-ischemia after surgery, lymphatic and capillary sclerosis from radiotherapy, and stagnant lymph flow following node dissection likely are factors in long-term predisposition to cellulitis.
8. Cellulitis following breast cancer surgery may occur years post-treatment. The source of infection is hypothesized to be endogenous flora introduced through the ductal system and residing in the parenchyma, which then serves as a nidus for overt infection.

C. History
   1. History of cancer and cancer treatment
   2. Current medications: Prescribed and over-the-counter
   3. History of presenting symptom(s): Precipitating factors, onset, location, and duration
   4. Changes in activities of daily living

D. Signs and symptoms
   1. Fever
   2. Chills and rigor
   3. Diffuse myalgia
   4. Headache
   5. Malaise
   6. Diffuse erythematous rash
   7. Localized area of hot, swollen, tender, erythematous skin
   8. Pain with mobility or ambulation

E. Physical exam
   1. Vital signs to evaluate for fever
   2. Skin exam

        a) Affected skin area is hot, swollen, tender, erythematous, and diffuse; edges are not well demarcated.

        b) Palpate for crepitus, which indicates gas production and suggests anaerobic involvement.

    3. Lymph node exam

        a) Regional draining lymph nodes usually are palpable and tender.

        b) After lymph node dissection or radiation therapy for breast cancer, the breast, or a portion of the breast, may be swollen, tender, erythematous, and warm to touch.

        c) Red streaks extending proximally and tender lymph nodes indicate lymphangitis.

IV. Diagnostic tests

  A. Laboratory

    1. Wound culture: Obtain a culture and aspirate or biopsy the leading edge of inflammation.

        a) For aspiration method, inject 0.5–1.0 ml of nonbacteriostatic saline, then aspirate and send for gram stain and culture.

        b) Because the number of organisms in the affected area usually is low, cultures often are inconclusive and not performed.

    2. Obtain blood cultures if patient has rigors, fever, or chills. If the patient has a central venous access device, obtain cultures from the device and percutaneously.

    3. Perform a complete blood count with differential (look for an elevated white cell count).

        a) Leukocytosis is early and marked in immunocompetent patients.

        b) In immunocompromised patients, leukocytosis appears later, is less marked, and disappears quickly.

    4. Erythrocyte sedimentation rate may be elevated.

    5. Possible necrotizing fasciitis requires immediate deep biopsy and frozen section for histopathology.

  B. Radiology: Plain x-ray of affected area if crepitus present to look for gas production indicating gangrene

V. Differential diagnosis

  A. Deep vein thrombosis or superficial thrombophlebitis (see Chapters 41 and 157)

  B. Early contact dermatitis (see Chapters 18 and 19)

  C. Acute urticarial plaque such as bee and insect bites

  D. Prevesicular herpes zoster (see Chapter 20)

  E. Necrotizing fasciitis and synergistic gangrene

  F. Diabetes mellitus (see Chapter 143)

  G. Allergic reaction

VI. Treatment

  A. The overall goal is resolution of infection with minimal tissue damage.

  B. Supportive care includes rest, immobilization and elevation of limbs, moist heat, and analgesia.

    C. Warm, moist compresses can be applied to the affected area for 20 minutes three to four times a day. To prevent burns and further tissue damage, do not use a heating pad or other electric heating device.

    D. Antibiotics: Because most cases are caused by group A beta-hemolytic streptococci or *Staphylococcus aureus*, antibiotic therapy should be directed at both organisms. Final determination of antibiotic therapy depends on the causative organism, sensitivity to the antibiotic, and overall patient response to therapy (see Appendix 1).

        1. For mild, early, uncomplicated cellulitis

            a) Augmentin® (amoxicillin/clavulanate potassium, SmithKline Beecham Pharmaceuticals, Philadelphia, PA) 875 mg po bid for 10 days

            b) Dicloxacillin 250 mg po q 6 hours for 10 days; higher doses may be given, depending on the severity of the infection, up to 500 mg to 1 g po every 6 hours.

            c) Erythromycin 250 mg po q 6 hours for 10 days; higher doses may be given, depending on the severity of the infection, up to 500 mg q 6 hours; may be used as an alternative for penicillin-allergic patients

            d) First-generation cephalosporins: Cephalexin 250–500 mg q 6 hours for 10 days

        2. For more severe cellulitis or neutropenia: Hospitalization and parenteral antibiotics are indicated.

            a) Penicillin 10 million units plus dicloxacillin 2 g tid IV; vancomycin 1.0–1.5 g per day IV is an alternative for penicillin-allergic patients.

            b) Subsequent antibiotic therapy should be modified according to response and culture.

        3. Necrotizing fasciitis and gangrene: Provide immediate referral to surgeon. Prompt surgical debridement and broad-spectrum IV antibiotics are crucial for survival.

  VII. Follow-up: Not indicated unless area is not healing

  VIII. Referrals: If cellulitis is suspected, refer to physician for complete evaluation.

    A. Infectious disease or surgical consult may be needed for definitive diagnosis.

    B. Pharmacology consult may be helpful in selecting and monitoring antibiotics.

References

Bodey, G.P., Rodriguez, S., Fainstein, V., & Elting, L.S. (1991). Clostridial bacteremia in cancer patients. *Cancer, 66,* 1928–1942.

El-Daher, N., & Magnussen, C.R. (1996). Skin and soft-tissue infections: Outpatient management and indications for hospitalization. *Consultant, 36,* 2563–2566, 2569–2570.

Gillen, P.B. (1995). Necrotizing fasciitis: Early recognition and aggressive treatment remain important. *Journal of Ostomy and Continence Nursing, 22,* 219–222.

Paley, P.J., Johnson, P.R., Adcock, L.L., Cosin, J., Chen, M.D., Fowler, J.M., Twiggs, L.B., & Carson, L.F. (1997). The effect of sartorius transposition on wound morbidity following inguinal-femoral lymphadenectomy. *Gynecologic Oncology, 64,* 237–241.

Rescigno, J., McCormick, B., Brown, A., & Myskowski, P.L. (1994). Breast cellulitis after conservative surgery and radiotherapy. *International Journal of Radiation Oncology, Biology, Physics, 29,* 163–168.

Simon, M.S., & Cody, R.L. (1992). Cellulitis after axillary lymph node dissection for carcinoma of the breast. *American Journal of Medicine, 93,* 543–549.

Yeavasis-Lupenko, E., Gill, V., & Chuna, B.A. (1995). Group G streptococcal cellulitis and bacteremia. *Heart and Lung, 24*(1), 89–90.

17. Decubitus Ulcer

Janet S. Fulton, PhD, RN

I. Definition: Also called bedsores; tissue destruction resulting from prolonged pressure; from Latin *decumbere,* to lie down or to recline

II. Pathophysiology: Decubitus ulcers are the manifestation of local tissue death.
   A. Death occurs when cellular metabolism is compromised by impaired circulation.
   B. Nutrients are denied, and waste products accumulate.

III. Clinical features: The development of pressure ulcers can be insidious and related to a number of interacting and seemingly unrelated factors. Pressure ulcers can develop over any bony prominence or any area of soft tissue subjected to prolonged pressure.
   A. Risk factors: Use a pressure risk assessment instrument for patients with limited mobility, regardless of cause (see Figure 17-1).
      1. Diminished ability to respond meaningfully to pressure and related discomfort
      2. Increased skin exposure to moisture, such as urine or perspiration
      3. Diminished physical activity
      4. Inability to change position or control position
      5. Inadequate fluid and nutritional intake
      6. Friction: Force created by two surfaces moving across one another; occurs with repositioning
      7. Shear: Mechanical force that is parallel to the skin; main effect on deep tissues
      8. Advanced age
      9. Other factors affecting circulation, such as smoking and elevated temperature
      10. Cancer cachexia or anorexia
      11. Pressure ulcers: Unequal distribution of weight makes the lower half of the body at greatest risk. Areas of risk include
         a) Supine position: Heels, sacrum, coccyx, ischial tuberosities, elbows, scapulae, C 7 prominence, occipital bone, and ears
         b) Lateral position: Lateral malleoli, medial malleoli, greater trochanters, ears, and sides of head
         c) Prone position: Toes, patellae, iliac crests, elbows, sternum, and ribs
         d) Sitting position: Plantar surfaces and heels of feet, ischial tuberosities, sacrum, coccyx, and elbows
         e) Pressure points located within the radiation field

Figure 17-1. Braden Scale for Predicting Pressure Sore Risk

	Patient's Name	Evaluator's Name		Date of Assessment				

Sensory perception
Ability to respond meaningfully to pressure-related discomfort

1. Completely limited:
Unresponsive (does not moan, flinch, or grasp) to painful stimuli, because of diminished level of consciousness or sedation
OR
limited ability to feel pain over most of body surface.

2. Very limited:
Responds only to painful stimuli; cannot communicate discomfort except by moaning or restlessness
OR
has a sensory impairment that limits the ability to feel pain or discomfort over half of the body

3. Slightly limited:
Responds to verbal commands but cannot always communicate discomfort or need to be turned
OR
has some sensory impairment which limits ability to feel pain or discomfort in one or two extremities

4. No impairment:
Responds to verbal commands; has no sensory deficit which would limit ability to feel or voice pain or discomfort

Moisture
Degree to which skin is exposed to moisture

1. Constantly moist:
Skin is kept moist almost constantly by perspiration, urine, etc. Dampness is detected every time patient is moved or turned

2. Moist:
Skin is often but not always moist. Linens must be changed at least once a shift.

3. Occasionally moist:
Skin is occasionally moist, requiring an extra linen change approximately once a day.

4. Rarely moist:
Skin is usually dry; linens require changing only at routine intervals.

Activity
Degree of physical activity

1. Bedfast:
Confined to bed

2. Chairfast:
Ability to walk severely limited or nonexistent; cannot bear own weight and/or must be assisted into chair or wheel chair

3. Walks occasionally:
Walks occasionally during day but for very short distances with or without assistance; spends majority of each shift in bed or chair

4. Walks frequently:
Walks outside the room at least twice a day and inside room at least once every two hours during waking hours

Mobility
Ability to change and control body position

1. Completely immobile:
Does not make even slight changes in body or extremity position without assistance

2. Very limited:
Makes occasional slight changes in body or extremity position but unable to make frequent or significant changes independently

3. Slightly limited:
Makes frequent though slight changes in body or extremity position independently

4. No limitations:
Makes major and frequent changes in position without assistance

Nutrition
Usual food intake pattern

1. Very poor:
Never eats a complete meal. Rarely eats more than one-third of any food offered; eats two servings or less of protein (meat or dairy products) per day; takes fluids poorly; does not take a liquid dietary supplement,
OR
is NPO[1] and/or maintained on clear liquids or IV[2] for more than five days

2. Probably inadequate:
Rarely eats a complete meal and generally eats only about half of any food offered; protein intake includes only three servings of meat or dairy products per day; occasionally will take a dietary supplement
OR
receives less than optimum amount of liquid diet or tube feeding

3. Adequate:
Eats more than half or most meals; eats a total of four servings of protein (meat, dairy products) each day; occasionally will refuse a meal but usually will take a supplement if offered
OR
is on a tube-feeding or TPN[3] regimen, which probably meets most nutritional needs

4. Excellent:
Eats most of every meal; never refuses a meal; usually eats a total of four or more servings of meat and dairy products; occasionally eats between meals; does not require supplementation

Friction and shear

1. Problem:
Requires moderate to maximum assistance in moving; complete lifting without sliding against sheets is impossible. Frequently slides down in bed or chair, requiring frequent repositioning with maximum assistance; spasticity, contracture, or agitation leads to almost constant friction.

2. Potential problem:
Moves feebly or requires minimum assistance; during a move, skin probably slides to some extent against sheets, chair, restraints, or other devices. Maintains relatively good position in chair or bed most of the time but occasionally slides down

3. No apparent problem:
Moves in bed and in chair independently and has sufficient muscle strength to lift up completely during move; maintains good position in bed or chair at all times

Total score

[1]NPO: Nothing by mouth; [2] IV: Intravenous; [3] TPN: Total parenteral nutrition

Source: Barbara Braden and Nancy Bergstrom. Copyright 1988. Reprinted with permission

B. Etiology of pressure ulcer (see Figure 17-2)
   1. Pressure
   2. Intensity: Amount of force exerted on a given area
   3. Duration: Length of time the force is applied
   4. Tolerance: Ability of the skin and supporting structures to endure pressure without adverse sequela
C. History
   1. History of cancer and cancer treatment
   2. Current medications: Prescribed and over-the-counter
   3. History of pressure sores: Precipitating factors, onset, location, and duration
   4. Changes in activities of daily living
D. Signs and symptoms
   1. Pain at pressure points: Patients often are unaware of the discomfort related to unrelieved pressure, especially if receiving large doses of pain medications.
   2. Weight loss
   3. Areas of erythematous or darkened skin
   4. Fever
   5. Abrasions, bleeding, or oozing from broken skin

Figure 17-2. A Conceptual Schema for the Study of the Etiology of Pressure Sores, Which Accounts for the Relative Contributions of the Duration and Intensity of Pressure and the Tissue Tolerance for Pressure

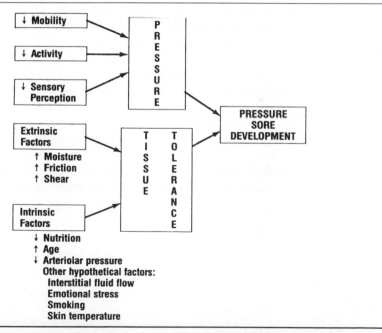

Note. From "A Conceptual Schema for the Study of the Etiology of Pressure Sores," by B. Braden and N. Bergstrom, 1987, *Rehabilitation Nursing, 12,* p. 9. Copyright 1987 by the Association of Rehabilitation Nurses. Reprinted with permission.

E. Physical exam
    1. Vital signs: Assess for fever.
    2. Integument system: Findings are summarized according to stage of pressure ulcer.
        a) Blanchable erythema
        b) The condition begins as an ill-defined erythematous patch at the point of pressure and varies in color from pale pink to bright red.
        c) Digital compression produces total blanching, and the erythema reappears promptly when the finger is lifted.
    3. Stage I
        a) Nonblanchable erythema of intact skin, the heralding lesion of skin ulceration
        b) In people with dark complexions, discoloration of the skin, warmth, edema, induration, or hardness may be indicators.
    4. Stage II
        a) Partial thickness skin loss involving epidermis, dermis, or both
        b) The ulcer is superficial and presents as an abrasion, blister, or shallow crater.
    5. Stage III
        a) Full-thickness skin loss involving damage to or necrosis of subcutaneous tissue that may extend down to, but not through, underlying fascia
        b) The ulcer presents clinically as a deep crater with or without undermining adjacent tissue.
    6. Stage IV
        a) Full-thickness skin loss with extensive destruction, tissue necrosis, or damage to muscle, bone, or supporting structures, such as tendons or joint capsules
        b) Undermining and sinus tracts also may be associated with stage IV ulcers.

IV. Diagnostic tests
    A. Laboratory: To assess nutritional status
        1. Serum transferrin and serum albumin are measures of visceral protein status.
        2. Creatinine: Height index is a method of estimating skeletal muscle mass.
        3. Hemoglobin levels can detect iron-deficiency anemia.
        4. Total lymphocyte count indicates both visceral protein status and cellular immune function.
        5. Do not use swab cultures to diagnose ulcer infections because all pressure ulcers are colonized. Swab cultures may not reflect the organism causing the infection.
    B. Radiology: Not indicated

V. Differential diagnosis
    A. Extravasation
    B. Tumor erosion
    C. Physical abuse

VI. Treatment
    A. Prediction and prevention
        1. Any patient with altered activity or mobility should be assessed for risk for pressure ulcer using a comprehensive scale, such as the Braden scale (see Figure 17-1).

2. Educate patient, primary caregiver, family members, and others about the risk factors, assessment parameters, and use of supportive devices to prevent or relieve pressure.
3. Maximize mobility/activity levels.
   a) For bed-bound patients
      (1) Reposition at least every two hours.
      (2) Use pillows or foam wedges to keep bony prominences from direct contact with bed.
      (3) Use devices that totally relieve pressure on the heels.
      (4) Avoid positioning the patient directly on the trochanter.
      (5) Elevate the head of the bed as little and for as short of a time as possible.
      (6) Use lifting devices to move rather than drag the individual during transfer and position change.
      (7) Use a pressure-reducing mattress.
   b) For chair-bound patients
      (1) Reposition at least every hour.
      (2) Have patient shift weight every 15 minutes, if able.
      (3) Use pressure-reducing devices for seating surfaces.
4. Perform good skin care.
   a) Use warm water and mild soap for bathing.
   b) Use moisturizers to prevent dry skin.
   c) Humidify environmental air (above 40%) to prevent dry skin.
5. Manage incontinence.
   a) Assess and treat urinary and stool incontinence.
   b) If incontinence cannot be controlled, use underpads or briefs made of materials that absorb moisture and keep the skin surface dry.
   c) Cleanse the skin with mild soap and warm water at the time of soiling.
   d) Apply a topical skin barrier.
6. Manage nutritional deficits.
   a) Maintain adequate hydration.
   b) Maintain adequate intake of protein, calories, and essential nutrients.
   c) Use nutritional supplements.
   d) Consider aggressive interventions, such as enteral or parenteral feedings (see Chapter 158).
   e) Use appetite stimulants (see Chapter 62)
   f) Consider adding vitamins and minerals, such as vitamin C and zinc, to enhance wound healing.
B. Treatment (see Figure 17-3)
   1. Debridement
      a) Surgical: A surgeon uses a scalpel, scissors, or laser to remove macroscopically identified necrotic tissue from the wound bed.
      b) Mechanical: Necrotic tissue is removed by applying a mechanical force (forced-stream water or whirlpool) or wet-to-dry dressings.
      c) Chemical: An enzymatic agent, such as collagenase (Collagenase Santyl® ointment, Knoll Laboratories, Mount Olive, NJ), fibrinolysin (Elase®, Fujisawa USA, Inc., Deerfield, IL), or Granulex® (Dow Hickam Pharmaceuticals, Sugar

Figure 17-3. Pressure Ulcer Flow Chart

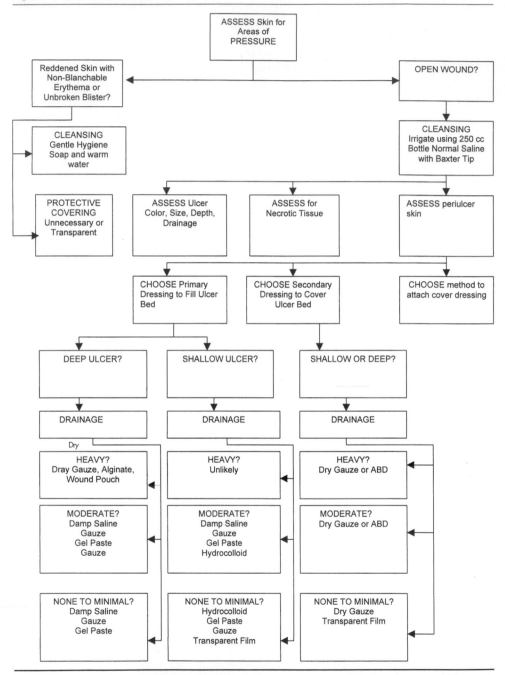

Note. From *Pressure Ulcers: Guidelines for Prevention and Nursing Management* (p. 286), by J.A. Maklebust and M. Siegreen, 1996, Springhouse, PA: Springhouse Corporation. Copyright 1996 by Springhouse Corporation.

Land, TX), which contains trypsin, a debriding agent, is used to selectively remove necrotic tissue.

d) Autolytic debridement: The body's own enzymes are used to digest devitalized tissue.

2. Cleaning: Removes inflammatory material on the wound surface

    a) Use 0.9% saline.

    b) Never use commercial cleansers on open wounds; they are toxic and can damage tissue.

3. Dressings: The primary purpose of a dressing is to maintain a wound environment supportive of healing and to contain exudate. See Table 17-1 for a summary of wound dressings.

4. Managing bacterial colonization and infection: Usually stage III and IV ulcers

    a) Minimize pressure ulcer colonization and enhance wound healing by effective wound cleansing and debridement.

    b) Topical antibiotic: Consider a two-week trial of a topical antibiotic for clean ulcers that are not healing or continue to produce exudate after two to four weeks of attentive care. The antibiotic should be effective against gram-negative, gram-positive, and anaerobic organisms. *Monitor for allergic sensitization.* Discontinue use in two weeks if no improvement or worsening of ulcer occurs.

        (1) Silver sulfadiazine 1% cream, applied topically to cleansed area(s) once or twice a day using a sterile gloved hand; apply to a thickness of approximately 16 mm, and reapply if removed by patient activity. Light gauze dressings may be used but are not required. Continue therapy as long as there is a threat of infection.

        (2) Triple antibiotic

            (a) Bacitracin applied topically to adequately cover a cleansed ulcer; available as an ointment, solution, or spray. Choose preparation that is easiest to apply to the area. Apply one to three times a day. Light gauze dressings may be used but are not required. Ointment is available 500 u/g; powder, 500 u/g; and spray (Polysporin® spray, Warner-Lambert Consumer Healthcare, Morris Plains, NJ), 120 u/g with polymixin B sulfate 2,350 u/g.

            (b) Neomycin sulfate applied to adequately cover a cleansed ulcer; available in cream or ointment, 0.5%. Apply one to three times a day and cover with a light gauze dressing. A high risk for allergic reaction to neomycin exists.

        (3) Do not use topical antiseptics, such as povidone iodine, iodophor, hydrogen peroxide, or acetic acid to reduce bacteria in wound tissue. These agents can retard growth of normal tissue.

        (4) Deep wounds can result in soft tissue infections and osteomyelitis requiring systemic antibiotics.

VII. Follow-up

    A. Short-term

      1. Monitor ulcer healing or progression of ulcer.

      2. Change interventions as needed.

Table 17-1. Properties of Commonly Used Dressing Materials

Dressing Category	Indications	Advantages	Disadvantages	Considerations
Polyurethane films	Protection of partial thickness red wounds; cover dressing for hydrophillic powder and paste preparations and hydrogels	Transparent; good adhesion; waterproof; reduces pain; minimizes friction forces to wound; time saving; easy to store	Adhesive injury to intact and new skin; nonabsorbent; some products difficult to apply; variable barrier function; can promote wound infection	Protect wound margins; avoid in wounds with infection, copious drainage, or tracts; change only if dressing leaks
Hydrocolloids	Protection of superficial and small, deep red wounds; autolytic debridement of small, noninfected yellow wounds*	Absorbent; nonadhesive to healing tissue; good barrier; waterproof; reduces pain; easy to apply; time saving; easy to store	Nontransparent; may soften and lose shape with heat or friction; odor and brown drainage on removal (melted dressing material)	Frequency of changes will depend on amount of exudate (change as needed for leakage); avoid in wounds with infection or tracts
Hydrogel sheets	Protection of superficial and moderately deep red wounds; autolytic debridement of small, noninfected yellow or black wounds*; del very system for topical antimicrobial creams (increases penetration)	Absorbent; nonadhesive; reduces pain; compatible with topicals; good conformity; easy to store	Poor barrier; semi-transparent; requires cover dressing to secure; can promote growth of *Pseudomonas* and yeast; expensive	Avoid in infected wounds; change every eight hours or as needed for leakage
Hydrophilic beads, powders, and pastes	Cleansing of draining yellow wounds; protection of deep draining and nondraining red wounds; autolytic debridement of noninfected black wounds*	Good "filler" for deep wounds; absorbs large amounts of exudate; rapid cleansing of yellow wounds; cost effective; helps control odor	Occasional pain on application; requires cover dressing; dressing material leaks out with position change if outer dressing not sealed; difficult to remove from tracts and deep pockets	Partially fill wound cavities to allow for expansion; avoid in wounds with fistulas or deep tracts; monitor electrolytes if copious drainage
Gel pastes	Protection of red wounds; autolytic debridement of noninfected yellow or black wounds*	Good "filler" for small, deep red wounds, easy to apply	Requires cover dressing; expensive; variable absorbency	Same as for hydrogels
Foams	Protection of red wounds; dressing for tracheostomy and drain sites	Insulates wound; provides some padding; nonadherent; easy to use; easy to store	Poor absorbency; poor barrier; nontransparent; requires sealing of edges with tape; poor conformability to deep wound	Change every 24 hours or as needed for leakage; avoid in draining wounds with viscous exudate

(Continued on next page)

Table 17-1. Properties of Commonly Used Dressing Materials (Continued)

Dressing Category	Indications	Advantages	Disadvantages	Considerations
Impregnated dressings	Protection of superficial infected and noninfected red wounds; "contact layer" for primarily closed wounds	Nonadherent (if gauze cover dressing used); antibacterial if medicated; easy to use; easy to store	Some products will adhere to wound if allowed to dry out; poor barrier if nonmedicated	Change at least every 24 hours (if nonadherent); if adherent, allow to separate spontaneously
Cotton and gauze dressings				
Wet to dry	Mechanical debridement of yellow wounds	Readily available; good mechanical debridement if properly used; cost effective "filler" for large wounds; effective delivery of topicals if kept moist	Delayed healing if used improperly; pain on removal (wet to dry); labor intensive	Use rolled gauze for packing large wounds (ensures complete removal); pack loosely (tight packing delays healing); use wide mesh gauze for debriding; use fine mesh gauze for protection; do not use cotton-filled materials on wound surface
Wet to damp	Mechanical debridement of red/yellow wounds	—	—	—
Continuous dry	Heavily exudating red wounds	—	—	—
Continuous moist	Protection of red wounds; autolytic debridement of yellow or black wounds*; delivery of topical medication	—	—	—

*Use with caution in critically ill patients who are leukopenic or have poor wound perfusion: avoid in patients with clinically infected wounds.

Note. From Pressure Ulcers: Guidelines for Prevention and Nursing Management (pp. 114–115), by J.A. Maklebust and M. Siegreen, 1996, Springhouse, PA: Springhouse Corporation. Copyright 1996 by Springhouse Corporation.

   B. Long-term
      1. Prevent additional ulcer formation.
      2. Continue periodic assessment of risk and intervene to minimize risks.

VIII. Referrals
   A. Physical therapy consult may help in determining daily exercise routines and positioning to maximize mobility and activity.
   B. Consult a registered dietitian for complete nutritional evaluation.
   C. Consult a certified enterostomal/wound care clinical nurse specialist for prevention and management strategies.
   D. Surgical consult may be needed for debridement of deep ulcers.
   E. Infectious disease consult may be helpful in treating infected wounds.

References

Agency for Health Care Policy and Research. (1992). *Clinical practice guideline, pressure ulcers in adults: Prediction and prevention.* AHCPR Publication No. 92–0047. Rockville, MD: Agency for Health Care Policy and Research, Public Health Service, U.S. Department of Health and Human Services.

Bergstrom, N., Braden, B., Boynton, P., & Brunch, S. (1995). Using a research-based assessment scale in clinical practice. *Nursing Clinics of North America, 30,* 539–551.

Braden, B., & Bergstrom, N. (1987). A conceptual schema for the study of the etiology of pressure sores. *Rehabilitation Nursing, 12,* 8–12.

Cowan, T., & Woollons, S. (1998). Dynamic systems for pressure sore prevention. *Professional Nurse, 13,* 387–394.

Dwyer, F.M., & Keeler, D. (1997). Protocols for wound management. *Nursing Management, 28*(7), 45–49.

Kanj, L.F., Wilking, S.V., & Phillips, T.J. (1998). Pressure ulcers. *Journal of the American Academy of Dermatology, 38,* 517–536.

Kozierowski, L. (1996). Treatment of sacral pressure ulcers in an adolescent with Hodgkin's disease. *Journal of Wound, Ostomy and Continence Nursing, 23,* 244–247.

Maklebust, J., & Siegreen, M. (1996). *Pressure ulcers: Guidelines for prevention and nursing management.* Springhouse, PA: Springhouse Corp.

McNees, P., Braden, B., Bergstrom, N., & Ovington, L. (1998). Beyond risk assessment: Elements for pressure ulcer prevention. *Ostomy and Wound Management, 44*(Suppl. 3A), 51S–58S.

Ovington, L.G. (1997). What is needed to monitor healing in the outpatient clinic setting? *Advances in Wound Care, 10*(5), 58–60.

Parish, L.C., Witkowski, J.A., & Crissey, J.T. (1997). *The decubitus ulcer in clinical practice.* New York: Springer.

Sacharok, C., & Drew, J. (1998). Use of a total quality management model to reduce pressure ulcer prevalence in the acute care setting. *Journal of Wound, Ostomy and Continence Nursing, 25,* 88–92.

Whittemore, R. (1998). Pressure-reduction support surfaces: A review of the literature. *Journal of Wound, Ostomy and Continence Nursing, 25,* 6–25.

Chapter

18. Atopic Dermatitis

Janet S. Fulton, PhD, RN

I. Definition: Also called eczema; is a superficial inflammatory skin reaction

II. Pathophysiology
   A. Atopic dermatitis probably is caused by combinations of immunologic dysregulation, epidermal barrier dysfunction, and increased genetic susceptibility.
   B. Dermatitis demonstrates increased capillary permeability, allowing easier movement of lymphocytes out of capillaries.
      1. T lymphocytes, stimulated by interleukin-1 (IL-1), will produce interleukin-2 (IL-2), which then acts as an autocrine stimulant of T lymphocyte proliferation.
      2. This developing inflammatory process proceeds by attracting "innocent bystanders," usually also T lymphocytes.
   C. Patients may have immunologic abnormalities, including elevated immunoglobulin E (IgE) levels, reduced cell-mediated immune responses, and slowed chemotaxis of neutrophils and monocytes.

III. Clinical features: Atopic dermatitis is a pruritic skin inflammation involving hypersensitivity that usually begins in childhood, as early as six weeks of age, with a variable course through adolescence. Symptoms tend to lessen with age; complete resolution in adulthood is common. In some patients, atopic dermatitis may persist into adulthood or may suddenly reappear after a long remission.
   A. Risk factors: Because atopic dermatitis is prone to exacerbations during periods of physical and emotional stress, patients undergoing cancer diagnosis and treatment may be considered to be at risk.
   B. Etiology: Most patients with atopic dermatitis have a positive family history of the atopic triad—dermatitis, asthma, and allergic rhinitis. Although the exact mode of inheritance is not known, autosomal dominance with varying penetration is suspected.
   C. History
      1. History of cancer and cancer treatment
      2. Current medications: Prescribed and over-the-counter
      3. History of presenting symptom(s): Precipitating factors, onset, location, and duration
      4. Changes in activities of daily living

5. Past medical history of asthma or allergic rhinitis
D. Signs and symptoms
   1. Severe, easily triggered itching is the outstanding feature of the disease.
   2. Other signs are related to scratching and rubbing of the skin.
      a) Scratching causes lichenification, which is cutaneous thickening and hardening from continued irritation and formation of papules that coalesce to form rough, scaly patches.
      b) Lichenification lowers the threshold for renewed itching.
E. Physical exam: Focuses on integument system
   1. Flexural involvement: Presence of lesions on back of neck, antecubital fossae, around wrists, behind knees, and around ankles
   2. Generalized dry skin
   3. Local signs of irritation and/or scratching
   4. Dry papules, excoriations, and/or lichenification in affected areas
   5. Follicular reactions common in dark-skinned patients
   6. Prominent lower eyelid folds, also called Dennie-Morgan folds, giving the appearance of being older than chronological age
   7. The cutaneous vasculature responds abnormally to stimulation; instead of normal "wheal and flare" response, firm rubbing of the skin elicits white dermographism, a simple white linear streak along the site of pressure with no erythema.

IV. Diagnostic tests: Diagnosis of atopic dermatitis is based on personal and family history of dermatitis and the presence of chronic, recurrent pruritic skin eruptions in classic locations.
   A. Laboratory: Usually not indicated
      1. May have elevated IgE; however, levels vary widely among individuals, so results are considered to be inconclusive.
      2. Allergy skin testing has not been considered to be especially helpful in diagnosis.
      3. Biopsy may be indicated if area does not respond to treatment.
   B. Radiology: Not indicated

V. Differential diagnosis
   A. Psoriasis
   B. Scabies
   C. Allergic contact dermatitis (see Chapter 19)
   D. Cutaneous T cell lymphoma

VI. Treatment
   A. The aim of treatment is to decrease trigger factors and pruritus, suppress inflammation, and lubricate the skin.
   B. Preventative measures
      1. Keep environmental temperature constant. Avoid excess humidity or extreme dryness. Humidifying indoor air may be helpful, especially in dry climates or during winter months.
      2. Wear absorbent, nonirritating cotton clothing. Avoid potentially offending fabrics (e.g., wool).

3. Use mild cleansers and warm water for bathing, and avoid friction when drying by patting the skin dry.
   a) Unscented Dove® (Lever Brothers Co., New York, NY) bath bar
   b) Unscented Neutrogena® (Neutrogena Corp., Los Angeles, CA) cleansing bar
   c) Oatmeal (e.g., Aveeno®, S.C. Johnson & Son, Inc., Racine, WI)
4. Lubricate the body daily immediately after bathing to trap water in the skin. Use unfragranced, lanolin-free moisturizers.
   a) Lubriderm® (Warner-Lambert Co., White Plains, NJ)
   b) Nutraderm® (Alcon Laboratories, Ft. Worth, TX)
   c) Eucerin® or Eucerin® Plus (Beiersdorf, Inc., Norwalk, CT)
   d) Moisturel® (Westwood-Squibb Pharmaceuticals, Buffalo, NY)
5. Wash clothing and towels in bland soap and thoroughly rinse.
   a) Ivory Snow® flakes (Proctor & Gamble Co., Cincinnati, OH)
   b) Cheer-Free® (Proctor & Gamble Co.)

C. Pharmacologic management of atopic dermatitis
   1. Exudative areas may benefit from drying with aluminum acetate (Burow's) solution compresses applied for 20 minutes, four to six times a day.
   2. Oatmeal (Aveeno) baths, while reducing dryness, also can be soothing, antipruritic, and anti-inflammatory.
      a) Mix one cup of Aveeno oatmeal and two cups of cold tap water; shake, and pour into tub half full of lukewarm water
      b) Soak in tub for 30 minutes.
   3. Topical corticosteroids: Treatment should be initiated with a high-potency steroid to quickly reduce symptoms and then should move to the lowest potency that will control symptoms.
      a) Ointments generally provide better biologic activity support for corticosteroids than creams or lotions but may be more difficult to apply.
      b) Lotions have a higher water content than creams, are easier to apply, and provide a protective, drying, and cooling effect.
      c) Topical corticosteroids should be applied to moist skin after bathing.
      d) Pharmacologic agents are listed in Appendix 14.
      e) Moderate disease—thicker or unresponsive areas: Medium-potency topical corticosteroid preparations
         (1) Triamcinolone 0.1% cream or ointment, two to three times a day, to control symptoms
         (2) Mometasone furoate 0.1% cream daily to control symptoms
      f) Mild disease: Low-potency topical corticosteroid preparations
         (1) Hydrocortisone 1%–2.5% cream
         (2) Desonide 0.05% cream
      g) Isolated lichenified lesions: Betamethasone dipropionate 0.05% cream or ointment twice a day for two to three weeks
   4. Oral corticosteroids
      a) Systemic steroids provide rapid relief in many cases; however, frequent use can lead to steroid dependence or rebound effect when discontinued. Systemic steroids should be limited to severe, acute episodes.

        b) Dosage for oral steroids is determined by severity of the episode. Suggest prednisone 0.5–1.0 mg/kg/day for a maximum of 7–10 days.

    5. Antibiotics

        a) Lesions often are colonized with *Staphylococcus aureus*. Antibiotic therapy may be helpful for persistent lesions or those with secondary infection. Treat with oral antibiotics that are effective against *Staphylococcus aureus* (see Appendix 1).

           (1) Cephalexin 250 mg po q 6 hours, or 500 mg q 12 hours (for uncomplicated infections) for 14 days

           (2) Dicloxacillin 125 mg po q 6 hours for 14 days; severe disseminated infections may require 250 mg po q 6 hours.

           (3) Erythromycin 250 mg po q 6 hours for 10 days.

        b) For limited involvement, topical antibiotics may be beneficial in place of oral antibiotics. Use mupirocin (Bactroban®, SmithKline Beecham Pharmaceuticals, Philadelphia, PA) 2% ointment three times daily for 10 days.

    6. Antiviral agents: Treat herpes infections aggressively. Patients with atopy are predisposed to more severe and disseminated infections (see Chapter 20).

        a) Herpes simplex: Valacyclovir (Valtrex®, Glaxo Wellcome, Inc., Research Triangle Park, NC) 500 mg orally bid for seven days.

        b) Varicella zoster: Valacyclovir 1,000 mg orally bid for seven days or famciclovir (Famvir®, SmithKline Beecham Pharmaceuticals) 500 mg po tid for seven days.

    7. Pruritus control

        a) Oral antihistamines

           (1) Hydroxyzine hydrochloride 10–50 mg po q 6 hours

           (2) Diphenhydramine hydrochloride 25–50 mg po q 4–6 hours

           (3) Cyproheptadine hydrochloride (Periactin®, Merck & Co., West Point, PA) 4 mg po tid, increasing the dosage to relieve symptoms but not to exceed 0.5 mg/kg daily.

           (4) Loratadine (Claritin®, Schering Corp., Kenilworth, NJ) 10 mg po qd

           (5) Cetirizine (Zyrtec®, Pfizer Inc., New York, NY) 5–10 mg po qd

        b) Other topical agents

           (1) Pramoxine hydrochloride (Prax®, Ferndale Laboratories, Ferndale, MI; Itch-X®, B.F. Ascher & Co., Lenexa, KS) (OTC): Follow label directions; may be used in addition to topical steroids

           (2) Doxepin cream 5% for short-term use (i.e., less than eight days); may be applied qid prn in addition to topical steroids; may also cause drowsiness

VII. Follow-up

    A. Short-term: Monitor patient for relief of symptoms and adjust therapies as needed.

    B. Long-term: Refer patient to dermatologist; adults with atopic dermatitis likely were diagnosed as children and should remain under the care of a dermatologist. New cases should be referred to a dermatologist for a complete evaluation and plan of care.

VIII. Referrals: Consult a dermatologist for comprehensive differential diagnosis.

References

Akiyama, H., Tada, J., Toi, J., Kanzaki, H., & Arata, J. (1997). Changes in *Staphylococcus aureus* density and lesion severity after topical application of povidone-iodine in cases of atopic dermatitis. *Journal of Dermatological Science, 16*(1), 23–30.

Boguniewicz, M. (1997). Advances in the understanding and treatment of atopic dermatitis. *Current Opinion in Pediatrics, 9,* 577–581.

el Samahy, M.H., & el-Kerdani, T. (1997). Value of patch testing in atopic dermatitis. *American Journal of Contact Dermatitis, 8*(3), 154–157.

Graham-Brown, R.A. (1997). Therapeutics in atopic dermatitis. *Advances in Dermatology, 13,* 3–31.

Guidelines of care for atopic dermatitis. (1992). *Journal of the American Academy of Dermatology, 26,* 485–488.

Halbert, A.R., Weston, W.I., & Morelli, J.G. (1995). Atopic dermatitis: Is it an allergic disease? *Journal of the American Academy of Dermatology, 33,* 1008–1018.

MacKie, R.A. (1997). *Clinical dermatology: An illustrated textbook* (4th ed.). New York: Oxford University Press.

Morren, A.A. (1994). Atopic dermatitis: Triggering factors. *Journal of the American Academy of Dermatology, 31,* 467–473.

Rothe, M.J., & Grant-Kels, J.M. (1996). Atopic dermatitis: An update. *Journal of the American Academy of Dermatology, 35,* 1–13.

Chapter

19.

Contact Dermatitis

Janet S. Fulton, PhD, RN

I. Definition: Any pruritic, reactionary skin disorder that results when a particular substance comes into contact with the skin; contact dermatitis may be divided into two types—irritant contact dermatitis and allergic contact dermatitis.

II. Pathophysiology
   A. Irritant contact dermatitis
      1. A nonallergic response of the skin occurs after exposure to irritating substances, which are defined as substances that nearly all people would have a reaction to if exposed in the concentration and for the duration of contact sufficient to elicit a reaction.
      2. The most common irritants are chemicals; physical and biologic agents are less frequently irritants. Irritants are classified as
         a) Mild to moderate: Substances that require repeated or prolonged exposure to produce inflammation
         b) Severe: Substances that injure skin immediately on contact (i.e., strong acids or alkalis)
      3. Irritants penetrate and disrupt the stratum corneum, which injures the epidermis resulting in an inflammatory reaction.
   B. Allergic contact dermatitis: A delayed hypersensitivity response that occurs from exposure to contact allergens
      1. Simple chemicals bind to an epidermal protein to form complete antigen, which then reacts with sensitized T lymphocytes.
      2. These lymphocytes then release mediators that attract an inflammatory infiltrate and form an eczematous response.

III. Clinical features
   A. Risk factors: Risk factors for patients with cancer include antiseptic solutions and ointments used in the care of this patient population.
      1. Solutions containing iodine and adhesive compounds on tapes and dressing materials are known to cause localized dermatitis consistent with the area of exposure.
      2. Latex allergies may manifest as contact dermatitis.
      3. Factors that contribute to the development of allergic contact dermatitis include genetic predisposition, duration of exposure, cutaneous permeability, and immune tolerance.

4. Friction, pressure, occlusion, maceration, and heat or cold may intensify the reaction.
   B. History
   1. History of cancer and cancer treatment
   2. Current medications: Prescribed and over-the-counter
   3. History of presenting symptom(s): Precipitating factors, onset, location, and duration
   4. Changes in activities of daily living
   5. Past medical history; exposure to known allergens or potential irritants, such as household cleaners, hair dyes, paint remover, or other chemical compounds; previous skin reactions
   C. Signs and symptoms
   1. Localized stiff-feeling skin
   2. Discomfort related to dryness
   3. Severe itching secondary to inflammation
   4. Pain related to fissures, blisters, or ulcers
   D. Physical exam: Complete skin exam (can affect any area of the body)
   1. Erythema, microvesiculation, and oozing in a circumscribed area are consistent with exposure to a known or potential irritant.
   2. Dry, thickened, fissured skin results from continued exposure to the irritant.
   3. Allergic reactions may include tense vesicles, blisters, and edema, including swelling of facial, periorbital, and genital areas.
   4. The affected area typically has a definite yet artificial pattern with sharp margins (e.g., a "square" consistent with a transparent adherent dressing, "stripes" consistent with tape, "spots" consistent with monitor leads).

IV. Diagnostic tests: Based on history of exposure
   A. Laboratory
   1. Patch testing for contact allergens is essential for specific identification of causative agents.
   2. No clinically useful methods are available to evaluate patients who are thought to have irritant dermatitis.
   B. Radiology: Not indicated

V. Differential diagnosis
   A. Latex allergy
   B. Atopic dermatitis (see Chapter 18)
   C. Hand dermatitis
   D. Nummular dermatitis
   E. Scabies

VI. Treatment: The aim of treatment is to eliminate contact with irritants or allergens, alleviate symptoms, and promote healing.
   A. Preventative measures
   1. Primary irritant dermatitis
      a) Decrease exposure to primary irritants—soaps, detergents, solutions, adhesives.
      b) Avoid using abrasive soaps and cleansing agents. Use of solvents, such as acetone, to cleanse the skin is one of the most frequent predisposing factors.

      c) Lubricate the skin with mild cream or lotion.
- (1) Lubriderm®
- (2) Nutraderm®
- (3) Eucerin® or Eucerin® Plus
- (4) Moisturel®

  2. Allergic contact dermatitis
      a) Avoid contact with known antigens whenever possible.
      b) Wash the area with mild soap and water after exposure to antigens.

B. Puritus management (see Chapter 14)
  1. Oral antihistamines (see Appendix 4)
      a) Hydroxyzine hydrochloride 10–50 mg po q 6 hours prn
      b) Diphenhydramine hydrochloride 25–50 mg po q 4–6 hours
      c) Cyproheptadine hydrochloride 4 mg po tid, increasing the dosage to relieve symptoms but not to exceed 0.5 mg/kg daily
      d) Doxepin 10–50 mg po q hs to control itching during sleep
  2. Topical lotions: Sarna® lotion (Stiefel Laboratories, Inc., Oak Hill, NY), Itch-X®, and Prax® lotion are available over-the-counter. Follow label directions.
  3. Drying agents: Exudative areas may benefit from drying with aluminum acetate (Burow's) solution compresses applied for 20 minutes four to six times a day.
  4. Soothing baths: Oatmeal (Aveeno®) baths, while reducing dryness, also can be very soothing, antipruritic, and anti-inflammatory. Mix one cup of Aveeno oatmeal and two cups of cold tap water; shake, and pour into tub half full of lukewarm water. Remain in tub for 30 minutes.
  5. Topical compresses: Cold, wet cloths may be soothing.
  6. Topical corticosteroids: Useful if involvement is limited; treatment should be initiated with a high-potency steroid to quickly reduce symptoms, then move to the lowest potency that will control symptoms. Ointments generally provide better biologic activity support for steroids than creams or lotions but may be more difficult to apply. Lotions have a higher water content than creams, are easier to apply, and provide a protective, drying, and cooling effect. Topical steroids should be applied to moist skin after bathing. Additional pharmacologic agents are listed in Appendix 14.
      a) Betamethasone dipropionate 0.05% cream bid (high potency)
      b) Triamcinolone 0.1% cream or ointment, two to three times a day, to control symptoms (medium potency)
      c) Hydrocortisone 1%–2.5% cream or ointment (low potency)
  7. Oral corticosteroids: Should be reserved for generalized allergic contact dermatitis (e.g., poison ivy) involving the face or groin or cases in which the itching cannot be controlled with local measures. Oral corticosteroids are inappropriate for use as chronic therapy. Dosage of oral corticosteroids is determined by severity of the episode. Suggest prednisone 0.5–1.0 mg/kg/day tapered over two to three weeks.

VII. Follow-up
A. Short-term
  1. Irritant dermatitis: Identify and eliminate the irritant.

      2. Monitor patient for relief of symptoms and adjust therapies as needed.

    B. Long-term: Refer to dermatologist for allergic dermatitis; patch testing may be necessary to identify the irritant.

VIII. Referrals: Consult a dermatologist for assistance in determining irritants and planning for long-term evaluation.

References

Drake, L.A., Dinehart, S.M., Goltz, R.W., Graham, G.F., Hordinsky, M.K., Lewis, C.W., Pariser, D.M., Skouge, J.W., Turner, M.L., Webster, S.B., et al. (1995). Guidelines of care for contact dermatitis. *Journal of the American Academy of Dermatology, 32,* 109–113.

Drake, L.A., & Millikan, L.E. (1995). The antipruritic effect of 5% doxepin cream in patients with eczematous dermatitis. *Archives of Dermatology, 131,* 1403–1408.

Scheinman, P.L. (1997). Is it really fragrance-free? *American Journal of Contact Dermatitis, 8,* 239–249.

Taylor, J.S., & Praditsuwan, P. (1996). Latex allergy: Review of 44 cases, including outcome and frequency association with allergic hand eczema. *Archives of Dermatology, 132,* 265–271.

Warner, M.R., Taylor, J.S., & Leow, Y.H. (1997). Agents causing contact urticaria. *Clinics in Dermatology, 15,* 623–635.

Wigger-Alberti, W., & Elsner, P. (1997). Preventive measures in contact dermatitis. *Clinics in Dermatology, 15,* 661–665.

Chapter

20. Herpes Zoster

Madonna K. McDermott, RN, MS, ANP, OCN®

I. Definition: Also called shingles; is a cutaneous infection produced by the reactivation of the varicella zoster virus (VZV) in the dorsal root ganglia

II. Pathophysiology
   A. The virus presumably remains latent in the dorsal root or cranial nerve ganglia following primary varicella (chicken pox) until reactivation.
   B. The infectious virus then reappears in the neurons and nerve-associated satellite cells and spreads to the skin through peripheral nerves.
   C. In acute herpes zoster, the skin is inflamed and already partially denervated and the dorsal-root ganglion shows inflammation, hemorrhagic necrosis, and neuronal loss.

III. Clinical features: Two clinical presentations can occur—primary infection (chicken pox) or reactivation (herpes zoster). Inflammation in the peripheral nerves may persist for weeks to months and usually leads to demyelination. Lesions usually involve a dermatone pattern with worsening of lesions for approximately seven days, then resolving, usually by day 14.
   A. Risk factors
      1. Most common in immunocompromised patients
         a) Hematologic malignancy
         b) Bone marrow transplantation
         c) Elderly
         d) Acute systemic illnesses
         e) HIV
      2. Emotional stress
   B. History
      1. History of cancer and cancer treatment
      2. Current medications: Prescribed and over-the-counter
      3. History of presenting symptom(s): Precipitating factors, onset, location, and duration
      4. Changes in activities of daily living
   C. Signs and symptoms
      1. A prodrome of one to four days of tingling, acute pain, tenderness, or itching in area of nerve involvement

2. Hyperesthesia: Abnormally increased sensitiveness
3. Hypoesthesia: Abnormally diminished sensitiveness

D. Physical exam: Examine entire skin for characteristic lesions and distribution.
   1. HEENT: Examine eyes for lesions
   2. Integument
      a) Vesiculopapular rash: Clear vesicles 3–5 mm in diameter on erythematous base
      b) Rash noted in dermatomal pattern
      c) Rash that stops at the midline

IV. Diagnostic tests
   A. The presumptive diagnosis of herpes zoster is made clinically.
   B. Tzanck smear can assist in diagnosis of herpetic infection but cannot distinguish herpes zoster from herpes simplex.
   C. Skin biopsy

V. Differential diagnosis
   A. Pleurisy
   B. Myocardial infarction (see Chapter 47)
   C. Cholecystitis
   D. Appendicitis
   E. Renal colic
   F. Ruptured intervertebral disc
   G. Herpes simplex (see Chapter 89)
   H. Impetigo
   I. Cellulitis (see Chapter 16)
   J. Contact dermatitis (see Chapter 19)

VI. Treatment: Aimed at symptomatic relief and decreasing the development of new lesions
   A. Mild to moderate cases: Antiviral agents
      1. Valacyclovir (Valtrex®) 1,000 mg po tid for seven days
      2. Oral acyclovir (Zovirax®, Glaxo Wellcome, Research Triangle Park, NC) 800 mg po five times a day for 7–10 days; must be initiated within 48 hours of cutaneous eruption to be beneficial
      3. Famciclovir (Famvir®) 500 mg po tid for seven days
   B. Severe cases: Parenteral agents given for severe cases in immunocompromised patients
      1. Acyclovir 12.4 mg/kg IV (one-hour infusion) every eight hours for five to seven days
      2. Vidarabine 10 mg/kg/day IV (12-hour infusion) for five to seven days
   C. Topical treatments promote drying of the lesions, and a topical antibacterial agent (e.g., bacitracin ointment) promotes healing and decreases the incidence of secondary infections.
   D. Acute herpes zoster pain and postherpetic neuralgia: Pain associated with shingles usually is neuropathic in nature and, therefore, is generally less responsive to mild analgesic drugs and narcotics; however, some patients do benefit from these drugs (see Appendix 10 a/b)
      1. Tricyclic antidepressant drugs

       a) Amitriptyline 10–25 mg po at bedtime, gradually increasing in increments of 10–25 mg every three to five days; usually to maximal effect at 100–150 mg po every night

       b) Nortriptyline 10 mg po every night, increasing by 10 mg every three days; usually to maximal effect at 50–100 mg po every night

  2. Anticonvulsant drugs: Can reduce the lancinating component of neuropathic pain; review individual drugs and monitoring information prior to initiating therapy.

       a) Gabapentin (Neurontin®, Parke-Davis, Morris Plains, NJ) gradual dose escalation by 100 mg po daily until effective pain relief is achieved; usually maximal effect at 300 mg po tid, 600 mg po tid, or 900 mg po tid

       b) Carbamazepine (Tegretol®, Novartis Pharmaceuticals, East Hanover, NJ) 200 mg po q 6–8 hours (up to 1,600 mg/day)

       c) Phenytoin (Dilantin®, Parke-Davis) 300 mg po every night

       d) Clonazepam (Klonopin®, Roche Laboratories, Nutley, NJ) 0.5 mg po q 12 hours or night-time dosing only because of sedation side effect

  3. Topical anesthetics

       a) Capsaicin cream 0.025% qid: Burning elicited with application may not be well tolerated; however, this side effect may diminish after repeated application.

       b) Aspercreme® (Chattem, Inc., Chattanooga, TN): Follow package directions

  4. Local injections of anesthetic drugs such as lidocaine, procaine, and mepivacaine

  5. Nonpharmacologic interventions

       a) Transcutaneous nerve stimulation (TENS) unit

       b) Acupuncture

       c) Biofeedback

VII. Follow-up: In one week for most patients; two to three days for patients who are immunocompromised, elderly, or debilitated

VIII. Referrals

  A. If the eye is involved, refer to an ophthalmologist urgently.

  B. If pain persists using conventional analgesic modalities, refer to a pain specialist.

References

Fitzgerald, E. (1994). Alleviating the pain of herpes zoster. *Emergency Medicine, 26*(3), 34–39.

Kost, R.G., & Straus, S.E. (1996). Postherpetic neuralgia—Pathogenesis, treatment, and prevention. *New England Journal of Medicine, 335,* 32–42.

Lamberg, S.I. (1995). Common problems of the skin. In L.R. Barker, J.R. Burton, & P.D. Zieve (Eds.), *Principles of ambulatory medicine* (4th ed.) (pp. 1439–1478). Baltimore: Williams & Wilkins.

Lawrence, J. (1994). Critical care issues in the patient with hematologic malignancy. *Seminars in Oncology Nursing, 10,* 198–207.

McMahon, M.A. (1994). Herpes zoster and the aging. *Journal of Gerontological Nursing 20*(12), 42–46.

Whitley, R.J. (1998). Varicella-zoster virus infections. In A.S. Fauci, E. Braunwald, K.J. Isselbacher, J.D. Wilson, J.B. Martin, D.L. Kasper, S.L. Hauser, & D.L. Longo (Eds.), *Harrison's principles of internal medicine* (14th ed.) (pp. 1086–1089). New York: McGraw-Hill.

Chapter

21. Skin Metastasis
Janet S. Fulton, PhD, RN

I. Definition: The extension of a neoplastic process from a primary site to the skin

II. Pathophysiology
   A. Vascular and lymphatic channels are considered to be the most common modes of metastasis for visceral carcinoma.
   B. For metastasis to occur, the primary neoplasm must be of sufficient size to release cells into the circulation.
   C. Other mechanisms of cutaneous metastasis include the following.
      1. Migration across the peritoneal cavity
      2. Iatrogenic implantation after surgical procedures
      3. Migration of cells along a central venous catheter tract
   D. Irradiated tissue can serve as a focus of metastatic implantation.
      1. Irradiation increases endothelial damage so that cancer cells are trapped and can persist for a long time, resulting in local implantations.
      2. Decreased immunologic surveillance in irradiated tissue probably enhances cancer cell survival and growth after implantation has occurred.

III. Clinical features
   A. Etiology
      1. Most frequent primary sites are visceral carcinomas (e.g., breast, stomach, lung, uterus, colon, kidney, prostate, ovary, liver).
      2. Skin metastasis generally is a late occurrence in the course of the disease.
      3. Occasionally, cutaneous metastases may be the presenting sign of malignancy.
         a) Cancers that become far advanced before symptoms are evident are more likely to demonstrate late sequelae, including cutaneous metastases, prior to diagnosis of the primary site.
         b) Cutaneous metastasis presenting as a tumor of unknown origin is rare.
   B. History
      1. History of cancer and cancer treatment
      2. Current medications: Prescribed and over-the-counter
      3. History of presenting symptom(s): Precipitating factors, onset, location, and duration
      4. Changes in activities of daily living

  5. Past surgical history that may produce iatrogenic introduction of cancer cells into cutaneous tissue

   a) Procedures: Skin grafts, needle biopsy, and thoracentesis

   b) Devices: Wound drains, prosthetic devices, chest tubes, or central venous access devices

 C. Signs and symptoms: The clinical appearance of cutaneous metastases is not distinctive and may include any of the following.

  1. Indurated or raised patches on the skin

  2. Localized thickened, firm areas on the skin; may have "orange peel" appearance

  3. Localized changes in skin color, including hyperpigmentation or redness

  4. Patches of scalp alopecia

 D. Physical exam

  1. Integument exam

   a) Localized lesion(s), often round or oval in appearance; may be a nodule, indurated or raised plaque, or thickened fibrotic area

   b) Usually flesh-colored; occasionally appear inflamed; may be pink to red

   c) Can be firm, solid, or rubbery on palpation. Nodules first may be detected at about 0.5 cm in diameter, although usually at 1–3 cm.

   d) Scalp lesions may form clusters, feeling like a bag of marbles when palpated.

   e) Lesions usually nonpainful, nontender to touch

    (1) May be freely movable or fixed

    (2) May be solitary, few, or multiple lesions

     (a) Multiple nodules occurring at a single site are considered a single metastasis.

     (b) Multiple metastases must involve more than one site.

     (c) Most often occur on cutaneous surfaces near the primary site: Distribution/characteristics

  2. Lymph node exam: May be palpable in regional lymphatics

  3. Types of skin metastasis

   a) Breast: Chest, abdomen, and scalp; occasionally resembles pig skin or orange peel

    1. Unique metastatic patterns (usually associated with breast cancer)

    2. Carcinoma erysipelatoides (inflammatory): Well-circumscribed, warm, tender, erythematous, and edematous patch with sharply elevated borders

    3. Carcinoma telangiectaticum: Involves multiple hemorrhagic papules on the skin overlying the site of a mastectomy for primary cancer of the breast

    4. Carcinoma en cuirasse

     (a) Initial appearance is scattered, hard papules or nodules over a red to red-blue, smooth surface.

     (b) Nodules later coalesce, forming a hard, well-defined, scleroderma-like plaque.

   b) Lung: Trunk and scalp; most commonly reddish nodules, symmetrical, along direction of intercostal vessels

   c) Hypernephroma: Scalp and operative scar; usually solitary lesion

   d) Ovarian: Abdomen and inguinal area; occasionally resembles pig skin or orange peel

   e) Bladder: Abdomen and inguinal area; occasionally resembles pig skin or orange peel

IV. Diagnostic tests: Laboratory: Suspected skin metastasis is confirmed by skin biopsy and histology.

V. Differential diagnosis
   A. Cellulitis (see Chapter 16)
   B. Lymphangioma: A benign tumor composed of lymphatic vessels
   C. Scarring alopecia
   D. Radiation dermatitis
   E. Hyperpigmentation and telangiectasia (see Chapter 12)
   F. Herpes zoster (see Chapter 20)

VI. Treatment
   A. Surgical excision may be indicated for solitary or few lesions.
   B. Radiation therapy may be used for convenience and tissue sparing. Radioresistant neoplasms and tissue radiotoxicity limit the usefulness of radiotherapy.
   C. Cryotherapy, or application of liquid nitrogen, may be used for *in situ* freezing of the lesions.
   D. Chemotherapy may be useful in decreasing the number of lesions and preventing further spread of disease.
   E. Odor can be controlled with topical metronidazole 0.75% applied daily to a clean, dry, nonstick dressing and covered with a sterile gauze.
   F. Treatment of aerobic infections of the skin (see Appendix 1)

VII. Follow-up
   A. In general, skin metastases are a poor prognostic sign.
   B. Death usually follows within one year of the identification of a metastatic skin lesion, with the exception of contiguous spread of breast cancer, which may last for years.
   C. If skin metastases are present, it is likely that the disease is widespread and that metastases to multiple other organs coexist.

VIII. Referrals: Refer to surgeon or dermatologist for biopsy confirmation of diagnosis and to enterostomal therapist for assistance with complex wound care management.

References

Bhandarkar, P., Green, K.M., & de Carpentier, J.P. (1997). Multiple cutaneous metastases from laryngeal carcinoma. *Journal of Laryngology and Otology, 111,* 654–655.

Caubet-Biayna, J., Morey-Mas, M., Ibarra, J., & Iriarte-Ortabe, J.I. (1998). Scalp metastases as the first manifestation of a lung adenocarcinoma. *Journal of Oral and Maxillofacial Surgery, 56,* 247–250.

Cohen, P.R. (1995). Skin clues to primary and metastatic malignancy. *American Family Physician, 51,* 1199–1204.

Finlay, I.G., Bowszyc, J., Ramlau, C., & Gwiezdzinski, Z. (1996). The effect of topical 0.75% metronidazole gel on malodorous cutaneous ulcers. *Journal of Pain and Symptom Management, 11,* 158–162.

Gage, I., Schnitt, S.J., Recht, A., Abner, A., Come, S., Shulman, L.N., Monson, J.M., Silver, B., Harris, J.R., & Connolly, J.L. (1998). Skin recurrences after breast-conserving therapy for early-stage breast cancer. *Journal of Clinical Oncology, 16,* 480–486.

Garcia-Gonzalez, E., Alverez-Paque, L., Loyla-Sarate, M., & Kisker-Melman, M. (1998). Seeding of gastric adenocarcinoma cells to the skin after invasive procedures. *Journal of Clinical Gastroenterology, 26,* 82–84.

Ichioka, S., & Yamada, A. (1994). Ultrasonographic demonstration of a skin metastasis of adenocarcinoma. *Journal of Dermatology, 21,* 690–692.

Kim, J.H., Benson, P.M., Beard, J.S., & Skelton, H.G. (1998). Male breast carcinoma with extensive metastases to the skin. *Journal of the American Academy of Dermatology, 38,* 995–996.

Strohl, R.A. (1998). Cutaneous manifestations of malignant disease. *Dermatology Nursing, 10*(1), 23–25.

Section **IV.**

Respiratory

Symptoms

Medical Diagnosis

Chapter

22. Cough

Madonna K. McDermott, RN, MS, ANP, OCN®

I. Definition
    A. A pulmonary protective reflex that is an important defense mechanism to clear the airways of both secretions and inhaled particles
    B. "Pathologic cough": Cough resulting from a disease process

II. Physiology/Pathophysiology
    A. Normal: Composed of three phases
        1. Deep inspiration
        2. Closure of the glottis accompanied by a rapid increase in pleural pressure
        3. Opening of the glottis with rapid release of pressure
    B. Pathophysiology: Neural mucosal receptors located within the nasopharynx, larynx, trachea, and bronchial tree initiate the cough reflex.
        1. Stimuli that activate these receptors are either chemical or mechanical irritation.
        2. Impulses are then conducted along afferent pathways via cranial nerves IX and X terminating at the cough center in the medulla.
        3. The cough reflex occurs through efferent pathways that cause forceful contraction of the diaphragm and other expiratory muscles.

III. Clinical features: Pathologic cough is of benefit when it results in the expulsion of secretions or other foreign material from the airways. Chronic cough lasts longer than three weeks. Potential complications of uncontrolled cough include rib fractures, syncope, urinary stress incontinence, hemoptysis, and rupture of superficial vessels.
    A. History
        1. History of cancer and cancer treatment
        2. Current medications: Prescribed and over-the-counter
        3. History of presenting symptom(s): Precipitating factors, onset, location, and duration
        4. Changes in activities of daily living
        5. Social history of smoking or exposure to occupational or environmental irritants
    B. Signs and symptoms
        1. May vary depending upon underlying cause
        2. Presence or absence of sputum production

C. Physical exam
1. Vital signs: Temperature and respiratory rate
2. Integument exam: Skin temperature, color, and peripheral edema
3. Oropharynx exam: Presence of mucus, erythema, or a "cobblestone" appearance to the mucosa, suggestive of postnasal drip
4. Pulmonary exam
    a) Check respiratory rate.
    b) Observe for accessory muscle use.
    c) Note any inspiratory stridor (suggestive of upper airway disease).
    d) Note rhonchi or expiratory wheezing (suggestive of lower airway disease).
    e) Observe for inspiratory crackles, described as "Velcro® dry" (suggestive of a process involving the pulmonary parenchyma, such as interstitial lung disease, alveolitis, pneumonia, or pulmonary edema)
    f) Crackles wet in the lung bases may be suggestive of congestive heart failure (CHF).
5. Cardiovascular exam: Jugular venous distention (JVD) and S_3 gallop, suggestive of CHF.

IV. Diagnostic tests: The following studies may be recommended if gastrointestinal reflux, CHF, and post-viral etiology are not suspected.
A. Laboratory: Sputum for cytology or gram and acid-fast stains
1. Cytology may be positive in presence of malignancy.
2. Gram and acid-fast stains may reveal infectious pathogen.
B. Radiology
1. Chest x-ray if no reversible airflow obstruction noted on pulmonary function tests
2. CT scan if chest x-ray suspicious of parenchymal lung disease
C. Other
1. Pulmonary function testing if asthma is suspected
2. Bronchoscopy if chest x-ray is suspicious of mass

V. Differential diagnosis
A. Medication-induced
1. Angiotensin converting enzyme (ACE) inhibitors (beginning one week after initiating treatment)
2. Ipratropium
3. Inhalation of nebulized water
B. Diseases
1. Asthma (see Chapter 28)
2. Infections
    a) Pneumonia (see Chapter 30)
    b) Bronchitis (see Chapter 28)
    c) Lung abscess
    d) Tuberculosis (see Chapter 34)
3. Gastroesophageal reflux (see Chapter 66)

      4. Postnasal drainage
      5. CHF (see Chapter 40)
      6. Tumors of the lung
      7. Lymphangitis
      8. Carcinomatosis (widespread dissemination of carcinoma in the body)
      9. Pleural effusion (see Chapter 29)
    10. Hypersensitivity pneumonitis
    11. Radiation pneumonitis
    12. Pericardial effusion (see Chapter 48)
    13. Vocal cord paralysis and spastic (spasmodic) dysphonia
    14. Motor neuron diseases (e.g., multiple sclerosis, stroke)
    15. Interstitial lung disease
    16. Aortic aneurysm
    17. Impacted cerumen
    18. Paraneoplastic syndrome—rare (see Appendix 12)
  C. Exposure to chemical or environmental irritants
  D. Chemical aspiration

VI. Treatment: Treatment is dependent on determining the underlying cause and then initiating appropriate therapy.
  A. Elimination of exogenous causative agents, such as cigarette smoke and ACE inhibitors
  B. Control of endogenous causative agents, such as postnasal drip (see Chapter 10) and gastroesophageal reflux (see Chapter 66)
  C. Treatment of specific respiratory tract infections
  D. Bronchodilators for reversible airflow obstruction with bronchiectasis (see Chapter 28)
  E. Treatment of lung tumors
  F. Treatment of interstitial lung disease
  G. Medication management (see Table 22-1) to suppress the cough if
      1. The cough performs no useful function
      2. Causes significant discomfort
      3. Treatment of the underlying process is not possible
      4. The cause of the cough is unknown.

Table 22-1. Examples of Oral Antitussives

Drug	Adults 12 Years and Older
Codeine	10–20 mg po every four to six hours (120 mg)/24 hours; available in elixir
Dextromethorphan	10–20 mg po every four to eight hours or 30 mg every eight hours (120 mg)/24 hours; lozenges or elixir
Benzonatate	100 mg po tid; do not chew
Guaifenesin	5–20 ml po every four hours
Hydrocodone	5 ml po every four to six hours

H. Humidified air for patients with a nonproductive cough in a dry environment

VII. Follow-up: Dependent upon definitive diagnosis and treatment plan
   A. Short-term
      1. Specific follow-up is determined by diagnosis.
      2. Viral tracheobronchitis usually resolves in two to four weeks. Return appointment for evaluation of symptoms within that time frame would be appropriate.
   B. Long-term
      1. Patients whose workup is essentially negative should be seen at least every one to three months if coughing persists.
      2. Evaluation and follow-up of patients with cancer who are experiencing cough is dependent upon the life expectancy of the patients.

VIII. Referrals: Not indicated unless symptoms persist; consult pulmonologist, cardiologist, or allergist for assistance in management.

References

Dudgeon, D.J., & Rosenthal, S. (1996). Management of dyspnea and cough in patients with cancer. *Hematology/Oncology Clinics of North America, 10,* 157–171.

Fouad, Y.M., Katz, P.O., Hatlebakk, J.G., & Castell, D.O. (1999). Ineffective esophageal motility: The most common motility abnormality in patients with GERD-associated respiratory symptoms. *American Journal of Gastroenterology, 94,* 1464–1467.

Hagen, N. (1994). Cough as a systemic manifestation of cancer. *Journal of Pain and Symptom Management, 9*(1), 3–4.

Irwin, R.S. (1999). Silencing chronic cough. *Hospital Practice, 34*(1), 53–60.

Irwin, R.S., Boulet, L.P., Cloutier, M.M., Fuller, R., Gold, P.M., Hoffstein, V., Ing, A.J., McCool, F.D., O'Byrne, P., Poe, P.H., Prakash, U.B., Pratter, M.R., & Rubin, B.K. (1998). Managing cough as a defense mechanism and as a symptom. A consensus panel report of The American College of Chest Physicians. *Chest, 115,* 602–603.

Ludviksdottir, D., Bjornsson, E., Janson, C., & Boman, G. (1996). Habitual coughing and its associations with asthma, anxiety, and gastroesophageal reflux. *Chest, 109,* 1262–1268.

Rousseau, P. (1996). Cough in the terminally ill: A brief synopsis. *American Journal of Hospice and Palliative Care, 13*(6), 45–46.

Smith, C.H., Loemann, J.A., Colangelo, L.A., Rademaker, A.W., & Pauloski, B.R. (1999). Incidence and patient characteristics associated with silent aspiration in the acute care setting. *Dysphasia, 14*(1), 1–7.

Chapter

23. Dyspnea
Madonna K. McDermott, RN, MS, ANP, OCN®

I. Definition: The subjective, abnormal, uncomfortable sensation of breathlessness

II. Pathophysiology
   A. No single mechanism is responsible for dyspnea.
   B. Dyspnea occurs when individual workload exceeds normal ventilation abilities.
   C. Neural receptors located in the upper respiratory tract, lungs, respiratory muscle, chest wall, and blood vessels send a message to the respiratory centers in the brain stem in response to changing levels of O_2 and CO_2.

III. Clinical features: Determine whether dyspnea is an acute or a chronic event.
   A. Etiologies: Causes of dyspnea are varied and numerous. Any disease resulting in impairment of the cardiovascular, respiratory, or hematologic system should be explored (see Figure 23-1).

Figure 23-1. Causes of Dyspnea in Patients With Cancer

Dyspnea as a result of cancer:
- Primary or metastatic cancer to the lung
- Pleural tumor
- Lymphangitic carcinomatosis
- Pericardial effusion
- Superior vena cava syndrome
- Paraneoplastic syndromes
- Hepatomegaly
- Pulmonary leukostasis
- Multiple tumor

Dyspnea as an indirect result of cancer:
- Anemia
- Pneumonia
- Electrolyte abnormalities
- Cachexia
- Pulmonary emboli
- Ascites

Dyspnea as a result of cancer treatment:
- Surgery
- Radiation therapy-induced
- Chemotherapy-induced pulmonary toxicity: Bleomycin, carmustine, mitomycin, busulfan, cyclophosphamide, methotrexate
- Cardiomyopathy

Dyspnea unrelated to cancer:
- Chronic obstructive pulmonary disease
- Asthma
- Pneumothorax
- Obesity
- Goiter
- Pulmonary hypertension
- Aspiration
- Congestive heart failure

B. History
1. History of cancer and cancer treatment
2. Current medications: Prescribed and over-the-counter
3. History of presenting symptom(s): Precipitating factors, onset, location, and duration
4. Changes in activities of daily living
5. Past medical history of asthma, bronchitis, pneumonia, heart disease, or anemia
6. Social history of smoking (packs/years)
C. Signs and symptoms: It can be described as the inability to get enough air, chest tightness, smothering feeling, tiredness in the chest, or choking.
1. Orthopnea: Dyspnea while in a supine posture
2. Trepopnea: Dyspnea occurring only in a lateral decubitus position; suggests heart disease
3. Paroxysmal nocturnal dyspnea (PND)
4. Platypnea: Dyspnea occurring only in the upright position; seen in patients with inadequate abdominal musculature
5. Sudden and unexpected dyspnea without exertion; may be suggestive of pulmonary emboli, spontaneous pneumothorax, evolving myocardial infarction, or anxiety
D. Physical exam: Dyspnea is a subjective experience; therefore, using visual analog scales similar to those used for pain assessment may be useful.
1. Vital signs: Respirations increased; weight status
2. Integument exam
    a) Pallor indicating anemia
    b) Cyanosis with a pulmonary origin
3. Cardiopulmonary exam
    a) Intercostal retraction
    b) Use of accessory muscles
    c) Peripheral edema and pulses
    d) Tachycardia
    e) Digital clubbing
4. Mental status exam to assess for hypoxia
    a) Memory or concentration problems
    b) Confusion
    c) Restlessness
5. Psychosocial exam
    a) Anxiety
    b) Fear
    c) Depression

IV. Diagnostic tests: The choice of appropriate diagnostic tests is guided by the rapidity of onset of symptoms, with acute symptoms requiring a more aggressive diagnostic workup.
A. Laboratory
1. Complete blood count: To evaluate for infection, neutropenia, anemia, and thrombocytopenia
2. Arterial blood gases (ABGs): To document presence of hypoxemia or hypercapnia, to characterize acid-base status, and to detect significant carboxyhemoglobin

B. Radiology
  1. Chest x-ray: Evaluate for infiltrates, interstitial lung disease, tumor, pleural effusion, pneumothorax, and cardiac enlargement.
  2. Echocardiogram: Assess right and left ventricular function or the presence of valvular heart disease.
  3. CT scan of chest to rule out obstruction, effusions.
  4. Ventilation/perfusion scan (V/Q scan), which demonstrates 100% sensitivity for pulmonary emboli; if V/Q scan is normal, pulmonary embolism is ruled out.
C. Other
  1. Pulmonary function tests
    a) Establish presence and severity of airway obstruction
    b) Serve as a baseline parameter in illness
    c) Assist in differentiation between emphysema and other forms of airway obstruction
    d) Evaluate reversibility of airway obstruction and results of therapy
  2. Pulse oximetry: O_2 less than 90% represents significant hypoxemia requiring ABGs and other studies.

V. Differential diagnosis
  A. Asthma, bronchitis (see Chapter 28)
  B. Pneumothorax (see Chapter 31)
  C. Pulmonary embolism (see Chapter 33)
  D. Pneumonia (see Chapter 30)
  E. Anaphylaxis
  F. Acute blood loss or hemolysis
  G. Pleural effusion (see Chapter 29)
  H. Pericardial effusion (see Chapter 48)
  I. Chronic obstructive pulmonary disease (COPD) (see Chapter 28)
  J. CHF (see Chapter 40)
  K. Electrolyte abnormalities (see Chapters 145–148)
  L. Anemia (see Chapters 112–118)
  M. Cachexia (see Chapter 62)
  N. Interstitial lung disease
  O. Anxiety (see Chapter 152)
  P. Obesity
  Q. Neuromuscular disorders
  R. Cancer-related
    1. Tumors
    2. Paraneoplastic syndromes (see Appendix 12)
    3. Surgery (e.g., pneumonectomy)
    4. Radiation therapy- or chemotherapy-induced pulmonary or cardiac disease

VI. Treatment: Designed to correct or treat the underlying cause and will be guided by findings obtained in the history and diagnostic studies
  A. Treat underlying etiology as appropriate.

1. Asthma, bronchitis (see Chapter 28)
2. Pneumothorax and pleural effusion relieved by thoracentesis procedure and oxygen therapy
3. Pulmonary embolism (see Chapter 33))
4. Pneumonia (see Chapter 30)
5. CHF (see Chapter 40)
6. Pericardial effusion (see Chapter 48)
7. Superior vena cava syndrome
8. COPD (see Chapter 28)
9. Electrolyte abnormalities (see Chapters 144–148)
10. Anemia (see Chapters 111–118)
11. Cachexia (see Chapter 62)
12. Cancer treatment for paraneoplastic syndromes—combination of these modalities
13. Interstitial lung disease
14. Anxiety (see Chapter 152)

B. Blood loss or hemolysis
1. Transfuse blood products as appropriate.
2. Determine cause and treat.

C. Obesity
1. Encourage activity and regular exercise.
2. Teach principles of balanced diet.

D. General guidelines regardless of cause
1. Administer O_2 therapy, 0.5–4 l/minute
2. Raise head of bed.
3. Administer morphine, 2–4 mg IV, for air hunger or nebulized in 5 cc of normal saline as ordered.
4. Provide cool environment.

VII. Follow-up: Based upon the diagnosis and treatment plan
A. Acute dyspnea may require hospitalization for aggressive diagnostic studies and interventions.
B. Less acute dyspnea may be followed-up in an ambulatory setting within 24–48 hours.

VIII. Referrals: To pulmonologist if symptoms do not resolve

References

Dudgeon, D.J., & Lertzman, M. (1998). Dyspnea in the advanced cancer patient. *Journal of Pain and Symptom Management, 16,* 212–219.

Dudgeon, D.J., & Rosenthal, S. (1996). Management of dyspnea and cough in patients with cancer. *Hematology/Oncology Clinics of North America, 10,* 157–171.

Escalante, C.P., Martin, C.G., Elting, L.S., Cantor, S.B., Harle, T.S., Price, K.J., Kish, S.K., Manzullo, E.F., & Rubenstein, E.B. (1996). Dyspnea in cancer patients. Etiology, resource utilization, and survival—Implications in a managed care world. *Cancer, 78,* 1314–1319.

Michelson, E., & Hollrah, S. (1999). Evaluation of the patient with shortness of breath: An evidence-based approach. *Emergency Medicine Clinics of North America, 17,* 221–237.

Parshell, M.B. (1999). Adult emergency visits for chronic cardiorespiratory disease: Does dyspnea matter? *Nursing Research, 48*(2), 62–70.

24. Hemoptysis

Sandra C. Henke, RN, MS, ANP, OCN®

I. Definition: Expectoration of blood that originates from the lower respiratory tract below the pharynx

II. Physiology/Pathophysiology
   A. Normal: The normal anatomy of the lung lends itself to the symptom of hemoptysis in various ways.
      1. The dual blood supply to the lung from the pulmonary and bronchial arterial systems, the proximity of all airways to vessels, and the diversity of conditions affecting the respiratory tract can lead to hemoptysis.
      2. Bleeding can originate from vascular disruption at any anatomic level, but the bronchial arterial system is the predominant source in most patients.
      3. Because the lung is, in effect, a sheet of blood, injury to either side of the alveolar-capillary membrane can cause varying degrees of hemoptysis.
   B. Pathophysiology
      1. Intermittent episodes of severe bleeding from bronchial artery-pulmonary vein channels develop in response to chronic inflammation.
      2. Bleeding occurs from superficial mucosal vessels in the proximal airways as a complication of an exacerbation of chronic bronchitis and bronchial irritation.

III. Clinical features: Hemoptysis signifies coughing up of an easily quantifiable amount of blood, either pure or mixed with sputum. The amount of bleeding indicates the severity of hemoptysis.
   A. History
      1. History of cancer and cancer treatment
      2. Current medications: Prescribed and over-the-counter
      3. History of presenting symptom(s): Precipitating factors, onset, and duration. Associated symptoms are cough, fever/night sweats, and recent weight loss
      4. Changes in activities of daily living
      5. Past medical history of recent exposures to respiratory infections, chest trauma
   B. Signs and symptoms
      1. General
         a) Anxiety

   b) Heart palpitations

   c) Fever

  2. Respiratory

   a) Spectrum ranges from blood-streaked sputum to frank pulmonary hemorrhage.

   b) Cough

   c) Dyspnea

 C. Physical exam

  1. Head, eyes, ears, nose, and throat (HEENT) exam

   a) Inspection of nose and mouth for any obvious bleeding source

   b) Poor dentition; gingivitis

   c) Pharyngeal erythema

   d) Cervical or supraclavicular adenopathy

  2. Pulmonary exam

   a) Asymmetric chest excursion may indicate bronchial obstruction.

   b) Dullness to percussion may indicate collapse or consolidation.

   c) Localized wheezing or stridor may indicate obstruction of airways.

   d) Absent or distant breath sounds indicate obstruction or collapse.

   e) Crackles may indicate pneumonia of infectious or inflammatory process or volume overload in CHF.

   f) Normal breath sounds are common.

  3. Cardiac exam

   a) Murmurs consistent with mitral stenosis

   b) Distant heart sounds

  4. Extremities

   a) Edema of lower extremities

   b) Unilateral edema/calf tenderness

IV. Diagnostic tests

 A. Laboratory

  1. Complete blood count (CBC) to rule out anemia

  2. Purified protein derivative skin test in cases of suspected tuberculosis

  3. Sputum analysis

   a) Acid-fast bacillus to confirm tuberculosis

   b) Culture and sensitivity to evaluate bronchial pneumonia

   c) Cytology to establish a diagnosis of lung cancer

  4. Coagulation tests: Prothrombin time/partial thromboplastin time and platelet count

  5. ABGs analysis: Estimates pulmonary reserve and the impact of bleeding

 B. Radiology

  1. Chest x-ray

   a) Apical cavitary disease may suggest tuberculosis.

   b) Central mass lesions are found with bronchogenic carcinoma.

   c) Focal consolidation might suggest bacterial pneumonia.

   d) Diffuse infiltrates suggest aspiration of blood or microvascular bleeding.

        e) Normal chest film does not necessarily mean that the source of bleeding is outside the thorax.

    2. CT scan as a noninvasive screening tool may be useful in identifying small lung cancers, diffuse interstitial disease, and bronchiectasis. Cardiac disease is suggested by enlarged left atrium or calcified mitral valve, suggesting mitral stenosis.

  C. Other: Bronchoscopy—examination of the upper and lower airways is indicated when hemoptysis is clinically significant; localizes bleeding and can identify conditions with specific and nonspecific manifestations. Procedure performed if

    1. Bleeding present for one week or longer
    2. Expectoration of more than 30 ml of blood daily
    3. Older age (more than 40 years)
    4. Abnormal chest radiographs
    5. Smoking history
    6. Chronic cough
    7. Anemia

V. Differential diagnosis

  A. Infection
    1. Pneumonia (see Chapter 30)
    2. Tuberculosis (see Chapter 34)
    3. Bronchiectasis
    4. Aspergillomas
    5. Lung abscess

  B. Neoplasm
    1. Primary bronchogenic carcinoma
    2. Lung metastasis

  C. Treatment-induced
    1. Bone marrow transplant
    2. Thrombocytopenia resulting in alveolar hemorrhage

  D. Cardiovascular disorders
    1. Mitral valve stenosis
    2. CHF (see Chapter 40)

  E. Chest trauma

  F. Pulmonary disorders
    1. Chronic bronchitis (see Chapter 28)
    2. Pulmonary embolism/pulmonary infarction (see Chapter 33)
    3. Pulmonary edema (see Chapter 32)
    4. Chemical bronchitis and/or pneumonia (see Chapter 30)

VI. Treatment
  A. Hemoptysis often stops spontaneously.
  B. Maintain patent airway.
  C. Manage underlying diagnosis.
  D. Provide symptom management (e.g., dextromethorphan with codeine elixir, one to two teaspoons every four to six hours to control cough)

VII. Follow-up
   A. Instruct patient to notify healthcare team should symptom recur or persist.
   B. Manage primary diagnosis/etiology of hemoptysis.

VIII. Referrals
   A. Pulmonologist for bronchoscopy
   B. Hospitalization for massive hemoptysis
   C. Referral for management of specific diagnosis
      1. Oncology referral for management of lung mass
      2. Infectious disease referral for management of identified infectious process

References

Barker, R.A., Knowles, G.K., & Sheppard, M.N. (1998). Breathlessness and profuse haemoptysis. *Lancet, 351*(9096), 108.

Cahill, B.C., & Ingbar, D.H. (1994). Massive hemoptysis. Assessment and management. *Clinics in Chest Medicine, 15*(1), 147–167.

Colice, G.L. (1996). Hemoptysis. Three questions that can direct management. *Postgraduate Medicine, 100*(1), 227–236.

Dweik, R.A., & Stroller, J.K. (1999). Role of bronchoscopy in massive hemoptysis. *Clinics in Chest Medicine, 210*(1), 89–105.

Hirshberg, B., Biran, I., Glazer, M., & Kramer, M.R. (1997). Hemoptysis: Etiology, evaluation, and outcome in a tertiary referral hospital. *Chest, 112*, 440–444.

Mroz, B.J., Sexauer, W.P., Meade, A., & Balsara, G. (1997). Hemoptysis as the presenting symptom in bronchiolitis obliterans organizing pneumonia. *Chest, 111*, 1775–1778.

Chapter

25. Orthopnea
Mary P. Pazdur, RN, MSN, AOCN®

I. Definition
   A. Respiratory discomfort (dyspnea) that occurs when patient is supine
   B. Paroxysmal nocturnal dyspnea (PND): Orthopnea that causes patient to awaken from sleep, with relief experienced upon sitting up

II. Pathophysiology: Change in position from supine to raised upper torso causes pulmonary excursion of diaphragm and enhances respiration in people with mechanical pressure, inflammation, or edema of respiratory tract.

III. Clinical features
   A. Etiologies
      1. Elevated pulmonary venous pressure
      2. Pulmonary edema
      3. Cor pulmonale
      4. Right-sided heart failure
      5. Increased venous return in people with a failing left ventricle
      6. In pulmonary- associated causes, occurs in advanced disease
         a) Lymphangitic spread
         b) Mediastinal tumor
         c) Extrinsic compression of airway with atelectasis
         d) Malignant pleural effusion
         e) Pericardial effusion
      7. Can be aggravated by other conditions
         a) Neuromuscular weakness
         b) Hypercapnia
         c) Pneumonia
         d) Metabolic acidosis
         e) Anemia
         f) Renal impairment
   B. History: Subjective history should focus on frequency and severity of dyspnea associated with orthopnea and should include the following.

1. History of cancer and cancer treatment
2. Current medications: Prescribed and over-the-counter
3. History of presenting symptom(s): Precipitating factors, onset, location, and duration. Associated symptoms are fever and chills, sputum production, chest pain, nocturnal palpitations, edema, and number of pillows used during sleep.
4. Changes in activities of daily living
5. Past medical history: Heart disease, hypertension, COPD, and pulmonary hypertension

C. Signs and symptoms
   1. Unable to sleep or rest in supine position (i.e., using more than two pillows)
   2. Signs of increased respiratory effort
      a) Muscle retraction (intercostals)
      b) Increased respiratory rate
      c) Nasal flaring
   3. Late signs of cyanosis: Circumoral or nail bed changes
   4. Cough
   5. Pleuritic pain
   6. Panic attacks

D. Physical exam
   1. Vital signs: Increased respirations and change in quality
   2. Pulmonary exam: Assess symmetry of pulmonary excursion; percussion (dullness over areas of pleural effusion)
      a) Wheezing or stridor, indicative of bronchial compression
      b) Rales, indicating CHF or pulmonary edema
   3. Cardiovascular exam
      a) Jugular venous distention, indicative of cardiomyopathy
      b) Left parasternal lift in left decubitus position, indicative of cardiomyopathy
      c) Murmurs, indicative of cardiopathy usually pansystolic
      d) S_3 or S_4, indicative of CHF
      e) Evaluate point of maximum intensity (PMI) for displacement associated with left ventricular hypertrophy.
      f) Hepatojugular reflux, indicative of CHF
      g) Peripheral edema

IV. Diagnostic tests
   A. Laboratory: CBC to rule out anemia
   B. Radiology: Chest x-ray to rule out pneumonia, effusion, and infiltrates
   C. Other
      1. Pulmonary function tests to evaluate lung capacity
      2. Echocardiogram and EKG to rule out cardiac etiology
      3. Digital pulse oximetry to evaluate oxygen saturation

V. Differential diagnosis
   A. Anterior mediastinal mass: Most common malignant tumor is thymoma.

    B. Pleural effusion (see Chapter 29)

    C. COPD (see Chapter 28)

    D. Pulmonary edema (see Chapter 32)

    E. Pulmonary hypertension (will precipitate right-sided heart failure)

    F. Cardiomyopathy with biventricular dilatation (see Chapter 39)

    G. Constrictive pericarditis (see Chapter 48)

    H. Pericardial effusion (see Chapter 48).

    I. Radiation-induced heart disease

VI. Treatment

    A. Treat underlying cause (see specific section).

      1. If cancer, chemotherapy or radiation therapy for sensitive tumors

      2. Pleural effusion: Thoracentesis or sclerosing pleurodesis (see Chapter 29)

      3. Pericardial effusion: Pericardiocentesis with sclerosis or pericardial window (see Chapter 48)

      4. Pulmonary edema and CHF: Depends on severity of symptoms and contributing factors; may require admission to an acute-care unit if unmanageable in the ambulatory setting (see Chapter 32)

      5. Left ventricular dysfunction management in ambulatory setting (subacute patients); pharmacologic management with physician collaboration

        a) Limit alcohol (no more than two ounces per day).

        b) Drug therapy should be individualized based on patient's tolerance and degree of symptom relief.

        c) Administer oxygen 2–4 l/minute as needed if pulse oximetry is 88% or lower.

      6. Correction of anemia with erythropoietin or RBC transfusion (see Chapters 111–117)

    B. Advanced cancer in palliative-care setting: Consider empiric measures if underlying mechanism not known or not amenable to other therapies; goal of care is supportive.

      1. Position individual to allow comfortable sleep.

      2. Comfort may be improved with the addition of cool air, such as from a fan.

      3. Administer opioids (e.g., oral hydrocodone) to treat dyspnea and promote comfort; nebulized morphine 2–4 mg in 5 ml normal saline as ordered.

      4. Administer albuterol (metered-dose inhaler or nebulizer) if underlying pulmonary process is suspected.

      5. Administer dexamethasone 4 mg po qid or prednisone 20 mg po qd

      6. Treat anxiety with relaxation methods or drug therapy (e.g., alprazolam 0.25 mg po q eight hours; increase as needed).

VII. Follow-up: Dependent on etiology

VIII. Referrals

    A. Homecare referral, if indicated, to teach caregiver and monitor effectiveness of interventions in patients with homebound status

    B. Physician or pulmonologist for collaboration in management

References

Abrahm, J.L. (1998). Promoting symptom control in palliative care. *Seminars in Oncology Nursing, 14,* 95–109

Cohn, J.N. (1996). The management of chronic heart failure. *New England Journal of Medicine, 335,* 490–498.

Ferguson, G.T., & Cherniack, R.M. (1993). Management of chronic obstructive pulmonary disease. *New England Journal of Medicine, 328,* 1017–1022.

Ripamonti, C., Fulfaro, F., & Bruera, E. (1998). Dyspnoea in patients with advanced cancer: Incidence, causes, and treatments. *Cancer Treatment Reviews, 24,* 69–80.

Thomas, C.R., & Bonomi, P. (1990). Mediastinal tumors. *Current Opinion in Oncology, 2,* 359–367.

Chapter

26. Wheezing
Madonna K. McDermott, RN, MS, ANP, OCN®

I. Definition: Abnormal lung sound described as a whistling sound

II. Pathophysiology: Wheezes are generated by the vibration of the bronchial wall resulting from narrowing of the lumen of a respiratory pathway from inflammation, edema, or obstruction.

III. Clinical features: Wheezing often is considered to be an essential feature of asthma; however, it is important to obtain a careful history to exclude other causes of wheezing. Failure to respond to bronchodilators is less likely to occur with asthma.
   A. Etiologies
      1. Bronchospasm
      2. Airway edema or collapse
      3. Intraluminal obstruction by neoplasm or secretions
      4. Asthma
      5. Croup
      6. Hay fever
      7. Mitral stenosis
      8. Pleural effusion
   B. History
      1. History of cancer and cancer treatment
      2. Current medications: Prescribed and over-the-counter
      3. History of presenting symptom(s): Precipitating factors, onset, and duration
      4. Changes in activities of daily living
      5. Past medical history: Bronchitis, pneumonia, or upper respiratory infections
   C. Signs and symptoms
      1. Asthma
         a) Nocturnal wheezing and/or dyspnea
         b) Wheezing triggered by irritants or allergens
      2. Stridor, or indicating obstruction
      3. Anxiety or restlessness
      4. Hemoptysis

     5. Pleuritic pain

     6. Dyspnea and cough

  D. Physical exam

     1. HEENT exam: Ears, pharynx, sinuses, and teeth to rule out local infection

     2. Lymph node exam for adenopathy, signifying infection

     3. Pulmonary exam

       a) Wheezes generally are more prominent during expiration than inspiration.

         (1) Localized areas of wheezing raises the suspicion of airway obstruction, possibly by tumor or foreign body.

         (2) Wheezing that is loudest in the laryngeal area is more indicative of upper airway obstruction.

       b) Barrel chest is seen more commonly in patients with emphysema than with asthma.

       c) Observe for accessory muscle usage indicating increased work-of-breathing.

     4. Integument exam

       a) Clubbing of the fingers indicative of a fibrotic lung disease (e.g., cystic fibrosis, interstitial lung disease)

       b) Cyanosis of the nail beds, indicating poor oxygenation

IV. Diagnostic tests

  A. Laboratory: ABGs to evaluate hypoxemia indicated by reduced PaO_2 (less than 80 mm Hg) in asthma and COPD

  B. Radiology

     1. Chest x-ray to evaluate obstruction, infiltrates

     2. High-resolution CT if bronchiectasis is suspected

  C. Other

     1. Spirometry before and after the patient uses an inhaled bronchodilator (FEV1: FVC [ratio of one-second forced expiratory volume to forced vital capacity] ratio less than 70% indicates airflow obstruction.)

     2. Allergen testing after diagnosis of asthma is confirmed

     3. Fiberoptic nasolaryngoscope exam if vocal cord dysfunction is suspected

     4. Bronchoscopy if central airway obstruction is suspected

V. Differential diagnosis

  A. Asthma (see Chapter 28)

  B. Vocal cord dysfunction

  C. Bronchiectasis

  D. Upper or central airway obstruction by laryngeal edema, bronchial stenosis, foreign-body aspiration, or tumor

  E. Bronchitis (see Chapter 28)

  F. Lung cancer

  G. Sarcoidosis

  H. Emphysema (seeChapter 28)

  I. Allergic reaction

  J. Drug-induced bronchospasm secondary to etoposide, paclitaxel, and docetaxel

VI. Treatment: Treatment is dependent on determining the underlying disease process and initiating appropriate therapy.
    A. Asthma (see Chapter 28)
    B. Vocal cord dysfunction: Patient education regarding disorder; speech therapy is primary intervention.
    C. Bronchiectasis: Treatment is dependent on cause of bronchiectasis. Causes include immunoglobulin deficiencies, recurrent aspiration, immotile cilia syndrome (Kartagener's syndrome), and postinfection conditions.
    D. Upper or central airway obstruction by laryngeal edema, bronchial stenosis, foreign-body aspiration, or tumor; treatment will be dependent upon etiology.
    E. COPD (see Chapter 28)

VII. Follow-up: Follow-up is determined by the rapidity, severity, and cause of the wheezing.

VIII. Referrals: Determined by etiology to a pulmonologist or allergist

References

Bodner, C.H., Ross, S., Little, J., Douglas, J.G., Legge, J.S., Friend, J.A., & Godden, D.J. (1998). Risk factors for adult onset wheeze: A case control study. *American Journal of Respiratory and Critical Care Medicine, 157*(1), 35–42.

den Otter, J.J., van Dijk, B., van Schayck, C.P., Molema, J., & van Weel, C. (1998). How to avoid underdiagnosed asthma/chronic obstructive pulmonary disease? *Journal of Asthma, 35,* 381–387.

27. Capillary Leak Syndrome

Susan A. Ezzone, MS, RN, CNP

I. Definition: Shift of intravascular fluid and albumin into the extravascular space

II. Pathophysiology
   A. Generalized capillary endothelial cell injury in multiple organs is responsible for the development of capillary leak syndrome (CLS).
   B. Cytokines such as IL-2 (interleukin) receptor-positive cells and CD8-positive lympho-cytes are present and may have a role in triggering CLS.
   C. A shift of fluid and albumin into body tissues occurs.
   D. An associated decreased peripheral vascular resistance, hypotension, and intravascular volume compound the fluid shift.

III. Clinical features
   A. Risk factors
      1. Bone marrow/peripheral stem cell transplant
         a) During preparative regimen
         b) During time of engraftment along with abnormalities in liver and renal function
         c) During rapid steroid tapers
         d) During infection or graft-versus- host disease
         e) During infusion of donor WBCs
         f) During infusion of marrow/blood stem cells
         g) Human leukocyte antigen (HLA)-mismatched bone marrow transplant recipient
         h) Oxygen toxicity
      2. Kidney transplant
      3. Liver transplant
      4. Biotherapy (especially interleukin and tumor necrosis factor)
      5. Chemotherapy
   B. History
      1. History of cancer and cancer treatment
      2. Current medications: Prescribed and over-the-counter
      3. History of presenting symptom(s): Precipitating factors, onset, location, and duration
      4. Changes in activities of daily living

C. Signs and symptoms
   1. Ascites
   2. Weight gain
   3. Edema and/or anasarca (generalized total-body edema)
   4. Chest pain
   5. Shortness of breath
   6. Productive or nonproductive cough
   7. Tachypnea
   8. Decreased urine output
   9. Fever
   10. Lethargy, malaise, or obtundation
   11. Confusion and restlessness
   12. Cyanosis and pallor of skin, lips, and nail beds
D. Physical exam
   1. Vital signs: Weight (signs of gain), blood pressure (hypotension), pulse (tachycardia)
   2. Pulmonary exam: Presence of rales and rhonchi on auscultation; dullness on percussion over consolidated areas
   3. Cardiac exam: Presence of S_3, S_4, murmur, or gallop; tachycardia; peripheral edema
   4. Abdomen exam: Ascites, tenderness, distention, softness or firmness, hepatomegaly, splenomegaly, presence or absence of bowel sounds

IV. Diagnostic tests
   A. Laboratory
      1. CBC with differential
         a) Elevated WBC count may increase suspicion of infection.
         b) Hemoconcentration may occur with an increased WBC count and hematocrit.
      2. Urinalysis
         a) Presence of leukocytes may be caused by infection.
         b) Presence of protein or casts may indicate renal failure or disease.
      3. Liver function tests, including total and direct bilirubin, to rule out hepatobiliary disease
      4. Renal function tests, including urea and creatinine, to evaluate renal function
      5. Serum albumin: May be decreased, leading to decreased oncotic pressure and edema
   B. Radiology: Chest radiograph to rule out noncardiogenic pulmonary edema, pleural effusion, pulmonary venous hypertension, interstitial infiltrates
   C. Other
      1. Bronchoscopy, with or without lung biopsy, can rule out infection, hemorrhage, or other causes of respiratory distress.
      2. ABGs may show hypoxia and CO_2 retention.
      3. Pulmonary function tests reveal decreased pulmonary compliance.
      4. Hemodynamic monitoring including pulmonary capillary wedge pressure (PCWP) and cardiac output (CO) to measure fluid status (normal PCWP = 6–12 mm Hg; normal CO = 4–8 l/minute)
         a) Decreased PCWP may indicate hypovolemia.
         b) Increased PCWP may indicate left ventricular failure or cardiac insufficiency.

      c) Cardiac output may be increased early in CLS, then decreased later in the syndrome.

V. Differential diagnosis
    A. Paraproteinemias or diseases/conditions with low protein levels
    B. Lymphoma
    C. Psoriasis
    D. Drug-induced, such as IV cyclosporine or amphotericin-B
    E. Viral syndrome, such as cytomegalovirus
    F. Pneumonitis
    G. Sepsis (see Chapter 140)
    H. Disseminated intravascular coagulation (see Chapter 119)

VI. Treatment: Supportive care until CLS resolves
    A. Administer glucocorticoids at high doses, then taper quickly as tolerated.
       1. Doses may be 0.5–2 mg/kg per day of IV methylprednisolone.
       2. Tapering schedules may depend on the duration of treatment.
       3. The dose may be decreased by 25% every three to four days.
    B. Provide IV fluid replacement.
       1. Infusion of colloids rather than crystalloids, such as blood or albumin
       2. Infusion of albumin
    C. Administration of diuretics is controversial because intravascular hypovolemia is present and acute renal failure may develop.
    D. Restrict oral fluids to 500–1,000 ml per day. Gradually increase fluids as condition improves.
    E. Hemodialysis may be necessary if acute renal failure occurs.
    F. Mechanical ventilation may be indicated if respiratory distress or failure occurs.
    G. Prophylactic antibiotics may promote growth of organisms and are not recommended.
    H. Administer vasopressors as needed for management of hypotension.
       1. Dopamine may be initiated at 5 mcg/kg/minute and titrated to a maximum of 20 mcg/kg/minute. Dosage range is 3–20 mcg/kg/minute.
       2. Dobutamine may be initiated at 5 mcg/kg/minute and titrated to a maximum of 20 mcg/kg/minute. It may be effective in increasing cardiac output. Dosage range is 2.5–20 mcg/kg/minute.
       3. Norepinephrine may be initiated at 5 mcg/kg/minute and titrated to desired effect. Dosage range is 8–30 mcg/minute.
    I. Provide nutritional support, such as enteral feedings or total parenteral nutrition, to maintain high caloric intake because of increased energy expenditure.

VII. Follow-up
    A. Inpatient hospitalization is necessary to manage the signs, symptoms, and complications of CLS.
    B. Perform daily monitoring of intake, output, weight, and renal and liver function.
    C. Perform frequent chest radiographs to monitor pulmonary edema.

VIII. Referrals
    A. Nephrology to evaluate acute renal failure and recommend management
    B. Pulmonologist consult to evaluate lung function, perform bronchoscopy, and recommend management

References

Amoura, Z., Papo, T., Ninet, J., Hatron, P.Y., Guillaumie, J., Piette, A.M., Bletry, O., Dequiedt, P., Talasczka, A., Rondeau, E., Dutel, J.L., Wechsler, B., & Piette, J.C. (1997). Systemic capillary leak syndrome: Report on 13 patients with special focus on course and treatment. *American Journal of Medicine, 103,* 514–519.

Bertorini, T.E., Gelfand, M.S., & O'Brien, T.F. (1997). Encephalopathy due to capillary leak syndrome. *Southern Medical Journal, 90,* 1060–1062.

Cahill, R.A., Spitzer, T.R., & Mazumder, A. (1996). Marrow engraftment and clinical manifestations of capillary leak syndrome. *Bone Marrow Transplantation, 18,* 177–184.

Cicardi, M., Berti, E., Caputo, V., Radice, F., Gardinali, M., & Agostoni, A. (1997). Idiopathic capillary leak syndrome: Evidence of CD8-positive lymphocytes surrounding damaged endothelial cells. *Journal of Allergy and Clinical Immunology, 99,* 417–419.

Hussein, M.M., Mooij, J.M.V., & El Tayeb, A.M. (1996). Pulmonary capillary leak syndrome associated with the use of intravenous cyclosporin. *Nephrology, Dialysis, Transplantation, 11,* 2342–2343.

Nurnberger, W., Willers, R., Burdach, S., & Gobel, U. (1997). Risk factors for capillary leakage syndrome after bone marrow transplantation. *Annals of Hematology, 74,* 221–224.

Roberts, S.L. (1990). High-permeability pulmonary edema: Nursing assessment, diagnosis, and interventions. *Heart and Lung, 19,* 287–298.

Schmidt, S., Hertfelder, H.J., Von Spiegel, T., Hering, R., Harzheim, M., Lassman, H., Deckert-Schulter, M., & Schlegel, U. (1999). Lethal capillary leak syndrome after a single administration of interferon beta-1b. *Neurology, 53,* 220–222.

White, B.S., & Roberts, S.L. (1990). High permeability pulmonary edema: Pathophysiology and mechanisms of injury. *Intensive Care Nursing, 6*(2),79–91.

28. Chronic Obstructive Pulmonary Disease

Sandra C. Henke, RN, MS, ANP, OCN®

I. Definition: Includes emphysema, chronic bronchitis, and asthma
   A. This diverse set of conditions shares the pathological common denominator of slowing of the expiratory flow rate and airway obstruction.
   B. The classic difference is that asthma is a reversible condition, while emphysema and chronic bronchitis are not.

II. Pathophysiology
   A. Emphysema is associated with a defect in the pulmonary elastic tissue, leading to destruction of alveolar as well as capillary beds within the alveolar wall.
      1. The loss of elastic tissue allows noncartilaginous airways to collapse during expiration.
      2. Inspiratory flow rates remain normal because airway caliber is not affected.
   B. Chronic bronchitis is inflammation of cells lining the bronchial wall produced by environmental triggers, resulting in edema, excessive mucus production, and loss of ciliary transport.
   C. Asthma likely is a genetically acquired disease precipitated by such factors as exercise, allergens, viral respiratory infections, and pollutants.
      1. Following an exposure, mediator-containing cells, such as mast cells, basophils, and macrophages, can be activated to release a variety of inflammatory compounds.
      2. These inflammatory compounds have a direct effect on the airway smooth muscle and capillary permeability.
      3. These stimuli then evoke increased airway responsiveness of the tracheobronchial tree, leading to narrowing of the airway passages.
   D. Chronic obstructive pulmonary disease (COPD) causes a reduced elastic recoil of the lung and results in increased intrathoracic pressure.
      1. Increased intrathoracic pressure during expiration results in the collapse and premature closure of the airways.
         a) Gas trapping and poor alveolar gas exchange during expiration result.
         b) A large residual volume at the end of expiration occurs because of early closure of airways (air trapping) and overdistended air spaces.
      2. The surface area for gas-exchange of the alveolar-capillary membrane is reduced as a result of disruption and destruction of alveolar walls.

3. Pulmonary diffusion is reduced because of a loss of alveolar surface area and pulmonary vasoconstriction, resulting in hypoxemia.

   a) Hypoxemia and pressure from adjacent distended alveoli decrease perfusion to normal alveoli, further reducing the capillary blood volume and the diffusing capacity.

   b) This is responsible for uneven mismatching of ventilation with blood flow and for the increased physiologic dead space and abnormal blood gas values common in emphysema.

4. The airflow obstruction generally is progressive, may be accompanied by airway hyperreactivity, and may be partially reversible.

III. Clinical features: Dyspnea is the hallmark symptom that brings the patient to medical attention. These diseases must be diagnosed and treated separately. Many patients present with features of all of these conditions (see Figure 28-1).

A. Risk factors

1. Cigarette smoking is well-established as the major risk factor for COPD; repeated irritation to the lung by tobacco smoke is the mechanism of lung tissue destruction.

2. Other environmental risk factors include air pollution, occupational exposures, infections, and familial and genetic factors.

3. A genetic deficiency of the enzyme 1-antitrypsin is associated with emphysema.

   a) Alveolar tissue normally contains both proteases and antiproteases.

   b) Neutrophil-derived elastase is the most essential protease.

   c) Alpha-antitrypsin is the most essential antiprotease.

      (1) Alveolar wall destruction is thought to result with decreased antitrypsin activity or increased elastase levels.

      (2) This particular genetic defect affects only 1%–2% of patients and is not associated with the more common pulmonary emphysema.

B. History: A careful history of the insidious onset of breathlessness on exertion, with or without a history of cough, sputum, or frequent lung infections, often provides direction to this diagnosis.

Figure 28-1. Clinical Features of Chronic Obstructive Pulmonary Disease

Emphysema
- Exertional dyspnea
- Pursed-lip breathing
- Barrel chest
- Digital clubbing
- History of tobacco use
- Possibly secondary to polycythemia

Chronic bronchitis
- Chronic cough with sputum production (for at least three months for two successive years)
- Post-tussive syncope
- Hemoptysis
- Frequent respiratory infections
- History of cigarette smoking common
- Severe obstruction, although not consistent

Asthma
- Chest tightness
- Wheezing
- Dyspnea
- Possible presence of allergy
- Possible exercise component
- Widespread airway obstruction
- Airway hyper-responsiveness
- Reversibility or partial reversibility
- Airway inflammation

1. History of cancer and cancer treatment
2. Current medications: Prescribed and over-the-counter
3. History of presenting symptom(s): Precipitating factors, onset, location, and duration. Associated symptoms are shortness of breath, cough (productive and nonproductive), and headache.
4. Changes in activities of daily living
5. Social history: Occupational history or chemical irritant exposure; a "pack year" history noting the number of packs of cigarettes smoked per day multiplied by the number of years the individual has smoked (e.g., two packs per day for 30 years is a "60-pack year" history.)
6. Past medical history: History of frequent upper respiratory infections, colds, or flu

C. Signs and symptoms
   1. Dyspnea with or without activity
      a) Dyspnea with physical activities that previously were accomplished without difficulty is identified.
      b) Dyspnea gradually increases with intensity of activity, but the rate of progression of dyspnea is variable.
   2. Cough
   3. Sputum described as thick, tenacious, or mucoid
   4. Difficulty clearing secretions
   5. Increased somnolence
   6. Headache resulting from chronic hypercapnia
   7. Cognitive and personality changes associated with hypoxemia
   8. Wheezing: Associated with asthma but can occur with chronic bronchitis

D. Physical exam
   1. Pulmonary exam
      a) Prolonged expiration/assessment of maximum expiratory flow
         (1) The patient exhales with maximal effort through an open mouth after a full inspiration.
         (2) The examiner listens with the bell of the stethoscope over the trachea in the suprasternal notch and records the time in seconds until airflow ceases.
         (3) Normal time to completely exhale is within four seconds.
         (4) A forced expiratory time greater than six seconds signifies significant expiratory obstruction.
      b) Hyperresonance to percussion (occurs as a result of hyperinflation)
      c) End expiratory wheeze and pursed-lip breathing pattern
      d) Diminished/distant breath sounds in advanced disease (caused by reduced flow and increased lung inflation)
      e) Increased anteroposterior diameter of the thorax resulting from hyperinflation of the lungs; dorsal kyphosis, prominent anterior chest, elevated ribs, and widening of costal angle, giving the chest the appearance of a barrel
      f) Increased use of accessory breathing muscles (neck and intercostals); the flattened diaphragm contributes less to inspiration, placing more burden on the accessory breathing muscles.

IV. Diagnostic tests
    A. Laboratory
        1. CBC to assess for polycythemia rubra vera
        2. Arterial blood gas analysis
            a) Typically normal early in the disease; indicated whenever a clinically important acid-base disturbance, hypoxemia, or hypercapnia is suspected
                (1) Hypoxemia (reduced arterial PO_2) is the most common abnormality.
                    (a) Normal PO_2 levels range from 70–100 mm Hg.
                    (b) PO_2 level below 70 indicates hypoxemia.
                    (c) Normal PO_2 level falls with increasing altitude.
                (2) Hypercapnia (elevated PCO_2): PCO_2 may become chronically elevated and/or may show an acute rise during an infection or other medical complications.
                    (a) Normal PCO_2 level ranges from 35–45 mm Hg.
                    (b) PCO_2 level above 45 indicates hypercapnia.
    B. Radiology: Chest radiograph
        1. Early in the disease, the chest film may be normal.
        2. With advanced COPD, the chest radiograph may reveal a low, flat diaphragm and an increase in the retrosternal space. Hyperinflation is apparent.
        3. Parenchymal bullae or subpleural blebs may be present, indicating lung tissue destruction.
    C. Other: Pulmonary function tests
        1. Objective measurement of the ability of the respiratory system to perform gas exchange by assessing its ventilation, diffusion, and mechanical properties
        2. Indications
            a) Evaluation of type and degree of pulmonary dysfunction
            b) Evaluation of symptoms of dyspnea and cough
            c) Detection of lung dysfunction
            d) Follow-up response to therapy
        3. Spirometry and measurement of lung volumes allow determination of the presence and severity of obstructive and restrictive pulmonary dysfunction.
            a) Obstructive dysfunction is identified as reduction in airflow rates.
            b) Restrictive pulmonary dysfunction is characterized by reduction in lung volumes.
            c) Forced expiratory volume in one second (FEV_1), the volume of gas expelled in the first second after maximal inspiration, is reduced in obstructive airway disease. FEV_1 is the measurement for disease severity and correlates with survival and degree of obstruction. Severe asthma may present during a respiratory crisis with decreased FEV_1. Use of bronchodilators results in prompt improvement.
            d) Forced vital capacity (FVC) is the volume of gas that can be forcefully expelled from the lungs after maximal inspiration
            e) Diffusing capacity of the lung (DLCO) is the measurement of the single-breath diffusing capacity for carbon monoxide, which reflects the ability of the lung to transfer gas across the alveolar/capillary interface.
                (1) Decreased values may help to confirm the diagnosis of airflow obstruction suspected from spirometry.

      (2) Emphysema causes a greater increase in total lung capacity than other obstructive diseases as well as reduced DLCO. However, DLCO is neither specific nor sensitive for emphysema.

V. Differential diagnosis
- A. Cancer treatment-related
  1. Interstitial infiltrative disease secondary to chemotherapeutic agents, which most often results in a diffuse interstitial fibrosis with a restrictive element
     - a) Bleomycin
     - b) Methotrexate
     - c) Busulfan
     - d) Carmustine
     - e) Mitomycin
  2. Surgical resection
     - a) Pneumonectomy
     - b) Lobectomy
  3. Radiation-induced pulmonary fibrosis
- B. Acute bronchitis
- C. Bronchiectasis

VI. Treatment
- A. Prevention of further damage
  1. Smoking cessation: Nicotine replacement therapy, preferably with bupropion
  2. Pneumovax injection every five years to prevent pneumococcal infections
  3. Annual administration of *Haemophilus influenzae* vaccine
- B. Bronchodilator therapy
  1. Ipratropium bromide (Atrovent®, Boehringer Ingelheim Pharmaceuticals Corp., Ridgefield, CT)
     - a) Slow onset but long duration of action
     - b) Metered-dose inhaler with spacer, three to six puffs four times per day
     - c) May be administered with saline as nebulized aerosol treatment for sputum expectoration
  2. Beta-adrenergic agonists: Provide faster action but for shorter duration; two to six puffs every three to six hours as needed
     - a) Metaproterenol (Alupent®, Boehringer Ingelheim Pharmaceuticals Corp.)
     - b) Albuterol (Ventolin®, Glaxo Wellcome Inc., Research Triangle Park, NC; Proventil®, Schering Corp., Kenilworth, NJ)
  3. Combination B agonist with ipratropium bromide (Combivent®, Boehringer Ingelheim Pharmaceuticals Corp.)
     - a) Faster action and long duration
     - b) Dosage: Two to four puffs every 12 hours
     - c) Side effects
       - (1) Tachycardia and skeletal tremor most common
       - (2) Should be discontinued if patient experiences these side effects
  4. Theophylline
     - a) Narrow therapeutic window with significant toxic effects

> *b)* Long-acting: 200–400 mg po at bedtime
> *c)* Maintain serum level at 8–12 mcg/ml.

C. Corticosteroid therapy
   1. Systemic corticosteroids
      a) These drugs are prescribed for patients with asthma and those with frequent exacerbation of symptoms.
      b) Prednisone: Administer 40 mg a day orally for 14 days, then taper.
      c) Discontinue after two to four weeks if no objective (spirometric) improvement is observed.
      d) Long-term therapy dose should be kept as low as possible to minimize side effects of muscle atrophy and depressed immune system function.
   2. Inhaled corticosteroids
      a) Patients are candidates for long-term inhaled corticosteroids if oral corticosteroids are found to be effective.
      b) The inhaled corticosteroids initially should be given in high doses (800 mcg beclomethasone per day) and then tapered as symptoms permit.
      c) Inhaled corticosteroids may permit discontinuance of systemic therapy.
      d) Inhaled application of steroids eliminates systemic side effects.

D. Pulmonary rehabilitation and oxygen therapy
   1. Education is aimed at assisting patients to understand the process of the disease, to modify risk factors, and to use medications properly.
   2. General exercise conditioning: Graded aerobic physical exercise programs (e.g., walking three times a week for 20 minutes) are helpful to prevent deterioration of physical condition.
   3. Breathing retraining
      a) Pursed-lip breathing to slow the rate of breathing
      b) Abdominal breathing exercises to relieve fatigue of accessory muscles of respiration
   4. Home oxygen therapy
      a) Prescribed for patients with COPD who have significant hypoxemia
      b) May be prescribed for continuous use, with exercise, or only at night
      c) Benefits include longer survival, reduced hospitalization, and improved quality of life
      d) A flow rate of 1–3 l/minute achieves a PO_2 of greater than 55 mm Hg.

E. Hospitalization
   1. Hospitalization is indicated for acute worsening of COPD that fails to respond to outpatient management.
   2. Pneumonia, pulmonary hypertension, cor pulmonale, and chronic respiratory failure characterize the end stage of COPD.
   3. Death usually occurs during an exacerbation of illness in association with acute respiratory failure.

VII. Follow-up
   A. Symptoms should improve with effective therapy, and patient should be seen frequently.
   B. Therapy may become ineffective over time and will need to be adjusted.
   C. Theophylline levels should be checked periodically.

VIII. Referrals
    A. Pulmonologist for diagnosis and initiation of therapy
    B. Hospitalization for acute exacerbations

References

Ferguson, G.T. (1998). Management of COPD. Early identification and active intervention are crucial. *Postgraduate Medicine, 103,* 129–134, 136–141.

George, R.B. (1999). Course and prognosis of chronic obstructive pulmonary disease. *American Journal of Medical Sciences, 318,* 103–106.

Magnussen, H., Richter, K., & Taube, C. (1998). Are chronic obstructive pulmonary disease and asthma different diseases? *Clinical and Experimental Allergy, 28,* 187–194.

Martinez, F.J. (1998). Diagnosing chronic obstructive pulmonary disease. The importance of differentiating asthma, emphysema, and chronic bronchitis. *Postgraduate Medicine, 103,* 112–117, 121–122, 125.

O'Byrne, P.M. (1999). The many faces of airway inflammation. Asthma and chronic obstructive pulmonary disease. *American Journal of Respiratory and Critical Care Medicine, 59*(5), 41–63.

Rennard, S.I. (1998). COPD: Overview of definitions, epidemiology, and factors influencing its development. *Chest, 113*(Suppl. 4), 235S–241S.

29. Pleural Effusion

Sandra C. Henke, RN, MS, ANP, OCN®

I. Definition: Accumulation of an abnormal quantity of fluid in the pleural cavity

II. Physiology/Pathophysiology
   A. Normal
      1. A small amount of fluid normally is present in the pleural space between the visceral and the parietal pleurae, serving as a lubricant for the pleural surfaces.
      2. Fluid passes continuously through this space and is exchanged at a rate of about 5–10 l/day.
   B. Pathophysiology
      1. Cancer cells may implant on the pleural surface and cause leakage into the pleural space. Cancer cells may obstruct the pleural or lymphatic channels and prevent reabsorption of fluid.
      2. Pleural effusion occurs when the usual balance between pleural fluid formation and resorption is disturbed because of increased secretion or impaired resorption.
         a) Fluid that accumulates in the pleural space restricts the lung's ability to expand, thereby altering air exchange and resulting in abnormal gas exchange and hypoxia.
         b) Pulmonary veins may become obstructed, causing an increase in capillary hydrostatic pressure in the visceral pleura.
         c) Increased osmotic pressure can reduce the ability of the visceral pleural capillaries to reabsorb fluid because of necrosis of the pleural space.

III. Clinical features: Effusions may be unilateral or bilateral.
   A. Risk factors
      1. CHF
      2. Pulmonary infection
      3. Neoplasm, particularly primary lung cancer or breast cancer
      4. Trauma or recent surgery
   B. Classifications
      1. Transudate production: Causes
         a) Disturbance of the balance between transcapillary pressure and plasma oncotic pressure

         b) Increased capillary pressure in heart failure and reduced plasma oncotic pressure in certain kidney or liver diseases

    2. Exudate: Increased fluid formation caused by increased capillary permeability

C. Etiology
1. Nonmalignancy-related
   a) CHF
   b) Hypoalbuminemia
   c) Atelectasis
   d) Inflammation
2. Paramalignant effusions; directly or indirectly caused by a tumor but not associated with pleural metastases
   a) Lymphatic obstruction as in mediastinal lymph node metastases
   b) Pneumonia or atelectasis related pleural effusion resulting from an obstructive bronchial tumor
   c) Chylothorax caused by invasion or obstruction of the thoracic duct
   d) Effusion resulting from chemotherapy or radiation treatment
3. Malignant effusions: Develop as a result of pleural metastases
   a) Breast cancer
   b) Lung cancer
   c) Lymphoma

D. History
1. History of cancer and cancer treatment
2. Current medications: Prescribed and over-the-counter
3. History of presenting symptom(s): Precipitating factors, onset, location, and duration
4. Changes in activities of daily living

E. Signs and symptoms: Degree of severity is related to the rapidity with which the fluid develops and accumulates.
1. May be absent or overshadowed by the underlying disease process
2. Dyspnea, gradually increasing over time
3. Pleuritic chest pain; occurs with parietal pleural inflammation
4. Cough; usually dry and nonproductive

F. Physical exam
1. Neck exam: Contralateral tracheal deviation with massive effusions
   a) Dullness to percussion at base and extending to the level of fluid accumulation
   b) Increased vocal fremitus over fluid collection
   c) Respiratory quality
      (1) Tachypnea
      (2) Labored breathing, use of accessory muscles
   d) Absent breath sounds over the fluid
   e) Restricted chest wall expansion
2. Pulmonary exam
3. Cardiovascular
   a) Jugular vein distention
   b) Poor capillary refill

IV. Diagnostic tests

  A. Laboratory: Pleural fluid analysis/thoracentesis: Determines etiology of the effusion

    1. Observation of fluid

      a) Pale yellow (straw) color indicates transudates.

      b) Red (bloody) color suggests malignancy/chest trauma/surgery.

      c) White color indicates chylothorax or lipid or fatty effusion.

      d) Brown color indicates longstanding bloody effusion.

      e) Purulent fluid indicates presence of empyema.

      f) Viscous fluid is suggestive of mesothelioma.

    2. Odor: Foul smell is consistent with empyema.

    3. pH

      a) Collect pleural fluid in a heparinized syringe.

      b) Exudate pleural pH ranges from 7.30–7.45.

      c) Transudate pleural pH ranges from 7.40–7.55.

    4. Serum and pleural fluid protein and lactate dehydrogenase (LDH) levels

      a) Elevation or presence of any one of these criteria indicates exudate.

      b) If absent, the fluid is typically a transudate.

        (1) Ratio of pleural fluid protein to serum protein 0.5

        (2) Ratio of pleural fluid LDH to serum LDH more than 0.6

        (3) Pleural fluid LDH more than two-thirds the upper limits of normal of the serum LDH

    5. Glucose

      a) Pleural fluid for glucose should be placed immediately in a tube containing sodium fluoride to stop glycolysis.

      b) Normal range is similar to that of serum glucose (60–100 mg/dl).

        (1) All transudates and most exudates have pleural fluid glucose concentrations similar to that of blood glucose.

        (2) The mechanism responsible for a low pleural fluid glucose level depends on the underlying disease.

        (3) Transport of glucose from blood to pleural fluid is decreased as in malignancy.

        (4) Use of glucose by constituents of pleural fluid, namely neutrophils, bacteria, and malignant cells, is increased.

        (5) When glucose is low, as in malignancy, range is 30–50 mg/dl.

    6. Cell count and differential

      a) Normal RBC count up to 100,000/mm

      b) Pleural WBC count diagnostic when greater than 10,000/mm

      c) Predominate neutrophils significant for acute inflammation

      d) Low cell count indicates transudate.

      e) High cell count indicates exudate.

      f) Greater than 50% lymphocytes consistent with malignancy or tuberculosis

    7. Specific gravity

      a) Low indicates transudate.

      b) High indicates exudate.

    8. Amylase

           a) Pleural fluid with elevated amylase (greater than the upper limits of normal for serum amylase) narrows the differential diagnosis of the exudative effusion.

           b) 10%–14% of patients with malignant pleural effusions have increased pleural fluid amylase.

           c) Adenocarcinoma of the lung is the most common malignancy causing increased amylase in pleural fluid, followed by adenocarcinoma of the ovary.

      9. Culture and sensitivity diagnose infectious etiology.

    10. Cytology: In more than 50% of pleural effusions caused by malignancy, cytology will be positive.

  B. Radiology: Chest radiograph reveals the following.

    1. Blunting at costophrenic angle, unilateral or bilateral

    2. Homogenous density in the dependent part of the hemithorax

    3. Density spreading upward and merging with the rest of the lung field in a meniscus shape over the lung base

    4. In massive pleural effusion, the entire hemithorax may be obscured by the fluid.

    5. In tension hydrothorax, the mediastinum is pushed to the opposite side.

    6. Decubitus chest views differentiate between free-flowing fluid and loculated fluid.

  C. Pleural biopsy

    1. Used only when diagnosis is urgently needed

    2. Used for diagnosis for tuberculous pleurisy and malignancy

V. Differential diagnosis

  A. Transudate

    1. CHF (see Chapter 40)

    2. Cirrhosis of the liver (rare without clinical ascites) (see Chapter 64)

    3. Kidney disease

    4. Constrictive pericarditis (see Chapter 48)

  B. Exudate

    1. Infections (bacterial, fungal, viral)

    2. Neoplasms (primary bronchogenic and metastatic breast cancer most commonly identified)

    3. Pulmonary embolism (see Chapter 33)

    4. Trauma and recent upper abdominal surgery

    5. Systemic connective tissue diseases (lupus erythematosus, rheumatoid arthritis) (see Chapter 108)

    6. Intra-abdominal diseases (subdiaphragmatic abscess, pancreatitis)

    7. Idiopathic

  C. Empyema

  D. Lupus pleuritis

  E. Esophageal rupture: High amylase, pleural fluid acidosis

  F. Chylothorax: Triglycerides (> 110 mg/dl)

  G. Hemothorax: Hematocrit (pleural fluid/blood ratio > 0.5)

  H. Peritoneal dialysis: Protein (< 1 g/dl), glucose (300–400 mg/dl)

  I. Intravascular migration of a central venous catheter

VI. Treatment
  A. Thoracentesis
    1. Symptom relief (dyspnea and pleuritic chest pain) will be achieved when pleural effusion is large enough to cause symptoms.
      a) Removal of part or all of the fluid will provide temporary relief and palliation while awaiting diagnosis to identify a more specific treatment.
      b) Obtain fluid for examination (see Diagnostic Tests, p. 163).
  B. Pleurodesis (sclerosing): Purpose of pleurodesis is to remove the pleural fluid and cause a chemical adhesion of the pleural surfaces, thereby preventing fluid from accumulating in the pleural space.
    1. May not be effectively treated with thoracentesis, such as in malignant pleural effusion
    2. Indicated when underlying disease causes effusion to reaccumulate rapidly following successful thoracentesis and effective disease treatment is not possible, as with progressive cancer
    3. Chest tube insertion with talc, tetracycline, or bleomycin for pleurodesis
      a) Obtain surgical consult for insertion and management of chest tube.
      b) Patient will be hospitalized for five to seven days for completion of procedure.
    4. Thoracoscopy with talc for pleurodesis
      a) Surgical consult for procedure
      b) Patient is placed under general anesthesia for procedure.
      c) Patient will be hospitalized for two to four days.
    5. Pleurex catheter
      a) Obtain surgical consult for placement of a permanent or semipermanent tube into pleural space for intermittent drainage of recurrent fluid.
      b) Procedure may be performed in ambulatory care center as outpatient.
      c) Instruct patient or care provider on fluid drainage procedures and insertion site care to be performed at home.
      d) By removing the fluid routinely, adhesion of the pleural surfaces also is achieved.
      e) When fluid decreases and is no longer being removed, the catheter may be removed in ambulatory care center.

VII. Follow-up: Short-term
  A. Thoracentesis
    1. Chest radiograph to evaluate for pneumothorax
    2. Results of pleural fluid analysis
    3. Referral for management of underlying diagnosis
  B. Recurrent pleural effusion: Referral for definitive management/pleurodesis

VIII. Referrals
  A. Specific to etiology of pleural effusion
    1. Internist for initial management of medical diagnosis
    2. Oncologist for positive cytology
  B. Surgery specialist (oncology or thoracic surgery)
    1. Pleural biopsy if etiology not determined by pleural fluid analysis
    2. Thoracentesis

References

Marchi, E., & Broaddus, V.C. (1997). Mechanisms of pleural liquid formation in pleural inflammation. *Current Opinion in Pulmonary Medicine, 3,* 305–309.

Robinson, R.D., Fullerton, D.A., Albert, J.D., Sorensen, J., & Johnston, M.R. (1994). Use of pleural Tenckhoff catheter to palliate malignant pleural effusion. *Annals of Thoracic Surgery, 57,* 286–288.

Rodriguez-Panadero, F. (1997). Current trends in pleurodesis. *Current Opinion in Pulmonary Medicine, 3,* 319–325.

Samuel, J.R. (1997). Management of recurrent spontaneous pneumothorax and recurrent symptomatic pleural effusion with chest tube pleurodesis. *Critical Care Nurse, 17*(1), 28–32.

Yim, A.P., Chung, S.S., Lee, T.W., Lam, C.K., & Ho, J.K. (1996). Thoracoscopic management of malignant pleural effusions. *Chest, 109,* 1234–1238.

Chapter

30. Pneumonia
Mary P. Pazdur, RN, MSN, AOCN®

I. Definition: Acute inflammation of the distal airways (alveoli)

II. Physiology/Pathophysiology
   A. Normal: Natural host defenses in the lung include phagocytosis of microorganisms, mucociliary action, and cough.
   B. Pathophysiology: Pneumonia occurs when an organism inoculates into the lungs and the host exhibits an inadequate response to rid the lungs of the organism

III. Clinical features
   A. Risk factors
      1. Elderly with decreased elasticity of lungs
      2. History of cigarette abuse causing decreased air exchange
      3. Chronic alcohol abuse (risk of aspiration)
      4. Chronic illnesses: Cardiac disease, diabetes mellitus, renal insufficiency, COPD
      5. Cancer-related causes (see Table 30-1)
         a) Obstruction of airway by tumor
         b) Myelosuppression related to cancer treatments or other immunosuppressive drugs
         c) Impaired gag reflex related to head and neck surgery or cranial nerve paresis
      6. Debilitation causing risk for aspiration or atelectasis
      7. Narcotic analgesia with suppression of cough reflex
      8. Mechanical ventilation
      9. AIDS
   B. Etiologies: Causative organisms: Bacteria, virus, fungus, or protozoa
      1. Community-acquired pneumonia (immunocompetent patient)
         a) Streptococcus pneumoniae
         b) Haemophilus influenzae
         c) Staphylococcus aureus
      2. Non-neutropenic pneumonia in critically ill patients
         a) Streptococcus pneumoniae
         b) Legionella
         c) Aerobic gram-negative bacilli

Table 30-1. Host Defects Predisposing to Specific Types of Pneumonia in Patients With Cancer

Host Defect	Underlying Disease Predisposing Factors	Microorganisms

Neutropenia	Acute leukemia
	Aplastic anemia
	Chemotherapy
	Radiation
		• Gram-negative bacilli
		  - *Escherichia coli*
		  - *Klebsiella pneumoniae*
		  - *Pseudomonas aeruginosa*, other sp.
		  - *Stenotrophomonas maltophilia*
		  - *Serratia marcescens*
		• Gram-positive cocci
		  - *Staphylococcus aureus*
		  - Coagulase-negative *Staphylococcus*
		  - Alpha-hemolytic *Streptococcus*
		• Fungi
		  - Yeast
		  - Candida
		  - Torulopsis
		  - Trichosporon
		  - Filariae
		  - Aspergillus
		  - Fusarium
		  - Agents of mucormycoses

Humoral immune dysfunction	Multiple myeloma	• *Pneumococcus, Haemophilus*
Splenectomy	CLL	• *Pneumococcus, Haemophilus*

Cellular immune dysfunction	Leukemia (ALL)
	Lymphoma (Hodgkin's)
	Organ transplant
	Corticosteroids
	Cyclosporine
	Fludarabine
		• Bacteria
		  - Legionella
		  - Nocardia
		  - Mycobacterium
		• Fungi
		  - *Cryptococcus neoformans*
		  - *Histoplasma capsulatum*
		  - *Coccidioides immitis*
		• Herpes viruses
		  - CMV, VZV, HSV, HHV-6
		• Parasites
		  - *Pneumocystis carinii*
		  - *Toxoplasma gondii*
		• Helminth
		  - *Strongyloides stercoralis*

Damage to anatomical barriers		
Mucositis, loss of ciliary function	Chemotherapy	• Organisms colonizing near the site of damage or obstruction
Loss of gag reflex	Head and neck tumors Analgesics	

(Continued on next page)

Table 30-1. Host Defects Predisposing to Specific Types of Pneumonia in Patients With Cancer *(Continued)*

Host Defect	Underlying Disease Predisposing Factors	Microorganisms
Local obstruction	Lung tumors	
	Lymphadenopathy	
Catheters	Endotracheal, nasogastric	
	Intravascular	• *Staphylococcus,* Candida, gram-negative bacilli
Defects being defined	Organ transplant	• Community respiratory viruses
	Leukemia	- Influenza, RSV - Parainfluenza, adenovirus

Note. From "Pneumonia in Cancer Patients" by E. Whimbey, J. Goodrich, and G. Bodey in J. Klastersly (Ed.), *Infectious Complications of Cancer*, 1995, p. 185. Boston: Kluwer Academic Publishers. Copyright 1995 by Kluwer Academic Publishers. Reprinted with permission.

    3. Neutropenic patients
      a) Gram-negative bacilli: *Pseudomonas aeruginosa, Escherichia coli, Klebsiella pneumoniae, Stenotrophomonas maltophilia, Serratia marcescens*
      b) Gram-positive cocci: *Staphylococcus aureus,* coag-negative staphylococcus, alpha-hemolytic streptococcus
      c) Miscellaneous: Yeast, fungi, aspergillus
    4. Severe and prolonged deficient cell-mediated immunity
      a) *Pneumocystis carinii*: Features characteristic cysts in sputum
      b) Bacteria: Legionella, nocardia, and mycobacterium
      c) Fungi: *Cryptococcus neoformans, Histoplasma capsulatum, Coccidioides immitis*
    5. Viral infection
      a) RNA viruses: Influenza A and B, parainfluenza respiratory syncytial viruses (RSV) in late fall, winter, and early spring
      b) Cytomegalovirus: Can occur between day 30 and day 100 after bone marrow transplant
  C. History
    1. History of cancer and cancer treatment
    2. Current medications: Prescribed and over-the-counter
    3. History of presenting symptom(s): Precipitating factors, onset, location, and duration
    4. Changes in activities of daily living
    5. Social history of smoking
    6. Past medical history: GERD, cardiac disease, diabetes mellitus, and renal insufficiency
  D. Signs and symptoms
    1. Fever is the predominant sign, but in patients receiving steroids or with chemotherapy-induced neutropenia, it may be absent. Shaking chills may accompany fever.
      a) High temperature with acute onset usually indicative of bacterial infection
      b) Low-grade temperature with gradual onset usually indicative of viral infection

    2. Dyspnea

    3. Cough: Productive of green or yellow sputum

    4. Tachypnea

    5. Tachycardia

    6. Pleuritic chest pain

    7. In elderly patients, subtle signs may be the only manifestations, including lethargy, fatigue, nausea, or change in mental status.

E. Physical exam

    1. Vital signs may show fever, tachypnea, and tachycardia.

    2. Pulmonary exam

       a) Chest expansion may be reduced on the affected side; if severe, respiratory compromise may reveal signs of cyanosis, intercostal muscle retractions, accessory muscle use, or nasal flaring.

       b) Tactile fremitus (increase over affected areas when patient says "ninety-nine") in sizable areas of consolidation

       c) Breath sounds decreased over affected area; bronchial breath sounds over areas of lobar pneumonia

       d) Adventitious sounds over affected area (e.g., crackles, sibilant wheezes)

IV. Diagnostic tests

A. Laboratory

    1. CBC with differential: Leukocytosis (may be absent in elderly or patients receiving chemotherapy); may also note increased bands

    2. Cultures: Often nondiagnostic

       a) Sputum: Sputum cultures should utilize material obtained in deep cough; in non-neutropenic patients, consider results only if field contains many polymononuclear (PMN) and no epithelial cells.

          (1) Gram stain may distinguish between gram-negative and gram-positive organisms but will not disclose specific organism.

          (2) Yield is specific for pathogen in only 25%–50% of community-acquired pneumonias.

          (3) Identity of microorganism takes 48–72 hours (longer with antibiotic sensitivities).

          (4) Sputum usually is contaminated by normal oral flora.

    3. Prior to initiating therapy, assess electrolytes, BUN, creatinine, serum albumin, and liver function studies for baseline values.

B. Radiology: Chest PA and lateral views (useful for documenting diagnosis, serving as a baseline for post-treatment follow-up, and providing data for differential diagnosis)

    1. Patchy, localized infiltrates most common finding; diffuse infiltrates in *Pneumocystis carinii* or viral pneumonias

    2. Lobar consolidations with air noted approximately 30%

    3. Pleural effusion is nonspecific finding; obtain lateral decubitus views if pleural effusion suspected

    4. Cavitary lesions associated with *Stapylococcus aureus*, anaerobes, fungi, and mycobacteria

    5. Hilar or mediastinal adenopathy in atypical mycobacterial pneumonias or pathogenic fungal pneumonias (histoplasmosis or coccidiosis)

    6. False-negative chest x-rays may be seen in dehydration, early stage (first 24 hours of infection), *Pneumocystis carinii,* or severe neutropenia

C. Other

    1. Fiberoptic bronchoscopy with bronchoalveolar lavage, especially in identification of microorganisms in patients with nosocomial infection

    2. Pulse oximetry if oxygen saturation questionable

V. Differential diagnosis

  A. COPD: Asthma, chronic bronchitis, or emphysema (see Chapter 28)

  B. Atelectasis

  C. Lung abscess

  D. CHF (see Chapter 40)

  E. Chemical inflammation from inhaled toxins (e.g., smoke)

  F. Pulmonary embolism (see Chapter 33)

  G. Cancer treatment-induced (radiation or chemotherapy)

VI. Treatment: Administer empiric therapy based on risk category and the high probability that the specific organism will not be identified. Patients increasingly are treated in ambulatory settings. Geographic variations in penicillin-resistant strep pneumonia will guide treatment (see Appendix 1).

  A. Patients less than 60 years old, without impaired immunity, and not on anticancer treatment: Likely pathogen *Streptococcus pneumoniae* or mycoplasma; treat with monotherapy.

    1. Oral macrolide therapy: Erythromycin 500 mg po qid, clarithromycin 500 mg po bid, or azithromycin 500 mg po for one day then 250 mg po qd for four days

    2. If penicillin-resistant strains low, penicillin VK 500 mg po qid

    3. Alternatives: Fluoroquinolones (levofloxacin, sparfloxacin, grepafloxacin, or trovafloxacin) or doxycycline

  B. Older than 60 years or comorbid condition (community-acquired)

    1. Erythromycin 500 mg po qid for seven days; azithromycin or clarithromycin are alternatives; amoxicillin and potassium clavulanate 875/125 mg po bid or oral second/third-generation cephalosporin

    2. Treatment should be based on institution's predominant organisms.

    3. Combination therapy indicated for broad coverage.

      a) Extended-spectrum beta-lactam antibiotic with carbapenems, aminoglycoside, quinolone, or trimethoprim and sulfamethoxazole

      b) Initial use of vancomycin is controversial; should be guided by practice setting

      c) Resistant strains of *Streptococcus pneumoniae* and *Haemophilus influenzae* are emerging; base therapy on susceptibility when known.

  C. Neutropenic patients with bacterial pneumonia are associated with high mortality directly related to low neutrophil count. Empiric therapy should start at onset of fever or respiratory symptoms, and opportunistic organisms (e.g., aspergillus) should be ruled out.

1. Ceftazidime 2 g IV every eight hours with clindamycin 600 mg IV every six hours
2. For penicillin allergy, aztreonam 2 g IV with clindamycin 600 mg every eight hours

D. Hospitalized, stable patient: Major pathogens include *Streptococcus pneumoniae, Haemophilus influenzae,* polymicrobes, aerobic gram-negative bacilli, Legionella, *Staphylococcus aureus, Chlamydia pneumoniae,* and viruses.
   1. Monotherapy with second-generation cephalosporin or third-generation cephalosporin, beta-lactamase inhibitor combined
   2. May add macrolide (po or IV for increased coverage); penicillin-resistant pneumococci will require vancomycin. If Legionella is suspected, add rifampin (see Appendix 1).

E. *Pneumocystis carinii*: Trimethoprim/sulfamethoxazole DS po three times per week for an indefinite time

F. In immunosuppressed patients who continue to have fever despite broad antimicrobial coverage: Fungus is suspected. Administer IV antifungal amphotericin B 1–15 mg/kg/day; vancomycin if gram stain shows gram-positive cocci in pairs or patient has venous access device.

G. Management considerations
   1. Indications for hospitalization: Pulse above 140, systolic B/P below 90, respiratory rate above 30, O_2 saturation less than 88%, altered mental status, comorbid conditions requiring simultaneous management
   2. Push fluids (six 8 oz glasses of fluid per day; more if febrile). Administer parenteral fluids for inadequate oral intake.
   3. Avoid cough suppressants if productive cough is present.
   4. Administer oxygen for O_2 saturation 88% or less.

VII. Follow-up: Prognosis dependent on etiologic organism, severity of infection, immunocompetence of host, coexisting diseases, stage of cancer
   A. Poor prognostic factors
      1. Advanced cancer refractory to cancer treatment
      2. Increased age
      3. Multi-lobar involvement
      4. Bacteremia
      5. Neutropenia
      6. Coexisting diseases: Diabetes mellitus, COPD, alcoholism
   B. Infiltrates on chest x-ray resolve more slowly than other parameters.
      1. In younger, healthier patients, x-ray clears in two to six weeks.
      2. Elderly or patients with bacteremia may take up to 12 weeks to clear.
   C. Prevention of pneumonia
      1. Careful handwashing
      2. Prophylactic antibiotics and antifungals for patients with prolonged and severe neutropenia is controversial.
      3. Splenectomized or elderly patients
         a) Influenza vaccine
         b) Pneumococcal vaccine (no live vaccines) dosage 0.5 ml IM or SC; may be given at same time but different site from influenza vaccine
         c) Colony-stimulating factors to reduce duration of neutropenia and prevent infections

VIII. Referrals
    A. Based on patient population and protocols for care
    B. Patients who do not respond to guidelines will need pulmonary or infectious disease
       consultation.

References

American Thoracic Society. (1993). Guidelines for the initial management of adults with community-acquired pneumonia: Diagnosis, assessment of severity, and initial antimicrobial therapy. *American Review of Respiratory Disease, 148,* 1418–1426.

Bartlett, J., & Mundy, L. (1995). Community acquired pneumonia. *New England Journal of Medicine, 333,* 1618–1624.

Gleason, P., Kapoor, W., Stone, R., Lave, J., Obrosky, D., Schultz, R., Singer, D., Coley, C., Marrie, T., & Fine, M. (1997). Medical outcomes and antimicrobial costs with the use of the American Thoracic Society guidelines for outpatients with community-acquired pneumonia. *JAMA, 278,* 32–39.

Mandel, L., & Campbell, D. (1998). Nosocomial pneumonia guidelines: An international perspective. *Chest, 113*(Suppl. 3), 188S–193S.

Shelhamer, J.H., Toews, G.B., Masur, H., Suffredini, A.F., Pizzo, P.A., Walsh, T.J., & Henderson, D.K. (1992). Respiratory disease in the immunosuppressed patient. *Annals of Internal Medicine, 117,* 415–431.

Stover, D., & Kaner, R. (1996). Pulmonary complications in cancer patients. *CA: A Cancer Journal for Clinicians, 46,* 303–320.

U.S. Public Health Service. (1997). Pneumococcus immunization prophylaxis: Recommendations for adults/older patients. *Nurse Practitioner, 21*(2), 110–113.

Whimbey, E., Goodrich, J., & Bodey, G. (1995). Pneumonia in cancer patients. In J. Klastersky (Ed.), *Infectious complications of cancer* (pp. 185–210). Boston: Kluwer Academic Publishers.

Chapter

31. Pneumothorax

Sandra C. Henke, RN, MS, ANP, OCN®

I. Definition: Accumulation of air or gas between the parietal and visceral pleura or pleural space

II. Pathophysiology: The amount of air or gas trapped in the intrapleural space determines the degree of lung collapse.
   A. Trapped air in the pleural space occupies the area normally used by the lung during respiration.
   B. The lung cannot expand fully because of the compression and begins to collapse.
   C. Ventilation of the collapsed lung becomes markedly reduced while the ventilation of the opposite lung is increased.
   D. Reduced oxygen and increased carbon dioxide tension cause decreased blood flow to the collapsed lung.
      1. To compensate, the contralateral lung receives a larger share of blood supply.
      2. Although this regulatory mechanism is not complete, it greatly improves the ventilation-perfusion relationship and prevents severe hypoxemia.
   E. When the communication between the pleural space and the atmosphere is sealed, the trapped air eventually undergoes absorption, resulting in gradual re-establishment of subatmospheric pressure and re-expansion of the lung.
   F. In some instances, the communication behaves as a one-way valve, allowing the air to enter the pleural cavity during elevation of intrathoracic pressure with cough or other expiratory efforts but preventing its exit.
      1. Under this circumstance, the pressure in the pneumothorax will become higher than that of the atmospheric pressure.
      2. Increased pressure may cause significant shift of the heart and other mediastinal structures to the opposite side, impairing both cardiac and lung function.
   G. If the pneumothorax is allowed to progress, elevated intrathoracic pressure may impede cardiac function by reducing venous return. Severe respiratory distress with profound hypoxemia and circulatory collapse are the consequences of this life-threatening medical emergency.

III. Clinical features: Patients diagnosed with pneumothorax are not always symptomatic. Symptoms may present slowly and increase gradually or may develop acutely and abruptly.
   A. Etiologies

    1. Spontaneous pneumothorax
        a) Spontaneous pneumothorax occurs without accidental or intentional trauma.
            (1) In young, otherwise healthy individuals, it may be caused by air leakage from ruptured congenital blebs adjacent to the visceral pleural surface, near the apex of the lung.
            (2) Most incidents of spontaneous pneumothorax are associated in those with a history of COPD.
                (a) Rupture of an emphysematous bulla during an episode of coughing or exercise commonly is reported.
                (b) Spontaneous pneumothorax often becomes a recurring condition requiring definitive medical management.
    2. Traumatic pneumothorax
        a) Traumatic pneumothorax results commonly as a consequence of chest injury.
            (1) Injury may result from laceration of the visceral pleura, often with a broken rib or as the result of a stab wound of the chest.
            (2) Injury may also develop as a result of a diagnostic intervention such as thoracentesis, pleural biopsy, or placement of a central venous catheter.

B. History
    1. History of cancer and cancer treatment
    2. Current medications: Prescribed and over-the-counter
    3. History of presenting symptom(s): Precipitating factors, onset, location, and duration. Associated symptoms are chest pain, dyspnea, and anxiety.
    4. Changes in activities of daily living

C. Signs and symptoms
    1. Dyspnea
    2. Chest pain, usually a sudden and sharp pleuritic pain exacerbated by breathing and coughing
    3. Anxiety

D. Physical exam: Abnormal physical findings not always present.
    1. Vital signs: Rapid pulse and hypotension
    2. Pulmonary exam
        a) Reduced or absent breath sounds over the collapsed lung
        b) Resonant percussion over affected hemithorax
        c) Asymmetrical or impaired chest wall movement
        d) Diminished or absent tactile fremitus
        e) Tracheal deviation: May be quite prominent
    3. Cardiovascular exam
        a) Weak and rapid pulse
        b) Neck vein distention
    4. Integument exam: Pallor

IV. Diagnostic tests
    A. Laboratory: Not indicated
    B. Radiology: Chest x-ray

1. Taken at full expiration, the chest film will accentuate the pneumothorax and demonstrate a small amount of air in the pleural cavity.
2. A visceral pleural line will be identified.
3. With significant pneumothorax, the entire lung will appear to have detached from the chest wall.
4. Because of reduction of its blood volume and presence of air around the lung, the density of a moderately collapsed lung usually will not be increased.
5. The absence of the vascular markings and the increased density of the lung help in detection of pneumothorax.
6. The extent of the pneumothorax is determined and reported as a percentage of lung collapse on the chest radiograph.

C. Other: Arterial blood gas analysis
   1. May be entirely normal with small pneumothorax
   2. Significant pneumothorax associated with the following results
      a) pH less than 7.35: Normal range of 7.35–7.45
      b) PaO_2 less than 80 mm Hg: Normal range of 80–100 mm Hg
      c) $PaCO_2$ above 45 mm Hg: Normal range of 35–45 mm Hg

V. Differential diagnosis
   A. Treatment-induced
      1. Thoracentesis
      2. Pleural biopsy
      3. Percutaneous or transbronchial lung biopsy
      4. Recent central line insertion
      5. Chest or neck surgery
      6. Post tracheostomy
   B. Emphysema with pleural bulla on chest radiographic (see Chapter 28)
   C. Chronic obstructive pulmonary disease exacerbation (see Chapter 28)
   D. Myocardial infarction (see Chapter 47)
   E. Pericarditis (see Chapter 48)
   F. Trauma
   G. Rib fracture
   H. Pleuritis
   I. Pneumonia (see Chapter 30)

VI. Treatment
   A. No treatment in small to moderate pneumothorax in which no signs of increased pleural pressure are seen, lung collapse is estimated at less than 30%, and the patient shows no signs of distress
      1. The pleural tear often will seal spontaneously, and the air in the pleural space will be absorbed.
      2. Resolution may require several days to weeks.
         a) Bed rest
         b) Monitoring vital signs for tachycardia and tachypnea
   B. Pneumothorax with more than 30% lung collapse

        1. Needle aspiration of air with a large-bore needle attached to a syringe
        2. Placement of a thoracostomy tube in the second or third intercostal space in the midclavicular line connected to an underwater seal or low suction pressure

    C. Symptomatic patients
        1. Require rapid evacuation of the air and re-expansion of the lung
        2. Require chest tube insertion immediately if evidence of respiratory distress, falling blood pressure, and a rising pulse rate exist

    D. Recurring spontaneous pneumothorax: Requires surgical evaluation
        1. Thoracoscopy or thoracotomy with pleural abrasion to prevent recurrence
        2. Pleurodesis with intrapleural sclerosing agents, such as talc or tetracycline; often considered in those patients with recurring spontaneous pneumothorax who also are poor surgical candidates
        3. Lung reduction surgery for excision of blebs or bullae in surgically eligible patients

VII. Follow-up
    A. Chest radiograph evaluation
        1. Identify stabilization or resolution of the pneumothorax with daily chest x-ray.
        2. Monitor re-expansion of the lung following removal of the pneumothorax.
    B. After the chest tube is placed and the lung has fully expanded, the medical team may consider alternative management approach.

VIII. Referrals
    A. Surgery or emergency referral for insertion of chest tube
    B. Thoracic surgical consultation for consideration of surgical approach for management of recurring spontaneous pneumothorax

References

Bauman, M.H., & Strange, C. (1997). The clinician's perspective on pneumothorax management. *Chest, 112,* 822–828.

Byrd, P., Fields-Ossorio, C., & Roy, T.M. (1999). Delayed chest radiographs and the diagnosis of pneumothorax following CT-guided fine needle aspiration of pulmonary lesions. *Respiratory Medicine, 93,* 379–381.

Gurley, M.B., Richli, W.R., & Waugh, K.A. (1998). Outpatient management of pneumothorax after fine-needle aspiration: Economic advantages for the hospital and patient. *Radiography, 209,* 717–722.

Martin, T., Gontana, G., Olak, J., & Ferguson, M. (1996). Use of pleural catheter for the management of simple pneumothorax. *Chest, 110,* 1169–1172.

Ponn, R.B., Silverman, H.J., & Federico, J.A. (1997). Outpatient chest tube management. *Annals of Thoracic Surgery, 64,* 1437–1440.

Chapter

32. Pulmonary Edema
Susan A. Ezzone, MS, RN, CNP

I. Definition: Clinical syndrome resulting in leakage of fluid from the pulmonary capillaries and veins into the interstitium and alveoli of the lungs

II. Physiology/Pathophysiology
   A. Normal: According to Starling's Law, the flow of fluid from the pulmonary capillaries to the lungs equals the removal of fluid by pulmonary lymphatics.
   B. Pathophysiology
      1. Pulmonary edema occurs when the pulmonary lymphatics are unable to remove fluid leaked into the lungs because of decreased intravascular oncotic pressure or increased interstitial oncotic pressure.
      2. Cardiogenic pulmonary edema may occur because of an increase in the hydrostatic pressure gradient associated with an altered hemodynamic status, such as in CHF.
      3. Noncardiogenic pulmonary edema is caused by leakage of fluid from pulmonary capillaries with a decrease in plasma oncotic pressure and elevation of capillary pressure, producing interstitial and intra-alveolar edema. This type of pulmonary edema is caused by an increased pulmonary capillary permeability.
      4. Direct damage to the epithelium of alveolar capillaries may cause leakage of fluid from the pulmonary capillaries.
      5. Decreased lung and small airway compliance may result in altered ventilation, hypoxia, and respiratory failure.

III. Clinical features
   A. Etiology: See Figure 32-1
   B. History
      1. History of cancer and cancer treatment
      2. Current medications: Prescribed and over-the-counter
      3. History of presenting symptom(s): Precipitating factors, onset, location, and duration
      4. Changes in activities of daily living
   C. Signs and symptoms
      1. Dyspnea, orthopnea
      2. Anxiety or feeling of impending doom
      3. Frothy-pink or salmon-colored sputum

Figure 32-1. Classification and Causes of Pulmonary Edema

Hemodynamic Edema
- Increased hydrostatic pressure
  - Left-sided heart failure
  - Mitral stenosis
  - Volume overload
  - Pulmonary vein obstruction
- Decreased oncotic pressure
  - Hypoalbuminemia
    - Nephrotic syndrome
    - Liver disease
    - Protein-losing enteropathies
- Lymphatic obstruction

Edema Due to Microvascular Injury
- Infectious agents: viruses, Mycoplasma, other
- Inhaled gases: oxygen, sulfur dioxide, cyanates, smoke
- Liquid aspiration: gastric contents, near-drowning
- Drugs and chemicals
  - Chemotherapeutic agents: bleomycin, other
  - Other medications: amphotericin B, colchicine, gold
  - Other: heroin, kerosene, paraquat
- Shock, trauma, and sepsis
- Radiation
- Miscellaneous
  - Acute pancreatitis; extracorporeal circulation; massive fat, air, or amniotic fluid embolism; uremia; heat; diabetic ketoacidosis; thrombotic thrombocytopenic purpura (TTP); disseminated intravascular coagulation (DIC)

Edema of Undetermined Origin
- High altitude
- Neurogenic

Note. From "The Lung" (p. 676) by L. Kobzik and F.J. Schoen in R.S. Cotran, V. Kumar, and T. Collins (Eds.), *Diseases of Vascular Origin*, 1994, Philadelphia: W.B. Saunders Company. Copyright 1994 by W.B. Saunders Company. Reprinted with permission.

4. Cough
5. Cyanosis, pallor
6. Diaphoresis
7. Unable to lie flat

D. Physical exam
1. Vital signs
   a) Tachypnea
   b) Tachycardia
   c) Hypotension
2. Integument exam: Skin pallor and livedo reticularis (skin discoloration with mottled appearance)
3. Pulmonary exam
   a) Abnormal breath sounds with occasional wheezing
   b) Abnormal breathing pattern or thoraco-abdominal dissociation (paradoxical movement of abdomen and thorax)
4. Cardiac exam
   a) Pulsus alternans, alternating weak and strong pulse, may be a sign of left ventricular failure in CHF
   b) Heart sounds with presence of S_3 and S_4
   c) Jugular venous distention
   d) Peripheral edema of extremities

IV. Diagnostic tests
A. Laboratory

1. Arterial blood gases
    a) Hypoxia (oxygen saturation < 90% and PaO_2 < 60 mm Hg)
    b) Hypercapnia (CO_2 > 45–55 mm Hg)
    c) Acidosis (pH < 7.35 nEq/liter). Early findings of pulmonary edema may be respiratory alkalosis because of hyperventilation.
2. Serum albumin: May be low (normal = 3.6–5.0 g/dl)
3. BUN and creatinine to evaluate kidney function to ensure that renal perfusion is occurring
4. Liver function tests to evaluate hepatic function (elevation in alanine aminotransferase [ALT], aspartate aminotransferase [AST] and bilirubin are seen with right ventricular failure and hepatic congestion)
B. Radiography: Chest radiograph
    1. Noncardiogenic: Bilateral consolidative pattern, interstitial edema
    2. Cardiogenic: Diffuse bilateral infiltrates, cardiomegaly
C. Other: Hemodynamic monitoring
    1. Pulmonary arterial pressure measurements with elevated pulmonary capillary wedge pressure (PCWP) (normal = 6–12 mm Hg)
    2. Systemic vascular resistance (SVR) may be elevated (normal=800–1,200 dynes/sec/m²)

V. Differential diagnosis
    A. CHF (see Chapter 40)
    B. Obstruction of pulmonary lymphatics by tumor compression
    C. Capillary leak syndrome (see Chapter 27)
    D. Neurogenic pulmonary edema
    E. Adult respiratory distress syndrome (ARDS)
    F. Early phase of septic shock (see Chapters 121 and 140)

VI. Treatment: Goal is to decrease pulmonary venous and capillary pressure, improve cardiac output, and correct underlying pathology. Patient is hospitalized for management.
    A. Drug therapy
        1. Use of loop diuretics (e.g., furosemide, bumetanide, torsemide) causes vasodilation and decreases pulmonary congestion. Doses of 0.5–1 mg/kg may be used.
        2. Administer metolazone (thiazide diuretic) 5–20 mg po once a day for treatment of CHF.
        3. Vasodilators cause vasodilation, therefore decreasing pulmonary vascular pressure.
            a) Nitroprusside is started at an IV infusion of 0.5 mcg/kg/minute and titrated to achieve the desired effect; average dose is 0.5–0.8 mcg/kg/minute.
            b) Nitroglycerin is started at an IV infusion of 10–20 mcg/minute, and the dose is increased by 5–10 mcg/minute every 5–10 minutes until the desired effect occurs.
        4. Morphine sulfate may be given to cause venous dilation at doses of 1–3 mg IV push. The dose is repeated every two to three hours as needed up to a total of 10–15 mg.
        5. Aminophylline may be given at 5 mg/kg IV infusion for symptoms of wheezing.
    B. Provide oxygen therapy and titrate dose based on patient response. Intubation and mechanical ventilation may be necessary.
    C. Position patient in semi-Fowler's position.

    D. Obtain daily weight to monitor fluid status.

    E. Obtain frequent intake and output measurements.

VII. Follow-up

    A. Daily physical assessment and evaluation of response to treatment is necessary.

    B. Diagnostic studies, such as chest radiograph and arterial blood gases, may be done to evaluate patient condition.

VIII. Referrals

    A. Pulmonary consult helpful to evaluate lung status and assist with medical management as needed.

    B. Respiratory therapy referral may be needed for oxygen therapy, ventilatory management, percussion, or respiratory treatments.

References

Beltrame, J.F., Zeitz, C.J., Unger, S.A., Brennan, R.J., Hunt, A., Moran, J.L., & Horowitz, J.D. (1998). Nitrate therapy is an alternative to furosemide/morphine therapy in the management of acute cardiogenic pulmonary edema. *Journal of Cardiac Failure, 4,* 271–279.

Fromm, R.E., Varon, J., & Gibbs, L.R. (1995). Congestive heart failure and pulmonary edema for the emergency physician. *Journal of Emergency Medicine, 13*(1), 71–87.

Hebra, J. (1996). Cardiovascular disorders. In J. Hebra & J.A. Kuhn (Eds.), *Manual of critical care nursing* (pp. 92–96). Boston: Little, Brown, & Co.

Kobzik, L., & Schoen, F.J. (1999). The lung. In R.S. Cotran, V. Kumar, & T. Collins (Eds.), *Diseases of vascular origin* (pp. 697–755). Philadelphia: Saunders.

LeConte, P., Coutant, V., N'Guyen, J.M., Touze, M.D., & Potel, G. (1999). Prognostic factors in acute cardiogenic pulmonary edema. *American Journal of Emergency Medicine, 17,* 329–332.

Thelan, L.A., Davie, J.K., Urden L.D., & Kritek, P.B. (1990). *Textbook of critical care nursing: Diagnosis and management.* St. Louis: Mosby.

33. Pulmonary Embolism

Sandra C. Henke, RN, MS, ANP, OCN®

I. Definition: The occlusion of the pulmonary artery or one or more of its branches by an embolus carried via the vascular system

II. Pathophysiology
   A. A common disorder that results from the migration of clots to the pulmonary circulation from distal veins, most often the vena cava and the large proximal vessels of the lower extremities
   B. Clot (thrombus) formation: Three factors facilitate clot formation in a vessel.
      1. Damage to the vessel wall causes platelets to adhere and activate clotting factors resulting in a thrombus.
      2. Venous stasis: Stagnation of blood flow, particularly in the lower extremities, predisposes clot formation as platelets aggregate and collect.
      3. Increased coagulability
   C. Embolism formation: Once detached from its original source, the blood clot (embolism) is carried with the blood flow. From the vein, it travels to the right side of the heart and then to the pulmonary artery.
   D. The embolus lodges in various parts of the pulmonary artery. A very large embolus may occlude the main pulmonary artery, whereas smaller ones will pass more distally.
   E. Mechanical occlusion of a pulmonary artery results in nonperfusion and loss of function of the lung supplied by that artery.
   F. Occlusion of a regional pulmonary artery results in changes of ventilation and perfusion to other lung regions.
      1. The blood is now diverted to nonoccluded branches of the pulmonary artery.
      2. Perfusion exceeds ventilation, resulting in pulmonary congestion of the affected lung regions.
         a) Lung volumes and compliance usually are reduced.
         b) Ventilation and perfusion are mismatched, and pulmonary shunting may cause hypoxemia.
         c) Pulmonary artery pressure may become elevated.
            (1) As the right ventricle is unable to generate high enough pressure, it may fail to maintain an adequate cardiac output if the pulmonary embolism (PE) is massive.
            (2) Reduced cardiac output aggravates hypoxemia, which, in turn, increases the pulmonary vascular resistance.

III. Clinical features: Depends on the size of the embolus and the patient's preexisting cardiopulmonary status; many emboli, mostly when small, produce little or no symptoms and are hardly suspected. A massive PE may cause acute right ventricular failure, systemic hypotension, and sudden death. No single symptom or sign or combination of clinical findings is pathognomonic of pulmonary thromboembolism.

   A. Risk factors
1. Surgery
2. Malignancy, specifically lung cancer
3. Trauma
4. Immobilization
5. Previous thrombosis
6. Antiphospholipid antibodies (associated with systemic lupus erythematosus)
7. Hypercoagulable state

   B. Etiologies
1. An embolus most commonly is a blood clot (thromboembolism); however, it may be a fat globule, air, tumor or other tissue fragment, or a foreign body.
2. Phlebitis, trauma, and inflammation are conditions in which local clotting takes place.
3. Conditions that promote venous stasis include prolonged bed rest; immobility resulting from pain, trauma, or surgery; general debility; and heart failure.
4. Medication-induced
   a) Tamoxifen and raloxifene may predispose development of PE.
   b) Amiodarone toxicity will display symptoms similar to PE.
   c) Estrogen therapy

   C. History
1. History of cancer and cancer treatment
2. Current medications: Prescribed and over-the-counter
3. History of presenting symptom(s): Precipitating factors, onset, location, and duration. Associated symptoms are shortness of breath and chest pain.
4. Changes in activities of daily living
5. Past medical history: Previous deep vein thrombosis, trauma

   D. Signs and symptoms: Do not generally differ between massive and less severe thromboembolism
1. Dyspnea with sudden onset: Severity out of proportion to clinical findings
2. Chest pain: Often anginal type at onset; later becomes pleuritic in nature
3. Hemoptysis (not common at presentation)
4. Apprehension
5. Diaphoresis
6. Cough

   E. Physical exam
1. Vital signs: Low-grade fever in approximately 40% of cases
2. Pulmonary exam
   a) Tachypnea
   b) Crackles: More prevalent in pulmonary infarction
   c) Wheezing: May be present
3. Cardiac exam

          a) Accentuation of the pulmonary component of the second heart sound

          b) Right-sided cardiac gallop

    4. Examination of extremities

          a) Thrombophlebitis evident: Warmth, erythema, cord-like

          b) Lower extremity pain, tenderness, or swelling

          c) Symptoms present in approximately 30% of cases

IV. Diagnostic tests

  A. Laboratory: Not indicated

  B. Radiology

    1. Ventilation/perfusion lung scan

      a) Most commonly used

      b) A vascular process, like PE, reduces lung perfusion without interfering with ventilation. Results are interpreted as being normal, low or intermediate (indeterminate) probability, or high probability for the presence of a pulmonary thromboembolism.

        (1) A normal perfusion scan rules out clinically significant pulmonary thromboembolism. No further studies are needed.

        (2) A low or indeterminate result indicates only a possibility of embolism. Further evaluation for deep vein thrombosis (see venous thrombosis studies) or a pulmonary arteriogram is indicated.

        (3) High probability result signifies immediate treatment is indicated.

    2. Chest radiograph

      a) Often determined to be abnormal, but findings often are related to medical history of COPD or cardiac disease and not of PE.

      b) Elevation of a hemidiaphragm and pulmonary infiltrates are identified most commonly.

    3. Venous thrombosis studies

      a) Ultrasonography or impedance plethysmography are the studies of choice for presence of a venous thrombosis.

      b) Presence of a thrombus in a deep vein will support the diagnosis of PE even when other studies are negative or nondiagnostic.

    4. Pulmonary angiography

      a) A highly sensitive test for diagnosis of PE that can detect emboli as small as 3 mm in diameter

      b) Expensive, invasive, and difficult to interpret

  C. Other

    1. Arterial blood gas analysis

      a) Typically normal

      b) Hypoxemia may be seen in massive PE. As this is present in many medical conditions, it remains nondiagnostic.

    2. EKG: Tachycardia and nonspecific ST-T wave changes are most common but nondiagnostic.

V. Differential diagnosis
   A. CHF (see Chapter 40)
   B. Myocardial infarction (see Chapter 47)
   C. Dissecting aortic aneurysm
   D. Pneumothorax (see Chapter 31)
   E. Pericarditis (see Chapter 48)
   F. Pneumonia (see Chapter 30)

VI. Treatment
   A. Prevention: Identify at-risk patients and institute preventive measures.
      1. Heparin
         a) Activates antithrombin III, which then inhibits both thrombin and activated factor X
         b) Prophylactic dose: 5,000 U SC every 8–12 hours
      2. Low molecular-weight heparin
         a) Requires less-frequent dosing of once per day
         b) Longer half-life
         c) Fewer bleeding complications
         d) Effective for patients undergoing orthopedic surgery, general medical patients, and patients with spinal cord injuries
      3. Lower extremity compression devices
         a) Enhance blood flow and may maintain fibrinolysis by applying pressure to the lower extremities
         b) Intermittent pneumatic compression and compression stockings: Effective and inexpensive
         c) No clear advantage to any one device
         d) Should be avoided in patients with known acute deep vein thrombosis who are most at risk of an embolic event
   B. Anticoagulation: The goal is to interrupt thrombosis and allow the lytic system to dissolve the clot.
      1. Heparin: First-line antithrombotic drug for PE because of its rapid onset of action
         a) Check baseline activated partial thromboplastin time (PTT).
         b) Administer initial IV bolus of 5,000–10,000 U.
         c) Provide continuous infusion at 1,000 U/hour.
         d) Check PTT six hours after infusion has begun.
         e) Maintain the PTT to 1.5–2.5 times the patient's control.
         f) Oral anticoagulant therapy may begin concurrently.
      2. Warfarin: Oral agent used for long-term anticoagulation after thromboembolism
         a) Dosage determined by measuring the prothrombin time (PT) and international normalized ratio (INR)—PT level of 1.25–1.5 times the patient's control value optimal or INR of 2.0–3.0
         b) Started concurrently with heparin
         c) Duration of warfarin therapy: Depends on clinical situation
            (1) Recommended duration is three to six months.
            (2) Longer treatment is advised if patient remains at risk for repeated embolism.
      3. Low molecular-weight heparin

a) May be preferred initial treatment of thrombosis
b) Also effective in those patients who are not candidates for therapy with warfarin
c) Longer half-life, administered subcutaneously
d) Less risk of bleeding for long-term therapy
C. Thrombolytic therapy
1. Promotes rapid resolution of emboli, but the role of thrombolysis for acute PE is not established.
2. Bleeding risks are increased and survival is not improved.
3. Clinical situations in which thrombolysis should be considered include patients with profound hypoxemia, patients who exhibit significant hemodynamic compromise, and patients with a large clot burden.
4. Contraindications include the presence of any active bleeding site or central nervous system disease within the preceding three to six months.
   a) Streptokinase, a foreign protein, combines with circulating plasminogen to form an activated complex that causes thrombolysis.
      (1) IV bolus of 250,000 U infused over 30 minutes
      (2) Maintenance dose of 100,000 U/hour for 12–48 hours
   b) Urokinase, a human protein, directly binds with circulating plasminogen and achieves a lytic state more rapidly than streptokinase.
      (1) IV bolus of 4,000 U/kg over 20 minutes
      (2) Maintenance dose of 4,000 U/kg for 12–24 hours
D. Embolectomy
1. Used for severely compromised patients who fail conventional therapy, including thrombolysis
2. Performed as a surgical procedure or as a catheter technique under radiographic guidance

VII. Follow-up
A. PTT is monitored and maintained at 2–2.5 times the patient's baseline control value for long-term heparin therapy. Standard duration of therapy is three months.
B. PT and INR are monitored and maintained at 1.5 times the patient's baseline control value and 2.0–3.0, respectively, for long-term warfarin therapy.

VIII. Referrals
A. Hospital admission in collaboration with physician and initial management in acute phase of care
B. Intensive care management in cases of massive emboli and severe cardiopulmonary compromise as seen with hypoxemia and hypercapnia
C. Surgery or interventional radiology referral if embolectomy is indicated

References

Arcasoy, S.M., & Kreit, J.W. (1999). Thrombolytic therapy of pulmonary embolism: A comprehensive review of current evidence. *Chest, 115,* 1695–1707.

Goldhaber, S.Z. (1999). Treatment of pulmonary thromboembolism. *Internal Medicine, 38,*620–625.

Grimm, K.J., & French, L. (1997). Low-molecular-weight heparin for PE. *Journal of Family Practice, 45,* 467–468.

Hull, R.D., Raskob, G.E., Brant, R.F., Pineo, G.F., & Valentine, K.A. (1997). The importance of initial heparin treatment on long-term clinical outcomes of antithrombotic therapy. *Archives of Internal Medicine, 157,* 2317–2321.

Miniati, M., Prediletto, R., Formichi, B., Marini, C., Di Ricco, G., Tonelli, L., Allescia, G., & Pistolesi, M. (1999). Accuracy of clinical assessment in the diagnosis of pulmonary embolism. *American Journal of Respiratory and Critical Care Medicine, 159,* 864–871.

Perrier, A., Buswell, L., Bounameaux, H., Didier, D., Morabia, A., de Moerloose, P., Slosman, D., Unger, P.F., & Junod, A. (1997). Cost-effectiveness of noninvasive diagnostic aids in suspected pulmonary embolism. *Archives of Internal Medicine, 157,* 2309–2316.

Raskob, G.E. (1995). Anticoagulants and thrombolysis in the treatment of pulmonary embolism. *Current Opinion in Pulmonary Medicine, 1,* 291–297.

Raskob, G.E. (1999). Heparin and low molecular weight heparin for the treatment of acute pulmonary embolism. *Current Opinion in Pulmonary Medicine, 5,* 216–221.

Raskob, G.E., & Hull, R.D. (1999). Diagnosis of pulmonary embolism. *Current Opinion in Hematology, 6,,* 280–284.

Schulman, S., Granqvist, S., Holmstrom, M., Carlsson, A., Lindmarker, P., Nicol, P., Eklund, S.G., Nordlander, S., Larfars, G., Leijd, B., Linder, O., & Loogna, E. (1997). The duration of oral anticoagulant therapy after a second episode of venous thromboembolism. *New England Journal of Medicine, 336,* 393–398.

34. Tuberculosis

Gena Schottmuller, RN, BA, CIC, and

Nancy C. Grandt, RN, CNP, MS, AOCN®

I. Definition: A bacterial infection caused by *Mycobacterium tuberculosis* (acid-fast bacillus)

II. Pathophysiology
   A. When a person inhales air that contains droplet nuclei expelled by an infected person, most of the larger particles become lodged in the upper respiratory tract. Infection is unlikely to develop; however, the droplet nuclei may reach the alveoli where infection may begin.
   B. Small numbers of bacilli may spread through lymphatic channels to lymph nodes and the bloodstream to more distant tissue and organs.
   C. Two to 10 weeks after exposure and subsequent infection, the immune system usually is effective in preventing the replication of the bacteria and further spread to active primary disease.
   D. Tuberculosis (TB) infection progresses to active TB (TB disease) when the tubercle bacilli overcome the immune system and begin to multiply.

III. Clinical features
   A. Risk factors
      1. Alcoholic or IV drug user
      2. Current or past prisoner
      3. Older than 65 years of age
      4. Foreign-born from countries with high prevalence of TB (e.g., southeast Asia, Africa, South America)
      5. Homeless
      6. Medically underserved
      7. High-risk racial/ethnic groups (Asians, southeast Asians, Pacific Islanders, African Americans, Hispanics, Native Americans)
      8. HIV infection (especially with failure of outpatient treatment for *Pneumocystis* or bacterial pneumonia—100 times greater risk)
      9. Immunocompromised (e.g., bone marrow depression, lymphoma, leukemia)
      10. Residents of long-term care facilities
      11. Close contact with individuals with infectious TB
      12. Diabetic (three times greater risk)
      13. Malnourished

B. Overview of TB
   1. TB is most likely to develop in the lungs (85%).
   2. TB can occur in the pleura, central nervous system, bones, and joints or may be disseminated (miliary) TB.
   3. More than 90% are asymptomatic at the time of primary infection with positive TB test.
   4. Four broad syndromes can be identified in the 10% that progress to symptomatic disease.
      a) Atypical pneumonia
      b) Tuberculous pleurisy
      c) Direct progression
      d) Early dissemination
   5. TB can take months to years to progress (most within two years).
      a) In the United States, 10% of individuals infected with TB go on to develop active disease at some point in their lives. Approximately 5% will develop disease in the first year or two, and another 5% will develop the disease in the later years of their lives.
      b) The remaining 90% will stay infected but disease-free for the rest of their lives.
   6. The tuberculin skin test (purified protein derivative [PPD] test, Mantoux test) is helpful in identifying those who may be infected with *Mycobacterium tuberculosis.*
      a) Most infected individuals will have a positive skin test 2–10 weeks after infection.
      b) Those with a positive skin test but who do not have active disease are not considered to be infectious to others.
      c) Once an individual has been infected and has a true positive skin test, the test usually will remain positive. Some people will lose reactivity with time.
C. History
   1. History of cancer and cancer treatment
   2. Current medications: Prescribed and over-the-counter
   3. History of presenting symptom(s): Precipitating factors, onset, location, and duration. Associated symptoms are hemoptysis, night sweats, weight loss, and loss of appetite.
   4. Changes in activities of daily living
   5. Past medical history: Diabetes mellitus, HIV, TB exposure or positive skin test
   6. Family history: TB
   7. Recent foreign travel (e.g., southeast Asia, Africa, South America)
D. Signs and symptoms
   1. Cough: Productive, prolonged, more than three weeks
   2. Hemoptysis
   3. Chest pain
   4. Fever
   5. Chills
   6. Nights sweats
   7. Easily fatigued
   8. Loss of appetite
   9. Weight loss greater than 10 pounds in six months

E. Physical exam
1. Cannot be used to confirm or rule out TB
2. Useful in providing information about patient's general condition and directs how TB is treated

IV. Diagnostic tests
A. Laboratory
1. Tuberculin skin test
   a) Traditional method of screening for infection with TB
   b) 0.1 ml of five tuberculin units PPD is administered intradermally into dorsal surface of forearm. A 6–10 mm wheal should develop.
   c) Reactions are read at 48–72 hours. Measure induration by inspection and palpation. Redness is not significant.
   d) Multiple puncture (tine) tests are not recommended to rule out TB or for individuals at high risk of developing TB. They may be used for screening large populations at low risk (e.g., preschoolers).
   e) Interpretation of PPD: Three different cut points for individuals with varying risk factors for TB (see Table 34-1)
2. In immunosuppressed individuals, delayed-type hypersensitivity responses (TB skin tests) may decrease or disappear (anergy).
3. Anergy may be caused by HIV infection, overwhelming miliary or pulmonary TB, severe or febrile illness, viral infections, Hodgkin's disease, sarcoidosis, live-virus vaccination, corticosteroids, or immunosuppressive drugs.

Table 34-1. Interpretation of Mantoux Skin Test

Reaction size (mm)	Result	Group
< 5	Negative reaction	—
≥ 5	Positive reaction	• Suspected or known HIV infection • Close contact of infectious case of TB • Persons who have a chest radiograph suggestive of previous TB • Persons who inject drugs (HIV status unknown)
≥ 10	Positive reaction	• Persons with certain medical conditions (e.g., COPD, lymphoma, leukemia) • Persons who inject drugs (if HIV negative) • Foreign-born persons from areas where TB is common • Medically underserved, low-income populations including high risk racial and ethnic groups • Residents of long-term care facilities • Children younger than four years of age • Locally identified high-prevalence groups (e.g., migrant farm workers or homeless persons)
≥ 15	Positive reaction	• All persons with no known risk factors for TB

Note. Based on information from Centers for Disease Control and Prevention, 1994.

4. Test for anergy by administering at least two other delayed-type hypersensitivity antigens (e.g., mumps, candida, or tetanus toxoid) in conjunction with TB skin test.
5. Reactions of ≥ 3 mm to any of the antigens (including TB) indicate that the individual is not anergic.
6. A negative test does not exclude the possibility of TB. 10%–20% of individuals with active TB have negative skin tests because of severe T cell immunodeficiency.
   a) Indications and/or recommendations for applying TB skin tests
      (1) Signs and symptoms of TB
      (2) Recent close contact of known TB case
      (3) Abnormal chest x-ray
      (4) High risk of TB
      (5) HIV infection
      (6) Immigrants from Africa, Asia, South America, and Oceania; inner-city populations; healthcare workers; residents in nursing homes, correctional institutions, or homeless shelters
   b) Booster effect
      (1) Some people with TB infection may have a negative skin test reaction when tested many years after infection.
      (2) The initial skin test may stimulate (boost) their ability to react to tuberculin.
      (3) Positive reactions to subsequent tests may be misinterpreted as new infection
      (4) Two-step testing is used to distinguish boosted reactions and reactions caused by new infection.
      (5) If the reaction to the first test is classified as negative, a second test should be performed one to three weeks later.
      (6) A positive reaction to the second test represents a boosted reaction and the person is classified as previously infected and treated accordingly (not a skin test conversion).
7. Sputum specimen collection for acid-fast bacillus (AFB)
   a) Examine at least three specimens by smear and culture.
   b) Obtain early-morning specimens on different days.
   c) Healthcare worker should supervise first specimen collections and instruct patient to do the following.
      (1) Clean and thoroughly rinse mouth with water.
      (2) Breathe deeply three times.
      (3) After third breath, cough hard and try to bring up sputum.
      (4) Expectorate sputum (at least one teaspoon) into sterile container.
      (5) Stay in room with door closed until coughing stops.
      (6) Aerosol induction may be necessary for patients having difficulty expectorating. While using a mist, breathe normally for 15 minutes, then cough hard.
   d) Smears positive for AFB may indicate active TB (usually takes 24 hours).
   e) Smears positive for AFB also may grow other atypical AFB.
   f) A culture that is positive and identified as *Mycobacterium tuberculosis* confirms the diagnosis of TB (typically available 10–14 days after collection, but may take four to six weeks).

B. Radiology: Chest x-ray, typically posterior-anterior or lateral view; CT scan may be necessary
 1. Abnormalities in apex of posterior segments of upper lobe or in superior segments of lower lobe, including infiltrates, mediastinal or hilar lymphadenopathy, and cavitation
 2. Unusual appearances in HIV-infected individuals with pulmonary TB
 3. Useful in ruling-out TB in individuals with positive skin test and no symptoms; however, cannot confirm TB
C. Other
 1. Bronchoscopy
  a) Useful when person is unable to cough up sputum
  b) Bronchial washings, brushings, and biopsies may be obtained.
 2. Gastric aspiration
  a) Used when unable to obtain sputum to analyze
  b) Uncomfortable and invasive
  c) Gastric acid is toxic to mycobacteria; must be processed immediately
 3. Tissue biopsy for extrapulmonary disease because sputum and gastric samples are usually negative

V. Differential diagnosis
 A. Pneumonia (see Chapter 30)
 B. HIV infection (see Chapter 156)
 C. COPD (see Chapter 28)
 D. Cancer of the lung

VI. Treatment
 A. Prevention for the healthcare worker for suspected or confirmed diagnosis
 1. Patient should wear a tight-fitting surgical mask when in the healthcare facility if facility does not have negative air ventilation.
 2. Healthcare worker should wear an N95 respirator mask when the patient is in a negative air room or when the patient is outside of the room and is unable to wear a surgical mask. (A HEPA-filtered or positive air purifier respirator [PAPR] also is acceptable.)
 3. Isolation precautions should be taken until the patient has been deemed not infectious by meeting all of the following criteria.
  a) Adequate therapy received for two to three weeks
  b) Favorable clinical response to therapy
  c) Three consecutive negative sputum smear results from sputum collected on different days
 B. Preventive pharmacologic therapy
 1. Isoniazid (INH), daily for 6–12 months, typically recommended
  a) Used for people who are infected with TB (positive skin test) but who do not have active disease
  b) Reduces the incidence of active disease by 55%–88%
 2. Alternative preventive therapy recommended when drug-resistant organisms are known (e.g., a combination of rifampin, pyrazinamide, and/or streptomycin) or for

patients with positive skin test and either silicosis or a chest x-ray demonstrating old fibrotic lesions with no evidence of current disease

   3. Monitor at least monthly for adverse reactions and compliance to prescribed therapy.

   4. Review for contraindications: Pregnancy, liver disease, previous drug reactions

   5. High-priority candidates for TB preventive therapy (see Figure 34-1)

C. Treatment of active disease

   1. Should include four drugs (typically): Isoniazid, rifampin, pyrazinamide, and either ethambutol or streptomycin. (Note: TB medications are provided free of charge by the health department.)

   2. The four-drug, six-month regimen is effective and should be used until drug susceptibility tests are completed.

   3. Three drugs may be adequate for initial regimen once resistance in the community is established.

   4. Isoniazid and rifampin for nine months is acceptable for people who are unable to or should not take pyrazinamide.

   5. Noncompliance is a major problem. Direct observation therapy may be necessary.

D. Monitoring individuals on therapy includes the following.

   1. Adherence to the prescribed protocol (counting medications and periodic urine tests)

   2. Observing for signs and symptoms of hepatitis and/or neurotoxicity

   3. Response to treatment

      a) For individuals with previously positive sputum cultures, obtain specimens for culture at least monthly until cultures convert to negative.

      b) When sputum is no longer positive for *Mycobacterium tuberculosis* after two months of treatment, obtain one additional sputum culture and smear.

Figure 34-1. High-Priority Candidates for Preventive Therapy

The following persons with a positive tuberculin test result should receive prophylactic treatment, *regardless of age*:

- Persons with known or suspected HIV infection
- Close contacts of persons with infectious, clinically active TB
- Persons who have a chest radiograph suggestive of previous TB and who have received inadequate or no treatment
- Injection drug users
- Persons with medical conditions that increase the risk of TB (diabetes mellitus, prolonged steroid therapy, immunosuppressive therapy)
- Recent tuberculin skin test converters
- Persons with a positive skin test reaction who are *younger than 35 years of age*
- Foreign-born from areas where TB is common
- Medically underserved, low-income populations, including high-risk racial and ethnic groups
- Residents of long-term care facilities
- Children younger than four years of age
- Locally identified high-prevalence groups (e.g., migrant farm workers or homeless persons)

Note. Based on information from Centers for Disease Control and Prevention, 1994.

VII. Follow-up
  A. Short-term
    1. Report positive TB test promptly to the local health department.
    2. Provide evaluation of close contacts, including skin tests.
    3. Educate patient and household contacts on transmission of disease, importance of therapy and compliance, and the necessity of reporting of noncompliance to health department.
    4. Provide a surgical mask for patient to use when in the healthcare system.
  B. Long-term
    1. Evaluate patient at regular intervals for medication compliance and toxicity.
    2. Assess for response to treatment.

VIII. Referrals
  A. Infectious disease specialist for management of drug therapy
  B. Pulmonologist for evaluation and treatment management
  C. Local health department to obtain free medications

References

Benenson, A.S. (1995). Tuberculosis. In A.S. Benenson (Ed.), *Control of communicable diseases manual* (16th ed.) (pp. 188–197). Washington, DC: American Public Health Association.

Centers for Disease Control and Prevention. (1994). *Core curriculum on tuberculosis. What the clinician should know* (3rd ed.). Atlanta: National Tuberculosis Training Initiative, cosponsored by the American Thoracic Society and Centers for Disease Control and Prevention.

Clark, P.A., Cegielski, J.P., & Hassell, W. (1997). TB or not TB? Increasing door-to-door response to screening. *Public Health Nursing, 14,* 268–271.

Guidelines for preventing the transmission of *Mycobacterium tuberculosis* in health care facilities. Centers for Disease Control and Prevention. (1994). *Morbidity and Mortality Weekly Report, 43*(RR-13), 1–132.

Tebas, P., Tapper, M.L., & Fraser, V.J. (1996). *Mycobacterium tuberculosis* and nontuberculosis mycobacteria. In R.N. Olmsted (Ed.), *APIC infection control and applied epidemiology: Principles and practice* (pp. 1–10). St. Louis: Mosby.

Tuberculosis morbidity: US 1996. (1997). *JAMA, 278,* 1309.

Chapter

35. Upper Respiratory Infection
Madonna K. McDermott, RN, MS, ANP, OCN®

I. Definition: Infection located in the upper respiratory tract

II. Physiology/Pathophysiology
   A. Normal: The head and neck form an anatomically complex region that includes the nose, paranasal sinuses, ears and mastoids, oral cavity, pharynx, and larynx.
      1. Functions
         a) Exchange and filtering of air
         b) The intake and separation of foods and liquids from the airway
         c) Functions of speech, taste, smell, and hearing
      2. Respiratory ciliated epithelium lines the areas involved in air exchange.
      3. Squamous cells line the oral cavity, tongue, and oropharynx.
   B. Pathophysiology
      1. A variety of pathogens may cause inflammation of the pharynx, larynx, and nasal mucosa or lymph tissue.
      2. Inflammation of the mucosal membranes of the nose usually is accompanied by edema or nasal discharge resulting in ostial obstruction.
      3. Transmission occurs by way of droplets or surface-to-surface contact in the common cold.

III. Clinical features: Upper respiratory infections (URIs) are the most common acute illnesses in the United States and the industrialized world. The common cold, pharyngitis, laryngitis, rhinitis, sinusitis, otitis externa, and otitis media are the most frequent infections that fall under the broader category of URIs.
   A. Etiologies: Usually viral in nature
      1. Common cold: Caused by a variety of viruses, including rhinoviruses (more commonly seen in early fall and mid to late spring), coronaviruses (occurring more in midwinter), influenza, parainfluenza, respiratory syncytial virus, and adenoviruses
      2. Pharyngitis
         a) Most often occurs as part of common colds caused by rhinovirus, coronavirus, or parainfluenza virus
         b) May be caused by infectious mononucleosis, herpangina, or group A streptococcus

   3. Laryngitis
      a) Most commonly associated with rhinovirus, influenza virus, parainfluenza virus, and adenovirus
      b) Occasionally associated with group A streptococcus, *Moraxella catarrhalis,* and Candida
   4. Rhinitis
      a) May be allergic or nonallergic
      b) May be triggered by seasonal pollens, molds, or mildew
B. History
   1. History of cancer and cancer treatment
   2. Current medications: Prescribed and over-the-counter
   3. History of presenting symptom(s): Precipitating factors, onset, location, and duration
   4. Changes in activities of daily living
   5. History of recent infections
C. Signs and symptoms (see Table 35-1)
D. Physical exam
   1. Common cold
      a) Absence of fever
      b) Exam of the pharynx, nasal cavity, ears, sinuses, and lungs are usually negative. Occasionally erythema or swollen nasal mucous membranes is noted.
      c) Possible enlarged cervical lymph nodes
   2. Pharyngitis
      a) Possible herpangina—small oral vesicles or ulcers on tonsils, pharynx, or posterior buccal mucosa
      b) Possible fever

Table 35-1. Signs and Symptoms of Common Upper Respiratory Infections

Signs/Symptoms	Common Cold	Pharyngitis	Laryngitis	Rhinitis
Malaise	+	+		
Rhinorrhea	+			+
Sneezing	+			+
Cough	+	+		+
Sore throat	+	+	+	+
Hoarseness	+		+	
Nasal congestion	+	+		+
Itchy eyes				+
Inflamed pharynx	(-)	+		
Fever	(-)	+		
Enlarged cervical lymph nodes	+	+		+

       c) Erythema of tonsils and pharynx

       d) Exudate in tonsillar area

       e) Enlarged and tender anterior cervical lymph nodes

    3. Laryngitis

       a) Hoarseness or loss of voice

       b) Presence of oral *Candida* in immunosuppressed patients

    4. Rhinitis

       a) Pale, boggy nasal mucosa with purulent discharge indicating infectious rhinitis or sinusitis

       b) Clear thin secretions indicating allergic and vasomotor rhinitis

       c) Enlarged inferior nasal turbinates

       d) Dark discoloration beneath both eyes ("allergic shiners")

       e) Occasional enlarged tonsils or adenoids, sore throat, and palatal petechiae

       f) Normal lung sounds

IV. Diagnostic tests: For the majority of URIs, no diagnostic tests are required.

  A. Laboratory

    1. Rapid strep test to rule out *Streptococcus* infection

    2. Throat culture to rule out *Streptococci, Neisseria gonorrhoeae, Neisseria meningitis, Neisseria lactamicus, Corynebacterium hemolyticum, Mycoplasma pneumoniae,* and chlamydia

    3. Mono spot test to rule out mononucleosis

    4. CBC with differential: Elevated WBC count in bacterial infections

    5. Cultures of any exudate or drainage, especially in neutropenic patients

  B. Radiology: Sinus x-rays; sinusitis will reveal fluid-filled sinus cavities.

  C. Other: Skin testing for allergies

V. Differential diagnosis: Immunocompromised patients are at increased risk for developing URIs; however, great care must be taken to exclude more serious and threatening illnesses and pathogens.

  A. Pharyngitis

    1. Stomatitis (see Chapter 11)

    2. Rhinitis (see Chapter 10)

    3. Sinusitis (see Chapter 10)

    4. Epiglottitis

    5. Mononucleosis

  B. Laryngitis

    1. Oral candidiasis

    2. Pharyngitis (see Chapter 4)

    3. Esophagitis

  C. Rhinitis

    1. Sinusitis (see Chapter 10)

    2. Otitis media (see Chapter 9)

    3. Deviated septum

    4. Nasal polyps or foreign body in nasal passage

     5. Hypothyroidism (see Chapter 150)

VI. Treatment: Treatment is dependent on identifying the underlying diagnosis, determining the causative agent, and then initiating appropriate therapy. Numerous over-the-counter drugs are available to treat URIs.
  A. Common cold: Symptomatic treatment
    1. Fever
      a) NSAIDs (avoid if history of bleeding ulcers, receiving anticoagulant therapy, and/or thrombocytopenic) (see Appendix 11)
      b) Acetaminophen (caution patients to avoid taking more than 4,000 mg of acetaminophen/24 hours)
    2. Congestion/runny nose
      a) Steam or cool mist to help to liquefy secretions
      b) Topical decongestants (limit use to five days to avoid rebound effect)
      c) Oral decongestants (see Table 35-2 and Appendix 6 and 7)
      d) Antihistamines (see Table 35-3 and Appendix 4 and 6)
      e) No evidence that expectorants are of benefit in URIs
  B. Pharyngitis (strep)
    1. Penicillin V 250 mg po tid–qid x 10 days
    2. Erythromycin 500 mg po bid x 10 days
    3. Doxycycline 150 mg po bid x 7–10 days
    4. Ciprofloxacin 500–750 mg po bid x 7–10 days
  C. Laryngitis
    1. Pain
      a) Acetaminophen (caution patients to avoid taking more than 4,000 mg of acetaminophen/24 hours)
      b) NSAIDs (avoid if history of bleeding ulcers, receiving anticoagulant therapy, and/or thrombocytopenic) (see Appendix 11)
    2. Group A streptococcus
      a) Penicillin V 250 mg po tid–qid x 10 days
      b) Erythromycin 250 mg po qid x 10 days
    3. *Moraxella catarrhalis*: Erythromycin 250 mg po qid x 10 days
  D. Rhinitis: Combination of decongestant and antihistamine H_1-receptor antagonist (e.g., Contac® [SmithKline Beecham, Philadelphia, PA], Comtrex® [Bristol-Myers Squibb, Princeton, NJ], Dimetapp® [American Home Products Corp., Madison, NJ]) (see Appendix 6)

Table 35-2. Recommended Dosage Guidelines for Nonprescription Oral Nasal Decongestants

Drug	Adults (12 years and older)
Phenylephrine	10 mg every 4 hours (60 mg/24 hours)
Phenylpropanolamine	25 mg every four hours or 50 mg every eight hours (150 mg/24 hours)
Pseudoephedrine	60 mg every four hours (360 mg/24 hours)

Table 35-3. Recommended Dosage Guidelines for Nonprescription Oral Antihistamines

Drug	Adults (12 years and older)
Brompheniramine maleate	4 mg every four to six hours (24 mg/24 hours)
Chlorcyclizine hydrochloride	25 mg every six to eight hours (75mg/24 hours)
Chlorpheniramine maleate	4 mg every four to six hours (24 mg/24 hours)
Dexbrompheniramine maleate	2 mg every four to six hours (12 mg/24 hours)
Dexchlorpheniramine maleate	2 mg every four to six hours (12 mg/24 hours)
Diphenhydramine citrate	38–76 mg every four to six hours (456 mg/24 hours)
Diphenhydramine hydrochloride	25–50 mg every six to eight hours (300 mg/ 24 hours)
Doxylamine succinate	7.5–12.5 mg every four to six hours (75 mg/24 hours)
Phenindamine tartrate	25 mg every four to six hours (150 mg/24 hours)
Pheniramine maleate	12.5–25 mg every four to six hours (150 mg/24 hours)
Pyrilamine maleate	25–50 mg every six to eight hours (200 mg/24 hours)
Triprolidine hydrochloride	2.5 mg every four to six hours (10 mg/24 hours)

VII. Follow-up

    A. Patients who are suspected of having acute bacterial or fungal infections should be seen in 24–48 hours if no significant improvement is noted.

    B. In patients whose symptoms do improve, schedule return visit for 10–14 days.

VIII. Referrals: Not indicated unless symptoms do not resolve; referral to pulmonologist or allergist may be indicated.

References

Brook, I. (1998). Microbiology of common infections in the upper respiratory tract. *Primary Care: Clinics in Office Practice, 25,* 633–648.

Green, K., Webster, H., Watanabe, S., & Fainsinger, R.L. (1994). Management of nosocomial respiratory tract infections in terminally ill cancer patients. *Journal of Palliative Care, 10*(4), 31–34.

Koster, F.T., & Barker, L.R. (1995). Respiratory tract infections. In L.R. Barker, J.R. Burton, & P.D. Zieve (Eds.), *Principles of ambulatory medicine* (4th ed.). Baltimore: Williams & Wilkins.

Moore, D.A., & Sharland, M.F. (1999). Upper respiratory tract infections. *Current Opinion in Pulmonary Medicine, 5,* 157–163.

Sokhandan, M., McFaddden, E.R., Huang, Y.T., & Mazanec, M.B. (1995). The contribution of respiratory viruses to severe exacerbations in asthma in adults. *Chest, 107,* 1570–1574.

Tietze, K.J. (1996). Cold, cough, and allergy products. In T. Covington (Ed.), *Handbook of nonprescription drugs* (11th ed.) (pp. 133–156). Washington DC: American Pharmaceutical Association.

Section V.

Cardiovascular

Symptoms

Medical Diagnosis

36. Angina
Cindy Jo Horrell, MS, CRNP, AOCN®

I. Definition: Discomfort in chest and/or adjacent substernal area, usually lasting longer than two minutes

II. Pathophysiology
   A. Symptomatic manifestation of myocardial ischemia brought on by exertion and associated with disturbance of myocardial function but without necrosis
   B. Angina occurs when oxygen demands exceed available vascular oxygen supply.
      1. The increased myocardial oxygen demands stem from norepinephrine release by adrenergic nerve endings in response to stress, physical exertion, or psychological distress.
      2. Restriction of coronary blood supply may be related to loss of normal endothelial vasoregulatory activity, resulting in coronary vasospasm.
   C. Angina is caused by transient reduction of oxygen supply from coronary artery constriction and previously narrowed vessels unable to supply adequate oxygen during increased oxygen demands.
      1. Stimuli alter the tone of the well-innervated coronary arterial bed.
      2. Severity of pain depends on underlying defect and change in coronary arterial tone.

III. Clinical features: A typical episode begins gradually and reaches maximum intensity over a period of a few minutes before dissipating. Angina is typically relieved by rest and/or use of sublingual nitroglycerin and/or oxygen.
   A. Etiology
      1. Atherosclerotic disease is most common etiology.
      2. Inadequate coronary perfusion from valvular stenosis or calcific obstruction
      3. Inappropriate vasoconstriction responses to autonomic and biochemical stimuli can increase total resistance and decrease myocardial perfusion called coronary microvascular dysfunction.
   B. History
      1. History of cancer and cancer treatment
      2. Current medications: Prescribed and over-the-counter
      3. History of presenting symptom(s): Precipitating factors, onset, location, and duration. Associated symptoms are diaphoresis, nausea/vomiting, dyspnea, palpitations, hemoptysis, and fever.

    4. Changes in activities of daily living
    5. Past medical history: Coronary artery disease, hyperlipidemia, hypercholesteremia, diabetes mellitus, angina, or myocardial infarction
    6. Family history of cardiac disease, diabetes
    7. Social history (smoking, occupation, exercise, illicit drug use)

C. Signs and symptoms: Women, diabetics, and elderly experience pain < 50% of the time, tending to have symptoms of dyspnea, nausea/vomiting, diaphoresis, and, in general, "feeling bad."
    1. Pain located substernal or retrosternal; radiation common down ulnar surface of left arm, neck, jaw, and right arm
    2. Dyspnea
    3. Faintness
    4. Fatigue
    5. Belching, dyspepsia
    6. Diaphoresis

D. Physical exam
    1. Vital signs: Measure blood pressure in both arms, assess for widening pulse pressure.
    2. Weight: Evaluate ideal body weight, presence of obesity.
    3. HEENT exam: Assess for xanthelasma, arcus senilis.
    4. Pulmonary exam: Auscultate lungs to rule out pulmonary etiology.
    5. Cardiovascular exam
        a) Presence of S_3 may indicate congestive heart failure (CHF) or anemia.
        b) Presence of pericardial friction rub could indicate pericarditis or early tamponade.
        c) Distant or muffled heart tones indicate pericardial effusion or tamponade.
        d) Rapid or irregular heart rate/rhythm could indicate atrial fibrillation or runs of ventricular tachycardia.
        e) Auscultate carotid arteries for bruits.
        f) Check jugular distention; reliable indicator of right atrial function to evaluate right-sided heart failure.
        g) Palpate peripheral pulses to assess vascular sufficiency; will be diminished in cardiac disease.
    6. Musculoskeletal exam: Palpate cervical and upper thoracic spine to rule out musculoskeletal origin.
    7. Abdominal exam: Auscultate abdomen for presence of bruit; palpate for hepatomegaly.

IV. Diagnostic tests
  A. Laboratory studies
    1. CBC: To rule out anemia; elevated white blood count suggests pneumonia, pleuritic origin.
    2. Cholesterol and full lipid profile: Elevated levels are risk factors for coronary artery disease; these values are rarely accurate in an acute setting and are low in stress states.
    3. Glucose: Check for presence of diabetes mellitus (a risk factor).
    4. Thyroid function: Elevated levels can cause atrial fibrillation.
    5. Homocysteine (intermediary amino acid in protein metabolism): Elevated level is a vascular risk factor. Consider drawing in young patients and patients with few or no identifiable risks; can be useful in patients known to have disease and/or risk factors.

B. Radiology: Chest x-ray to rule out pulmonary origin of pain, presence of aortic dissection

C. Other

1. 12-lead EKG: To evaluate dysrhythmia that could increase oxygen demand

2. Chemical (Persantine® [Boehringer Ingelheim Pharmaceuticals, Inc., Ridgefield, CT] or adenosine or thallium) stress test

   a) To evaluate angina with no clear etiology, to measure perfusion; if results equivocal, send for exercise stress test.

   b) Radionuclide perfusion study can identify fixed versus variable heart muscle defect.

V. Differential diagnoses

A. Cardiac origin

1. Myocardial infarction (see Chapter 47)

2. Aortic dissection

3. Pericarditis (see Chapter 48)

4. Prolapsed mitral valve

5. Atherosclerotic disease

6. Coronary vasospasm

7. Aortic stenosis

8. Radiation-induced valvular stenosis

9. Chemotherapy-induced cardiomyopathy (see Chapter 39)

B. Gastrointestinal origin

1. Gastroesophageal reflux (see Chapter 66)

2. Esophageal motility disorders

3. Peptic ulcer disease (see Chapter 73)

4. Biliary disease

C. Pulmonary origin

1. Pneumonia (see Chapter 30)

2. Bronchitis (see Chapter 28)

3. Pleurisy

4. Pneumothorax (see Chapter 31)

5. Pulmonary embolus (see Chapter 33)

D. Musculoskeletal origin

1. Cervical radiculopathy

2. Costochondritis

3. Myositis

4. Osteoarthritis (see Chapter 106)

E. Other

1. Anemia (see Chapters 111–116)

2. Hyperventilation/anxiety (see Chapter 152)

3. Herpes zoster, left chest (see Chapter 20)

4. Drug abuse (e.g., amphetamines, cocaine)

5. Hyperthyroidism (see Chapter 149)

VI. Treatment
  A. Identify and treat underlying disease (e.g., anemia, drug abuse)
  B. Lifestyle adjustments/decrease or eliminate risk factors
    1. Management of hypertension (see Chapter 45)
    2. Cessation of cigarette smoking
    3. Management of dyslipidemia (see Chapter 42)
    4. Estrogen replacement therapy in postmenopausal women (see Chapter 151)
    5. Initiation of exercise program
    6. Diet modification
  C. Pharmacologic therapy
    1. Nitrates are drugs of choice for acute anginal episode. They relax vascular smooth muscle causing a decrease in venous return and a decrease in arterial pressure decreasing myocardial oxygen demand.
      a) Also indicated in the prophylaxis of angina and treatment of angina unresponsive to recommended doses of beta-blockers or calcium channel blockers.
      b) Relatively contraindicated in patients with severe anemia, postural hypotension, increased intracranial pressure, and aortic stenosis.
      c) Can decrease the pharmacologic effect of heparin.
      d) Examples include
        (1) Sublingual nitroglycerin 0.15–1.2 mg every 5 minutes x 3 doses
        (2) Isosorbide dinitrate sublingual 2.5–5 mg until pain relieved
        (3) Nitroglycerin ointment 1–1.5 inches every 4 hours
        (4) Nitroglycerin transdermal patch 10–25 mg qd
    2. Beta-adrenergic blockers are antianginal, antiarrhythmic, and antihypertensive; competitively block receptors in the heart. Decreases excitability, decreases workload, and decreases oxygen consumption of the heart.
      a) Indicated for angina caused by coronary atherosclerosis and to manage stress-related angina, syncope, and palpitations.
      b) Contraindicated in sinus bradycardia, second- or third-degree heart block, CHF, and chronic obstructive pulmonary disease (COPD).
      c) Use cautiously in patients with diabetes mellitus or hepatic dysfunction.
      d) Examples include
        (1) Metoprolol 50 mg po bid or sustained release of 50 mg, 100 mg, or 200 mg po; may increase to 450 mg per day
        (2) Atenolol 50 mg po every day; may increase to 200 mg per day
        (3) Nadolol 40 mg po every day; may increase to 160–240 mg per day
    3. Calcium channel blockers are antianginal and antihypertensive.
      a) Indicated for angina caused by coronary artery spasm and chronic stable angina. Inhibits movement of calcium ions across membranes of cardiac and arterial muscle cells.
      b) Contraindicated in sick sinus syndrome, heart block, and ventricular dysfunction because it slows velocity of cardiac impulse conduction and depresses myocardial contractility and dilation of coronary arteries.
      c) Increased effects reported with cimetidine and ranitidine.
      d) Examples include

       (1) Verapamil 80–160 mg po every 8 hours

       (2) Diltiazem 30–80 mg po every 6 hours

       (3) Amlodipine 5–10 mg po every day

       (4) Nicardipine 20–40 mg po every 8 hours

       (5) Nifedipine 20–40 mg po every 8 hours

       (6) All available in daily sustained release form

4. For hyperhomocysteinemia: Reduce homocysteine by breaking it down, allowing it to be cleared by bloodstream.

   a) Folic acid 1–5 mg po per day

   b) B_{12} and B_6 standard supplements orally

5. Anti-inflammatory agents for pericarditis, pleurisy, and pneumothorax (see Appendix 11)

6. H_2 blockers, antacids, antibiotics: For esophageal pain and biliary colic

7. Analgesics and anti-inflammatory agents: For musculoskeletal pain (see Appendices 8 a/b and 11)

8. Invasive therapy: Patients for whom other therapy fails

   a) Angioplasty: For single- or multivessel disease

   b) Coronary artery bypass surgery: For left-main or triple-vessel disease

VII. Follow-up

  A. Frequent return visits until dose adjustments have finalized

  B. Routine return visits: To monitor blood pressure, presence/absence of symptoms, side effects of pharmacologic therapy (e.g., kidney, hepatic function)

VIII. Referrals

  A. Cardiologist

    1. Refer when basic therapies are ineffective.

    2. Refer complicated patients with comorbid disease or with risk factors.

  B. Dietitian: For diet modification (essential component)

References

Beattie, S. (1999). Management of chronic stable angina. *Nurse Practitioner, 24*(5), 44, 49, 53–54, 59–61.

Braunwald, E. (1997). Part 1: Examination of the patient. In E. Braunwald (Ed.), *Heart disease: A textbook of cardiovascular medicine* (vol. 1, 5th ed.) (pp. 3–7). Philadelphia: Saunders.

Gersh, B.J., Braunwald, E., & Rutherford, J.D. (1997). Chronic artery disease. In E. Braunwald (Ed.), *Heart disease: A textbook of cardiovascular medicine* (vol. 1, 5th ed.) (pp. 1290–1301). Philadelphia: Saunders.

Jackson, G. (1993). The management of stable angina. *Hospital Practice, 28*(1), 59–63, 67–70, 75.

Meyer, N. (1999). Using physiologic and pharmacologic stress testing in the evaluation of coronary artery disease. *Nurse Practitioner, 24*(4), 70, 72, 75–76, 78, 81–82.

Moghadasian, M.H., McManus, B.M., & Frohlich, J.J. (1997). Homocysteine and coronary artery disease. Clinical evidence and genetic and metabolic background. *Archives of Internal Medicine, 157,* 2299–2308.

Parker, J.D., & Parker, J.O. (1998). Nitrate therapy for stable angina pectoris. *New England Journal of Medicine, 338,* 520.

Parmley, W.W. (1997). Optimal treatment of stable angina. *Cardiology, 88*(Suppl. 3), 27–31.

Refsum, H., Ureland, P.M., Nygard, O., & Vollset, S.E. (1998). Homocysteine and cardiovascular disease. *Annual Review of Medicine, 49,* 31–62.

Savonitto, S., & Ardissino, D. (1998). Selection of drug therapy in stable angina pectoris. *Cardiovascular Drugs and Therapy, 12*(2), 197–210.

Seager, L. (1995). Diagnosis of chest pain. *Postgraduate Medicine, 97*(2), 131–136, 139–140, 143–145.

Thadani, U., & Chohan, A. (1995). Chronic stable angina pectoris. *Postgraduate Medicine, 98*(6), 175–176, 179–183, 187–188.

Warner, C. (1997). Triaging & interpreting chest pain. *Journal of Cardiovascular Nursing, 12*(1), 84–92.

37. Palpitations

Brenda K. Shelton, RN, MS, CCRN, AOCN®

I. Definition: Subjective sensation described by some patients as heart skipping, fluttering, pounding, or racing

II. Pathophysiology
   A. Increase in stroke volume or contractility, sudden change in heart rate or rhythm, or unusual cardiac movement within the thorax may stimulate palpitations
   B. Excess adrenergic stimulation results in increased contractility.
   C. High levels of circulating catecholamines (e.g., from anxiety) can stimulate the myocardial cells.

III. Clinical features: The clinical significance of palpitations depends greatly on whether they arise from sinus, atrial, or ventricular dysrhythmias. Palpitations should be evaluated to determine whether they are related to a life-threatening dysrhythmia; however, in many cases they are not treated. Continuous palpitations are present for several minutes or more. Intermittent palpitations are present for seconds.
   A. Etiology
      1. Rapid heart rates (usually exceeding 150 beats/minute) may reflect dysrhythmia, such as sinus tachycardia (rarely exceeds 160 beats/minute), atrial flutter, atrial fibrillation, supraventricular tachycardia, and ventricular tachycardia.
      2. Intermittent palpitations may occur with premature atrial, junctional, or ventricular contractions.
      3. Isolated single palpitations
         a) Premature atrial or ventricular beats
         b) Blocked beats
      4. Paroxysmal episode with abrupt onset and resolution
         a) Paroxysmal atrial fibrillation
         b) Paroxysmal atrial tachycardia with variable block
         c) Frequent premature atrial or ventricular beats
         d) Multifocal atrial tachycardia
         e) Supraventricular tachycardia
      5. Paroxysmal episodes with less abrupt onset
         a) Exertion

    b) Emotion

    c) Drug-induced: Sympathomimetic, theophylline

    d) Stimulant use: Coffee, tobacco

    e) Insulin reaction

    f) Pheochromocytoma

   6. Persistent palpitations at rest

    a) Aortic or mitral regurgitation

    b) Large ventricular septal defect

    c) Bradycardia

    d) Severe anemia

    e) Hyperthyroidism

    f) Pregnancy

    g) Fever

    h) Marked volume depletion

    i) Anxiety

 B. History: Palpitations may be the first or only manifestation of dysrhythmias; however, a thorough health history can reflect other vague signs and symptoms that were previously overlooked.

   1. History of cancer and cancer treatment

   2. Current medications: Prescribed and over-the-counter

   3. History of presenting symptom(s): Precipitating factors, onset, location, and duration

   4. Changes in activities of daily living

   5. Past medical history: Heart defects, angina, myocardial infarction, palpitations, rheumatic fever, endocarditis

   6. Family history: Heart disease

   7. Social history: Nicotine consumption (e.g., cigarettes, chewing tobacco, pipe smoking) and illicit drug use

 C. Signs and symptoms

   1. Sensation of fluttering or skipping

   2. Sensation of continuous fluttering or racing, usually rapid heart rate

   3. Shortness of breath

   4. Chest tightness/discomfort

   5. Dizziness

   6. Tinnitus

 D. Physical exam: Focus on cardiac exam

   1. Apical heart rate: Fast or irregular

   2. Pulse deficit: Difference in the rate between the apical and radial pulse (radial lower); more indicative of premature beats than a rapid heart rate

   3. Heart sounds: Gallops or murmurs may be present in some conditions

   4. Finger clubbing: Sign of long-term perfusion deficits

   5. Presence of jugular venous pulsation: Indicates cardiac decompensation

IV. Diagnostic tests

 A. Laboratory:

   1. CBC: To identify anemia

2. Electrolytes: To rule out imbalances
3. Free T4 and TSH: To rule out hypothyroidism and hyperthyroidism
B. Radiology: Echocardiogram provides valuable information regarding valvular function, ventricular size, ventricular dilatation, or the estimated cardiac output with that rhythm.
C. Other
1. An electrocardiogram (EKG) rhythm strip in leads II, AVF, and V1: These leads clearly define a particular portion of the normal P, QRS, and T waves; will help to discern one rhythm from another, as P waves or QRS direction are highlighted.
2. 12 lead EKG: Will better define the rhythm disturbance and determine whether there is accompanying ischemia. If the rhythm is not always present, an exercise stress test may be performed in attempt to trigger the rhythm disturbance and plan treatment.
3. 24-hour Holter™ (Johnson & Johnson, New Brunswick, NJ) monitor: Provides 24 hours of continuous rhythm monitoring that is particularly helpful if the rhythm disturbance is intermittent. The patient also keeps a diary that will aid in identifying clinical symptoms that are directly related to the rhythm disturbance.
4. Event monitors: May be used with holter monitoring; criteria- and/or patient-triggered
5. Electrophysiologic (EP) testing: For life-threatening dysrhythmias; may need to "map" the source of the dysrhythmia and provide an avenue for definitive treatment.

V. Differential diagnosis
A. Coronary artery disease
B. Myocardial infarction (see Chapter 47)
C. Mitral valve prolapse
D. Wolff-Parkinson-White syndrome
E. Cardiomyopathy: Dilated, hypertrophic (see Chapter 39)
F. Pulmonary embolism (see Chapter 33)
G. Hyperthyroidism (see Chapter 149)
H. Electrolyte imbalance (see Chapters 144–148)

VI. Treatment: The treatment of palpitations depends on the etiologic factors, patient's tolerance, and aggressiveness of planned support.
A. Do NOT treat palpitations if all of the following are true.
1. Cause of rhythm is known (e.g., drug- , caffeine- , anxiety-induced)
2. No symptoms of instability
3. Rhythm is unlikely to disintegrate into a life-threatening unstable rhythm
B. Emergency management of palpitations
1. Provide supplemental oxygen and IV fluids if not contraindicated. Many of the etiologies of palpitations respond well to one of these two measures.
2. Determine patient's instability (e.g., hypotension, shock-like symptoms).
3. Correct underlying etiology or risk factors, if known.
   a) Discontinue medications that may increase risk of dysrhythmias.
   b) Eliminate smoking, alcohol, and caffeine.
   c) Control fevers and factors that increase metabolic rate (e.g., stress, pain).

4. Regulate metabolic balance (e.g., electrolytes, hormones).
5. Definitive treatment, as indicated by etiology.

VII. Follow-up
  A. Patients with untreated palpitations that resolve spontaneously may not need formalized follow-up.
  B. Patients should indefinitely avoid cardiac stimulants (e.g., caffeine, tobacco, black licorice).
  C. Patients under medical treatment for dysrhythmias may have a variety of cardiac tests performed on a periodic basis, depending on the type and etiology of the dysrhythmia.
    1. 24-hour Holter monitor
    2. 12 lead EKG (periodically, usually annually)
    3. Echocardiogram
    4. Multiple gated acquisition (MUGA) scan
    5. Antidysrhythmia medication serum level

VIII. Referrals
  A. Cardiologist: For evaluation of dysrhythmias of unknown origin or when patient is refractory to treatment; will determine whether an interventional cardiologist or dysrhythmia expert is needed.
  B. Pharmacist: To advise patients in correct administration of antidysrhythmic medications; many of these agents have altered absorption with food, pH levels, or other concomitant medications.
  C. Dietitian: Refer patients on antidysrhythmic therapy who must monitor their intake of certain electrolytes, particularly sodium and potassium.

References

Cummins, R.O. (Ed). (1994). *Textbook of advanced cardiac life support* (4th ed). Dallas: American Heart Association.

Howard, M. (1995). Cardiac disorders. In C. Paradiso (Ed.), *Lippincott's review series. Pathophysiology* (pp. 25–52). Philadelphia: J.B. Lippincott.

McLachlan, S.A., Millward, M.J., Toner, G.C., Guiney, M.J., & Bishop, J.F. (1994). The spectrum of 5-fluorouricil cardiotoxicity. *Medical Journal of Australia, 161*(3), 207–209.

Rinkenberger, R. (1991). Cardiac rhythm in the critical care setting: Pathophysiology and diagnosis. In D.R. Dantzker (Ed.), *Cardiopulmonary critical care* (2nd ed.) (pp. 437–498). Philadelphia: W.B. Saunders.

Chapter

38. Peripheral Edema
Mary Ann Winokur, CRNP, MSN

I. Definition: Accumulation of fluid within the interstitial spaces

II. Pathophysiology
   A. Edema is caused by an imbalance between the forces containing fluid within the vasculature and those forcing fluid through the vascular wall.
   B. Increased hydrostatic pressure, increased capillary permeability, decreased plasma oncotic pressure, and lymphatic or venous obstruction forces fluid to move through the blood vessel wall.

III. Clinical features: Edema is a problem of fluid distribution and does not always indicate fluid excess.
   A. Etiology
      1. Unilateral extremity edema indicates a local inflammatory or obstructive response.
      2. Bilateral lower extremity edema most often is the result of a systemic disease or condition or medication-induced with drugs such as estrogen, NSAIDs, lithium, oral contraceptives, tricyclic antidepressants, calcium channel blockers, and nitrates.
      3. Unilateral upper extremity edema is rare and usually is the result of obstruction of the subclavian vein or innominate vein by a malignancy or thrombosis such as lymphedema and cellulitis.
      4. Bilateral upper extremity edema is rare and usually is the result of obstruction of the superior vena cava by a malignancy or thrombosis.
   B. History
      1. History of cancer and cancer treatment
      2. Current medications: Prescribed and over-the-counter
      3. History of presenting symptom(s): Precipitating factors, onset, location, and duration. Associated symptoms are pain, numbness, tingling, swelling, or cramping of extremities, shortness of breath at rest and with activity, chest discomfort at rest and with activity, constipation, cold intolerance, and warmth of extremity.
      4. Changes in activities of daily living
      5. Past medical history: Myocardial infarction (MI), deep venous thrombosis, hypertension, murmur
   C. Signs and symptoms

1. Bilateral lower extremity edema
    a) CHF symptoms
        (1) Dyspnea on exertion
        (2) Orthopnea
        (3) Paroxysmal nocturnal dyspnea
        (4) Sudden weight gain
    b) Nephrotic syndrome symptoms: Most frequently occur in children
        (1) Frequent urination
        (2) Edema
    c) Liver failure symptoms: Generally the result of cirrhosis
        (1) Abdominal girth enlargement
        (2) Change in skin color (yellow)
        (3) Itching skin
        (4) Right upper quadrant fullness or pain
        (5) Anorexia
        (6) Weight loss
        (7) Fatigue
        (8) Nausea
        (9) Flatulence
        (10) Change in bowel habits
        (11) Easy bruising or bleeding
2. Unilateral lower extremity edema
    a) Varicose veins
    b) Redness of lower extremity
    c) Pain of lower extremity
    d) Warmth of lower extremity
    e) Low-grade fever
D. Physical exam
    1. Bilateral lower extremity edema
        a) CHF findings
            (1) Cardiovascular exam
                (a) S_3 or S_4
                (b) Elevated jugular venous pulsation (JVP)
                (c) Tachycardia
                (d) Hypertension
            (2) Pulmonary exam: Rales
            (3) Abdominal exam
                (a) Hepatomegaly
                (b) Hepatojugular reflux
        b) Nephrotic syndrome findings
            (1) Generalized edema (anasarca)
            (2) Hypertension
        c) Liver failure findings
            (1) Abdominal exam
                (a) Ascites

     (b) Spider telangiectasis
   (2) Integument exam: Jaundice
   (3) Neurologic exam: Altered mental status
 2. Unilateral lower extremity edema
  a) Vital signs: Fever
  b) Integument exam
   (1) Skin color and appearance
   (2) Warmth, redness, and tenderness
   (3) Pitting edema: Painless edema in women > age 40 could represent gynecologic cancer.
   (4) Decreased mobility of affected extremity
   (5) Peau d'orange skin involving the foot and dorsal hump representing chronic stasis

IV. Diagnostic tests
 A. Laboratory
  1. Nephrotic syndrome indications
   a) Serum albumin: Decreased < 3.0 g/dl
   b) Total protein: Decreased < 6 g/dl
   c) Urine protein excretion: > 3.5 g/24 hours
   d) Serum creatinine and BUN: Increased
  2. Cholesterol: Fasting cholesterol > 200 g/dl
  3. Serum creatinine: Increased in nephrotic syndrome
  4. Antinuclear antibody (ANA): Increased may indicate systemic lupus erythematosus inducing nephrotic syndrome
  5. Liver function tests (LFTs): Elevated AST and ALT, alkaline phosphatase, bilirubin, indicating liver-induced condition
  6. Prothrombin time: Prolonged indicates liver-induced condition
  7. Serum protein electrophoresis: Serum protein levels decreased in liver disease
 B. Radiology
  1. Chest x-ray: Kerley B lines (increased interstitial edema), cardiac enlargement indicating heart failure
  2. Echocardiogram: Decreased left ventricular ejection fraction, valvular disease, hypertrophy, chamber size suggestive of heart failure
  3. Duplex ultrasonography: To rule out thrombophlebitis or deep venous thrombosis
 C. Other
  1. Renal or liver biopsy: To make a definitive diagnosis, if needed
  2. Paracentesis: To make a definitive diagnosis or for comfort measures, if needed

V. Differential diagnosis
 A. Unilateral extremity edema: Indicates a local inflammatory response
  1. Lymphedema (see Chapter 110)
  2. Venous insufficiency
  3. Thrombophlebitis (see Chapter 157)
  4. Cellulitis (see Chapter 16)

    5. Ruptured Baker's cyst

    6. Gynecologic cancer with obstruction

    7. Deep venous thrombosis (see Chapter 41)

  B. Bilateral lower extremity edema

    1. CHF (see Chapter 40)

    2. Nephrotic syndrome

    3. Liver failure

    4. Acute glomerulonephritis

    5. Dependent edema

  C. Unilateral upper extremity edema

    1. Lymphedema (see Chapter 110)

    2. Obstruction of innominate or subclavian vein

  D. Bilateral upper extremity edema: Superior vena cava obstruction

VI. Treatment: Depends on the underlying etiology of the edema

  A. CHF (see Chapter 40)

  B. Nephrotic syndrome

    1. Reduce protein intake: 0.5–0.6 g/kg/day

    2. Angiotensin-converting enzyme (ACE) inhibitors (e.g., captopril, lisinopril, enalapril): Frequently will reduce the amount of proteinuria

    3. Dietary salt restriction: Key to management of edema < 1 g/day

    4. Diuretics: Thiazide diuretics (e.g., hydrochlorothiazide) for mild edema; loop diuretics (e.g., Lasix®, Hoechst Aktiengesellschaft, Frankfurt, Germany) for more refractory edema

    5. Low-fat/low-cholesterol diet (<30% of total calories) and lipid-lowering medication

    6. Heparin/Coumadin® (Dupont Pharmaceutical Company, Wilmington, DE) therapy: If thrombosis occurs (see Chapter 41)

  C. Liver failure

    1. Abstinence from alcohol or other hepatotoxic agents (e.g., acetaminophen)

    2. Bedrest: Helps to mobilize ascites; activity can be increased when diuresis is initiated.

    3. Dietary sodium restriction: < 1 g/day with adequate caloric intake; restriction can be increased to 1–2 g/day when diuresis initiated.

    4. Fluid restriction: If serum sodium < 130 of approximately 1–1.5 liters/day.

    5. Diuretics: Spironolactone (Aldactone®, G.D. Searle & Co., Chicago, IL) is used in patients who fail to diurese with sodium restriction and bed rest.

      a) Goal: Daily weight loss of 0.5–1.0 kg/day

      b) Aldactone: 25 mg po bid to maximum of 150 mg po qid

      c) Loop diuretics

        (1) Can be added if Aldactone fails to initiate diuresis

        (2) Metolazone (Zaroxolyn®, Medeva Pharmaceuticals, Inc., Rochester, NY): 30 minutes prior to standard loop diuretics can be beneficial.

    6. Large volume paracentesis: If respiratory compromise occurs or for comfort measures.

    7. Vitamins: Folic acid and thiamin

  D. Venous insufficiency

       1. Bed rest with leg elevated
       2. Intermittent elevation of legs during day
       3. Avoidance of prolonged standing
       4. Support hose
   E. Thrombophlebitis (see Chapter 157)
   F. Lymphedema (see Chapter 110)
   G. Deep venous thrombosis (see Chapter 41)

VII. Follow-up: As indicated by the underlying disease process

VIII. Referrals
   A. Cardiologist: For CHF, MI, valvular heart disease, longstanding or poorly controlled hypertension
   B. Vascular surgeon: For venous insufficiency, peripheral vascular disease
   C. Dietitian: For dietary interventions (low-fat, low-cholesterol, low-sodium diet)
   D. Gynecologist: If unilateral painless lower extremity edema is present to rule out pelvic tumor causing obstruction (women)
   E. Renal specialist: For nephrotic syndrome
   F. Gastroenterologist: For liver failure

References

Ellison, D.H. (1994). Diuretic drugs and the treatment of edema: From clinic to bench and back again. *American Journal of Kidney Diseases, 23,* 623–643.

Morrison, R.T. (1997). Edema and principles of diuretic use. *Medical Clinics of North America, 81,* 689–704.

Powell, A.A. (1997). Peripheral edema. *American Family Physician, 55,* 1721–1726.

Seller, R. (Ed.). (1993). *Differential diagnosis of common complaints.* Philadelphia: W.B. Saunders.

Williams, A.V., & Holmstrom, T.F. (1996). Three edemas. *Journal of the South Carolina Medical Association, 92,* 306–310.

Chapter

39. Cardiomyopathy

Martha E. Langhorne, MSN, RN, FNP

I. Definition: A group of heterogenous cardiac diseases characterized by myocardial dysfunction not caused by atherosclerosis, valvular disease, or hypertension

II. Pathophysiology
   A. Dilated (congestive) cardiomyopathy is a disease of the heart muscle in which the cardiac chambers have been dilated, resulting in decreased ventricular contractility.
      1. Decreased contractility leads to decreased ejection fraction, decreased stroke volume, and increased end-diastolic and residual volumes.
      2. Morphologic findings in dilated cardiomyopathy are usually nonspecific.
      3. Cardiac cellular membrane damage, calcium overload, and energy depletion occur.
      4. The compensatory adrenergic mechanisms from heart failure cause further heart muscle damage.
      5. Increases in cardiac wall tension and wall stress produce cellular hypertrophy and fibrosis in an already dilated heart.
         a) The degree of fibrosis will vary from an average of 4% to as high as 20% of the total cardiac tissue volume.
         b) In most cases, the degree of fibrosis does not cause any change in diastolic or systolic function.
      6. Because of the effect of the chamber dilation, tricuspid and mitral regurgitation are common.
   B. Restrictive cardiomyopathy involves a restrictive filling of one or both of the ventricles, usually caused by endomyocardial fibrosis and development of thrombosis of the inflow tracts. This process has been described as occurring in three distinct phases: necrotic, thrombotic, and fibrotic.
      1. Necrotic stage: An acute inflammatory reaction characterized by elevated eosinophils, causing myocardial abscesses
         a) Eventually, these abscesses may cause arteritis, causing necrosis of the cardiac muscle.
         b) Over time, the endocardium becomes thickened and mural thrombi develop.
      2. Thrombotic stage: Thrombi form in the myocardium.
         a) Thrombi can become massive, causing restriction of ventricular filling, which causes high intraventricular pressures and low cardiac output.

      b) The risk of systemic emboli increases, and the patient often does not survive this stage.

    3. Fibrotic stage: Hyaline fibrous tissue develops in attempt to heal the myocardium.

      a) No further inflammation occurs at this point.

      b) The degree of damage is determined by the effect of the thickening of the myocardium on ventricular filling and atrioventricular valve function.

C. Hypertrophic (i.e., idiopathic hypertrophic subaortic stenosis): Distinctive feature is a disproportionate thickening of the intraventricular septum, but it may involve all ventricular segments equally.

    1. The heart may appear to be normal size; however, a thickened septum results.

    2. An already hypertrophied myocardium will cause a malposition of the mitral valve leaflet during systole.

      a) The poor fit of the leaflet over a previously stretched septum will cause a narrowing of the aortic area, which results in left ventricular outflow obstruction.

      b) Myocardial ischemia occurs and is likely caused by myocardial oxygen supply-demand mismatch.

III. Clinical features: Majority of cases of dilated cardiomyopathy are idiopathic. Cardiomyopathy is classified as dilated, restrictive, or hypertrophic.

A. Etiologies

    1. Dilated cardiomyopathy is most often seen in

      a) Black men

      b) Alcoholics

      c) Peripartum women

      d) Patients suffering from an infectious process.

    2. Restrictive cardiomyopathy can result from

      a) Myocardial infiltrative diseases (e.g., amyloidosis, sarcoidosis)

      b) Storage diseases (e.g., hemachromatosis, glycogen storage disease)

      c) Endomyocardial disease (e.g., cardiac metastasis)

      d) Radiation or chemotherapy-induced (anthracyclines)

      e) A tropical form (more common)

    3. Hypertrophic cardiomyopathy usually carries a better prognosis; however, it can overlap with the other classifications.

      a) Many cases have a genetic component with mutations in the myosin heavy-chain gene that is an autosomal dominant transmission.

      b) An acquired form occurs in the elderly with chronic hypertension.

B. History

    1. History of cancer and cancer treatment

    2. Current medications: Prescribed and over-the-counter

    3. History of presenting symptom(s): Precipitating factors, onset, location, and duration. Associated symptoms are shortness of breath at rest, when active, or both; shortness of breath relieved with stop in activity; orthopnea, fatigue, palpitations, ankle or periorbital edema, chest discomfort, and leg cramping.

    4. Changes in activities of daily living

C. Signs and symptoms

1. Dilated cardiomyopathy
   a) Dyspnea on exertion
   b) Orthopnea
   c) Palpitations
   d) Fatigue, weakness
   e) Chest pain, not anginal in nature
2. Restrictive cardiomyopathy
   a) Dyspnea
   b) Fatigue
   c) Peripheral edema
3. Hypertrophic
   a) Dyspnea or breathlessness on exertion
   b) Syncope with exercise
   c) Angina (may be lessened when recumbent)
   d) Palpitations

D. Physical exam
1. Dilated cardiomyopathy
   a) Vital signs: Blood pressure will reveal a narrow pulse pressure of < 30 mm Hg.
   b) Pulmonary exam: Assess for rales, indicating pulmonary congestion.
   c) Cardiac exam
      (1) Extra heart sounds (e.g., S_3 and S_4) are commonly present.
      (2) Holosystolic murmur with plateau-shaped intensity, high-pitch, harsh blowing heard best at the apex and radiating to the left axilla indicates mitral regurgitation, which is common.
      (3) Holosystolic murmur heard best at the left lower sternum that increases with inspiration is indicative of tricuspid regurgitation, which is less common
      (4) Assess for peripheral edema.
2. Restrictive cardiomyopathy
   a) Pulmonary exam: Assess for rales and rhonchi, indicating pulmonary congestion.
   b) Cardiac exam
      (1) Regurgitation murmurs, as described above, may be present.
      (2) Apical impulse will be prominent.
      (3) Assess for jugular vein distention.
   c) Abdominal exam: Assess for hepatomegaly or ascites, indicating systemic congestion.
3. Hypertrophic cardiomyopathy
   a) Physical exam often unremarkable
   b) Cardiac exam
      (1) Coarse ejection systolic murmur at the left sternal border that radiates to the mitral or aortic area, not to the axilla or neck, and changes with Valsalva maneuver indicates decrease in preload.
      (2) Loud S_4 may be heard.
      (3) Double or triple forceful apical impulse may be present.
      (4) Bisferious (having two beats) carotid pulse indicates obstruction.

IV. Diagnostic tests
   A. Laboratory: CBC to rule out anemia
   B. Radiology: Chest x-ray
      1. May reveal cardiac enlargement or interstitial pulmonary edema indicative of dilated or hypertrophic cardiomyopathy.
      2. Chest x-ray revealing moderate cardiomegaly, pleural effusions, and pulmonary vascular congestion indicates restrictive cardiomyopathy.
   C. Other
      1. EKG
         a) Dilated: Left bundle branch block or right bundle branch block with ST-T wave abnormalities
         b) Restrictive: Low voltage, sinus tachycardia, ST-T wave abnormalities, frequent dysrhythmias, atrial fibrillation
         c) Hypertrophic: Prominent septal Q waves in lead 1, aVL, V5–6, atrial fibrillation, ventricular tachycardia
      2. Echocardiogram
         a) Dilated: Low ejection fraction < 40%
         b) Restrictive: Increased ventricular wall thickness, bilateral atrial enlargement, thickened cardiac valves
         c) Hypertrophic: Ventricular hypertrophy, asymmetrical septal hypertrophy, and a > 1.3 thickness of the left ventricular posterior walls
      3. Cardiac catheterization and MRI: Useful in distinguishing between restrictive cardiomyopathy and restrictive pericarditis.
         a) Restrictive pericarditis usually involves both ventricles, whereas restrictive cardiomyopathy impairs the left ventricle more than the right.
         b) MRI: Used to determine thickness of pericardium.

V. Differential diagnosis
   A. Endocarditis (see Chapter 44)
   B. Pericarditis (see Chapter 48)
   C. Rheumatoid arthritis (see Chapter 108)
   D. Systemic lupus erythematosus
   E. Chemical-induced: Cobalt, lead, phosphorus, carbon monoxide, mercury, cocaine, heroin, chemotherapy
   F. Duchenne's muscular dystrophy
   G. Mediastinum radiation
   H. Nutritional deficiencies (e.g., thiamin)
   I. Valvular disorder

VI. Treatment
   A. Treat underlying disease or cause
   B. Dilated cardiomyopathy
      1. Medications (dysrhythmic agents) are given to increase ventricular compliance (see Chapter 43).

    2. Symptomatic therapy is used to treat the heart failure, mainly by prescribing digoxin, diuretics, and ACE inhibitors (see Chapter 40).

    3. Long-term anticoagulant therapy is used to prevent thromboembolism (see Chapter 41).

    4. Heart transplant may be a consideration for those no longer responsive to medical therapy.

C. Restrictive cardiomyopathy

    1. Diuretics for pulmonary and systemic congestion

    2. Digoxin if left ventricular systolic dysfunction

D. Hypertrophic cardiomyopathy

    1. Avoidance of strenuous activity

    2. Medical therapy

        a) Beta-adrenergic agonist: To decrease myocardial contractility and heart rate (propranolol 160–320 mg po every day)

        b) Calcium channel antagonists: To augment diastolic ventricular filling

            (1) Verapamil 80–160 mg po every 8 hours; sustained release 120–240 mg po every day

            (2) Diltiazem 30–80 mg po every 6 hours; sustained release 60–300 mg po every day

        c) Potassium-sparing diuretics: To improve pulmonary congestion without sacrificing electrolyte balance

    3. Dual chamber pacing: To minimize left ventricular outflow tract obstruction

    4. Anticoagulation: If paroxysmal or chronic atrial fibrillation develops

    5. Surgery: Useful in treating symptoms

        a) Septal myotomy

        b) Mitral valve replacement

VII. Follow-up

A. Short-term: Ongoing evaluation and management of anticoagulation therapy

    1. Measure monthly electrolyte levels when using diuretics (especially with non-potassium-sparing medications).

    2. Monitor weight and status of water weight gain.

B. Long-term: To monitor treatment regime and progression of cardiac dysfunction

VIII. Referrals: Cardiologist for treatment plan

References

Conti, J., & Curtis, A. (1993). Antiarrhythmic therapy in patients with congestive heart failure. *Postgraduate Medicine, 94*(5), 121–137.

Farrar, D., Chow, E., & Brown, C. (1995). Isolated systolic and diastolic ventricular interactions in pacing-induced dilated cardiomyopathy and effects of volume loading and pericardium. *Circulation, 92,* 1284–1290.

Habib, F., Springall, D., Davies, G., Oakley, C., Yacoub, M., & Polak, J. (1996). Tumor necrosis factor and inducible nitric oxide synthase in dilated cardiomyopathy. *Lancet, 347,* 1151–1154.

Kato, R., Yokota, M., Ishihara, H., & Sobue, T. (1996). Correlation between left ventricular contractility and relaxation in patients with idiopathic dilated cardiomyopathy. *Clinical Cardiology, 19,* 413–418.

Man, A., Schwarz, Y., & Greif, J. (1998). Case report: Cardiac tamponade following fine needle aspiration (FNA) of a mediastinal mass. *Clinical Radiology, 53,* 151-152.

Martel, M.K., Sahijdak, W.M., Haken, R.K.T., Kessler, M.L., & Turrisi, A.T. (1998). Fraction size and dose parameters related to the incidence of pericardial effusions. *Journal of Radiation Oncology, Biology, Physics, 40,* 155–161.

Olivetti, G., Abbi, R., Quaini, F., Kajstura, J., Cheng, W., & Nitahara, J. (1997). Apoptosis in the failing heart. *New England Journal of Medicine, 336,* 1131–1141.

Shan, K., Lincoff, M., & Young, J.B. (1996). Anthracycline-induced cardiotoxicity. *Annals of Internal Medicine, 125,* 47–58.

Chapter

40. Congestive Heart Failure

Mary Ann Winokur, CRNP, MSN

I. Definition: A clinical syndrome or condition characterized by signs and symptoms of intravascular and interstitial volume overload when the heart is unable to generate a cardiac output sufficient to meet the body's metabolic needs

II. Physiology/Pathophysiology
   A. Normal
      1. In the normal individual, the cardiovascular system adjusts the total cardiac output to meet the metabolic demands of the peripheral tissues.
         a) These adjustments include alterations in ventricular rate and stroke volume.
         b) The product of these two parameters results in the cardiac output.
      2. Ventricular rate is primarily controlled by the autonomic nervous system.
         a) The parasympathetic system reduces the heart rate through cholinergic mechanisms mediated by the vagus nerve.
         b) The sympathetic nervous system increases heart rate by local and humoral release of catecholamines.
      3. Stroke volume is a function of innate cardiac contractility as well as the end diastolic pressure or preload and the impedance to flow or afterload.
         a) Increasing preload by increasing cardiac filling results in an increased stroke volume. This relationship is known as the Frank Starling Law Curve.
         b) Decreasing afterload increases stroke volume.
         c) Increasing contractility increases cardiac stroke volume.
   B. Pathophysiology
      1. The initial event in the development of heart failure is myocyte damage or overload caused by increased pressure or volume. These two factors result in increased wall tension.
      2. Ischemia results in decreased compliance secondary to scarring, asyncronous left ventricular (LV) relaxation, and remodeling
      3. Heart failure can be the result of systolic dysfunction (pump failure) and/or diastolic dysfunction (increased resistance to filling and reduced compliance).

III. Clinical features: Congestive heart failure (CHF) is a serious and common condition affecting an estimated three million Americans, resulting in average mortality rates of 10%

at one year and 50%–60% five years after diagnosis. Approximately 400,000 new cases of heart failure develop each year.

A. Etiology
1. Coronary artery disease (CAD): Underlying cause (myocardial infarction [MI] or ischemia) in 50%–75% of patients with heart failure
   a) Systolic dysfunction generally results from CAD.
   b) Diastolic dysfunction results from uncontrolled or poorly controlled hypertension.
2. Uncontrolled or poorly controlled hypertension
3. Cardiomyopathy: Idiopathic, alcohol-induced, illicit drug use, myocarditis, infiltrative processes, and some chemotherapeutic agents (anthracyclines).
4. Valvular heart disease from mitral regurgitation (MR) and aortic stenosis (AS)
5. Congenital heart disease: Accounts for only a small portion
6. Aging process

B. Functional classifications of heart disease: New York Heart Association Classification
1. Class I: No limitation of physical activity; normal activity does not cause increased fatigue, dyspnea, or anginal pain.
2. Class II: Slight limitation of physical activity is experienced; normal physical activity does cause symptoms.
3. Class III: Marked limitation of physical activity is noted; patients are comfortable at rest, but less than normal activity results in symptoms.
4. Class IV: Patients are unable to participate in any physical activity without discomfort; symptoms may be present at rest.

C. History
1. History of cancer and cancer treatment
2. Current medications: Prescribed and over-the-counter
3. History of presenting symptom(s): Precipitating factors, onset, location, and duration. Associated symptoms are shortness of breath, fatigue, chest discomfort, extremity edema, orthopnea, syncope, and paroxysmal nocturnal dyspnea.
4. Changes in activities of daily living
5. Past medical history/family history of heart disease

D. Signs and symptoms
1. Many patients with significantly impaired left ventricle (LV) function have no symptoms of heart failure.
2. Approximately 20% of patients with left ventricular ejection fractions (LVEF) of less than 40% (normal LVEF 55% or greater) meet none of the clinical criteria for heart failure.
3. Approximately 40% of patients with LVEF < 30% have dyspnea on exertion (DOE).
4. Systolic dysfunction
   a) Paroxysmal nocturnal dyspnea (PND)
   b) Orthopnea
   c) Dyspnea on exertion (DOE), which is progressive
   d) Bilateral lower extremity edema or sacral edema if bedridden (dependent edema)
   e) Decreased exercise tolerance; easy fatigability
   f) Unexplained confusion, altered mental status, or fatigue in an elderly patient
   g) Abdominal symptoms associated with ascites/hepatic engorgement

              (1) Distended abdomen
              (2) Nausea/vomiting

     5. Diastolic dysfunction
        a) DOE
        b) Orthopnea
        c) PND
        d) Weight gain: Rapid over short period of time (i.e., three to four pounds in one to three days)

E. Physical exam: Focus on cardiac and pulmonary exam
     1. Systolic dysfunction
        a) Elevated jugular venous distention (JVD)
        b) S_3
            (1) Most sensitive finding
            (2) Found in approximately 65% of patients with LVEF < 30%
        c) Laterally displaced apical impulse
        d) The above listed physical signs are the most specific and are virtually diagnostic in a patient with compatible symptoms (e.g., DOE, PND, orthopnea).
        e) Pulmonary rales that do not clear with cough
        f) Peripheral edema not caused by venous insufficiency
        g) Hepatojugular reflux
     2. Diastolic dysfunction: As many as 30%–40% of patients with heart failure have normal systolic function; however, all patients with systolic dysfunction have some degree of diastolic dysfunction.
        a) Minimally displaced, forceful point of maximal impulse (PMI) without an S_3
        b) S_4: Indicates normal left atrial pressure, a decreased rate of relaxation, and early filling; may be present for years before symptoms develop.
        c) Diastolic blood pressure > 105 and the absence of elevated JVD

IV. Diagnostic tests
  A. Laboratory
     1. CBC: Anemia as contributing factor or anemia of chronic disease
     2. Electrolytes: To evaluate for imbalances
     3. BUN/creatinine: To evaluate for evidence of impaired renal perfusion
     4. Urinalysis: Evidence of target organ disease (TOD) (proteinuria)
     5. Liver function tests (LFTs): Elevated liver enzymes indicative of hepatic congestion
     6. Prothrombin time prolonged: Indicative of hepatic congestion
     7. Thyroid function test: T_4, TSH to rule out hyperthyroidism
  B. Radiography: Chest x-ray to evaluate for cardiomegaly, left ventricle hypertrophy (LVH), pulmonary edema, pulmonary hypertension, pleural effusion
  C. Other
     1. EKG to evaluate for
        a) LVH
        b) Evidence of ischemia/infarction
     2. Echocardiography: Evaluate LV size/function, ejection fraction, rate of contraction, and changes in wall thickness to assist in confirming diagnosis.

3. Radionuclide ventriculogram: The majority of patients with heart failure have moderate to severe LV dysfunction and LVEF < 35%–40%
4. Stress testing: Evaluate ischemia as possible cause for CHF
5. Cardiac catheterization to evaluate for
   a) Evidence of pulmonary hypertension
   b) Valvular disease
   c) Coronary artery disease
   d) Pulmonary wedge pressure
6. Dysrhythmia screening evaluations: Not routinely warranted for patients with heart failure
   a) Ventricular dysrhythmias are common in patients with heart failure, and sudden death as a result of these dysrhythmias occurs in approximately 50% of patients.
   b) Atrial fibrillation is present in 10%–15% of patients and may occur in up to 50% of patients with Class III–IV heart failure.

V. Differential diagnosis
   A. Chronic obstructive pulmonary disease (COPD) (see Chapter 28)
   B. Valvular heart disease
   C. Hyperthyroidism (see Chapter 149)
   D. Angina (see Chapter 36)
   E. Renal disease
   F. Liver disease
   G. Venous insufficiency
   H. Medications
      a) Chemotherapy-induced
         (1) Anthracyclines
         (2) High-dose cyclophosphamide
         (3) 5-fluorouracil
         (4) Paclitaxel
      b) Biotherapy-induced
         (1) Alpha interferon
         (2) Interleukin
      c) Prolonged use of diuretics with recent noncompliance with medications
   I. Malnutrition: Thiamin deficiency
   J. Pelvic tumors
   K. Radiation-induced
   L. Myocardial and pericardial metastases

VI. Treatment
   A. Determine and treat underlying etiology of CHF.
   B. Systolic dysfunction
      1. Nonpharmacologic: Patient and family education and counseling on nature of disease process, signs and symptoms, treatment plan, dietary restrictions (e.g., sodium 1–2 g/day), risk factor reduction, smoking cessation, cardiac rehabilitation, compliance issues, activity recommendations, and prognosis.

2. Pharmacologic
   a) Diuretics (see Chapter 45)
      (1) Patients presenting with signs/symptoms of significant volume overload should be started immediately on a loop diuretic.
      (2) Moderate to severe overload should be treated with loop diuretics.
      (3) Mild overload can be treated with thiazide diuretics.
   b) ACE inhibitors (see Chapter 45): Use the maximum dose tolerated by the patient.
      (1) Patients with heart failure caused by left ventricular systolic dysfunction should begin taking an ACE inhibitor unless there are specific contraindications, such as history of intolerance or adverse reactions, serum potassium > 5.5 that is refractory to reduction, and symptomatic hypotension (systolic blood pressure < 90).
      (2) Start patients with serum creatinine > 3.0 on half of the usual dose, as hyperkalemia is more likely in patients with some degree of renal insufficiency.
      (3) Administration of ACE inhibitors reduces blood pressure and systemic vascular resistance (SVR) and significantly reduces left and right atrial pressures. This is accompanied by a modest increase in cardiac output, increased exercise tolerance, and improved well-being and quality of life.
   c) Inotropic agents (e.g., digoxin, dobutamine, vesnarinone, milrinone)
      (1) Digoxin: 0.125–0.25 mg/day po
         (a) Effective for patients with atrial fibrillation with a rapid ventricular response.
         (b) Can prevent clinical deterioration and improve symptoms.
         (c) Should be used routinely in patients with severe heart failure; add to therapy for patients with mild or moderate failure who remain symptomatic after optimal management with ACE inhibitors and diuretics.
      (2) Dobutamine, vesnarinone, and milrinone
         (a) Reserve for patients who no longer benefit from other inotropic agents
         (b) Start under the supervision of a cardiologist.
   d) Vasodilators: Arteriolar vasodilators (e.g., hydralazine)
      (1) A major component of heart failure is an excess increase in systemic vascular resistance (SVR); hydralazine decreases SVR and increases cardiac output.
      (2) Cardiac output increases approximately 50% along with a similar degree of reduction of SVR.
   e) Venodilators (nitrates)
      (1) Nitrates reduce atrial pressures by dilating peripheral veins and redistributing blood so that more is present in the peripheral veins and less is in the chest.
      (2) Nitrates also increase exercise tolerance.
      (3) Arteriolar vasodilators increase cardiac output and venodilators decrease filling pressures. Combining these groups of drugs has been proven to prolong life in patients with moderate heart failure (V–HeFT studies).
      (4) Hydralazine/isosorbide dinitrate (isosorbide 10–40 mg po tid/hydralazine 25 mg po tid, titrating up to 75 mg tid) also is an appropriate alternative therapy for patients with contraindications or intolerance to ACE inhibitors.
   f) Anticoagulation: Routine anticoagulation is not recommended unless patient has

a history of systemic or pulmonary embolism, recent atrial fibrillation, or a mobile LV thrombus (see Chapter 41).

g) Special considerations for systolic dysfunction
   (1) For patients with systolic dysfunction and angina who are not candidates for revascularization, nitrates and aspirin are the drugs of choice.
   (2) As a result of their negative inotropic effect, calcium channel blockers and beta-blockers should be used only under the supervision of a cardiologist.
   (3) One beta-blocker (carvedilol) and two calcium channel blockers (felodipine, amlodipine) currently are approved and recommended for the treatment of CHF.

C. Diastolic dysfunction
   1. Control heart rate and maintain normal sinus rhythm: Tachycardia will reduce cardiac output by decreasing filling time and will increase ischemic episodes. Beta–blockers and calcium channel blockers are the drugs of choice for diastolic dysfunction, as they decrease oxygen consumption and ischemia, thereby improving relaxation.
   2. Inotropic (digoxin): May worsen diastolic dysfunction by increasing oxygen consumption and decreasing the filling time.
   3. Prevent/reduce LV hypertrophy: Treat the underlying condition (e.g., antihypertensive, valve replacement).
   4. Prevent ischemia: Use beta-blockers, calcium channel blockers, nitrates, and revascularization.
   5. Relieve venous congestion: Vigorous diuresis will result in decreased filling pressures and is not tolerated in patients with diastolic dysfunction, as they require higher filling pressures. Cautious use of diuretics is prudent.

VII. Follow-up
   A. Telephone or return clinic visit: Within 24 hours of initiating treatment
   B. Return clinic appointment: Within two weeks until patient's weight stabilizes and symptoms resolve, then every three to six months.
   C. Laboratory follow-up: Depends on therapy initiated
      1. Potassium levels: For patients starting diuretics and ACE inhibitors; weekly during titration
      2. Serum creatinine: For patients started on diuretics and ACE inhibitors
      3. Digoxin levels: 7–10 days after treatment initiated and, if stable, every three to six months
         a) Repeat levels for worsening heart failure.
         b) Repeat levels if deterioration in renal function.
         c) Repeat levels if signs of toxicity (e.g., confusion, nausea, visual disturbances) are present.
         d) Concomitant use of digoxin can alter the plasma level of numerous drugs (e.g., quinidine, verapamil, amiodarone, antibiotics, calcium channel blockers, erythromycin, phenobarbital, anticholinergic agents); check digoxin levels one week after initiation of any of these medications.
      4. During exacerbation, monitor PT because of increased incidence of bleeding.

    E. Patient education: Signs and symptoms requiring immediate attention

    F. Home-health referral: For homebound patients

VIII. Referrals

    A. Emergency room and cardiologist: Immediately refer for

        1. Cardiogenic shock

           a) Most commonly seen postmyocardial infarction.

           b) Other causes include acute mitral regurgitation, myocarditis, dilated cardiomy-opathy, dysrhythmia, and pericardial tamponade.

        2. Pulmonary edema.

    B. Internist/cardiologist

        1. Newly diagnosed patients

        2. Patients with heart failure with complicating conditions (e.g., renal failure, liver failure)

        3. Patients with signs/symptoms of dysrhythmias

        4. Patients who deteriorate after stabilization

References

Baker, D.W., Konstam, M.A., Bottorff, M., & Pitt, B. (1994). Management of heart failure: Pharmacologic treatment. *JAMA, 272,* 1361–1366.

Beattie, S., & Pike, C. (1996). Left ventricular diastolic dysfunction: A case report. *Critical Care Nurse, 16*(2), 37–50.

Carson, P.E., Johnson, G.R., Dunkman, W.B., Fletcher, R.D., Farrell, L., & Cohn, J.N. (1993). The influence of atrial fibrillation on prognosis in mild to moderate heart failure. The V-HeFT studies. The V-HeFT VA cooperative study group. *Circulation, 87,* 1102–1110.

Cash, L.A. (1996). Heart failure from diastolic dysfunction. *Dimensions in Critical Care, 15*(4), 170–177.

Edwards, V. (1991). Recognition and management of heart failure in the primary care setting. *Nurse Practitioner Forum, 2*(1), 42–47.

Lilly, L.S. (1993). Heart failure. In L.S. Lilly (Ed.), *Pathophysiology of heart disease* (pp.147–165). Philadelphia: Lea & Febiger.

Packer, M., & Cohen, J. (1999). Consensus recommendations for the management of chronic heart failure. On behalf of the membership of the Advisory Council to Improve Outcomes Nationwide in Heart Failure (Review). *American Journal of Cardiology, 83*(2A), 1A–38A.

Sullivan, M.J. & Hawthorne, M.H. (1996). Non-pharmacologic interventions in treatment of heart failure. *Journal of Cardiovascular Nursing, 10*(2), 47–57.

U.S. Department of Health and Human Services. (1994). *Heart failure: Evaluation and care of patients with left-ventricular systolic dysfunction. Clinical practice guideline, no. 11* (AHCPR Publication No. 94-0612). Washington, DC: Author.

Wilson, B.E., & Newmark, S.R. (1994). Thyrotoxicosis-induced congestive heart failure in an urban hospital. *American Journal of the Medical Sciences, 308,* 344–348.

Wright, J.M. (1995). Pharmacologic management of congestive heart failure. *Critical Care Nursing Quarterly, 18*(1), 32–44.

Chapter

41. Deep Vein Thrombosis

Kristine Turner Story, RN, MSN, ARNP

I. Definition: A thrombus in the deep veins that obstructs blood flow and may produce emboli

II. Pathophysiology
   A. A thrombus starts as a clot nidus in the setting of stasis, endothelial injury, and a hypercoagulable state (Virchow's triad).
   B. The clot nidus, composed of RBCs, fibrin, and platelets, propagates to fill the vein lumen, causing partial or complete obstruction of blood flow, or may shed emboli.
   C. The thrombus may float freely in the blood vessel, leading to embolization.

III. Clinical features: Classic physical findings in deep vein thrombosis (DVT) include a unilateral swollen, erythematous, warm extremity. The most common sites include anterior and posterior tibial veins, peroneal veins, popliteal veins, and superficial and deep femoral veins. Diagnosis based on clinical findings alone is accurate only 50% of the time. A statistically significant correlation exists between idiopathic DVT and later symptomatic development of cancer.
   A. Risk factors
      1. A model for predicting DVT has recently been identified and is outlined in Figure 41-1.
      2. Other risk factors include
         a) Sepsis
         b) Presence of a vascular access device
         c) Cardiac disease
         d) Obesity
         e) Antithrombin III deficiency
         f) Protein S and protein C deficiency
         g) Activated protein C resistance (factor V Leiden)
         h) Dysfibrinogenemia
         i) Thrombocytosis
         j) Systemic lupus erythematosus
         k) Presence of antiphospholipid antibodies
         l) Polycythemia vera
         m) Recent surgery

Figure 41-1. Clinical Predictors for Deep Vein Thrombosis

Major Factors
- Active cancer
- Paralysis or recent casting of a lower limb
- Recently bedridden for more than three days and/or major surgery within four weeks
- Localized tenderness along the deep venous system
- Swollen calf or thigh by measurement
- Calf swelling of more than 3 cm in symptomatic leg
- Strong family history of deep venous thrombosis (DVT)

Minor Factors
- Hospitalization in the last six months
- Leg trauma in the last 60 days
- Findings in symptomatic leg only
  - Pitting edema
  - Dilated superficial veins
  - Erythema

Probability of DVT Based on Clinical Predictors
- High probability: 85%
  no alternative diagnosis with $\geq$ three major factors
  or
  $\geq$ two major factors + $\geq$ two minor factors
- Moderate probability: 33%
  all patients without a high or low probability of DVT
- Low probability: 5%
  no alternative diagnosis with one major factor + $\leq$ one minor factors
  or
  no alternative diagnosis with no major factors and $\leq$ two minor factors
  or
  has alternative diagnosis with one major factor and $\leq$ two minor factors
  or
  has alternative diagnosis with no major factors and $\leq$ three minor factors

Note. From "Accuracy of Clinical Assessment of Deep Vein Thrombosis" by P.S. Wells, J. Hirsh, D.R. Anderson, A.W. Lensing, G. Foster, C. Kearon, J. Weitz, R. D'Ovidio, A. Cogo, & P. Prandoni, 1995, *Lancet, 345*, pp. 1326–1330. Copyright 1995 by *The Lancet Ltd.* Reprinted with permission.

B. History
 1. History of cancer and cancer treatment
 2. Current medications: Prescribed and over-the-counter
 3. History of presenting symptom(s): Precipitating factors, onset, location, and duration. Associated symptoms are chest pain and shortness of breath.
 4. Changes in activities of daily living
 5. Past medical history of DVT, cardiac disease
C. Signs and symptoms
 1. A dull ache, tight feeling, or frank pain in the calf, especially with walking
 2. Distention of the superficial venous collateral vessels
 3. Slight fever possible
 4. Tenderness over the involved vein
D. Physical exam
 1. Vital signs: Fever and tachycardia
 2. Integument exam
  a) Skin cyanotic: If severe obstruction
  b) Skin pale and cool: If reflex arterial spasm is superimposed
 3. Extremities exam
  a) Unilateral edema in the involved extremity (may not have obvious swelling if early)
  b) Warmth and erythema of involved extremity
  c) Thigh or calf tenderness to palpation
  d) Tender palpable venous cord of involved vein
  e) Homan's sign: Positive in less than 50% of cases and has high incidence of false-positives (calf pain produced with dorsiflexion of the foot)

IV. Diagnostic tests
   A. Laboratory
       1. D-dimer test: A negative result has shown a high negative predictive value for DVT in patients without cancer but does not reliably exclude DVT in patients with cancer.
       2. Consider obtaining antithrombin III, protein C and S, and antiphospholipid antibodies if recurrent disease or no risk factors.
   B. Radiology
       1. Doppler ultrasonography: Measures venous patency by detecting the movement of red blood cells through the vein.
           a) Has a sensitivity and specificity of 95% with a skilled operator, is noninvasive and inexpensive.
           b) Is less reliable for diagnosing DVT in calf veins than contrast venography.
       2. Impedance plethysmography: Measures changes in the venous volume of the leg and detects impaired venous emptying.
           a) Has a sensitivity and specificity of 95% with a skilled operator; is noninvasive and inexpensive.
           b) Is less reliable for diagnosing DVT in calf veins than contrast venography.
           c) At least one study has shown decreased sensitivity and specificity of impedance plethysmography in patients with cancer as compared to patients without cancer.
       3. Contrast venography: Determines presence of DVT by use of contrast material infused into the venous system by a catheter in the foot.
           a) Is the gold standard for diagnosing DVT.
           b) Is expensive, invasive, and is difficult to perform in the critically ill patient, patients with edema or cellulitis, and patients with well-developed collateral circulation.
           c) Equipment is not portable.
       4. Radionuclide scintigraphy: Uses various radiopharmaceuticals to detect DVT.
           a) Less reliable in the calf and cannot differentiate intrinsic from extrinsic compression.
           b) Not as reliable in recurrent DVT.
           c) Expensive and requires delayed imaging after nucleotide injected.
           d) May complement negative or equivocal doppler studies, especially in surgical patients and in patients with low or intermediate probability lung scans.

V. Differential diagnosis
   A. Calf muscle strain or tear
   B. Intramuscular hematoma
   C. Cellulitis (see Chapter 16)
   D. Superficial phlebitis (see Chapter 157)
   E. Obstruction of lymphatics by tumor, from irradiation, or lymph node dissection
   F. Acute arterial occlusion
   G. Ruptured Baker's cyst
   H. Chronic venous insufficiency
   I. Lymphangitis/fibrositis
   J. Kidney, liver, or heart disease: Usually has bilateral edema
   K. Hypoalbuminemia

VI. Treatment
    A. Prevention of DVT in high-risk patients
        1. Elevation of foot of bed 15°–20° with slight knee flexion
        2. Frequent leg exercises: Every two hours if bedridden to improve venous flow
        3. Use of elastic stockings or intermittent pneumatic compression devices
        4. Aspirin: 81–325 mg po qd
        5. Low-dose SC heparin: 5,000 units two hours preoperative, then q 8–12 hours for lower abdominal, pelvic, and lower extremity surgeries. Consult surgeon prior to prescribing.
        6. Low-molecular weight heparin: For lower abdominal, pelvic, and hip or knee replacement surgeries
            a) Enoxaparin (Lovenox®, Rhône-Poulenc Rorer Pharmaceuticals, Inc., Collegeville, PA): 40 mg SC two hours preoperative, then qd for 7–10 days for abdominal/pelvic surgery, 30 mg SC bid, starting 12–24 hours postop for 7–10 days for hip/knee replacement. Consult surgeon prior to prescribing.
            b) Ardeparin (Normiflo®, Wyeth-Ayerst Pharmaceuticals, Philadelphia, PA): 50 U/kg SC q 12 hours for 14 days, starting evening or day following surgery; indicated for knee replacement only.
            c) Danaparoid (Orgaran®, Organon, Inc., West Orange, NJ): 750 anti-Xa units SC bid for 7–10 days, starting one to four hours preoperative; indicated only for hip replacement surgery. Consult surgeon prior to prescribing.
            d) Dalteprin (Fragmin®, Pharmacia & Upjohn, Peapack, NJ): 2,500 IU SC qd for 5–10 days, starting one to two hours preoperative; use 5,000 IU for patients with malignancy; indicated only for abdominal surgery. Consult surgeon prior to prescribing.
    B. Treatment of existing DVT
        1. Continuous IV infusion of heparin is the gold standard to anticoagulate, prevent distal migration of thrombus, and decrease future thrombi (see Figures 41-2 and 41-3).

Figure 41-2. Guidelines for Anticoagulation: Unfractionated Heparin

---

Disease suspected:
- Obtain baseline activated partial thromboplastin time (APTT), prothrombin time, CBC.
- Check for contraindication to heparin therapy.
- Give heparin 5,000 U IV push, and order imaging study.

Disease confirmed:
- Rebolus with heparin 80 IU/kg IV, and start maintenance infusion at 18 U/kg.
- Check APTT q six hours to maintain in a range that corresponds to a therapeutic blood heparin level.
- Check platelets daily.
- Start warfarin therapy on day one at 5 mg, and adjust subsequent daily dose according to PT/international normalizing ratio (INR).
- Stop heparin therapy after approximately four to five days of combined therapy when INR is >2.0 for two consecutive days.
- Anticoagulate with warfarin for at least three months at an INR of 2.0 to 3.0.

Note. From "Antithrombotic Therapy for Venous Thrombolic Disease" by T.M. Hyers, G. Agnelli, R.D. Hull, J.G. Weg, T.A. Morris, M. Samama, and V. Tapson, 1998, *Chest, 114*(Suppl. 5), p. 565S. Copyright 1998 by the American College of Chest Physicians. Reprinted with permission.

Figure 41-3. Body Weight-Base Dosing of IV Heparin

Heparin 25,000 IU in 250 ml D$_5$W, infused at a rate dictated by body weight through an infusion apparatus calibrated for low flow rates

Activated partial thromboplastin time (APTT)	Dose Change (U/kg/h)	Additional Action	*Next APTT
< 35 (< 1.2 x mean normal)	+4	Rebolus with 80 IU/kg	Six hours
35–45 (1.2–1.5 x mean normal)	+2	Rebolus with 40 IU/kg	Six hours
47–70 (1.5–2.3 x mean normal)	0	0	Six hours
71–90 (2.3–3.0 x mean normal)	-2	0	Six hours
> 90 (> 3 x mean normal)	-3	Stop infusion for one hour	Six hours

*During the first 24 hours, repeat APTT every six hours; thereafter, monitor APTT once every morning unless it is outside the therapeutic range.

Note. From "Antithrombotic Therapy for Venous Thrombolic Disease" by T.M. Hyers, G. Agnelli, R.D. Hull, J.G. Weg, T.A. Morris, M. Samama, and V. Tapson, 1998, *Chest, 114*(Suppl. 5), p. 565S. Copyright 1998 by the American College of Chest Physicians. Reprinted with permission.

2. Recurrence or progression of DVT is 15 times more frequent when therapeutic APTT is not reached within the first 48 hours of treatment.
3. Heparin is contraindicated in the following conditions.
    a) Underlying coagulopathy (e.g., von Willebrands disease, hemophilia, vitamin K deficiency)
    b) Surgical procedure in the preceding two weeks
    c) Thrombocytopenia
    d) Trauma
    e) CNS disease (e.g., stroke, arteriovenous malformation, brain metastasis)
    f) Severe, uncontrolled hypertension
    g) Active bleeding
    h) Heparin allergy
4. Initiate warfarin (Coumadin®, Dupont Pharmaceuticals Company, Wilmington, DE) therapy (see Figure 41-4), and discontinue heparin when the therapeutic PT/INR is reached.
    a) Warfarin is not as effective as initial therapy because anticoagulation takes several days.
    b) Without initial heparinization, cutaneous necrosis can occur in individuals deficient in protein C and S when warfarin is started initially.
    c) The duration of warfarin therapy varies based on clinical and patient factors (see Figure 41-5).
    d) Monitor dosages more closely in patients receiving concomitant medications that may affect warfarin (see Table 41-1).
5. Low-molecular weight heparin (LMWH) rather than IV heparin is gaining favor as a treatment for DVT in selected patients with uncomplicated DVT in an outpatient setting (see Table 41-2).

Figure 41-4. Initiation and Dose Adjustment of Warfarin in Deep Vein Thrombosis

- Start warfarin and heparin on the same day, if possible.
- Obtain baseline prothrombin time (PT)/international normalizing ratio (INR).
- Start with 5 mg po qd.
- Repeat PT/INR the next day.
- Repeat warfarin dose if PT/INR unchanged.
- Obtain daily PT/INR until value is in therapeutic range.
- Reduce warfarin dose when PT/INR starts to rise.
- Overlap heparin with warfarin until at least two consecutive PT/INR values are in the therapeutic range.

Adjust total weekly warfarin dose using the following guidelines

INR	Adjustment
1.1–1.4	Day 1: Add 10%–20% of total weekly dose (TWD) of warfarin. Weekly: Increase TWD by 10%–20%. Return: One week for PT/INR
1.5–1.9	Day 1: Add 5%–10% of TWD. Weekly: Increase TWD by 5%–10%. Return: Two weeks for PT/INR
2.0–3.0	No change. Return: Four weeks for PT/INR
3.1–3.9	Day 1: Subtract 5%–10% of TWD. Weekly: Reduce TWD by 5%–10%. Return: Two weeks for PT/INR
4.0–5.0	Day 1: No warfarin. Weekly: Reduce TWD by 10%–20%. Return: One week for PT/INR
> 5.0	Stop warfarin; monitor INR until 3.0 is reached. Weekly: reduce TWD by 20%–50%. Return: Daily for PT/INR

Recommended INR levels

1.2–1.5	For indwelling devices
2.0–3.0	To prevent thrombus in high-risk situations (e.g., high-risk surgery, chronic recurrent DVT, atrial fibrillation)
2.5–3.5	To prevent recurrent thrombus in patients with mechanical valves

Note. From "Antithrombotic Therapy for Venous Thrombolic Disease" by T.M. Hyers, G. Agnelli, R.D. Hull, J.G. Weg, T.A. Morris, M. Samama, and V. Tapson, 1998, *Chest, 114*(Suppl. 5), p. 565S. Copyright 1998 by the American College of Chest Physicians. Reprinted with permission.

    a) Enoxaprin is currently the only LMWH approved by the U.S. Food and Drug Administration (FDA) for this indication.

    b) Correct dosing in extremely obese patients and in patients with renal insufficiency is unclear.

    c) Further studies are necessary to validate this therapy in high-risk patients.

  6. Placement of a vena cava filter to prevent pulmonary embolism in recurrent DVT has been advocated, but a recent study suggests that the filters may not be beneficial and may actually increase the risk of recurrent DVT.

Figure 41-5. Duration of Warfarin Therapy

Three to six months
- Reversible or time-limited risk factors and a first event
- Heterozygous activated protein C resistance

At least six months
- Idiopathic etiology and a first event

Twelve months to lifetime
- Recurrent disease for any etiology
- First event with the following etiologies:
  - Cancer, until resolved
  - Homozygous activated protein C resistance
  - Antiphospholipid antibody, until resolved
  - Deficiency of antithrombin, protein C or S

Note. From "Antithrombotic Therapy for Venous Thrombolic Disease" by T.M. Hyers, G. Agnelli, R.D. Hull, J.G. Weg, T.A. Morris, M. Samama, and V. Tapson, 1998, *Chest, 114*(Suppl. 5), p. 568S. Copyright 1998 by the American College of Chest Physicians. Reprinted with permission.

Table 41-1. Drug and Food Interactions with Warfarin by Level of Supporting Evidence

Level of Evidence	Potentiation	Inhibition
I.	Alcohol (if concomitant liver disease), amiodarone, anabolic steroids, cimetidine, clofibrate, cotrimoxazole, erythromycin, fluconazole, isoniazid, metronidazole, miconazole, omeprazole, phenylbutazone, piroxicam, propafenone, propranolol, sulfinpyrazone	Barbiturates, carbamazepine, chlordiazepoxide, cholestyramine, griseofulvin, nafcillin, rifampin, sucralfate, high Vitamin K-content foods or enteral feedings, large amounts of avocados
II.	Acetaminophen, chloral hydrate, ciprofloxacin, dextropropoxyphene, disulfiram, itraconazole, quinidine, phenytoin, tamoxifen, tetracycline, flu vaccine	Dicloxacillin
III.	Acetylsalicylic acid, disopyramide, 5-fluorouracil, ifosfamide, ketoprofen, lovastatin, metolazone, moricizine, nalidixic acid, norfloxacin, ofloxacin, propoxyphene, sulindac, tolmetin, topical salicylate	Azathioprine, cyclosporine etretinate, trazadone
IV.	Cefamandole, cefazolin, gemfibrozil, heparin, indomethacin, sulfisoxazole	

Level I: Highest level of evidence based on research
Level IV: Lowest level of evidence based on historic cohort studies

Note. From "Anticoagulants: Mechanisms of Actions, Clinical Effectiveness, and Optimal Therapeutic Range" by J. Hirsh, J.E. Dalen, D.R. Anderson, L. Poller, J. Bussey, J. Ansell, D. Deykin, and J.T. Brandt, 1998, *Chest, 114*(Suppl. 5), p. 448S. Copyright 1998 by the American College of Chest Physicians. Reprinted with permission.

      7. The Fifth ACCP Consensus Conference on Antithrombotic Therapy (1998) recommends use of warfarin 1 mg po qd in patients with long-term indwelling central venous catheters to prevent axillary-subclavian venous thrombosis.

VII. Follow-up
    A. Short-term
       1. Frequent dose adjustments of warfarin may be necessary; follow guidelines in Figure 41- 4.

Figure 41-6. Guidelines for Anticoagulation: Low-Molecular Weight Heparin

---

Disease suspected:
• Obtain baseline activated partial thromboplastin time (APTT), prothrombin time (PT), CBC.
• Check for contraindication to heparin therapy.
• Give unfractionated heparin 5,000 U IV, and order imaging study.

Disease confirmed:
• Give enoxaprin (Lovenox®, Rhône-Poulenc Rorer Pharmaceuticals, Inc., Collegeville, PA) 1 mg/kg subcutaneously every 12 hours.
• Start warfarin therapy on day one at 5 mg po, and adjust the subsequent daily dose according to international normalizing ratio (INR).
• Consider checking a platelet count between days three and five.
• Stop low molecular weight heparin therapy after at least four to five days of combined therapy when INR is > 2.0 for two consecutive days.
• Anticoagulate with warfarin for a least three months at an INR of 2.0 to 3.0.

Note. From "Antithrombotic Therapy for Venous Thrombolic Disease" by T.M. Hyers, G. Agnelli, R.D. Hull, J.G. Weg, T.A. Morris, M. Samama, and V. Tapson, 1998, *Chest, 114*(Suppl.5), p. 567S. Copyright 1998 by the American College of Chest Physicians. Reprinted with permission.

---

    2. If patient is symptomatic and high-risk with a negative impedance plethysmography or Doppler ultrasound, possibly repeat testing in four to six days.

    3. Monitor for the serious complication of heparin-induced thrombocytopenia (HIT).

       a) Suspect if the platelet count falls by > 50%.

       b) HIT typically develops at a median of 10 days (ranges from 3–15 days) after exposure to heparin but may occur earlier in patients who have been previously sensitized to heparin.

B. Long-term

    1. A postphlebotic syndrome characterized by some combination of chronic vascular insufficiency, chronic pain, venous stasis, recurrent cellulitis, and ulceration can occur in up to 50% of people with DVT. This syndrome may be disabling in a minority of patients.

    2. Recurrence of DVT is common; instruct patients to immediately report signs and symptoms of recurrence.

    3. Consider long-term heparin therapy if a patient cannot take oral medications or if the thrombus is refractory to warfarin (paraneoplastic syndrome), peptic ulcer disease, alcoholism, or hepatic disorders.

    4. Discontinue anticoagulants three to five days prior to invasive procedures.

VIII. Referrals: Vascular surgeon for complicated cases or if chronic sequelae exist.

References

Banerjee, A. (1997). The assessment of acute calf pain. *Postgraduate Medical Journal, 73,* 86–88.

Barloon, T.J., Bergus, G.R., & Seabold, J.E. (1997). Diagnostic imaging of lower limb deep venous thrombosis. *American Family Physician, 56,* 791–801.

Bergqvist, D. (1996). Low molecular weight heparins. *Journal of Internal Medicine, 240,* 63–72.

Berry, B.R., & Nantel, S. (1996). Heparin therapy, current regimens and principles of monitoring. *Postgraduate Medicine, 99*(6), 64–76.

Brigden, M.L. (1996). Oral anticoagulant therapy, practical aspects of management. *Postgraduate Medicine, 99*(6), 81–102.

Decousus, H., Leizorovicz, A., & Parent, F. (1998). A clinical trial of vena caval filters in the prevention of pulmonary embolism in patients with proximal deep vein thrombosis. *New England Journal of Medicine, 338,* 409–415.

Eftychioou, V. (1996). Clinical diagnosis and management of the patient with deep venous thrombosis and acute pulmonary embolism. *Nurse Practitioner, 21*(3), 50–69.

Gould, M.K., Dembitzer, A.D., Sanders, G.D., & Garber, A.M. (1999). Low-molecular weight heparins compared with unfractionated heparin for treatment of acute deep venous thrombosis. A cost effectiveness analysis. *Annals of Internal Medicine, 130,* 789–799.

Hirsh, J., Dalen, J.E., Anderson, D.R., Poller, L., Bussey, J., Ansell, J., Deykin, D., & Brandt, J.T. (1998). Anticoagulants: Mechanisms of actions, clinical effectiveness, and optimal therapeutic range. *Chest, 114,* 445S–469S.

Hyers, T.M., Agnelli, G., Hull, R.D., Weg, J.G., Morris, T.A., Samama, M., & Tapson, V. (1998). Antithrombotic therapy for venous thrombolic disease. *Chest, 114,* 561S–578S.

Keefe, D.L., Roistacher, N., & Pierri, M.K. (1994). Evaluation of suspected deep vein thrombosis in oncologic patients. *Angiology, 45,* 771–775.

Koopman, M.M.W., Prandoni, P., Piovella, F., Ockelford, P.A., Brandjes, D.P.M., Van der Meer, J., Gallus, A.S., Simmonneau, G., Chesterman, C.H., Prins, M.H., Bossuyt, P.M.M., de Haes, H., Van den Belt, A.G.M., Sagnard, L., D'Azemar, P., & Buller, H.R. (1996). Treatment of venous thrombosis with intravenous unfractionated heparin administered in the hospital as compared with subcutaneous low-molecular weight heparin administered at home. *New England Journal of Medicine, 334,* 682–687.

Lee, A.Y.Y., Julian, J.A., Levine, M.N., Weitz, J.I., Kearon, C., Wells, P.S., Ginsberg, J.S. (1999). Clinical utility of a rapid whole-blood D-dimer assay in patients with cancer who present with suspected acute deep venous thrombosis. *Annals of Internal Medicine, 131,* 417–423.

Levine, M., Gent, M., Hirsh, J., LeClerc, J., Anderson, D., Weitz, J., Ginsberg, J., Turpie, A., Demers, C., Kovacs, M., Geerts, W., Kassis, J., Desjardins, L., Cusson, J., Cruickshank, M., Powers, P., Brien, W., Haley, S., & Willan, A. (1996). A comparison of low-molecular-weight heparin administered primarily at home with unfractionated heparin administered in the hospital for proximal deep vein thrombosis. *New England Journal of Medicine, 334,* 677–681.

Prandoni, P., Lensing, A.W.A., Buller, H.R., Cogo, A., Prins, M.H., Cattelan, A.M., Cuppini, S., Noventa, F., & Ten Cate, J.W. (1992). Deep-vein thrombosis and the incidence of subsequent symptomatic cancer. *New England Journal of Medicine, 327,* 1128–1133.

Selig, P.M. (1996). Management of anticoagulation therapy with the international normalized ratio. *Journal of the American Academy of Nurse Practitioners, 8,* 77–80.

Stephen, J.M., & Feied, C.F. (1995). Venous thrombosis, lifting the clouds of misunderstanding. *Postgraduate Medicine, 97,* 36–47.

Wells, P.S., Hirsh, J., Anderson, D.R., Lensing, A.W., Foster, G., Kearon, C., Weitz, J., D'Ovidio, R., Cogo, A., & Prandoni, P. (1995). Accuracy of clinical assessment of deep-vein thrombosis. *Lancet, 345,* 1326–1330.

42. Dyslipidemia

Diane G. Cope, PhD, ARNP-CS, AOCN®

I. Definition: Disorders characterized by an elevation in serum cholesterol, low-density lipoprotein (LDL), or triglyceride concentrations or a decrease in the high-density lipoprotein (HDL)

II. Physiology/Pathophysiology
   A. Normal physiology: Serum cholesterol is a measure of normal body production of cholesterol plus dietary intake of cholesterol.
      1. Lipids, such as cholesterol and triglycerides, are complex proteins (i.e., lipoproteins) that circulate in the blood.
      2. Lipoprotein-protein components are known as apoproteins, which have a structural and functional role.
      3. Four major classes of lipoproteins are based on density.
         a) Chylomicrons: Derived from dietary fat and carry triglycerides
            (1) Low-density
            (2) Lipoprotein lipase removes triglyceride.
            (3) Patients deficient in this enzyme have high triglyceride levels and increased risk for pancreatitis.
         b) Very low density lipoproteins (VLDL): Triglyceride-rich and acted on by lipoprotein lipase
            (1) Function to carry triglycerides synthesized in the liver and intestines to capillary beds in adipose tissue and muscle where they are hydrolyzed.
            (2) After triglyceride removal, VLDL is further metabolized to LDL.
            (3) VLDLs serve as recepters of cholesterol transferred from HDL, which is mediated by the enzyme cholesterol ester transfer protein (CETP).
            (4) Has no role in atherogenesis
         c) LDLs: Major carriers of cholesterol
            (1) Most clearly implicated in atherogenesis
            (2) When LDLs exceed, they traverse the endothelial wall and become trapped in the arterial intima.
         d) HDLs: Believed to function in peripheral tissues as receptors of free cholesterol
            (1) Cholesterol is esterified and stored in the central core of HDL.
            (2) HDL cholesterol concentration is most predictive of coronary heart disease (CHD).

B. Pathophysiology: High blood cholesterol levels are a result of hepatic dysfunction in the production of LDL receptors, which facilitate absorption of LDL and circulating cholesterol.

III. Clinical features: Dyslipidemia may be asymptomatic or may be associated with other disorders. Therefore, clinical manifestations may be present as a result of other symptom disorders.
    A. Etiology: See Figure 42-1
    B. Risk factors: See Figure 42-2
        1. Increased dietary fat
        2. Genetic variations in lipoprotein structures, receptors, and metabolic enzymes
        3. Obesity
        4. Sedentary lifestyle
    C. History
        1. History of cancer and cancer treatment
        2. Current medications: Prescribed and over-the-counter
        3. History of presenting symptom(s): Precipitating factors, onset, location, and duration

Figure 42-1. Etiology of Secondary Dyslipidemia

Increased LDL Level	Increased Triglyceride Level	Decreased HDL Level
• Diabetes mellitus	• Alcoholism	• Cigarette smoking
• Hypothyroidism	• Diabetes mellitus	• Diabetes mellitus
• Nephrotic syndrome	• Hypothyroidism	• Hypertriglyceridemia
• Obstructive liver disease	• Obesity	• Menopause
• Steroids	• Renal insufficiency	• Obesity
• Progestin	• Beta-adrenergic blockers	• Uremia
• Beta-adrenergic blockers	• Estrogens	• Steroids
• Thiazides	• Ticlopidine	• Beta-adrenergic blockers
		• Progestins

Figure 42-2. Coronary Heart Disease Risk Factors

Positive Risk Factors	Negative Risk Factor
• Men: ≥ 45 years	• High HDL level: ≥ 60 mg/dl
• Women: ≥ 55 years or postmenopausal without estrogen replacement therapy	
• Family history of premature coronary heart disease: Myocardial infarction in father before age 55 or in mother before age 65	
• Cigarette smoking	
• Hypertension: Blood pressure > 140/90 mm Hg or taking antihypertensive medications	
• HDL level < 35 mg/dl	
• Diabetes mellitus	
• Stress: Job, family, personal	

Note. Subtract one positive risk factor if negative risk factor is present.

Note. Based on information from Blake & Triplett, 1995; Expert Panel on Detection, Evaluation, and Treatment of High Blood Cholesterol in Adults, 1993; LaRosa, 1998.

4. Changes in activities of daily living
5. Family history: Heart disease, endocrine disorders
6. Social history: Tobacco use, alcohol intake, diet
D. Signs and symptoms: Nonspecific
E. Physical exam
1. Vital signs: Blood pressure may be increased.
2. Cardiac exam: May note carotid or aortic bruits or cardiac murmurs.

IV. Diagnostic tests
A. Laboratory
1. Measure total cholesterol and HDL levels in a nonfasting state every five years beginning at age 20 in patients without evidence of CHD or positive risk factors.
2. If cholesterol, HDL, or triglyceride concentrations are elevated in a patient without known CHD, perform a lipoprotein analysis (see Table 42-1).
3. Diagnosis is based on repeat measurements of lipids; a single measurement of cholesterol is insufficient.
B. Radiology: Not indicated

V. Differential diagnosis
A. Diabetes mellitus (see Chapter 143)
B. Laboratory error

VI. Treatment
A. Initiation of treatment is based on the LDL level and the presence of CHD risk factors (see Table 42-2).
B. Patients with no history of CHD but with multiple risk factors or patients with known CHD and less than 100 mg/dl, LDL level should be treated by diet modifications, regular physical activity program, and smoking cessation.
C. Diet therapy: Evaluate cholesterol levels of patients on Step I diet at six and 12 weeks of Step I diet therapy. If no reduction in levels, move to Step II diet.
1. Step I diet
   a) Saturated fats: 8%–10% of total calories
   b) Cholesterol intake: < 300 mg/day

Table 42-1. Lipoprotein Analysis

Classification	Total Cholesterol Level	LDL Level	HDL Level	Triglycerides
Desirable	200 mg/dl	< 130 mg/dl	≥ 60 mg/dl	< 200 mg/dl
Borderline high-risk	200–239 mg/dl	130–159 mg/dl	35–59 mg/dl	200–400 mg/dl
High-risk	≥ 240 mg/dl	≥ 160 mg/dl	< 35 mg/dl	400–1,000 mg/dl

Note. Based on information from Blake & Triplett, 1995; Expert Panel on Detection, Evaluation, and Treatment of High Blood Cholesterol in Adults, 1993; LaRosa, 1998.

Table 42-2. Treatment Initiation and Target Low Density Lipoprotein Levels

Classification	LDL Treatment Initiation Levels		Target Levels
	Diet Therapy	Drug Therapy	
No coronary heart disease (CHD); < two risk factors	> 160 mg/dl	> 190 mg/dl	< 160 mg/dl
No CHD; > two risk factors	> 130 mg/dl	> 160 mg/dl	< 130 mg/dl
CHD or other atherosclerotic disease	> 100 mg/dl	> 130 mg/dl	< 100 mg/dl

Note. Based on information from Blake & Triplett, 1995; Expert Panel on Detection, Evaluation, and Treatment of High Blood Cholesterol in Adult, 1993; LaRosa, 1998.

   2. Step II diet
      a) Saturated fats: < 7% of total calories
      b) Cholesterol intake: < 200 mg/day
   D. Regular physical activity program
      1. Individualized program
      2. Aerobic exercise for 30 minutes four or more times/week
   E. Weight reduction program with goal of ideal body weight
   F. Drug therapy
      1. Consider patients with an elevated LDL level after six months of diet therapy.
      2. Obtain baseline LFTs, as drug therapy can increase liver function enzymes.
         a) Bile acid-binding resins
            (1) Cholestyramine (Questran®, Mead Johnson & Company, Evansville, IN): 4 g po bid
            (2) Colestipol (Colestid®, Pharmacia & Upjohn, Peapack, NJ): 5 g po bid
         b) HMG-CoA reductase inhibitors (statins)
            (1) Atorvastatin (Lipitor®, Parke-Davis, Morris Plains, NJ): 10–80 mg po per day
            (2) Cerivastatin (Baycol®, Bayer Corporation Pharmaceutical Division, West Haven, CT): 0.3 mg po in the evening
            (3) Fluvastatin (Lescol®, Novartis Pharmaceuticals Corporation, East Hanover, NJ): 20 mg or 40 mg po at bedtime (hs)
            (4) Lovastatin (Mevacor®, Merck & Co., Inc., West Point, PA): 20 mg, 40 mg, or 80 mg po with evening meal
            (5) Pravastatin (Pravachol®, Bristol-Myers Squibb Company, Princeton, NJ): 10 mg, 20 mg, or 40 mg po at hs
            (6) Simvastatin (Zocor®, Merck & Co., Inc.): 5 mg, 10 mg, 20 mg, or 40 mg po at hs
         c) Fibric acid analog
            (1) Gemfibrozil (Lopid®, Parke-Davis): 600 mg po bid
            (2) Nicotinic acid (Niacor®, Upsher-Smith Laboratories, Minneapolis, MN): 1.5–6 g po daily in divided doses

VII. Follow-up
    A. Measure LDL level and LFTs six and 12 weeks after the initiation of drug therapy.
    B. If the LDL target level is reached, monitor follow-up levels every six to 12 months.
    C. Annually follow-up lipoprotein analysis for patients with CHD.

VIII. Referrals: Cardiologist if no reduction in LDL level after three months of drug therapy or if patient is classified as high-risk.

References

Blake, G.H., & Triplett, L.C. (1995). Management of hypercholesterolemia. *American Family Physician, 51,* 1157–1166.

Expert Panel on Detection, Evaluation and Treatment of High Blood Cholesterol in Adults. (1993). Summary of the second report of the National Cholesterol Education Program (NCEP) Expert Panel on Detection, Evaluation and Treatment of High Blood Cholesterol in Adults. *JAMA, 269,* 3015–3023.

Foody, J., & Sprecher, D. (1998). Current concepts in preventive cardiology. *The Clinical Advisor for Nurse Practitioners, 1*(6), 56–62.

LaRosa, J.C. (1998). Cholesterol and atherosclerosis: A controversy resolved. *Advance for Nurse Practitioners, 6*(5), 36–41.

The Scandinavian Simvastatin Survival Study Group. (1994). Randomised trial of cholesterol lowering in 4444 patients with coronary heart disease: The Scandinavian Simvastatin Survival Study. *Lancet, 344,* 1383–1389.

43. Dysrhythmias

Brenda K. Shelton, RN, MS, CCRN, AOCN®

I. Definition: Abnormal rate or rhythm of the heart classified by the region of the heart in which they arise, resulting in sinus, atrial, nodal, or ventricular dysrhythmias

II. Pathophysiology: The pathophysiology mechanism can predict the rhythm disturbance or the patient's level of stability (see Table 43-1).

III. Clinical features: Clinical implications of dysrhythmias vary between individuals, but the severity generally is determined by whether the patient is "stable" or "unstable" by symptomatology and the potential for rhythm disturbance to disintegrate into a life-threatening rhythm. Clearly identified life-threatening rhythms include frequent sinus pauses, ventricular tachycardia, ventricular fibrillation, second-degree heart block type II, third-degree heart block, and asystole. Other rhythm disturbances may present as stable or unstable and require further evaluation.
   A. Risk factors: Typical dysrhythmias are associated with physiologic disorders, medications, cancer-related, and electrolyte disorders (see Table 43-2 and 43-3).
   B. Etiology (see Table 43-1 and 43-3)
   C. History
      1. History of cancer and cancer treatment
      2. Current medications: Prescribed and over-the-counter
      3. History of current symptoms: Precipitating factors, onset, location, and duration
      4. Changes in activities of daily living
   D. Signs and symptoms: All symptoms of reduced blood flow are important to note; however, those considered indicative of cardiovascular "instability" resulting from the rhythm disturbance are marked with an asterisk (*).
      1. Palpitations
      2. Anxiety
      3. *Chest discomfort: May radiate to left arm, shoulder, or jaw
      4. *Dyspnea
      5. Headache
      6. Dizziness: More pronounced when sitting or standing
      7. Tinnitus
      8. *Mental status changes

Table 43-1. Pathophysiologic Mechanisms of Specific Dysrhythmias

Mechanism of Dysrhythmia	Examples of Resulting Dysrhythmias	Etiologies of Physiologic Alteration
Myocardial irritability	• Atrial flutter • Premature ventricular contraction/beats (PVC/PVB) • Ventricular tachycardia • Ventricular fibrillation	• Hypoxemia • Myocardial ischemia • Electrolyte disturbances • Pain • Fear, anxiety
Conduction pathway blockage or slowing through the atrioventricular (AV) node	• First-degree AV block • Second-degree AV block (Type I or Type II) • Third-degree AV block	• Medications: Digoxin and derivatives, beta-blockers, calcium channel blockers • Acidosis • Cardiac exposure to radiation • Myocardial ischemia
Alternate conduction pathways	• Supraventricular tachycardia (SVT)	• Congenital condition • Wolff-Parkinson-White (WPW) syndrome • Mitral valve prolapse • Atrial enlargement • Pulmonary disease
Catecholamine dependence	• Sinus tachycardia • Supraventricular tachycardia • Premature ventricular contractions	• Catecholamine medications (e.g., dopamine, levodopa, inhalant sympathomimetics) • Prolonged stress or anxiety • Fever
Vagal stimulation	• Sinus bradycardia • Sinus pauses • Junctional rhythm • Second-degree heart block, Type I	• Vomiting • Intractable coughing • Right coronary artery disease • Hepatic disease
Normal variants	• Sinus arrhythmia	

9. Reduced urine output
10. Anorexia
11. Nausea

E. Physical exam: Focused on determining whether the rhythm disturbance is stable or unstable
    1. Stable rhythms do not demonstrate significantly compromised cardiac output; therefore, no outward physical signs.
    2. Unstable rhythms have the potential to be life-threatening and demonstrate that the rhythm is unable to sustain adequate perfusion to the vital organs.
    3. If abnormal clinical findings of the heart, lungs, and brain are present, the rhythm is considered unstable and should be treated immediately, possibly with electrical intervention.
    4. Physical exam: Cardiac exam
       a) Pulse strength and equality: Evaluate at several sites (e.g., apical, carotid, radial, femoral, pedal) and compare to normal; determine the apical/peripheral pulse

Table 43-2. Risk Factors for Dysrhythmias

Risk Factor/Concomitant Diseases	High-risk Dysrhythmias	Etiology of Rhythm Disturbance
Acid-base imbalances (acidosis)	• Sinus or junctional bradycardia • Heart block	Acidosis slows conduction throughout the heart, producing bradydysrhythmias.
Adrenal insufficiency	• All tachycardias (sinus, SVT, VT) • Premature ventricular contractions	Adrenal insufficiency causes hypotension that may be compensated for by a rise in heart rate. The nature of the rhythm is sinus, unless other physical disturbances are present. In severe adrenal insufficiency, hyperkalemia produces irritability with ventricular rhythms (see Table 43-3).
Cardiomyopathy	• All atrial rhythms • Premature ventricular contractions, ventricular tachycardia	Cardiac hypertrophy results in less efficient myocardial contraction, reduced cardiac output, and ventricular irritability.
Diabetes mellitus	• All bradycardia rhythms • All tachycardia rhythms	Autonomic neuropathies of diabetes cause a multitude of conduction disturbances, with some patients exhibiting both rapid and slow rhythms. Atrial disturbances may also occur.
Electrolyte disorders	• See Table 43-3.	Electrolytes are important in the depolarization and repolarization of myocardial tissues. Alterations in serum electrolytes result in slower or faster conduction and rhythm disturbances.
Gastrointestinal disease	• See Table 43-3.	GI disease affects fluid and electrolyte absorption and may cause dysrhythmias from these imbalances.
Infection/sepsis	• All tachycardias • Sinus bradycardia, junctional rhythms, or heart block • See Table 43-3.	The predominant dysrhythmia associated with infection is tachycardia, as increased metabolic rate requires a higher cardiac output. Bradycardic rhythms occur rarely but relate to specific pathogens (e.g., nocardia, toxoplasmosis) or acidosis.
Ischemic heart disease	• Any dysrhythmia	Ischemia of the myocardium may disrupt the normal conduction pathway or promote irritability in any area of the heart. All rhythm disturbances are seen, but life-threatening rhythms are of particular concern.
Mitral valve prolapse	• Supraventricular tachycardia	Valvular prolapse causes atrial/junctional irritation that stimulates an alternate conduction pathway.

(Continued on next page)

Table 43-2. Risk Factors for Dysrhythmias (Continued)

Risk Factor/Concomitant Diseases	High-risk Dysrhythmias	Etiology of Rhythm Disturbance
Pain	• Sinus tachycardia • Increased rate of any other baseline rhythm	Pain precipitates the release of catecholamines that increase the baseline rate of any rhythm.
Pulmonary embolism	• Sinus tachycardia • Atrial rhythms • Premature ventricular contractions	The initial response to pulmonary embolism and its associated hypoxemia is tachycardia. In most patients, this is sinus tachycardia. Severe hypoxemia may lead to ventricular dysrhythmias, particularly premature ventricular contractions. Pre-existing pulmonary disease or atrial rhythms (after resolution of the acute pulmonary embolism) are problematic.
Pulmonary parenchymal disease	• All atrial rhythms	Pulmonary injury leads to inflammation, edema, and back-pressure of blood from the lungs to the right heart. Right heart failure and, particularly, atrial enlargement lead to atrial rhythms.
Renal failure	• See Table 43-3.	Renal failure causes dysrhythmias from electrolyte or acid-base imbalances.
Wolff-Parkinson-White (WPW) syndrome	• Supraventricular tachycardia	WPW syndrome is a congenital disorder in which an established alternate pathway bypasses the AV node. This re-entry mechanism enhances the risk of tachydysrhythmias.
Cancer-related therapy		
Amsacrine	• All ventricular rhythms	Amsacrine has been associated with increased incidence of PVCs and ventricular tachycardia, but the mechanism for this disorder is unknown.
Antitumor antibiotics (except bleomycin)	• Ventricular rhythm disturbances • Tachycardia	Myocardial cells are damaged and become atrophied, hypertrophied, and less able to initiate coordinated muscle contraction. Myopathy induced by these agents causes congestive heart failure and associated rhythm disturbances.
Biotherapeutic agents (interferon or interleukin-2)	• All tachycardias • Premature ventricular contractions • Ventricular tachycardia	Cytokines increase the body's metabolic rate and enhance catecholamine release. Dysrhythmias associated with certain biotherapeutic agents are defined, but the exact physiologic mechanism remains unclear.

(Continued on next page)

Table 43-2. Risk Factors for Dysrhythmias (Continued)

Risk Factor/Cancer Related Therapy	High-risk Dysrhythmias	Etiology of Rhythm Disturbance
Bone marrow reinfusion	• Sinus bradycardia • Junctional rhythm • First-degree heart block	Preservatives or marrow treatments (e.g., DMSO, citrate) cause bradycardia during bone marrow reinfusion.
Chest irradiation > 60 Gy	• Conduction disturbances (e.g., sinus pauses, junctional rhythm, heart block, idioventricular rhythm)	Radiation damage to the normal conduction pathway leads to alternated pacemakers of the heart, often lower in the conduction system.
Cisplatin, bleomycin, vinblastine for testicular cancer	• Supraventricular tachycardia • Ventricular dysrhythmias	This drug combination is thought to cause coronary artery vasospasm with dysrhythmias. Symptoms and signs of cardiac ischemia (e.g., chest pain) often accompany EKG rhythm disturbances.
Cytosine arabinoside	• All ventricular rhythms	Mechanism is unknown but is dose-dependent.
5-fluorouracil	• Any tachycardia or premature beats • Ischemic ST and T wave changes	5-fluorouracil is associated with a 1.7% risk of cardiotoxicity that resembles unstable angina and its associated EKG changes. Reversible cardiac failure occurs in a small number of these patients.
Paclitaxel	• Sinus bradycardia • Junctional rhythm • First-degree heart block	Paclitaxel is preserved in cremophor, known to cause bradycardic rhythms.
Pheresis	• Sinus bradycardia • Junctional rhythm	Citrate preservative used in pheresis procedure binds with calcium, making patient hypocalcemic causing dysrhythmias.
Vinca alkaloids	• All tachycardias • All bradycardias	Autonomic neuropathies associated with vinca alkaloids are less well-defined than peripheral neuropathies. Autonomic neuropathy of the vagus nerve is thought to occur with these agents and cause disruption of the homeostatic mechanism of heart rate regulation by this nerve.

(Continued on next page)

Table 43-2. Risk Factors for Dysrhythmias (Continued)

Risk Factor/Concomitant Diseases	High-risk Dysrhythmias	Etiology of Rhythm Disturbance
Recent surgery		
Anesthesia	• All dysrhythmias	Most anesthetic agents are cardiac suppressants, commonly slowing the heart rate and reducing inotropic force that can lead to compensatory tachycardia.
Pneumonectomy	• Sinus tachycardia • Supraventricular tachycardia	Right pneumonectomy procedures often require accompanying pericardial dissection for attainment of an adequate vascular margin surrounding the tumor or repair of the major pulmonary artery.
Medications (taken within past three days or one week if patient has renal or hepatic compromise)		
Antidepressants especially tricyclic	• All tachycardias	Many of these drugs are CNS stimulants that increase heart rate and automaticity.
Antidiarrheals (e.g., lomotil), especially those containing parasympatholytic agents, such as atropine	• All tachycardias	See explanation for antidiarrheals.
Antiemetics	• Premature beats • All tachycardias	Medications alter nervous system response to excessive peristaltic waves and also may enhance or suppress cardiac conduction. Parasympatholytic medications to slow peristalsis also inhibit the vagus nerve, leading to tachycardia.
Catecholamines or their precursors (e.g., epinephrine, dopamine, levodopa)	• All tachycardias • Premature ventricular contractions	Catecholamines increase heart rate and cardiac cell automaticity. While useful for fight-or-flight mechanisms, they may cause dysrhythmias.
Medications preserved in cremophor-phenytoin	• Sinus bradycardia • Junctional rhythm • First-degree heart block	Cremophor slows cardiac conduction. It is dose-dependent, so slower infusions or reduced cremophor in suspension will decrease incidence of dysrhythmia.
Recreational drugs, especially cocaine	• All tachycardias • Ventricular irritability	Drugs are CNS stimulants that increase heart rate and automaticity.

Table 43-3. Acid-Base and Electrolyte Abnormalities and EKG Rhythm Disturbances

Electrolyte Abnormality	Dysrhythmia/EKG Abnormality
Hypokalemia	• Increased irritability, premature beats • Flattening of T wave or appearance of U wave

Hyperkalemia	• Increased irritability, premature beats
	  - Decreased ability to generate action potential
	  - Tall, peaked T waves in precordial leads
	  - Decreased amplitude of R wave
	  - Widening of QRS complex
	  - Widening of PR complex until P wave disappears
	  - QRS complex blends into T wave
	• Ventricular fibrillation

Hypocalcemia	• Increased irritability, premature beats • Heart block • Ventricular fibrillation • Prolonged QT intervals
Hypercalcemia	• Shortened QT interval
Hypomagnesemia	• Increased irritability, premature beats • Increased conduction through AV node (tachycardia)
Acidosis	• Slowed conduction (bradycardia, junctional rhythm, and heart block)

Note. Based on information from Evanoff & Weinman, 1991; Rinkenberger, 1991.

deficit, evidence of weak or thready pulses at one site, or pulsus alternans (i.e., alternating strong and weak pulse).

b) Heart sounds: S_3, S_4, split heart sounds, and summation gallops are particularly important to note because they may indicate cardiovascular incompetence resulting from the dysrhythmia.

   (1) S_3 gallop: Slow or rapid heart rates and ventricular dysrhythmias may cause heart failure that may present with this abnormal heart sound. Sound is most often heard with the bell of the stethoscope at the 4th–5th intercostal space, midclavicular line.

   (2) S_4 gallop: Indicates decreased compliance of the left ventricle, which can occur with aortic stenosis, systemic hypertension, pulmonic stenosis, pulmonary hypertension, and coronary artery disease.

   (3) Summation gallop: S_3 and S_4 are present and overlap during a tachydysrhythmia.

   (4) Split S_2 heart sounds: Clinically significant in tachydysrhythmia.

c) Blood pressure: A systolic BP < 90 mm Hg, mean BP < 60 mm Hg, or more than a 40 mm Hg drop from baseline systolic are indicative of hypotension and should be considered as a potential outcome of the rhythm disturbance, although sometimes poor cardiac output is the cause of the rhythm and not the consequence.

d) Jugular venous pulsations (JVPs): Greater than 2 cm above the clavicle when cardiac output is compromised; more pronounced and appear as a large wave moving up the neck when ventricular tachycardia is present.

e) Capillary refill: Longer than three seconds is considered indicative of compromised cardiac output when other obvious causes or peripheral vascular disease are not present.

5. Integument exam: Skin color, temperature, and appearance; cyanosis, mottling, cool/clammy skin are signs of poor perfusion.

6. Neurologic exam: Quick mini-mental exam; wakefulness, orientation, appropriateness, and visual acuity provide data to reflect brain perfusion.

7. Pulmonary exam: Respiratory rate and effort; increased when perfusion is inadequate.

IV. Diagnostic tests
    A. Laboratory
        1. CBC: To identify anemia as a potential cause of dysrhythmia
        2. Electrolytes: To rule out imbalances; magnesium, calcium, and potassium
        3. Free T_4 and TSH: To rule out hyperthyroidism and hypothyroidism
    B. Radiology: Not indicated
    C. Other: EKG rhythm strip in leads II, AVF, and V1 each clearly define a particular portion of the normal P, QRS, and T waves. It will help discern one rhythm from another, as P waves or QRS direction are highlighted. Table 43-4 includes a grid for differentiating rhythm disturbances.
        1. Recommended order for examining the rhythm
            a) Determine rate: < 60, 60–100, > 100
            b) Determine regularity: Regular, irregular with a pattern, grossly irregular
            c) Determine if P waves precede every QRS or some QRS or if no P waves are present.
            d) Measure PR interval if present, and compare to normal value of 0.12–0.20 seconds.
                (1) Note if PR interval varies with a pattern or is totally erratic.
                (2) Note early beats with or without a P wave even if the QRS complex is unchanged.
            e) Measure QRS interval, and compare to normal value of 0.04–0.10 seconds.
                (1) Note all varied appearances of the QRS.
                (2) Measure each different QRS.
                (3) Determine if QRS complexes all go in the same direction and, if not, whether specific variants go in the opposite direction.
        2. The 12 lead EKG will better define the rhythm disturbance and determine whether there is accompanying ischemia.
            a) Newer variations of the 12 lead EKG are the 15 and 18 lead EKG and are more important for detection of myocardial infarction than dysrhythmia interpretation.
            b) If the rhythm is not always present, an exercise stress test may be performed in attempt to trigger the rhythm disturbance and plan treatment.
        3. 24- or 48-hour Holter™ (Johnson & Johnson, New Brunswick, NJ) monitor provides 24 or 48 hours of continuous rhythm monitoring that is particularly helpful if the rhythm disturbance is intermittent. The patient also keeps a diary that

Table 43-4. Differentiating EKG Rhythm Disturbances

EKG Rhythm	Rate not identifiable	Rate <60	Rate 60–100	Rate >100	Irregular	Regularly irregular	Regular	Normal P waves	No P waves	PR interval constant	PR interval varies	QRS interval normal	QRS interval wide
Normal sinus rhythm (NSR)			X				X	X		X		X	
Normal sinus bradycardia (NSB)		X					X	X		X		X	
Sinus pauses/arrest		X	X		X			X		X		X	
Normal sinus tachycardia (NST)				X			X	X		X		X	
Atrial fibrillation (AF)		X	X	X	X				X			X	
Atrial flutter (Afl)		X	X	X		X			X			X	
Supraventricular tachycardia (SVT)				X			X		X			X	
Junctional (nodal) rhythm		X					X		X			X	
Accelerated junctional (nodal) rhythm			X				X		X			X	
Premature ventricular contractions (PVCs)		X	X	X		X		X		X			X
Ventricular tachycardia (VT)				X			X		X				X
Ventricular fibrillation (VF)	X												

(Continued on next page)

Table 43-4. Differentiating EKG Rhythm Disturbances *(Continued)*

EKG Rhythm	Rate not identifiable	Rate <60	Rate 60-100	Rate >100	Irregular	Regularly irregular	Regular	Normal P waves	No P waves	PR interval constant	PR interval varies	QRS interval normal	QRS interval wide
Asystole	X												
First-degree atrioventricular block (1° AVB)		X	X				X	X		X			
Second-degree atrioventricular block, Type I (2° AVB-I)		X	X			X		X			X	X	
Second-degree atrioventricular block, Type II (2° AVB-II)		X	X			X		X		X		X	X
Third-degree atrioventricular block (3° AVB)		X					X	X			X		X

Note. Some categories vary with the rhythm (i.e., rate can be slow, normal, or rapid in atrial fibrillation); therefore, some rhythms may have more than one criteria within the same category.

will help to identify clinical symptoms that are directly related to the rhythm disturbance.

4. Event monitoring allows patient to have a Holter with a marker to identify time periods when symptoms are present.

5. Life-threatening dysrhythmias may require electrophysiologic (EP) testing to "map" the source of the dysrhythmia and provide an avenue for definitive treatment.

6. Echocardiogram is not used to diagnose dysrhythmias but provides valuable information regarding the cause of the rhythm or the estimated cardiac output with that rhythm.

V. Differential diagnosis
   A. Cardiovascular disease
   B. Pulmonary embolism (see Chapter 33)
   C. Acid-base imbalance
   D. Electrolyte disturbance (see Chapters 144–148)
   E. Drug overdose or idiosyncratic reaction
   F. Medication-induced

VI. Treatment: The treatment of dysrhythmias depends on the etiologic factors, patient's tolerance, and aggressiveness of planned support.
   A. Do not treat a dysrhythmia if all of the following are true.
      1. Cause of rhythm is known and treatable.
      2. There are no symptoms of instability.
      3. The rhythm is unlikely to disintegrate into a life-threatening unstable rhythm.
   B. Emergency management of dysrhythmias
      1. Determine patient tolerance.
      2. Correct underlying etiology.
      3. Regulate metabolic balance (e.g., electrolytes, hormones).
      4. Definitive treatment as indicated
         a) Management of tachydysrhythmias
            (1) Vagal maneuvers (e.g., coughing, bearing down as if to have a bowel movement, manual carotid massage) will frequently break paroxysmal supraventricular tachycardia.
            (2) Whether patient is stable or unstable, administer adenosine if it is readily available. It has a short half-life, has few adverse effects, and may break the rhythm or identify flutter waves that definitively diagnose the rhythm.
            (3) Stable: Medical therapy (see Tables 43-5 and 43-6)
            (4) Electrical therapy: Synchronized cardioversion
         b) Management of bradydysrhythmias
            (1) Asymptomatic/stable: Medical therapy
            (2) Pacemaker: Automatic external, temporary transvenous, permanent

VII. Follow-up
   A. Holter monitor: Performed periodically (usually once every year) as follow-up to ascertain whether the antidysrhythmic treatment is effective.

Table 43-5. Antidysrhythmia Therapy for Supraventricular Tachycardia

Drug	Dose	Category	Miscellaneous
Adenosine	6 mg by rapid IV push; wait 1–2 minutes, if no response 12 mg by rapid IV push	Purine nucleoside	Can cause several seconds of asystole; patient may experience crushing chest pain; supraventricular tachycardia will recur 50–60% of time; half –life less than five seconds; patients on theophylline may require larger doses, whereas dipyridamole potentiates its effects.
Digoxin	10–15 μ/kg lean body weight	Digitalis glycoside	Rate and conduction effect seen within 5–30 minutes; peak effect within 1½ –3 hours; correct hypokalemia immediately; toxicity increases with increased calcium levels and decreased potassium/magnesium levels.
Diltiazem	Bolus: 0.25 mg/kg over 2 minutes; if not controlled after 15 minutes, may give additional 0.35 mg/kg over 2–5 minutes Follow with 5–15 mg/hour continuous infusion	Calcium channel blocker	Load and follow with maintenance infusion; less myocardial depression than verapamil
Esmolol	Load with 250–500 μg/kg for one minute followed by continuous infusion of 25–50 μg/kg per minute at 5–10 minute intervals to max of 300 μg/kg per minute	Beta-adrenergic blocker	Very rapid onset and short duration; should be diluted to 10 mg/ml before administration; do not use in patients with significant atrio-ventricular (AV) block or bradycardia.
Propranolol	1–3 mg IV push over 2–5 minutes (no faster than 1 mg/minute); may repeat after two minutes to total dose of 0.1 mg/kg	Beta-adrenergic blocker nonselective	Watch for signs and symptoms of bronchospasm with nonselective beta blockers; treat with sympathomimetics and aminophylline; do not use in patients with significant AV block or bradycardia
Verapamil	5 mg IV push over 2 minutes, 5–10 mg after 15–30 minutes Maximum dose: 30 mg	Calcium channel blocker	Watch blood pressure; 2–4 mg dosing over three to four minutes for elderly or patients with low-normal blood pressure; reverse with calcium chloride, 0.5–1 g slowly IV; watch use in patients with Wolff-Parkinson-White syndrome.

Table 43-6. Classification and Mechanism of Action of Antidysrhythmics

Group	Mechanism of Action	Currently Approved Drugs	Investigational Agents
Ia	• Depress Na⁺ conductance, increase action potential duration, decrease membrane responsiveness • Prolong QRS interval	Quinidine, procainamide, disopyramide	Aprindine, pirmenol, acecainide hydrochloride cifenline succinate
Ib	• Natural blockade, increase K⁺ conductance, decrease action potential duration and effective refractory period. Do not significantly alter EKG levels	Lidocaine, phenytoin, mexiletine, tocainide	Pirmenol, aprindine
Ic	• Natural blockade, marked depression of phase 0 through profound slowing of conduction. Have a slight effect on conduction. Prolong PR and QRS intervals.	Flecainide, propafenone	Lorcainide
Miscellaneous			
I	• Has local anesthetic properties. Interferes with fast inward depolarizing current carried by sodium ions.	Moricizine	
II	• Interfere with Na⁺ conductance (closes the slow Na⁺ channel), depress cell membrane, decrease automaticity and increase effective refractory period of the AV node. Have little effect on conduction. Slow the exit of K⁺ out of the cell.	Propranolol, acebutolol, esmolol	Practolol
III	• Interfere with norepinephrine, increase action potential duration and effective refractory period. Prolong repolarization.	Amiodarone, bretylium, ibutilide, sotalol	
IV	• Ca⁺⁺ antagonist, increase AV nodal effective refractory period.	Verapamil, bepridil	Gallopamil, tiapamil
Unclassified	Opens K⁺ channels	Adenosine	

B. Medication blood levels: Monitored with every dose change when regulating the appropriate dose, then every three months if the patient's physical condition remains unchanged. Normal levels for commonly monitored medications are listed in Table 43-7.

C. Implanted pacemaker/defibrillator tests and battery changes

VIII. Referrals

A. Cardiologist: For evaluation of dysrhythmias of unknown origin or when patient is refractory to treatment; to determine if an interventional cardiologist or dysrhythmia expert is needed.

B. Pharmacists: To advise patients regarding correct administration of antidysrhythmic medications, as many of these agents have altered absorption with food, pH levels, or

Table 43-7. Laboratory Reference Ranges for Antidysrhythmic Levels

Medication	Normal Range	Defined Toxicity Level	Variables Affecting Accuracy
Amiodarone	0.5–2.5 mcg/ml	> 2.5 mcg/ml	• Stored longer than 24 hours falsely reduces value.
Digoxin	0.5–2.0 ng/ml	> 2.0 ng/ml	• Be certain digoxin, not digitoxin, level is requested. • Radioactive tracers administered within previous 24 hours falsely elevate. • Levels are elevated with hypokalemia, hypocalcemia, hypomagnesemia.
Flecainide	0.2–1.0 mcg/ml	> 1.0 mcg/ml	• Indicate concomitant propranolol or quinidine on laboratory requisition when sending specimen. • Must be processed by lab within two hours
Lidocaine	1.5–6.0 mcg/ml	6–8 mcg/ml	• Do not send in serum separator tube, as it may absorb lidocaine and falsely lower levels.
Procainamide	4.9–12 mcg/ml	16–20 mcg/ml	• Hemolyzed or hyperlipidemic specimens falsely lower levels.
Propranolol	50–100 ng/ml	> 500 ng/ml	• Do not insert blood through laboratory tube stopper, as the stopper may falsely reduce levels. • Smoking decreases plasma concentration.
Quinidine	2–6 mcg/ml	> 10 mcg/ml	

Note. Based on information from Chernecky & Berger, 1997.

other concomitant medications. The pharmacist also will advise the patient regarding use of over-the-counter medications that may interfere with antidysrhythmics or act as cardiac stimulants (e.g., cold and allergy remedies).

C. Dietitian: Refer patients on antidysrhythmic therapy who must monitor their intake of certain electrolytes. The nutritionist also may advise the patient about food substances that contain caffeine or other cardiac stimulants (e.g., cola, chocolate).

D. Tobacco cessation program: Refer patients who use tobacco, as nicotine replacement products are contraindicated in patients with dysrhythmias.

References

Chernecky, C.C., & Berger, B.J. (1997). *Laboratory tests and diagnostic procedures* (2nd ed.). Philadelphia: W.B. Saunders.

Cummins, R.O. (Ed.). (1997). *Textbook of advanced cardiac life support* (4th ed.). Dallas: American Heart Association.

Evanoff, G.V., & Weinman, E.J. (1991). Fluid and electrolyte disorders. In D.R. Dantzker (Ed.), *Cardiopulmonary critical care* (2nd ed.) (pp. 161–198). Philadelphia: W.B. Saunders.

Harpole, D.H., Liptay, M.J., DeCamp, M.M., Jr., Mentzer, S.J., Swanson, S.J., & Sugarbaker, D.J. (1996). Prospective analysis of pneumonectomy: Risk factors for major morbidity and cardiac dysrhythmias. *Annals of Thoracic Surgery, 61,* 977–982.

Howard, M. (1995). Cardiac disorders. In C. Paradiso (Ed.), *Lippincott's review series. Pathophysiology.* Philadelphia: J.B. Lippincott.

Huff, J., Doernbach, D.P., & White, R.D. (1993*). EKG workout. Exercises in arrhythmia interpretation* (2nd ed.). Philadelphia: J.B. Lippincott.

Jakacki, R.I., Larsen, R.L., Barber, G., Heyman, S., Fridman, M., & Silber, J.H. (1993). Comparison of cardiac function after anthracycline therapy in childhood. Implications for screening. *Cancer, 72,* 2739–2745.

McLachlan, S.A., Millward, M.J., Toner, G.C., Guiney, M.J., & Bishop, J.F. (1994). The spectrum of 5-fluorouricil cardiotoxicity. *Medical Journal of Australia, 161,* 207–209.

Rinkenberger, R. (1991). Cardiac rhythm in the critical care setting: Pathophysiology and diagnosis. In D.R. Dantzker (Ed.), *Cardiopulmonary critical care* (2nd ed.) (pp. 437–498). Philadelphia: W.B. Saunders.

Schober, C., Papageorgiou, E., Harstrick, A., Bokemeyer, C., Mugge, A., Stahl, M., Wilke, H., Poliwoda, H., Hiddemann, W., & Kohne-Wompner, C.H. (1993). Cardiotoxicity of 5-fluorouracil in combination with folinic acid in patients with gastrointestinal cancer. *Cancer 72,* 2242–2247.

Thomas, P., Giudicelli, R., Guillen, J.C., & Fuentes, P. (1994). Is lung cancer surgery justified in patients with coronary artery disease? *European Journal of Cardiothoracic Surgery, 8,* 287–291.

Chapter

44. Endocarditis

Brenda K. Shelton, RN, MS, CCRN, AOCN®

I. Definition: A general term used to describe inflammation of the endocardial lining or valves of the heart.

II. Pathophysiology
   A. Endocarditis is an inflammatory disorder that results from injury to the endocardial surface of the heart.
      1. Turbulent blood flow or the presence of pathogenic organisms are the most common causes of endothelial injury.
      2. The injury initiates thrombus formation to protect the injured site.
      3. In patients who are hypercoagulable, the degree of injury required to initiate a thrombus is less than in other patients, increasing the risk of "sterile thrombus" production or precipitation of nonbacterial thrombotic endocarditis (NBTE).
   B. In bacterial endocarditis, the pathogens adhere to the injured endocardial surface and are incorporated into the thrombus.
      1. The growth of these pathogens produce "fern-like" deposits known as vegetation.
      2. Vegetations are most likely to be present on rough surfaces or in areas of turbulent, high-velocity blood flow (e.g., near the cardiac valves).
      3. It is postulated that hypermetabolic states that increase heart rate and cardiac output may enhance the risk of this disorder.
      4. Vegetations may break off and embolize any area of the body, leading to great variation in the clinical signs and symptoms of this disease.
      5. They also may affect valve integrity (e.g., leaky valves).

III. Clinical features: Endocarditis is classified by its acuity of presentation (acute versus subacute) and whether it is infective or noninfective (see Table 44-1). Endocarditis is not uncommon, affecting as many as one in one thousand patients admitted to hospitals. Mortality rate is approximately 10%–20% of cases. Endocarditis is not a commonly reported manifestation of malignant disease; however, as many as 1.2% of autopsied patients with cancer had noninfective endocarditis, suggesting a greater prevalence than reported.
   A. Risk factors
      1. Most common risk factors in the general population
         a) Structural heart disease

Table 44-1. Infectious Causes of Endocarditis

Risk Factor	Microorganism
Early after prosthetic valve replacement	Staphylococcus coagulase-positive or -negative: 50% Gram-negative: 20% Fungal: 10% Other: 20%
Late after prosthetic valve replacement	Alphahemolytic streptococcus: 35% Staphylococcus coagulase-negative: 20% Staphylococcus coagulase-positive: 10% Gram-negative: 10% Other: 25%
IV drug abuse	Staphylococcus coagulase-positive: 50% Streptococcus (alpha and beta): 15% Other: 35%
Immunosuppressed patients (i.e., those who have undergone solid organ transplant or bone marrow transplant, those who are HIV-positive not IV-drug using, those with autoimmune disease on corticosteroids)	Staphylococcus coagulase-positive or -negative: 50% Streptococcus (alpha and beta): 20% Fungal: 10% Opportunistic: 5% Other: 5%

Note. Based on information from Kukuckova et al., 1996; Trilla & Miro, 1995; & Weyman, Rankin, & King, 1977.

        (1) Congenital heart disease
        (2) Mitral valve prolapse
        (3) Prosthetic valves
        (4) Rheumatic heart damage
    b) Autoimmune systemic illness
        (1) Systemic lupus erythematosus (SLE)
        (2) Scleroderma
    c) IV drug abuse
    d) Recent cardiac surgery: Coronary artery bypass or valve replacement
    e) Male gender: Not supported in studies of patients with malignancy and endocarditis
  2. Long-term indwelling catheters (especially central venous): Tunneled external catheters, pheresis catheter, peripherally inserted central catheter (PICC), Swan Ganz, implantable ports
  3. Cancers
    a) Intestinal tumors
    b) Tumors metastasizing to the heart cause endocarditis
        (1) Less than 2% of the time
        (2) Tumor types identified as causing right-sided valvular disorders (e.g., tricuspid, pulmonic): Kidney, testes, thyroid, melanoma
        (3) Tumor types identified as causing left sided valvular lesions (e.g., mitral, aortic): Bronchogenic

    c) Leukemia and myeloproliferative disorders (Loeffler's endocarditis) caused by eosinophilic infiltration cardiomyopathy

    d) Nonbacterial thrombotic endocarditis

      (1) Occurs because of excess thrombotic potential

      (2) Tumor types (especially adenocarcinoma)

        (a) Pancreatic cancer (38%): Most likely to cause vegetations

        (b) Lymphoma (26%)

        (c) Carcinoma of GI tract (20%)

        (d) Carcinoma of lung (16%)

  4. Bone marrow transplantation

    a) Incompetent immune system

    b) Treatment regimen results in extensive endothelial wall injury

  5. Other diseases

    a) Intestinal diseases

    b) Hypercoagulable conditions

      (1) Trousseau's syndrome

      (2) Protein C deficiency

      (3) Protein S deficiency

      (4) Antithrombin III deficiency

      (5) Disseminated intravascular coagulation (DIC)

    c) Carcinoid syndrome, especially right-sided valves

B. Etiology: Most common source is bacteremia

  1. Bacteremia can cause endocarditis, even on a normal, healthy, and intact endocardium. The most common infectious organisms associated with endocarditis are

    a) Alpha-hemolytic streptococcus

    b) Beta-hemolytic streptococcus

    c) *Staphylococcus aureus*

    d) Gram-negative bacilli

    e) Diphtheroid

    f) Rickettsiae

    g) Chlamydia

    h) Polymicrobials

  2. Infectious etiologies by population group (see Table 44-1)

C. History

  1. History of cancer and cancer treatment

  2. Current medications: Prescribed and over-the-counter

  3. History of presenting symptom(s): Precipitating factors, onset, location, and duration. Associated symptoms are recent fever or chills, recent loss of appetite, fatigue, chest pain, weight loss, visual loss, and painful nodules on fingers.

  4. Changes in activities of daily living

  5. Past medical history: Heart murmur, heart disease, rheumatic fever, lupus

  6. Social history: IV drugs for therapy or recreation

D. Signs and symptoms (see Table 44-2)

  1. Flu-like syndrome

    a) Arthralgia

    b) Myalgia

Table 44-2. Clinical Presentation of Acute and Subacute Bacterial Endocarditis

Clinical Feature	Acute Endocarditis	Subacute Endocarditis
Onset	< six weeks onset	> six weeks onset
Organisms	*Staphylococcus aureus* Beta-hemolytic streptococcus	Alpha streptococcus
Virulence	Very virulent	Less virulent
Valvular status before disorder	Previously normal valves	Previously damaged valves
Valves involved	Tricuspid; pulmonic	Mitral
Valvular presentation	Valve perforation common Large friable vegetations with high tendency to embolize	Valve perforation rare Smaller, thicker vegetations

Note. Based on information from Raad, Luna, & Khalil, 1994; Rosen & Armstrong, 1973.

      c) Low-grade fever
      d) Chills
      e) Anorexia
      f) Weakness, fatigue
      g) Night sweats: Depend on organism
  2. Angina: From cardiac dysfunction resulting from inflammation of endocardium or valves, effects on contractility, or embolization to coronary artery
  3. Mental status changes: Usually reflect embolic stroke (less focal if caused by hypoxemia).
      a) Usually sudden onset
      b) Upper extremity weakness
  4. GI symptoms
      a) Abdominal pain: Occurs with decreased perfusion (cardiac dysfunction) but may also signal embolization to the GI organs
      b) Anorexia
      c) Nausea
      d) Constipation
  5. Genitourinary dysfunction
      a) Oliguria
      b) Dark, concentrated urine
  6. Joint and bone pain: Indicative of osteomyelitis
E. Physical exam
  1. Vital signs: Fever, hypotensive
  2. Integument exam
      a) Petechiae of skin, oral mucosa, conjunctivae
      b) Oslers nodes: Painful, red, tender subcutaneous nodules in the finger pads
      c) Janeway lesions: Flat, small, painless, irregular, nontender red spots on the palms of hands and soles of feet
      d) Splinter hemorrhage of fingernails

3. HEENT exam
   a) Roth's spots: Retinal hemorrhages characterized by white or yellow center surrounded by a red irregular halo
   b) Conjunctival hemorrhage
   c) Visual field cuts: Noted by point discrimination testing; are present after embolic stroke.
   d) Decreased finger-to-nose testing in visual field
4. Pulmonary exam
   a) Peripheral tissue hypoxemia indicated by presence of
      (1) Skin cyanosis
      (2) Cool extremities
      (3) Generalized hypoxemia: Present if cardiac dysfunction is present.
   b) Central cyanosis indicated by presence of
      (1) Bluish inner eyelids
      (2) Bluish oral mucosa.
   c) Chronic hypoxemia indicated by presence of
      (1) Finger clubbing
      (2) Dark spots on the skin.
5. Cardiac exam
   a) Pansystolic murmur heard best at base of heart
   b) Full bounding point maximal impulse (PMI)
   c) Vascular exam
      (1) Weak, thready pulses
      (2) Weaker distal pulses
6. Abdominal exam
   a) Splenomegaly: Tenderness is present if an acute episode and previous embolic infarctions have not occurred.
   b) Hepatomegaly: Tenderness is present in an acute episode.
   c) Diffuse abdominal pain to palpation: May be present as a result of bowel ischemia, hepatomegaly, or splenomegaly.
7. Neurologic exam
   a) Mental status changes
   b) Paresis: Noted by bilateral strength testing; usually unilateral weakness
   c) Aphasia

IV. Diagnostic tests
  A. Laboratory
    1. CBC: To rule out
       a) Normocytic, normochromic anemia
       b) Leukocytosis
       c) Increased erythrocyte sedimentation rate.
    2. Blood cultures: To identify bacteremia organism (may require three or more sets before organism is isolated)
  B. Radiology: Chest x-ray may show enlarged heart.

C. Other
1. Echocardiogram is the definitive diagnostic tool when endocarditis involves valve abnormalities (> 90% of cases), yet does not rule out endocarditis if negative.
   a) Presence of valvular vegetations or perforation: Vegetations < 3 mm cannot be detected on traditional echocardiogram, and may require transesophageal echocardiogram (TEE).
   b) Some clinicians advocate use of TEE exclusively in monitoring treatment response with this disease process because small vegetations still require ongoing antimicrobial therapy but may not be detected by traditional echocardiogram.
   c) Assess competence of valves.
   d) Global myocardial hypokinesis may be seen in the absence of valvular abnormalities and can be used with blood culture results to confirm diagnosis of endocarditis.
2. Dysrhythmias and EKG abnormalities: Conduction disturbances (e.g., heart block, bradycardia, prolonged PR interval, left bundle branch block)

V. Differential diagnosis
   A. Bacteremia/septicemia
   B. Congestive heart failure (see Chapter 40)
   C. Myocardial abscesses
   D. Myocardial infraction (see Chapter 47)
   E. Pericarditis (see Chapter 48)
   F. New or primary cardiac valvular disorder

VI. Treatment
   A. Antibiotics: Based on organisms of high-risk or positive blood cultures (see Table 44-3)
      1. Must be IV for at least 14 days
      2. Usually four to six weeks of antibiotic therapy (possibly several weeks of oral therapy after IV)
      3. If blood cultures are still positive after 21 days (or if the patient becomes more acutely ill), remove permanent indwelling catheters.
   B. Anticoagulation: To prevent embolization of vegetations (see Chapter 41)
      1. Weight-based heparin: To achieve partial thromboplastin time 1.3 to 1.5 times control
      2. Conversion to oral anticoagulant: After clear echocardiogram, unless patient has known malignancy-associated hypercoagulable state
   C. Valve replacement: May be indicated in disease-free patients
      1. Valvular replacement surgery: More complex, requiring significant cardiopulmonary bypass time and is associated with more complications than coronary artery bypass surgery
      2. Valvuloplasty: Not usually the surgical procedure of choice because of the need to prevent future valvular vegetations

VII. Follow-up
   A. Prolonged antimicrobial therapy: Requires frequent medical follow-up with physical exam that includes heart sounds, assessment for heart failure, and skin assessment; will assist in determining whether the selection of antimicrobial therapy is appropriate.

Table 44-3. Antimicrobial Treatment of Endocarditis

Infecting Organism	Antimicrobial Treatment
Staphylococcus aureus	Oxacillin 2 g IV q four hours for six weeks plus gentamycin or tobramycin 1.5–2.0 mg/kg IV q eight hours
Staphylococcus epidermis	Vancomycin 1 g IV q 12 hours with rifampin 300 mg po q eight hours for six to eight weeks with gentamycin 1 mg/kg IV q eight hours for first two weeks of therapy
Streptococci	Penicillin-G 2 million units IV q four hours for four weeks or penicillin with an aminoglycoside for two weeks
Group A beta-hemolytic streptococci and *Streptococcus pneumoniae*	Penicillin-G 3–5 million units IV q four hours in combination with gentamycin 1.0–1.5 mg/kg IV q eight hours for four to six weeks. If allergic to penicillin, vancomycin with an aminoglycoside
Gram-negative (*Haemophilus influenzae,* actinobacillus, cardiobacterium, eikenella, Kingella)	Penicillin or ampicillin with an aminoglycoside for four weeks

Note. Based on information from Bochud, Eggiman, Calandra, VanMelle, & Saghafi, 1994; Kukuckova et al., 1996; Specer, 1995; Trilla & Miro, 1995.

    B. Echocardiogram: Perform monthly while patient is on antimicrobial therapy and then at least yearly, as one episode of endocarditis is a risk factor for repeated episodes.

    C. After a person has had any episode of endocarditis, prophylactic antimicrobial treatment is prescribed for all procedures that pose risk for embolization.

        1. Dental work

        2. Bladder catheterization

        3. GI scope procedures

        4. Surgery of any type

        5. Vaginal delivery

VIII. Referrals

    A. Cardiologist: Consult if endocarditis is complicated by multiple embolization episodes or if echocardiogram does not return to normal with therapy.

    B. Anticoagulation clinic: Some patients on long-term anticoagulation therapy are referred for monitoring and dose adjustments.

References

Bochud, P.Y., Eggiman, P., Calandra, T., VanMelle, G., & Saghafi, L. (1994). Bacteremia due to viridans streptococcus in neutropenic patients with cancer: Clinical spectrum and risk factors. *Clinical Infectious Disease, 18*(1), 25–31.

Edoute, Y., Haim, N., Rinkevich, D., Brenner, B., & Reisner, S.A. (1997). Cardiac valvular vegetations in cancer patients: A prospective echocardiographic study of 200 patients. *American Journal of Medicine, 102,* 252–258.

Fujishima, S., Okada, Y., Irie, K., Kitazono, T., Saku, Y., Utsunomiya, H., Sugihara, S., Sadoshima, S., Fujishima, M. (1994). Multiple brain infarction and hemorrhage by nonbacterial thrombotic endocarditis in occult lung cancer-case report. *Angiology, 45*(2), 161–166.

Goumas, P.D., Naxakis, S.S., Rentzis, G.A., Tsiotos, P.D., & Papadas, T.A. (1997). Lateral neck abscess caused by Streptococcus bovis in a patient with undiagnosed colon cancer. *Journal of Laryngology & Otology, 111,* 666–668.

Hanfling, S.M. (1960). Metastatic cancer to the heart: Review of the literature and report of 127 cases. *Circulation, 22,* 474.

Kukuckova, E., Spanik, S., Ilavska, I., Helpianska, L., Oravcova, E., Lacka, J., Krupova, I., Grausova, S., Koren, P., Bezakova, I., Grey, E., Balaz, M., Studena, M., Kunova, A., Torfs, K., Trupl, J., Korec, S., Stopkova, K., & Krcmery, V. (1996). Staphylococcal bacteremia in cancer patients: Risk factors and outcome in 134 episodes prior to and after introduction of quinolones into infection prevention in neutropenia. *Supportive Care in Cancer, 4,* 427–434.

Meehan, S., Schmidt, M.C., & Mitchell, P.F. (1996). Infective endocarditis in a patient with Hodgkin's lymphoma: A case report. *Specialty Care Dentist, 14*(2), 57–60.

Raad, I.I., Luna, M., & Khalil, S.A. (1994). The relationship between the thrombotic and infectious complications of central venous catheters. *JAMA, 271,* 1014–1016.

Rosen, P., & Armstrong, D. (1973). Nonbacterial thrombolic endocarditis in patients with malignant neoplastic diseases. *American Journal of Medicine, 54,* 23.

Schuchter, L., Hendricks, C., Holland, K., Shelton, B.K., Hutchins, G.M., Baughman, K.L., & Ettinger, D.S. (1989). Eosinophilic myocarditis associated with high dose interleukin therapy. *American Journal of Medicine, 88,* 439–440.

Spencer, R.C. (1995). The emergence of epidemic, multiple-antibiotic-resistant stenotrophomonas (xanthomonas) maltophilia and burkholderia (pseudomonas) cepacia. *Journal of Hospital Infection, 30*(Suppl.), 453–464.

Trilla, A., & Miro, J.M. (1995). Identifying high risk patients for Staphlococcal aureus infections: Skin and soft tissue infections. *Journal of Chemotherapy, 7*(Suppl. 3), 37–43.

Weyman, A.E., Rankin, R., & King, H. (1977). Loeffler's endocarditis presenting as mitral and tricuspid stenosis. *American Journal of Cardiology, 40,* 438.

Chapter

45. Hypertension

Mary Ann Winokur, CRNP, MSN

I. Definition: A systolic blood pressure > 140 plus/minus a diastolic pressure > 90 mm Hg on more than three occasions

II. Physiology/Pathophysiology
  A. Normal
    1. Blood pressure is maintained as the result of the continuous regulation of cardiac output (CO) and systemic vascular resistance (SVR). This regulation takes place at the site of the heart, pre- and post-capillary venules, and the kidneys.
    2. The overall regulation of these sites is stimulated or suppressed by the autonomic nervous system and humoral influences, such as the renin-angiotensin-aldosterone system.
      a) Renin is secreted by the juxtaglomerular apparatus in response to a number of stimuli, including a decrease in intravascular volume, decreased perfusion pressure, beta-adrenergic stimulation, and hypokalemia.
      b) Renin acts on angiotensinogen to form angiotensin 1 (a substance with no known biologic activity), which is converted in the lung to angiotensin II by angiotensin-converting enzyme (ACE).
        (1) Angiotensin II is a potent vasoconstrictor that acts on the adrenal cortex to release aldosterone.
        (2) Aldosterone increases sodium and water reabsorption in the distal tubule of the nephron.
      c) Renin production is inversely proportional to effective blood volume. Stimuli that increase effective blood volume suppress renin; stimuli that decrease effective blood volume stimulate renin.
    3. Catecholamines affect blood pressure regulation centrally by the vasomotor centers in the brain and peripherally through the action of the sympathetic nervous system.
  B. Pathophysiology
    1. The pathogenesis of essential/primary hypertension is multifactorial.
    2. Catecholamines elevate blood pressure by increasing peripheral resistance and increasing cardiac output (e.g., as in pheochromocytoma).
    3. Increased calcium appears to increase vascular tone, which can lead to increased blood pressure.

III. Clinical features: As many as 50 million Americans (25% of the adult population) have hypertension. The majority of patients are unaware of their condition; only a minority are adequately controlled. More than 90% of hypertension is idiopathic (primary or essential hypertension), while 2%–5% is the result of other identifiable causes (secondary hypertension).

A. Risk factors

1. Modifiable contributing factors to the development of primary hypertension
   a) Obesity
   b) Excessive use of alcohol
   c) Cigarette smoking: Acutely raises blood pressure
   d) Polycythemia
   e) NSAID: Can raise blood pressure 5 mm Hg; hypertensive patients should avoid
   f) Increased salt intake
      (1) Salt alone may not be enough to significantly raise normal blood pressure; however, a genetic predisposition to salt sensitivity may be enough to significantly raise blood pressure.
      (2) African Americans and the elderly population have a high prevalence of salt sensitivity

2. Nonmodifiable risk factors for the development of primary hypertension
   a) Age: Risk increases after age 60.
   b) Gender: Men have a greater incidence of hypertension than premenopausal women.
   c) Race: In African Americans, incidence and earlier onset of hypertension is increased; the severity of hypertension is greater with an increased incidence of target organ disease (TOD).

3. Secondary hypertension: Suspect in patients
   a) Whose age, history, physical exam, severity of hypertension, or initial laboratory findings are not consistent with essential hypertension.
   b) In whom blood pressure responds poorly to drug therapy.
   c) With previously well-controlled hypertension and current increase in blood pressure.
   d) In whom blood pressure is accelerating or who have malignancy.
   e) Who present with sudden onset of hypertension.

B. Classification: According to the Joint National Committee on Detection, Evaluation, and Treatment of High Blood Pressure (JNC-VI); classification includes all adults age 18 years and older.

1. Normal blood pressure: < 130 systolic and < 85 diastolic
2. High normal blood pressure: Includes 130–139 systolic and/or 85–89 diastolic
3. Hypertension: Further classified by stages
   a) Stage I hypertension: 140–159 systolic and/or 90–99 diastolic
   b) Stage II hypertension: 160–179 systolic and/or 100–109 diastolic
   c) Stage III hypertension: Systolic > or = 180 mm Hg systolic and or diastolic > or = 110 mm Hg

C. The goal of evaluation is threefold.

1. To determine if there is a secondary cause for the blood pressure elevation

   2. To assess TOD
   3. To asses other cardiac risk factors
D. History
   1. History of cancer and cancer treatment
   2. Current medications: Prescribed and over-the-counter
   3. History of presenting symptom(s): Precipitating factors, onset, and duration. Associated symptoms are jittery, nervous, sweaty for no reason, or experiencing heart palpitations
   4. Changes in activities of daily living
   5. Family history: Hypertension, premature coronary artery disease (CAD) (i.e., myocardial infarction [MI] before age 55 in father or first-degree male relative or before age 65 in mother or first-degree female relative), stroke, other cardiovascular disease, diabetes mellitus, dyslipidemia
   6. Past medical history: Cardiovascular disease, cerebrovascular disease, renal disease, diabetes mellitus, dyslipidemia, gout, hypertension
   7. Social history of tobacco and alcohol use
   8. History of diet: Fat and cholesterol intake
E. Signs and symptoms
   1. Patients with mild to moderate primary hypertension are generally asymptomatic
   2. Patients with severe or poorly controlled hypertension may present with symptoms of TOD (e.g., CHF, nephropathy, retinopathy, stroke).
F. Physical exam: According to the JNC-VI guidelines, assess the involvement or damage of the target organs (i.e., heart, brain, kidneys, eyes, peripheral arteries).
   1. Vital signs
      a) Hypertension should not be diagnosed on the basis of a single measurement.
         (1) Confirm elevated readings on at least two subsequent visits during a one- to several-week period of time (unless systolic blood pressure is 180 and diastolic blood pressure is > 110), with average levels of systolic readings of 140 mm Hg or > and/or diastolic readings averaging 90 mm Hg or > to diagnose hypertension.
         (2) Take blood pressure in both arms with patient in same position; document the higher reading. Always take blood pressure in the same manner to achieve accurate readings.
         (3) JNC guidelines recommend taking blood pressures with the patient seated and arm free of clothing and supported at heart level. The patient should not have smoked or ingested caffeine within 30 minutes of measurement.
      b) Height and weight: To assess for overweight status
      c) Osler's maneuver to rule out pseudohypertension (see Appendix 13)
   2. HEENT/Fundoscopic exam indicating retina TOD
      a) Arteriolar narrowing
      b) Arteriovenous nicking
      c) Hemorrhages
      d) Exudate
      e) Papilledema
      f) Retinopathy

   3. Neck exam
- *a)* Carotid bruits
- *b)* Distended jugular veins
- *c)* Enlarged thyroid: To evaluate for hypo- or hyperthyroidism

   4. Cardiac exam: May indicate CAD, CHF, cardiomyopathy if present
- *a)* Increased rate
- *b)* Increased size by percussion
- *c)* Precordial heave
- *d)* Clicks
- *e)* Murmurs
- *f)* Arrhythmias
- *g)* S_3 indicating CHF
- *h)* S_4
- *i)* Suspect pseudohypertension when TOD is absent in spite of high blood pressure and can be confirmed by Osler's maneuver.
  - (1) Palpate radial or brachial artery, and inflate cuff above systolic blood pressure.
  - (2) Determine palpable artery, even though it is pulseless.
  - (3) Positive when artery is palpable; negative if artery not palpable.

   5. Pulmonary exam: Rales, coarse sounds indicating CHF

   6. Abdominal exam
- *a)* Bruits: Aortic, renal
- *b)* Enlarged kidneys
- *c)* Masses
- *d)* Abnormal aortic pulsation
- *e)* Hepatomegaly

   7. Extremity exam indicating peripheral vascular disease
- *a)* Diminished or absent pulses
- *b)* Bruits (femoral)
- *c)* Edema

   8. Neurologic exam: General exam to evaluate for any focal defects

IV. Diagnostic tests
  A. Laboratory
    1. CBC: To evaluate for anemia
    2. Urinalysis: To evaluate nephropathy (e.g., proteinuria)
    3. Fasting glucose: To rule out diabetes mellitus
    4. Potassium
- *a)* Baseline value before initiating diuretic or ACE inhibitor
- *b)* Hypokalemia: May elevate blood pressure or adrenal precipitate aldosteronism or Cushing's disease

    5. Calcium: Deficiencies are associated with an increased prevalence of hypertension.
    6. Creatinine and BUN: Will be elevated in those with renal TOD
    7. Uric acid: Frequently elevated in patients with hypertension and may reflect decreased renal blood flow
    8. Fasting cholesterol profile (total, HDL, LDL, triglycerides); cardiovascular risk profile data

B. Radiology
   1. Chest x-ray
      a) Cardiac enlargement
      b) Evidence of pulmonary edema/CHF
   2. Echocardiogram: Not routinely performed on hypertensive patients unless there is evidence of TOD
C. Other: EKG
   1. Evidence of left ventricular hypertrophy (LVH) indicating target organ damage
   2. Evidence of previous MI or current ischemia

V. Differential diagnosis
  A. Diseases
    1. Paraneoplastic syndrome (see Appendix 12).
    2. Secondary diseases
       a) Renal artery stenosis
       b) Adrenal aldosteronism and Cushing's syndrome
       c) Pheochromocytoma
       d) Coarctation of the aorta
       e) Renal parenchymal diseases
       f) Thyroid disorders (see Chapters 149 and 150)
       g) Hyperparathyroidism
  B. Medication-induced
    1. Oral contraceptives
    2. Steroids
    3. NSAIDs
    4. Nasal decongestants
    5. Cough suppressants
    6. Cyclosporine
    7. Erythropoietin
    8. Tricyclic antidepressants
    9. MAO inhibitors
  C. White coat hypertension
    1. Elevated blood pressure when in doctor's office
    2. May indicate hypertensive tendency; patients should have blood pressure checked outside of office for a period of 7–10 days and report levels if elevated.
  D. Pseudohypertension
    1. Present in the elderly
    2. Caused by rigid brachial arteries that do not compress by sphygmomanometer cuff; gives false high readings
    3. Can be caused by incorrect cuff size.

VI. Treatment
  A. Goals: Prevention of morbidity and mortality most frequently related to strokes, MI, CHF, and renal failure; control of blood pressure by the least intrusive means possible.

B. Therapies to lower blood pressure: Require intensive, lifelong commitments to lifestyle modification and, possibly, drug therapy.
   1. Tobacco avoidance
   2. Weight reduction
   3. Moderation of alcohol intake: Limit to no more than one ounce of ethanol per day
   4. Physical activity: Regular aerobic activity can reduce systolic blood pressure by approximately 10 mm Hg.
   5. Moderation of dietary sodium intake: < 2 g per day
   6. Increase in potassium intake: Maintain normal plasma levels.
   7. Increase in calcium intake to recommended daily allowance (800–1,200 mg per day).
   8. Dietary reduction of fats: < 30% total calories per day
C. Pharmacologic treatment
   1. Depends on the patient's cardiac risk profile and the degree of hypertension
   2. Initiate drug therapy only after establishing a lifestyle modification program (see Table 45-1).
   3. For high-normal blood pressure and stage I hypertension with no major risk factors and no evidence of TOD, lifestyle modification for up to one year is recommended.
   4. For high normal blood pressure and stage I hypertension with at least one cardiovascular risk factor with evidence of TOD, lifestyle modification for three to six months is recommended.
   5. For high normal blood pressure and stage I hypertension with a high cardiovascular risk profile, drug therapy should begin immediately along with lifestyle modification.
   6. For all patients in stages II and III hypertension, drug therapy should begin immediately with lifestyle modifications.
   7. Hypertensive urgencies are those situations in which it is desirable to reduce blood pressure within 24 hours (e.g., SBP > 240, DBP > 130). Hypertensive urgencies include accelerated or malignant hypertension without severe symptoms or progressive TOD, as previously defined.
   8. Hypertensive emergencies are those situations that require immediate blood pressure reduction within minutes (not necessarily to normal limits) to prevent or limit TOD (e.g., DBP > 130).
      a) Hypertensive encephalopathy
      b) Intracranial hemorrhage
      c) Acute left ventricular failure with pulmonary edema
      d) Dissecting aortic aneurysm
      e) Eclampsia
      f) Unstable angina
      g) Acute myocardial infarction
   9. Initial therapy should be monotherapy
      a) If blood pressure remains elevated for one to three months after initiating monotherapy, consider
         (1) Substituting another agent from another class
         (2) Increasing the dose of the initial drug
         (3) Adding a second agent from another class.

Table 45-1. Drugs for Hypertension

Type	Action	Special Considerations
Diuretics:		
Thiazide: Hydrochlorothiazide	Decreased plasma volume	More effective antihypertensive than loop diuretics
	Decreased extravascular fluid volume	Preferred diuretic
	Decreased cardiac output followed by decreased peripheral resistance with normalization of cardiac output	May decrease potassium, sodium, chloride, magnesium
		May increase calcium, uric acid, blood sugar, and triglyceride
Loop: Bumetanide	As above	Causes greater potassium loss, resulting in enhanced effect of digoxin
Furosemide	As above	Causes calcium loss
Potassium-sparing: Spironolactone	Aldosterone antagonist	Use in combination with other diuretics to avoid/reverse hypokalemia
Cardiac selective beta-blockers:		
Atenolol, bisoprolol, metoprolol	Decreased cardiac output and increased total peripheral resistance	Aggravates asthma
	Decreased plasma renin activity	May mask hypoglycemia
	Decreased AV node conduction	May alter blood sugar
		May cause muscle weakness or fatigue
		May exacerbate peripheral vascular disease
		Decreases heart rate
Alpha-beta-blockers:		
Labetalol	Similar to beta-blockers	May be more effective in African Americans than other beta-blockers
	Vasodilation	May cause postural hypotension. Titration should be based on standing blood pressure

(Continued on next page)

Table 45-1. Drugs for Hypertension *(Continued)*

Type	Action	Special Considerations
ACE inhibitors: Enalopril*, lisinopril*, benazepril, fosinopril, capoten, quinapril* (*also used in CHF)	Inhibits the formation of angiotensin II, resulting in direct decrease in arterial pressure and indirect decrease in venous pressure	Side effects may include absence of taste, cough, rash, hyperkalemia, neutropenia, renal failure
		May increase or decrease digoxin levels
		May be necessary to decrease or discontinue diuretics during titration of ACE inhibitor to prevent hypotension
		Decrease dose in patients with serum creatinine > 2.5 mg/dl
		Follow serum potassium, creatinine, BUN, weekly during initiation/titration
		Can cause acute renal failure in patients with bilateral renal artery stenosis or severe stenosis in a single artery
Calcium channel blockers: Nondihydropyridines: diltiazem	Blocks inward movement of calcium ions across cell membranes, resulting in smooth muscle relaxation	Also blocks slow channels in the heart and can reduce sinus rate and produce heart block
		May exacerbate or precipitate CHF
Dihydropyridines: amlodipine,* felodipine,* nifedipine (*worsening of CHF may be less with these agents)	Same as other calcium channel blockers	More potent peripheral vasodilators than diltiazem and may result in increased dizziness, headache, peripheral edema, and tachycardia
Central sympatholytic: Clonidine	Reduces sympathetic outflow, resulting in decreased blood pressure	Side effects include dry mouth, drowsiness, dizziness, sedation, constipation, depression
		Do not discontinue therapy abruptly; may cause severe rebound hypertension
		May cause orthostatic hypotension
Direct vasodilators: Hydralazine	Direct smooth muscle vasodilation	May exacerbate angina
		Should be used in combination with beta-blockers and diuretics because of fluid retention and reflex tachycardia

Note. This is not a complete list of all available medications but rather a representative sample.

b) Diuretics and beta-blockers have been shown to reduce cardiovascular morbidity/mortality.
c) ACE inhibitors
  (1) Effective and generally well-tolerated
  (2) Less effective, but not ineffective in African Americans
  (3) No adverse effects on plasma lipid concentration or glucose tolerance
  (4) Some have been shown to prolong survival in patients with heart failure or left ventricular dysfunction, after myocardial infarction, and to preserve renal function in patients with diabetes mellitus.
  (5) Patients with high levels of plasma renin activity may experience excessive hypotensive responses to ACE inhibitors.
  (6) Cough is a common side effect.
  (7) Hyperkalemia can occur, especially in patients taking potassium supplements or potassium-sparing diuretics or those with reduced renal function.
d) Angiotensin receptor antagonist
  (1) Interferes with binding of angiotensin II to angiotensin I
  (2) May prove to be as effective as ACE inhibitors without cough
  (3) Like ACE inhibitors, may be less effective in African Americans
e) Beta-adrenergic blocking agents
  (1) Less effective in African Americans
  (2) Decreased mortality in patients with hypertension and in patients who have had an MI
  (3) Usually not recommended for patients with heart failure
  (4) May mask hypoglycemia
  (5) May increase or decrease blood glucose levels
  (6) May increase serum triglycerides and decrease HDL
  (7) May induce bronchospasm
  (8) May exacerbate peripheral arterial insufficiency
  (9) May decrease heart rate significantly
f) Labetalol: Mixed alpha- and beta-blocker
  (1) Prompt decrease in blood pressure
  (2) Orthostatic hypotension more frequent than with other beta-blockers
  (3) Equally effective in African Americans and Caucasians
  (4) Does not alter serum lipids
g) Calcium channel blockers
  (1) Verapamil and diltiazem prolong AV nodal conduction; therefore, must be used with caution in patients also taking beta-blockers.
  (2) All calcium channel blockers except amlodipine and felodipine should be used cautiously in patients with CHF; these drugs have a negative inotropic effect on the heart, especially the left ventricle.
  (3) No effect on lipid concentrations
h) Diuretics
  (1) Like beta-blockers, have been shown to decrease mortality in patients with hypertension.
  (2) Elderly patients can be effectively treated with small doses.

          (3) Loop diuretics can be used to treat hypertension in patients with renal insufficiency (creatinine > 1.5).

          (4) Can cause hypokalemia, hyponatremia, hypochloremia, and hypomagnesemia

          (5) Can cause hypercalcemia, hyperuricemia, and hyperglycemia

          (6) Can increase serum triglycerides and cholesterol

      i) Alpha-adrenergic blocking agents

          (1) Cause arterial and venous dilatation

          (2) Frequently cause postural hypotension, especially after first dose (increased incidence in elderly)

          (3) Do not adversely affect blood lipids and may increase HDL

          (4) Symptomatic relief of prostatism

      j) Central sympatholytic: Frequently causes sedation, dry mouth, and depression

D. Special considerations

    1. All drugs approved for the treatment of hypertension are effective in lowering blood pressure. Diuretics, beta-blockers, ACE inhibitors, and calcium channel blockers are, perhaps, the best tolerated.

    2. Only beta-blockers and diuretics have been shown in large-scale controlled clinical trials to reduce mortality in hypertensive patients.

    3. ACE inhibitors, calcium channel blockers, and alpha-adrenergic blockers have a more favorable effect on some cardiovascular risk factors.

    4. Diuretics and calcium channel blockers are more effective than beta-blockers or ACE inhibitors in African Americans.

    5. Diabetic patients, especially those with nephropathy, may benefit most from an ACE inhibitor.

    6. For patients with hyperlipidemia, an ACE inhibitor, alpha-blocker, or calcium channel blocker may be a good choice.

    7. Patients with CHF may have extra benefit from an ACE inhibitor.

    8. Beta-blockers may be indicated for hypertensive patients with angina, post myocardial infarction, or those with migraines.

VI. Follow-up

    A. Recheck blood pressure in two years for initial readings of < 130 and < 85.

    B. Recheck readings in one year for high normal blood pressures.

    C. For blood pressure 140–159/90–99, confirm within a two-month period.

    D. Reevaluate within one month for blood pressure 160–179/100–109.

    E. Reevaluate within one week for blood pressure > = 180/110.

VII. Referrals

    A. Cardiologist: Refer patients with

        1. Hypertension at any stage with evidence of TOD

        2. Hypertension resistant to treatment

        3. Well-controlled blood pressure now resistant to treatment

        4. Hypertensive emergencies or urgencies.

    B. Nephrologist: Refer patients with evidence of renal TOD.

    C. Ophthalmology: Refer patients with evidence of TOD of retina.

    D. Neurology: Refer patients with history of stroke and/or TIA.

References

American Pharmaceutical Association (APhA) & American Academy of Physician Assistants (AAPA). (1998). *Special report: A review of the Sixth Report of the Joint National Committee on Prevention, Detection, Evaluation, and Treatment of High Blood Pressure.* Alexandria, VA: AAPA.

Carlson, R.W. (1992). Reducing the cardiotoxicity of the anthracyclines. *Oncology, 6*(6), 95–100.

Felicetta, J.V. (1996). Hypertension in the elderly. *Clinical Geriatrics, 4*(10), 87–93.

National Institute of Mental Health. (1993). *The fifth report of the Joint National Committee on Detection, Evaluation, and Treatment of High Blood Pressure* (NIH Publication No. 93-1088). Washington, DC: U.S. Government Printing Office.

Hamet, P. (1996). Cancer and hypertension. *Hypertension, 28,* 321–324.

Lily, L.S. (1993). Hypertension. In L.S. Lily (Ed.), *Pathophysiology of heart disease* (pp. 208–266). Philadelphia: Lea & Febiger.

Ofili, E.O. (1995). Managing high blood pressure and hypertensive cardiovascular disease in blacks. *Urban Cardiology, November/December,* 20–25.

Porsche, R. (1995). Hypertension: Diagnosis, acute antihypertension therapy and long term management. *AACN Clinical Issues, 6,* 515–525.

46. Hypotension
Mary Ann Winokur, CRNP, MSN

I. Definition: An abnormally low blood pressure when compared to the patient's baseline pressure and associated systemic symptoms; in general, a systolic blood pressure < 90 mm Hg and a diastolic pressure < 60 mm Hg is considered to be within the lower limits of normal.

II. Physiology/Pathophysiology
   A. Normal
      1. Blood pressure is maintained as the result of the continuous regulation of cardiac output (CO) and systemic vascular resistance (SVR).
      2. This regulation takes place at the sites of the heart, pre- and postcapillary venule, and the kidneys.
      3. The overall regulation of these sites is stimulated or suppressed by the autonomic nervous system and humoral influences.
   B. Pathophysiology: Hypotension results from the disruption of CO and SVR or the malfunction of the other regulatory systems; therefore, perfusion cannot meet the metabolic needs of the end organs.

III. Clinical features
   A. Etiology
      1. Vascular and cardiac etiologies
      2. Distributive etiologies (i.e., sepsis and drug-induced)
      3. Obstructive (i.e., pneumothorax, emboli, stenosis)
      4. Neoplastic
   B. History
      1. History of cancer and cancer treatment
      2. Current medications: Prescribed and over-the-counter
      3. History of presenting symptom(s): Precipitating factors, onset, location, and duration. Associated symptoms are dizziness, lightheadedness, syncope, chest discomfort, shortness of breath, vomiting, diarrhea, fever, chills, and melena.
      4. Changes in activities of daily living
      5. Recent history of infection
   C. Signs and symptoms
      1. Dizziness/lightheadedness

       2. Nausea/vomiting

       3. Diarrhea

       4. Fever/chills

       5. Chest pain

       6. Shortness of breath

       7. Weakness

       8. Fatigue

   D. Physical exam

       1. Vital signs

         a) Hypotension

         b) Fever indicating sepsis

         c) Orthostatic changes in vital signs: A drop of 10–20 mm Hg or more of systolic or diastolic blood pressure along with a pulse rate increase of 10–15 beats/minute

       2. Integument exam: Evaluate for

         a) Temperature: Hypo/hyperthermia

         b) Color: Pale, cold, clammy

         c) Poor skin turgor or dry mucous membranes indicating dehydration.

       3. Neurologic exam: Altered mental status

         a) Restlessness

         b) Agitation

         c) Confusion

         d) Lethargy

         e) Coma

       4. Cardiac exam

         a) S_3: Indicative of CHF

         b) S_4: May be present in MI

         c) Murmurs for valvular disease

         d) Jugular vein distention (JVD) in heart failure

       5. Pulmonary exam

         a) Rales: Pulmonary edema

         b) Rhonchi: Pneumonia

         c) Bilaterally equal breath sounds: Pneumothorax, hemothorax

       6. Examination of extremities: Assess for

         a) Weak or absent pulse

         b) Cool or mottled extremities

         c) Presence of edema

       7. Rectal exam if bleeding suspected to guaiac stool

 IV. Diagnostic tests

   A. Laboratory

       1. CBC with differential: To assess for

         a) Anemia

         b) Leukocytosis

       2. BUN/creatinine to rule out sepsis: Increased values indicate dehydration, metabolic acidosis, acute renal failure.

      3. Cultures: As indicated to rule out sepsis
        a) Visible wounds
        b) Urine
        c) Blood
  B. Radiology
      1. Chest x-ray: Assess for
        a) Heart size
        b) Evidence of CHF (i.e., cardiomegaly)
        c) Pulmonary edema
        d) Pneumonia (i.e., infiltrates)
      2. Echocardiogram: To evaluate
        a) Effectiveness of left ventricle
        b) Valve status
  C. Other: EKG to assess for
      1. Acute changes indicative of myocardial infarction/ischemia
      2. Left ventricular hypertrophy
      3. Dysrhythmia secondary to MI or electrolyte imbalances

V. Differential diagnosis
  A. Cardiac and vascular
      1. Hypovolemia
      2. Pump failure
      3. Valvular dysfunction
  B. Distributive
      1. Sepsis
      2. Anaphylactic shock
      3. Drug-induced
        a) Angiotensin-converting enzyme (ACE) inhibitors
        b) Diuretics
        c) Nitrates
        d) Beta-blockers
        e) Central sympatholytics
        f) Alpha-adrenergic blocking agents
        g) Tricyclic antidepressants
        h) Steroids from acute withdrawal
      4. Neurogenic
      5. Acute adrenal insufficiency
  C. Obstructive
      1. Pneumothorax (see Chapter 31)
      2. Pericardial tamponade (see Chapter 48)
      3. Pulmonary emboli (see Chapter 33)
      4. Pulmonary hypertension
      5. Aortic or mitral stenosis
  D. Neoplastic
      1. Spinal lesions

2. Biotherapy (cytokines)
   a) Interleukin-2
   b) Interferon
   c) Tumor necrosis factor

VII. Treatment
  A. Place patient in Trendelenburg or supine position with legs elevated.
  B. Use of oxygen
     1. Depends on arterial blood gases (ABGs) and patient's baseline pulmonary function, although may be initiated immediately if patient is hypovolemic.
     2. Two liters by nasal cannula would be helpful and rarely affects CO_2 retention.
  C. Monitor urine output.
     1. Patient may be oliguric or nonoliguric.
     2. Use Foley catheter.
     3. Urine output should be maintained at least 25–30 cc/hour.
  D. Volume replacement: Determine by blood pressure, electrolyte status, and cardiovascular status.
  E. Vasoactive drugs
     1. Dopamine 1–2 mg/kg/minute IV: Dose will stimulate dopaminergic receptors and increased renal blood flow.
     2. Dobutamine: A synthetic catecholamine with greater inotropic effect than dopamine
     3. Diuretics: Used only when volume deficits are corrected.
  F. Corticosteroids (e.g., hydrocortisone): Used to treat acute adrenal insufficiency.
  G. Antibiotics if sepsis (see Appendix 1)

VII. Follow-up: Frequent to intermittent, depending on cause of hypotension and whether condition becomes problematic.

VIII. Referrals
  A. Cardiologist: If patient is not responding to treatment
  B. Infectious disease specialist: For sepsis
  C. Nephrologist: For acute renal failure secondary to shock

References

American Pharmaceutical Association (APhA) & American Academy of Physician Assistants (AAPA). (1998). Special report: A review of the Sixth Report of the Joint National Committee on Prevention, Detection, Evaluation, and Treatment of High Blood Pressure. Alexandria, VA: AAPA.

Hravnak, M., & Boujoukos, A. (1997). Hypotension. *AACN Clinical Issues, 8,* 303–318.

47. Myocardial Infarction

Brenda K. Shelton, RN, MS, CCRN, AOCN®, and
Lisa Keel, RN, MSN, CNS

I. Definition: Total occlusion of a coronary artery, resulting in ischemia, injury, and necrosis of the myocardium

II. Pathophysiology
   A. Pathophysiology involves coronary artery occlusion, direct cardiac compromise, and sympathetic stimulation.
   B. Initially after occlusion (first 24 hours), platelets and fibrin adhere to the rough edges of the occlusion, potentially "extending" the area of ischemia.
   C. Coronary artery occlusion leads to ischemia, injury, and, then, necrosis if circulation is not restored.
      1. The "wave of injury" is the term used to describe which of these three changes has occurred in the myocardium.
      2. The wave of injury predicts the depth of myocardial damage.
   D. Ischemia leads to the release of toxic metabolites (e.g., arachidonic acid, oxygen-free radicals) that enlarge the area of ischemia and injury.
   E. Cardiac muscle or other structures (e.g., papillary muscle, conduction pathway, valves) deprived of oxygen lead to cell death and clinical manifestations typical of myocardial infarction (MI) (necrosis).
   F. Mediastinal radiation therapy at any dose causes microvascular changes that interfere with coronary blood flow.

III. Clinical features: The clinical manifestations of MI are indicative of hypoxemic muscle damage, conduction pathway disruption, and poor pumping capabilities. The majority of MIs involve the left ventricle. If approximately 40% of the left ventricle is damaged, expect a high mortality rate. The greatest mortality occurs within two hours after the onset of symptoms and is related to sudden arrhythmic death. Most MIs occur when the person is at rest (51%); only a few occur with heavy exertion (13%). Asymptomatic (silent) MIs occur in about 10% of cases.
   A. Risk factors
      1. Typical risk factors for heart disease
         a) Older age: > 60 years
         b) Family history: First-degree relative with an MI age < 60 years

   c) Hyperlipidemia: Cholesterol > 200 mg/dl, triglycerides > 200
       (1) Familial hypercholesterolemia
       (2) Glomerulonephritis
   d) Obesity: > 15% above ideal body weight
   e) Hypertension
   f) Smoking
   g) Stress: Particularly anger
   h) Sedentary lifestyle
   i) Increased homocystine levels
   j) Diabetes mellitus
2. Dysrhythmia
3. Recreational drug use: Particularly stimulants (e.g., cocaine, speed balls, high-dose caffeine)
4. Other health problems: Increase risk of hypertension or coronary artery disease (CAD)
   a) Adrenal cancer: Possibly caused by abnormal cortisol secretion
   b) Anemia: Hematocrit < 25% increases risk, particularly if pre-existing CAD is present; it may occur with even lower RBC counts with more severe or symptomatic CAD.
   c) Colorectal cancer and CAD: Jointly associated in men > 60 years and women < 50 years of age
   d) Endometrial cancer: Possibly caused by hormonal imbalance
   e) Esophageal and gastric cancer: Unknown mechanism
   f) Survivor of childhood cancer: Thought to be related to decreased growth hormone
5. Medications
   a) Levodopa, dopamine, epinephrine: Increase sympathetic stimulation, increasing workload on the heart
   b) Nonselective beta-blockers: Increase cholesterol
   c) Birth control pills, excess vitamin K: Enhance hypercoagulability
   d) Postchemotherapy for testicular cancer: Agents alone do not cause cardiac disease, but Einhorn regimen is associated with late cardiovascular abnormalities (e.g., Raynaud's syndrome, hypertension).
B. Etiology
   1. Coronary artery occlusion occurs from major mechanisms.
      a) Vasospasm
      b) Rupture of atheromatous plaque with thrombus > 80%
      c) Embolus
      d) Unknown
   2. A combination of changes in the coronary artery usually accompanies infarction
      a) Atheromatous plaques involving about 50%–75% artery occlusion produce exertional, symptomatic, stable angina.
      b) Ruptured atheromatous plaques involving existing lesions worsen coronary blood flow.

  c) A combination of plaque development, ruptured plaque, and platelet adhesion to a roughened endothelial lining leads to 95%–98% coronary artery occlusion and unstable angina.

C. Myocardial classification

 1. MI is classified by depth of myocardial injury. The depth of injury predicts the severity of cardiac dysfunction.

  a) Epicardial: Term not commonly used among cardiovascular specialists

  b) Subendocardial: Non-Q-wave MI

  c) Transmural: Full thickness, Q-wave MI

 2. MI is classified by portion of the heart damaged from ischemia, which will predict clinical manifestations, diagnostic test findings, complications, and prognosis.

  a) Anterior

  b) Lateral

  c) Septal

  d) Inferior

  e) Posterior

 3. MI also is classified by the severity of left ventricular dysfunction. The Killip classification was developed in the 1960s and is still used today.

  a) Killip Class I: Uncomplicated MI, perhaps few crackles on lung auscultation

  b) Killip Class II: Mild heart failure, bilateral crackles on lung auscultation

  c) Killip Class III: Pulmonary edema, with or without intubation

  d) Killip Class IV: Cardiogenic shock

D. History

 1. History of cancer and cancer treatment

 2. Current medications: Prescribed and over-the-counter

 3. History of presenting symptom(s): Precipitating factors, onset, location, and duration

 4. Changes in activities of daily living

 5. Family history: Cardiovascular disease (e.g., hypertension, CAD, aneurysms, peripheral vascular disease, MI)

 6. Risk factors for CAD and MI (see pp. 291–292)

E. Signs and symptoms

 1. Pain

  a) Most common symptom (72%)

   (1) Chest (80%)

   (2) Epigastric, shoulder, or arm (20%)

   (3) Shoulder, neck, or jaw (8%)

  b) Typically severe, lasting 30 minutes or longer and not relieved by rest or sublingual nitroglycerin

  c) Lack of pain or atypical pain does not exclude an MI, especially in a diabetic patient or woman.

 2. Irregular heart beat

 3. Dyspnea

 4. Diaphoresis

 5. Nausea

      6. Dizziness

      7. Weakness

      8. Abdominal pain

      9. Anxiety

    10. Restlessness

F. Physical exam

  1. Vital signs

    a) Heart rate: Varies

      (1) Location of MI may cause bradycardia, tachycardia, or irritable rhythms.

      (2) Persistent tachycardia is a particularly poor prognostic sign.

      (3) Affected coronary artery influences heart rate and rhythm.

        (a) RCA occlusion causes bradycardia and heart block.

        (b) LCA occlusion causes ventricular rhythms (particularly ventricular fibrillation) and high-level heart block (e.g., complete heart block).

    b) Blood pressure: Normotensive but may be altered

      (1) In patients with acute infarction, blood pressure normally is elevated.

      (2) Progressive hypotension, particularly with a narrow pulse pressure (< 30 mm Hg), is a sign of severely compromised cardiac output with catecholamine-induced vasoconstriction.

      (3) Measure blood pressure in both arms to rule out the possibility of aortic dissection as the etiology of symptoms.

    c) Tachypnea: Occurs as the body attempts to compensate for reduced cardiac function and decreased cardiac output.

    d) Low-grade fevers: Often are present and represent an inflammatory response to tissue ischemia and injury.

  2. Cardiac exam

    a) Auscultation of heart sounds

      (1) May be normal

      (2) Irregular rhythm: May indicate ventricular ectopy

      (3) S_4 gallop: Often present and indicates an extensive anterior MI

      (4) S_3 gallop: May be present if CHF is present

      (5) Split S_1: Often normal, but split S_2 usually indicates papillary muscle rupture

      (6) Blowing systolic murmur: Indicates mitral regurgitation and is more often present in an extensive anterior MI

      (7) Holosystolic murmur: Most often heard with inferior MI with papillary muscle rupture

      (8) Pericardial friction rub

        (a) Heard as early as 24 hours after MI but usually 48–72 hours after MI; late onset (10–14 days after MI) usually indicates Dressler syndrome (postmyocardial pericarditis). Rub usually lasts for several days.

        (b) May represent transmural infarction

        (c) Is frequently transient and intermittent

    b) Jugular vein distention (JVD): Considered positive at > 2 cm above the clavicle when patient is in 30° upright position indicating right heart failure.

    c) Pulses

        (1) Point of maximal impulse (PMI) at heart apex
            (a) May be shifted laterally from left midclavicular line
            (b) May be below fifth intercostal space as a result of cardiomegaly or dyskinesia
            (c) Lift or thrill may be palpable with severe murmurs.
            (d) Large area of dyskinetic myocardium may cause systolic bulge along the left sternal border.
            (e) S_4 may be palpable.
        (2) Peripheral pulses may be weaker.
            (a) Equal but weaker indicates decreased cardiac output.
            (b) Pulsus alternans (alternating one strong, one weak) indicates high thoracic pressure or pericardial effusion.
            (c) Pulsus paradoxus (systolic decreases with inspiration) indicates high thoracic pressure, pericardial effusion, or tamponade.
            (d) Weak and thready pulses indicate myocardial dysfunction with poor contractility.
    d) Pallor or cyanosis, coolness, clamminess, or capillary refill less than three seconds indicate inadequate peripheral tissue perfusion.
  3. Pulmonary exam
    a) Chest excursion: May have shallow respirations but is usually equal
    b) Tachypnea: Common
    c) Labored respirations with nasal flaring: Use of sternocleidomastoid muscles is possible
    d) Breath sounds
        (1) End inspiratory fine crackles are characteristic of left ventricular dysfunction.
        (2) The location of the lung fields in which fine crackles are found correlates with the severity of the left ventricular dysfunction (i.e., further "up," more severe).
        (3) Coarser crackles or wheezes may be present with pulmonary edema.
  4. Neurologic exam: Abnormalities may reflect pain, fear, poor perfusion, or impaired mentation.
  5. Abdominal exam: Commonly manifests abnormalities, as blood shunts away from this system during acute MI
    a) Abdominal pain
        (1) Mesenteric ischemia-related abdominal pain is severe, diffuse, and not exacerbated by palpation.
        (2) Rebound tenderness indicates bowel infarction.
    b) Altered bowel motility: Decreased bowel sounds are common manifestations of reduced blood flow.
    c) Right upper quadrant discomfort and hepatomegaly may be present.
        (1) Relates to congestive failure
        (2) Prevalent after severe hypotensive episode

IV. Diagnostic tests
  A. Laboratory

1. CBC to assess for anemia
2. Cardiac enzymes (see Table 47-1)
   a) Creatine phosphokinase (CPK) total: > 115
      (1) Peaks in 24 hours
      (2) Marks cardiac muscle death
   b) CPK-MB isoenzymes (> 5% of total CPK significant for MI)
      (1) Begins to rise in 8–10 hours, peaks in 12–18 hours
      (2) Returns to normal in 72–96 hours
      (3) Specific for myocardial injury
   c) Lactic dehydrogenase (LDH) total and isoenzyme are seldomly used because of the availability of more specific enzyme tests that remain elevated for longer periods of time.
   d) Cardiac troponin-I
      (1) Unique myocardial protein: More sensitive than CPK
      (2) Rises in three to six hours
      (3) Diagnostic window is longer (four to nine days).
      (4) Increased specificity and longer diagnostic window promote use of this enzyme rather than use of LDH enzyme tests.
   e) Cardiac troponin-T: Similar to cardiac troponin-I; however, too many false positives result
   f) Myoglobin levels: Myoglobin released early from injured cardiac cells (two to four hours) and peaks at 3–15 hours. May also be elevated with any other muscle injury in the body. Seldom used because of lack of sensitivity.
B. Radiology
   1. Chest x-ray: Cannot detect MI, although can detect complications (e.g., CHF, pericardial effusion)
   2. Nuclear and tomographic imaging
      a) Technetium-99 pyrophosphate scan: Shows cardiac "hot spots" with excess uptake of nuclear substance

Table 47-1. Cardiac Enzyme Changes with Acute Myocardial Infarction

Enzyme	Onset	Peak	Return to Normal	Normal or Significant Value
CPK	4–6 hours	24 hours	2–3 days	Normal = < 100 mcg/ml
CPK-MB	4–6 hours	12–30 hours	2–3 days	Sig[a] = > 10% of total
Cardiactroponin-I	3–6 hours	2–4 days	4–9 days	Sig = > 300 mcg/ml
LDH	8–12 hours	2–4 days	7–10 days	Normal = 150–300 U/ml
LDH-1	6–24 hours	3–4 days	3–4 days	Sig = > 30–35% of total
SGOT	8–12 hours	3–6 days	3–6 days	Normal = 8–40 U/ml

[a] Significant value for abnormal

Note. Laboratory units of measurement and normal values vary among institutions.

        b) Thallium-201 scan (myocardial perfusion scan): Shows "cold spots" of poor uptake of nuclear substance

           (1) Tests useful when EKG is inconclusive and enzyme levels have returned to normal

           (2) Abnormal 12–36 hours after MI; remains abnormal for four to seven days

           (3) May be used to evaluate heart function prior to discharge

        c) Nuclear scans: May be abnormal after any radiation to the heart region and may not be useful when symptoms of myocardial infarction require evaluation.

    C. Other

        1. EKG: See Table 47-2 for typical ischemia, injury, prior infarct changes; see Table 47-3 for lead and location of infarct

        a) Rhythm analysis in the frontal plane: Will show clear evidence of ST changes on the anterior heart but may miss lateral, inferior, or posterior injury. Signal average cardiac monitoring helps to eliminate artifact and enhance accuracy of alarms.

        b) 12-lead EKG: Shows ischemia and injury in a transmural MI of the left ventricle but may miss a significant right ventricular infarction

        c) 15-lead EKG or right-sided EKG: Uses the usual EKG leads but adds right-sided leads that will aid in diagnosis of right ventricular infarction (rarely used)

           (1) Approximately 30%–50% of inferior infarctions involve the right ventricle.

           (2) Right ventricular infarctions produce different clinical symptoms and complications and require different treatment plans.

Table 47-2. EKG Changes of Ischemia, Injury, Prior Injury

EKG	Onset	Resolution
Reversible ischemia		
T wave inversion or flat, depressed T wave	With stress	Return to baseline with rest or medication (nitroglycerin)
Reversible injury		
ST segment elevation	Within one to two hours	Two to three days (persistent elevation may indicate LV aneurysm)
Infarction		
T wave elevation	Very early	Several hours
T wave inversion	Within one to two hours	Several days to weeks (may be permanent)
ST segment elevation and T wave inversion	Within one to two hours	Several hours to days
Q wave	Three hours to several days	Permanent

Table 47-3. Common Types of Myocardial Infarction and EKG Changes With Myocardial Infarction

Location	Type of Infarct	Artery Involved	Leads Involved	Signs and Symptoms, Clinical Findings
Left ventricle	Anterior wall	Left anterior descending (LAD)	I, aVL and V_{1-4} (ST elevation/T wave inversion)	• Hypotension • Left-sided S_3 • Tachycardia • Increased pulmonary artery wedge pressure (PAWP) and central venous pressure (CVP) • Pulmonary congestion, CHF • Ventricular arrhythmias • Cardiogenic shock
	Lateral wall	LAD and left circumflex (LCX)	I, aVL and V_{4-6} (ST elevation/T wave inversion)	• Same as anterior wall; usually associated with anterior wall involvement. • Monitor for posterior wall extention.
Right ventricle	Inferior wall	Right coronary artery (RCA), LCX, if dominant	II, III, aVF (ST elevation/T wave inversion)	• Nausea/vomiting • Bradycardia • Sinoatrial (SA) / Atrioventricular (AV) node conduction disturbances
	Right ventricular (occurs with 33%–45% of inferior wall myocardial infarctions)	RCA (proximal segment)	ST elevation in II, III, aVF also V_4R–V_6R with ST elevations; if lead III changes are > II, significant for right ventricle MI	• Hypotension • Bradycardia: 50%–75% have complete heart block • Clear lung fields unless in left ventricle failure • Right-sided S_3 or possible S_4 • Increased jugular venous distension (JVD), increased CVP, and decreased cardiac output
Both	Posterior wall	RCA, LCX	V_{1-4} reciprocal changes; depressed ST segments Tall "T" waves in V_{1-4}	• Hypotension • Bradycardia • Conduction defects

(3) Right V_4 lead is most sensitive for right ventricular infarction.
2. Cardiac catheterization: Gold standard of diagnosis; if this technology is immediately available and the patient is stable enough to tolerate the procedure, perform as an immediate diagnostic and therapeutic treatment modality.
    a) Criteria
        (1) EKG changes that show acute injury (ST elevation)
        (2) Suspicious symptoms
    b) Permits immediate access to potentially reopen vessel with angioplasty, coronary stent, or laser therapy

V. Differential diagnosis
  A. Cardiac
    1. Angina (see Chapter 36)
    2. Aortic dissection
    3. Cardiac contusion
    4. Pericardial effusion/tamponade (see Chapter 48)
    5. Dysrhythmia (see Chapter 43)
    6. Endocarditis (see Chapter 44)
    7. Pericarditis (see Chapter 48)
    8. Superior vena cava syndrome
  B. Pulmonary
    1. Pulmonary embolism (see Chapter 33)
    2. Pneumonia: Pleuritic chest pain common with certain microorganisms (see Chapter 30)
  C. GI
    1. Cholecystitis
    2. Esophagitis
    3. Pancreatitis (see Chapter 72)
    4. Peptic ulcer disease (see Chapter 73)
  D. Other: Pectoral muscle injury/costochondritis

VI. Treatment: Listed in order of priority for most patients. When interventional cardiology is immediately available, medications may be delayed until cardiac catheterization or percutaneous transvenous coronary angioplasty can be performed (see Table 47-4).
  A. Goals of treatment
    1. Elimination of chest discomfort
    2. Restoration of blood flow
  B. Oxygen therapy: Higher PaO_2 than usual desired to reduce risk of myocardial ischemia
  C. Rest: Decreases oxygen demand and consumption
  D. Analgesics
    1. Reduced pain will decrease oxygen consumption, potentially preserving myocardium.
    2. Morphine sulfate is often used.
      a) Potent analgesic effects
      b) Easily reversible

Table 47-4. Treatment of Myocardial Infarction

Treatment	Rationale	Nursing Guidelines
Medications		
Oxygen	Myocardial oxygen consumption is increased with MI, making increased delivery or availability desirable.	• Use ABG and oxygen saturation to guide dose. • Hypoxia may occur with extensive MIs.
Nitrates (Nitroglycerin)	Nitrates selectively dilate coronary arteries and mesenteric arteries, both of which are compromised with MI. Dilating these vessels increases available oxygen. Nitrates also venodilate, decreasing preload and decreasing workload on the heart.	• Doses titrated until pain-free or the mean arterial pressure is below 60 mm Hg. • Sublingual doses require adequate salivation for melting and absorption.
Aspirin (Antiplatelet therapy)	Reduces platelet aggregation at site of ruptured plaque or roughened endothelium where coronary artery occlusion is occurring.	• Aspirin should be chewed for maximal absorption.
Thrombolytics	Agents lyse existing clots in the coronary arteries, immediately restoring circulation to the myocardium. This action reperfuses the myocardium, restoring circulation to ischemic tissue, which in turn reduces infarct size, preserves left ventricular function, and decreases mortality.	• See Table 47-5, Thrombolytic Therapy.
Weight-based heparin	Heparin follows thrombolytic therapy or replaces it when thrombolytics are contraindicated. It serves to maintain patency of the coronary artery after thrombolytic or interventional procedures and prevents complete thrombosis of a partially occluded coronary artery.	• Weight-based heparin reduces risk of bleeding while optimizing anticoagulant benefits.
Beta-blockers	Reduces myocardial oxygen consumption.	• Given to all patients unless clearly contraindicated (e.g., pulmonary edema). • Beta-selective agents ensure cardiac action more than vascular effects. • Dose determined by stable heart rate 50–60/minute without hypotension.
Angiotensin-converting enzyme (ACE) inhibitors or ACE II blockers	Decreases constrictive effects of angiotensin, decreasing afterload, and decreasing workload on the heart.	• Used cautiously in conjunction with beta-blockers.
Morphine sulfate	Primarily used to reduce pain and alleviate anxiety, but added benefits include histamine stimulation with venodilation and decreased preload and bronchodilation permitting better oxygenation.	• Dose adjusted for hypotension. • Some patients experience too much histamine stimulation and actually present with bronchoconstriction.

(Continued on next page)

Table 47-4. Treatment of Myocardial Infarction (Continued)

Treatment	Rationale	Nursing Guidelines
Medications		
IIB and III A platelet inhibitors (e.g., ticlopidine hydrochloride [Ticlid®, Roche Laboratories, Nutley, NJ])	Interferes with platelet membrane function by inhibiting fibrinogen binding, reducing platelet aggregation, and improving coronary stent survival.	• May inhibit other hematologic cell function (e.g., neutropenia). • Ticlopidine dose: 250 mg po bid with food.
Interventional Cardiology		
Intra-aortic balloon pump	Increases coronary artery perfusion, decreases left ventricular workload, and decreases afterload.	• Requires continuous nurse monitoring for appropriate timing and amount of support. • Likely to induce thrombocytopenia. • Requires concomitant anticoagulation.
Percutaneous transluminal coronary angioplasty (PTCA)	Opens occluded arteries with local pressure from an expanded balloon at the point of narrowing.	• Ideally performed immediately and prior to thrombolytic administration. • Reocclusion during hospitalization not uncommon. Requires immediate availability of coronary artery bypass graft (CABG) in case complications occur.
Coronary artery stent	Placement of small synthetic bypass links permit rechanneling coronary blood flow past the site of small obstructions in easy-to-access areas of the coronary arteries.	• May be performed with minimally invasive surgery techniques. • Requires postoperative anticoagulation. • High reocclusion rate.
CABG surgery	Host vessel or synthetic mesh grafts replace occluded coronary arteries by circumventing occluded area.	• Concerns that bypass machine filters enhance hematogenous spread of cancer. • Requires post-operative anticoagulation.

  c) Enhances histamine release, decreasing venous tone, causing venodilation and decreased preload, which decrease pulmonary artery pressure.

  d) Bronchodilator properties may enhance oxygenation.

 E. Antiplatelet therapy

  1. Indicated in unstable angina or evolving myocardial infarction.

  2. One or two baby aspirin (80 mg) or one adult aspirin (325 mg chewable, nonenteric coated tablet) administered immediately (even before confirmed diagnosis) serves to reduce platelet aggregation at the occlusion site, preventing worsening ischemia and extension of MI. Aspirin MUST be chewed for immediate absorption.

  3. Other antiplatelet drugs used include: Ticlid® (Roche Laboratories, Nutley, NJ)

   a) Act late in clotting process

   b) Have less risk of reocclusion

 F. Thrombolytic therapy (see Table 47-5)

  1. Goals

Table 47-5. Thrombolytic Therapy

Agent	Mechanism of Action	Advantages	Disadvantages	Administration Guidelines
Streptokinase	• Coagulant from beta-hemolytic streptococci that forms complex with plasminogen and results in fibrinolysis	• Low-cost; extensive clinical research exists • Highly effective	• Potential allergic reaction • Hypotension • Lytic state lasts approximately 36 hours; may require repeat infusions	• Dose: 1.5 million units IV bolus dose over 60 minutes • Intracoronary dose: 20,000 units directly into vessel, then maintenance dose of 2,000 U/minute for 60 minutes
Anisoylated plasminogen streptokinase activator (APSAC) (Eminase®, Roberts Pharmaceutical Corporation, Eatontown, NJ; anistreplase)	• Same as above	• Shorter acting than streptokinase • Easy administration	• Expensive • Potential allergic reactions	• Dose: 30 units IV rapidly over five minutes; half-life is 90 minutes
Urokinase	• Produced by the human kidney and isolated in the urine. • In response to thrombus, it converts fibrin-bound plasminogen to plasmin on the clot surface.	• Nonantigenic • No hypotension	• Only approved for intracoronary use in MI • Long lytic state • Expensive	• Dose: 3 million units IV over 90 minutes • Intracoronary dose: 6,000 units/minute for up to two hours • Continue infusion until artery maximally opened or 15–30 minutes after initial opening. • Heparin is administered IV prior to urokinase.
Tissue plasminogen activator (TPA)	• Naturally secreted by the endothelium • In response to thrombus, converts fibrin-bound plasminogen to plasmin on the clot surface	• Clot-specific • Nonantigenic • No hypotension • Short duration of effect	• Slightly greater incidence of strokes compared to streptokinase • Expensive	• Dose: 100 mg IV infusion over three hours
Recombinant t-PA (R-tPA)	• Same as above	• Less dependent upon market availability	• More expensive	• Same as above
Reteplase recombinant (Retavase®, Centocor, Inc., Malvern, PA)	• Recombinant fibrinolytic form	• Fast-acting • Easily administered • Early trial indicates more complete clot lysis and reperfusion. • Few allergic reactions	• More expensive	• Dose: 10 units IV bolus x 2 given 30 minutes apart

        a) Decrease infarct size

        b) Decrease mortality

        c) Preserve left ventricular function

        d) Establish reperfusion and coronary artery patency

  2. Patient candidate criteria

        a) Chest pain less than six hours duration (individual institutions may extend to 12 hours; benefit lasts up to 12 hours)

        b) ST elevations on EKG in two consecutive leads of 1 mm or more

  3. Contraindications

        a) Active internal bleeding

        b) Intracranial/intraspinal surgery within prior two months

        c) Intracranial neoplasm, arterial venous malformation, or aneurysm

        d) Uncontrolled hypertension with diastolic blood pressure > 120 mm Hg

        e) Severe blood dyscrasia

        f) Other possible contraindications: Surgery within prior 10 days, previous stroke, recent CPR, hemorrhagic retinopathy

  4. Intracoronary may be given when occluded vessel is visualized on catheterization.

  5. Usually given IV when immediate cardiac catheterization is not available

  6. Symptoms/signs of myocardial reperfusion in thrombolytic therapy: Successful reperfusion in 75%–80% of MIs

        a) Rapid and early rise and peak of enzymes

        b) Normalization of ST segment

        c) Reperfusion dysrhythmia

           (1) Particularly ventricular fibrillation or multifocal ventricular tachycardia

           (2) Seen 10–20 minutes and up to two to four hours after administration

           (3) Result of showered lactic acid throughout myocardium where coronary artery feeds

        d) Immediate relief of chest pain

G. Nitroglycerin (NTG)

  1. Initially administered sublingually. Be certain patient has adequate salivation to melt tablet. Use caution with patients who have had radiation to head and neck area.

  2. Start IV NTG as soon as possible.

  3. Titrate to effect unless adverse effects are not tolerated.

        a) Prophylactic dose in patients with relieved chest pain is 10–50 mcg/minute.

        b) Therapeutic dose routinely is 1 mcg/kg/minute (50–150 mcg/minute).

        c) No maximum dose. Advanced cardiovascular disease awaiting bypass surgery may require 300–600 mcg/minute.

        d) May limit drug when hypotension occurs.

H. Weight-based heparin therapy: Bolus followed by continuous infusion

I. Beta-blocker

  1. Decreases myocardial oxygen consumption

  2. Decreases catecholamine effects on heart

  3. Beta-1 selective agents preferred (e.g., metoprolol)

  4. Loading dose given until heart rate 50–65 beats per minute; watch blood pressure. Usually give 5 mg IV every five minutes for three doses, then orally.

   5. Maintenance oral or IV bolus doses given to sustain beta-blockade for four to seven days.
J. Percutaneous transvenous coronary angioplasty (PTCA), balloon angioplasty
   1. Requires left heart catheterization
   2. Intracoronary thrombolytic given concomitantly whenever possible
   3. Followed by heparin infusion
   4. Arterial line sheath usually left in place for 8–24 hours in case repeat PTCA is required
K. Coronary artery bypass graft surgery (CABG): Indicated for refractory ischemia or when PTCA has been unsuccessful
   1. Therapy is controversial because it is thought that the heart-lung bypass may cause unintentional hematogenous spread of malignancy.
   2. New bypass filters currently are being researched to prevent hematogenous spread of malignancy.
   3. Cases of straightforward (i.e., short OR time) CABG performed with concomitant cancer surgery for lung, esophageal, and gastric cancers are documented.
L. Coronary artery stent
   1. Newer multilink stents can cover longer part of coronary artery.
   2. Reocclusion may occur during the inpatient stay or within six months outpatient, presenting with acute and dramatic MI symptoms.
M. Unique treatment for right ventricular infarction
   1. Fluid loading: Up to 10 liters to achieve adequate preload volume
   2. Diuresis: Maybe required after the infarction is complete
   3. Atropine: 0.5 mg IV for symptomatic bradycardia
   4. Transcutaneous pacing: Early if atropine does not work
N. Manage complications of MI
   1. Dysrhythmia
   2. Cardiogenic shock (high death rate)
   3. CHF
   4. Hypoxemia
   5. Bleeding secondary to antiplatelet/thrombolytic therapy
   6. Shock (high death rate)
   7. Renal failure

VII. Follow-up
   A. Serial physical exam, 12 lead EKG, and exercise stress test: Perform at least annually
   B. Therapeutic drug monitoring: Required every three to four months after stabilization of dose for antidysrhythmias or anticoagulants
      1. Anticoagulants: Coagulation profile usually every two to four weeks until stable, then every four to six months
      2. Antidysrhythmics: CBC every six months; rarely can these agents induce aplastic anemia.
      3. Lipid-lowering drugs: Liver function tests at one month initially, then every six months
      4. Beta-blockers: Evaluate glucose every 6–12 months for glucose intolerance.

VIII. Referrals
    A. Electrophysiologist: Consult if refractory dysrhythmia is present.
    B. Dietitian: To advise patient how to alter risk factors (e.g., obesity, hyperlipidemia)
    C. Preventive cardiologist: May consult for risk-factor analysis and modification
    D. Cardiac rehabilitation: Consultation ensures gradual return to activities of daily living while monitoring limitations from cardiovascular disease.

References

Akchurin, R.S., Davidov, M.I., Partigulov, S.A., Brand, J.B., Shiriaev, A.A., Lepilin, M.G., & Dolgov, I.M. (1997). Cardiopulmonary bypass and cell-saver technique in combined oncologic and cardiovascular surgery. *Artificial Organs, 21,* 763–765.

Berger, C.C., Bokemeyer, C., Schneider, M., Kuczyk, M.A., & Schmoll, H.J. (1995). Secondary Raynaud's phenomenon and other late vascular complications following chemotherapy for testicular cancer. *European Journal of Cancer, 31A*(13–14), 2229–2238.

Boehringer Mannheim Corporation. (1996). Retavse™ (Reteplase, recombinant), prescribing information. Gaithersburg: Author, Therapeutics Division.

Bokemeyer, C., Berger, C.C., Kuczyk, M.A., & Schmoll, H.J. (1996). Evaluation of long-term toxicity after chemotherapy for testicular cancer. *Journal of Clinical Oncology 14,* 2923–2932.

Clem, J.R. (1995). Pharmacotherapy of ischemic heart disease. *AACN Clinical Issues, 6,* 404–417.

Effat, M.A. (1995). Pathophysiology of ischemic heart disease: An overview. *AACN Clinical Issues, 6,* 367–374.

Gunnar, R.M., Passmania, E.R., & Bourdillon, P.D. (1990). Guidelines for the early management of patients with acute myocardial infarction: A report of the American College of Cardiology/American Heart Association Task Force on Assessment of Diagnostic and Therapeutic Cardiovascular Procedures (subcommittee to develop guidelines for early management of patients with acute myocardial infraction). *Journal of American College of Cardiology, 16,* 249–260.

Gyenes, G., Fornander, T., Carlens, P., Glas, U., & Rutqvist, L.E. (1997). Detection of radiation-induced myocardial damage by technetium-99m sestamibi scintigraphy. *European Journal of Nuclear Medicine, 24*(3), 286–292.

Gyenes, G., Fornander, T., Carlens, P., Glas, U., & Rutqvist, L.E. (1996). Myocardial damage in breast cancer patients treated with adjuvant radiotherapy: A prospective study. *International Journal of Radiation Oncology, Biology, Physics, 36,* 899–905.

Louie, E.K., & Langholtz, D. (1994). Strategies for re-establishing coronary blood flow during acute phase of MI. *Chest, 105,* 574–584.

Murphy, M.J., & Berding, C.B. (1999). Use of measurements of myoglobin and cardiac troponins in the diagnosis of acute myocardial infarction. *Critical Care Nurse, 19*(1), 58–65.

Neugut, A.I., Jacobson, J.S., Sherif, G., Ahsan, H., Garbowski, G.C., Waye, J., Forde, K.A., & Treat, M.R. (1995). Coronary artery disease and colorectal neoplasia. *Diseases of the Colon and Rectum, 38*(8), 873–877.

Ogowa, A., Kanda, T., Sugihara, S., Masumo, H., & Kobayashi, I. (1995). Risk factors for myocardial infarction in cancer patients. *Journal of Medicine, 26*(5–6), 221–233.

Pepine, C.J. (1994). Adjunctive pharmacologic therapy for acute MI. *Clinical Cardiology, 17*(Suppl. 1), 110–114.

Randall, D.C., & Jones, D.L. (1997). Eliminating unnecessary lactate dehydrogenase testing. A utilization review study and national survey. *Archives of Internal Medicine, 157,* 1441–1447.

Scherck, K.A. (1997). Recognizing a heart attack: The process of determining illness. *American Journal of Critical Care, 6,* 267–273.

Stewart, J.R., Fajardo, J.F., Gillette, S.M., & Constine, L.S. (1995). Radiation injury to the heart. *International Journal of Radiation Oncology, Biology, Physics, 31,* 1205–1211.

Stewart, S.L. (1992). Acute MI: A review of pathophysiology, treatment, and complications. *Journal of Cardiovascular Nursing, 6,* 1–25.

Talvensaari, K.K., Lanning, M., Tapanainen, P., & Knip, M. (1996). Long-term survivors of childhood cancer have an increased risk of manifesting the metabolic syndrome. *Journal of Endocrinology and Metabolism, 81,* 3051–3055.

Takahashi, T., Nakano, S., Shimazaki, Y., Kaneko, M., Nakahara, K., Miyata, M., Kamiike, W., & Matsuda, H. (1995). Concomitant coronary bypass grafting and curative surgery for cancer. *Surgery Today, 25*(2), 131–135.

48. Pericarditis/Pericardial Effusion/ Cardiac Tamponade

Brenda K. Shelton, RN, MS, CCRN, AOCN®

I. Definition
   A. Three terms are used to describe the clinical conditions of increased pericardial pressure: pericarditis, pericardial effusion, and pericardial tamponade.
   B. Pericarditis is inflammation of the lining surrounding the heart. It is termed pericarditis when exudate is present but is termed constrictive pericarditis when fibrous bands restrict cardiac movement.
   C. Pericardial effusion involves purulent, bloody, or malignant fluid accumulation within the pericardial sac.
   D. Pericardial tamponade (cardiac tamponade) is fluid accumulation in the pericardial sac that is so great that normal contraction and ejection capabilities fail.

II. Physiology/Pathophysiology
   A. Normal: The intrapericardial pressure is subatmospheric, which allows the inflow of low-pressure venous blood into the right heart.
   B. Pathophysiology: When the pericardium is constricted by fibrous bands or filled with fluid, the pressure in the pericardial sac is raised to a level that exceeds the normal filling pressure of the ventricle.
      1. Initially, the primary pathophysiology is venous congestion caused by obstruction to the inflow of blood into the heart.
      2. Later, when ventricular filling is more severely restricted, symptoms of left ventricular failure prevail.

III. Clinical features: Approximately 10%–30% of patients with cancer experience some variation of this syndrome during the course of illness, although the severity and reversibility will vary with different clinical indicators. Multiple studies suggest that the mean life expectancy after diagnosis of malignant pericardial disease is two to five months.
   A. Classifications of pericardial effusion: Pericardial effusions are further classified by exudate type.
      1. Transudative effusions are the result of abnormal capillary permeability, LDH < 200, protein < 35, fluid to serum LDH ratio 0.6, and protein ratio 0.5.
      2. Exudative effusions occur when there is an inflammatory stimulus and are characterized by LDH > 200, protein > 35, fluid to serum LDH ratio 0.6, and fluid to protein ratio > 0.3.

B. Risk factors
   1. Malignancy involving the chest
      a) Bronchogenic cancer: 80% of cases
      b) Lymphoma
      c) Breast cancer
      d) Others: Renal cell, melanoma, gastric, ovarian, primary cardiac myxoma
   2. Thoracic lymphatic obstruction
   3. Radiation of at least 3,000 cGy to more than 33% of the heart region or fraction sizes greater than 300 cGy/day
   4. Chemotherapy (usually high-dose) or biotherapy agents that cause capillary permeability
      a) Cytosine arabinoside
      b) Cyclophosphamide
      c) Interferon
      d) Interleukin-2 and interleukin-11
      e) Granulocyte-macrophage-colony-stimulating factor
C. Etiology
   1. Most common causes of pericardial diseases in patients with cancer are drug- or treatment-induced capillary permeability and malignant cell invasion of the pericardium. Table 48-1 summarizes the most common etiologies of pericardial disorders.
   2. Traumatic injury may be accompanied by hemorrhagic tamponade.
   3. Infectious diseases also may cause this syndrome (uncommon). Fluid collection related to infection may be purulent and harboring infective organisms or serous and related to the inflammatory response of the pericardium.
D. History
   1. History of cancer and cancer treatment
   2. Current medications: Prescribed and over-the-counter
   3. History of presenting symptom(s): Precipitating factors, onset, location, and duration
   4. Changes in activities of daily living
   5. Past medical history: CHF, thoracic lymphatic obstruction, systemic lupus erythematosus, bacterial endocarditis, bacteremia, renal dysfunction
E. Signs and symptoms: Table 48-2 compares and contrasts key symptoms with each disorder.
   1. The severity of signs and symptoms often reflect the chronicity of the problem.
   2. Rapidly developing effusions may present symptomatically with as little as 50–80 ml of fluid accumulation.
   3. Patients with slow-developing effusions compensate for progressive reduction in cardiac output as the effusion occurs and may not demonstrate signs or symptoms until there is more than 1,000 ml of fluid in the pericardial sac.
F. Physical exam: Findings depend on whether the patient is experiencing pericarditis, pericardial effusion, or pericardial tamponade. Table 48-3 compares and contrasts key physical exam findings with each disorder.

IV. Diagnostic tests
   A. Laboratory: Not indicated except to test pericardial fluid. Some advocate obtaining serum values of LDH, protein, and glucose to compare with pericardial fluid.

Table 48-1. Etiologies of Pericardial Disease

Pathophysiologic Mechanism	Examples of Etiologies
Capillary permeability-induced fluid extravasation into the pericardium	• Cytosine arabinoside • Inflammatory cytokines given as anticancer therapy (e.g., interleukin-2, tumor necrosis factor) • Leukemia • Rheumatoid arthritis • Systemic lupus erythematosus
Severe chest venous congestion and obstruction of normal lymphatic fluid removal	• Cardiomyopathy • Myocardial infarction • Thoracic lymphatic duct obstruction from pulmonary infection or pulmonary tumor
Hemorrhage into the pericardium	• Chemotherapy-induced cardiomyopathy (e.g., cyclophosphamide) • Renal failure • Postcardiac surgery • Severe thrombocytopenia • Traumatic injury (e.g., motor vehicle accident)
Pericardial inflammation with exudative fluid response	• Myocardial infarction • Radiation exposure • Renal failure (e.g., uric acid-related inflammation)
Infectious disorder	• Nocardia • Serratia • Toxoplasmosis • Tuberculosis
Malignant involvement	• Breast cancer • Head and neck cancer • Hodgkin's and non-Hodgkin's lymphomas • Lung cancer
Unknown mechanism	• Leukemia

Note. From "Cardiac Tamponade" (p. 390) by B.K. Shelton, in C.A. Ziegfeld, B.G. Lubejko, and B.K. Shelton (Eds.), *Oncology Fact Finder. Manual of Oncology Nursing,* 1998, Philadelphia: J.B. Lippincott. Copyright by J.B. Lippincott. Adapted with permission.

    B. Radiology: Chest x-rays
        1. Symmetrical cardiac enlargement (> one-half the diameter of the chest)
        2. Widened mediastinum or water bottle silhouette of the heart and major vessels
        3. Clear lung fields
    C. Other
        1. Echocardiogram: Definitive diagnostic tool for confirmation of pericardial disease
            a) When effusion or tamponade are present, fluid is visible within the pericardial sac.
            b) Restricted ventricular filling present with impending cardiac tamponade, with right ventricular abnormalities occurring earlier in the disease process.
            c) Distorted or inadequate ventricular expansion is characteristic with all pericardial syndromes.
        2. EKG

Table 48-2. Symptoms of Pericarditis, Pericardial Effusion, and Pericardial Tamponade

Symptom	Pericarditis	Pericardial Effusion	Pericardial Tamponade
Chest pain	• Severe, sharp, and localized • Exacerbated by movement, deep breathing, or lying flat • May be relieved, in part, by sitting up and leaning forward	• Dull and diffuse • Less positional	• More often described as chest "heaviness" or absent
Cough	• Not present	• From congestive heart failure • Characterized by pulmonary congestion	• Severity depends on degree of left ventricular failure
Dyspnea	• Mild to moderate • From chest discomfort	• Moderate to severe • From congestive heart failure	• Severe air hunger From low cardiac output and hypoxemia

a) Pericarditis: Low-voltage QRS complexes, tachycardia, ST elevation in all precordial leads

b) Pericardial effusion: Low-voltage QRS complexes, tachycardia with early effusion, and bradycardia/heart block in late effusion or impending tamponade

c) Pericardial tamponade: Electrical alternans (alternating positive and negative deflected QRS complexes) occurs in a small number of patients but almost always signifies impending cardiac tamponade.

V. Differential diagnosis
   A. CHF (see Chapter 40)
   B. Superior vena cava syndrome
   C. Myocardial infarction (see Chapter 47)
   D. Dissecting aortic aneurysm
   E. Tension pneumothorax (see Chapter 31)
   F. Cardiac metastasis

VI. Treatment: Definitive treatment of pericarditis is very different from treatment of pericardial effusion and tamponade.
   A. Pericarditis
      1. Anti-inflammatory treatments: Because pericarditis is an inflammatory process, anti-inflammatory agents are administered once hemorrhagic pericarditis is ruled out. Therapy is usually continued until symptoms subside, or approximately two weeks.
         a) Moderate-dose aspirin: 650 mg po every four hours
         b) Moderate-dose nonsteroidal anti-inflammatory agents (e.g., ibuprofen 400–600 mg po tid)
         c) Corticosteroids: Patients with pericarditis refractory to nonsteroidal anti-inflammatory agents or who are terminally ill may use for symptomatic relief; rapid-

Table 48-3. Physical Exam Findings With Pericarditis, Pericardial Effusion, and Pericardial Tamponade

Signs	Pericarditis	Pericardial Effusion	Pericardial Tamponade
Heart sounds	• Pericardial rub	• Muffled heart sounds	• Absent heart sounds
Point of maximal impulse	• Normal	• Shifted to the left (toward the axilla) or downward (toward sixth intercostal space)	• Barely discernible but shifted laterally and downward if palpable
Strength and equality of pulses	• Decreased peripheral pulses • More diminished in lower extremities	• Decreased peripheral pulses • More diminished in lower extremities	• Minimal carotid pulse • Absent lower extremity pulses
Jugular venous distention (JVD) and jugular venous pulsation (JVP)	• Slight increase in JVD and JVP (two to four cm above clavicle)	• Bulging neck veins (JVD) and JVP near mandible	• Bulging neck veins (JVD) JVP prominently produces a large continuous wave up the neck and to the chin (i.e., cannon a waves).
Central venous pressure	• Normal to slight elevation (10–12 cm of H_2O or 6–8 mm Hg)	• Moderate elevation (15–18 cm of H_2O or 8–12 mm Hg)	• Extremely high (18–26 cm of H_2O or 12–22 mm Hg), becoming close to ventricular or pulmonary artery pressures if a PA catheter is in place
Peripheral edema	• Trace-dependent edema initially noted • Peripheral (especially lower extremities) and dependent edema will increase with progression of cardiac dysfunction.	• Moderate 2+ to 3+ edema of the extremities (especially lower) with slow fluid accumulation • Rapidly developing effusions produce minimal edema.	• Severe upper and lower extremity edema may be present but actually reflects the severe effusion, not tamponade. • Rapidly developing effusions produce minimal edema.
Hepatomegaly and splenomegaly	• Rarely present • When noted, usually mild size change but produces discomfort	• Reflects degree of venous congestion • Common finding in conjunction with slow-developing or chronic effusions	• Reflects degree of venous congestion • Common finding in conjunction with slow-developing effusions leading to tamponade
Blood pressure	• Narrow pulse pressure (rising diastolic rather than dropping systolic)	• Hypotension: Diastolic blood pressure rises first, then the systolic pressure decreases (narrowing pulse pressure). • The presence of a pulsus paradoxus > 10 mm Hg signifies resistance to the inflow of blood into the heart.	• Frank systolic hypotension with narrow pulse pressure or large pulsus paradoxus • Pulmonary artery pressures become nearly equal because of equalization of the pressure within and around the heart.

(Continued on next page)

Table 48-3. Physical Exam Findings With Pericarditis, Pericardial Effusion, and Pericardial Tamponade *(Continued)*

Signs	Pericarditis	Pericardial Effusion	Pericardial Tamponade
Cardiac rhythm	• Normal sinus rhythm • Low QRS voltage on EKG	• Tachycardia is the earliest heart rate response to decreased cardiac output. • Low QRS voltage more prominent than with pericarditis. Bradycardia or heart block may occur with high thoracic pressure and poor coronary blood flow during inspiration.	• High thoracic resistance leads to poor ventricular filling, particularly during inspiration. • Bradycardia, heart block, or short periods of asystole may occur during inspiration. • Electrical alternans (QRS alternating above and below isoelectric line) occurs in about 15% of patients.
Mental status	• Normal	• Awake, alert, oriented • Anxious, restless	• Alterations in mental status may be present if blood flow to the brain is impaired.
Urine output	• Normal	• Oliguria often is an early indicator of compromised cardiac output.	• Anuria

acting agents (e.g., dexamethasone 4–10 mg po or IV tid or hydrocortisone 125 mg IV qid) usually are prescribed for a few weeks.

2. Observation alone: May be the treatment of choice for mild or moderate pericardial effusion when the effusion is expected to resolve spontaneously.

3. Vigorous IV fluid administration (200–500 ml/hr): Despite clinical symptoms of heart failure, this is essential in impending tamponade to increase venous pressure above pericardial pressure, enhancing venous return.

B. Pericardial effusion/tamponade

1. Fluid removal: Severe pericardial effusion or tamponade with evidence of collapsed ventricles requires aspiration of pericardial fluid.

   a) The method of fluid removal is based on the etiology and patient's hemodynamic status.

   b) See Table 48-4 for an overview of several therapies used to remove pericardial fluid.

2. Radiation: When malignant pericardial effusions are confirmed and slow-growing (e.g., breast cancer) tumors and tumors amenable to radiation therapy are present, 100–200 Gy mediastinal radiation daily for three to four weeks may be administered.

3. Chemotherapy: When malignant pericardial effusions are confirmed and amenable to chemotherapy, specific antitumor antineoplastic therapy is given (e.g., for small cell lung cancer). Some advocate administration of chemotherapeutic agents into the pericardial sac, although the physician usually administers these at the time of fluid removal via pericardial catheter or pericardiocentesis.

4. Some authors advocate diuretic therapy for removal of excess circulating fluid, encouraging osmotic shifting of fluid out of spaces, such as the pericardial sac.

Table 48-4. Treatment of Neoplastic Cardiac Tamponade

Treatment	Indications	Methodology	Nursing Implications
Pericardial catheter (may use to drain and remove or may leave in for several days)	Short-term emergent removal of slow- or rapid-developing effusion. Can be performed emergently with echocardiogram or fluoroscopic guidance.	Fluoroscopic directed pericardial catheter with drainage and/or sclerosing	• Preprocedural preparation: Administer minor sedation, at bedside or in procedure room; light meal permitted if clinical condition warrants. • Maintain catheter patency. • Maintain a closed system. • Account for drainage quantity, color, and consistency at each shift. • Keep drainage bag below the level of the heart. • Sudden cessation of drainage may indicate misplacement or clotting of the catheter; observe the patient for recurrent tamponade. • Sudden increase in catheter drainage may indicate clotting abnormality; report to the physician. • Flushing the catheter with approximately 3 cc of preservative-free normal saline may be performed by physician or nursing staff every four to eight hours as needed. If the drainage is extremely bloody, low-dose heparin may be used. • Exit site care: Catheter is not sutured in place but has a curled tip that should stay in the pericardial sac. Maintain a sterile dressing over the exit site. • Nursing during administration of sclerosing agent: Administer pain medication if doxycycline is used. • Administer antipyretics if bleomycin is used. Clamp catheter for two to four hours after administration of sclerosing agent.
Balloon pericardiotomy	Short term emergent removal of slow- or rapid-developing effusion.	Catheter inserted into pericardial sac and balloon inflated to open a hole in the pericardial sac; catheter is immediately removed, and pericardial fluid drains into the mediastinum	• Preprocedure preparation: Same as pericardial catheter. • Monitor for recurrent tamponade symptoms.
Pericardio-peritoneal shunt	Palliative management of recurrent malignant effusions, particularly with limited life expectancy.	Local anesthesia used for percutaneous subxiphoid insertion of a Denver shunt that drains pericardial fluid into the abdomen	• Preprocedural preparation: Same as pericardial catheter. • Monitor for recurrent tamponade from occlusion of the shunt.

(Continued on next page)

Table 48-4. Treatment of Neoplastic Cardiac Tamponade *(Continued)*

Treatment	Indications	Methodology	Nursing Implications
Pericardial window	Chronic, severe effusions in a patient with otherwise good performance status. Must be able to tolerate a thoracoscopic procedure.	Thoracotomy or thoracotomy surgical wound with resection of lower section of pericardial sac; screen-like grid placed to allow pericardial fluid drainage into mediastinum	• Preoperative preparation: Regular operative procedure with anesthetic. • Postoperative thoracotomy: Prevent pulmonary complications by encouraging coughing and deep breathing. • Mediastinal chest tube care: Monitor drainage (no bubbling from a mediastinal chest tube; tube is positioned in the epigastric region); usual chest tube exit site care. • Inform patient/significant other about symptoms of occlusion and reaccumulation.
Pericardectomy	Chronic, severe effusions in a patient with otherwise good performance status. Must be able to tolerate a thoracotomy procedure. Used only after catheter or balloon fluid removal and pericardial window have failed.	Pericardial resection or stripping so there is no place for pericardial fluid to accumulate	• Rarely performed with other therapeutic options readily available. Most commonly used with fibrous pericarditis, which occurs after radiation exposure to the heart. • Chronic congestive failure symptoms may be present after pericardectomy.
Pericardiocentesis	Life-threatening cardiac tamponade in presence of moderate-large pericardial effusion when open procedure cannot be performed promptly.	Emergency bedside insertion of a needle into pericardial sac for removal of fluid; long cardiac needle attached to alligator clamp that is connected to V chest lead of the EKG machine. Needle inserted subxiphoid and pointed toward the left shoulder; when injury curve occurs on EKG machine, needle backed off and fluid aspirated	• Keep emergency equipment (e.g., crash cart, defibrillator) nearby during procedure. • Use EKG machine and alligator clip for evidence of position whenever possible (helps to avoid removal of intracardiac blood). • Save aspirated fluid; pericardial fluid should not clot but will clot if it is withdrawn from the ventricle. • Monitor return or strengthening of pulses during fluid removal.

Note. From "Cardiac Tamponade" (pp. 393–395) by B.K. Shelton in C.A. Ziegfeld, B.G. Lubejko, & B.K. Shelton (Eds.), *Oncology Fact Finder. Manual of Oncology Nursing,* 1998, Philadelphia: J.B. Lippincott. Copyright by J.B. Lippincott. Adapted with permission.

     a) These advisements have not been clinically researched and are not supported by our pathophysiologic knowledge of effusions or cardiac tamponade.

     b) Undertake procedure with extreme care and constant monitoring for worsening cardiac output.

VII. Follow-up

  A. Pericarditis is followed clinically by physical exam with heart sounds, pulses, jugular venous distention, PMI assessment, and an EKG. When the patient has repeated exposure to the triggering factor, frequent physical examinations (daily to weekly) and serial EKGs are monitored.

  B. Patients with pericardial effusion or a history of tamponade will have echocardiograms at one month after treatment, then at least every 6–12 months, depending upon the rate of accumulation during the first episode.

VIII. Referrals

  A. Home nurse visitation: Intermittent visits required by many patients with effectively treated pericardial effusions for evaluation of symptoms signaling recurrence. These visits, in conjunction with routine clinic appointments, should detect pericardial effusion before impending tamponade.

  B. Hospice: May refer patients in whom pericardial effusion is a manifestation of severe recurrent metastatic disease with a poor prognostic outcome; patients still should receive aggressive symptomatic support.

  C. Cardiologist or thoracic surgeon: May be appropriate to assist with treatment and management

References

Beauchamp, K.A. (1998). Pericardial tamponade: An oncologic emergency. *Clinical Journal of Oncology Nursing, 2,* 85-95.

Colombo, A., Olson, H.G., Egan, J., & Gardin, J.M. (1988). Etiology and prognostic implications of a large pericardial effusion in men. *Clinical Cardiology, 11,* 389–394.

Cormican, M.C., & Nyman, C.R. (1990). Intrapericardial bleomycin for the management of cardiac tamponade secondary to malignant pericardial effusion. *British Heart Journal, 63,* 61–62.

Dragonette, P. (1998). Malignant pericardial effusion and cardiac tamponade. In C.C. Chernecky & B.J. Berger (Eds.), *Advanced and critical care oncology nursing: Managing primary complications* (pp. 425–443). Philadelphia: W.B. Saunders.

Groeger, J.S., & Keefe, D. (1991). Cardiac tamponade. In J.S. Groeger (Ed.), *Critical care of the cancer patient* (2nd ed., pp. 250–259). St. Louis: C.V. Mosby.

Hamel, W.J. (1998). Care of patients with an indwelling pericardial catheter. *Critical Care Nurse, 18*(5), 40–53.

Hancock, E.W. (1990). Neoplastic pericardial disease. *Cardiolgy Clinics, 8*(4), 673–682.

Joiner, G.A., & Kolodychuk, G.R. (1991). Neoplastic cardiac tamponade. *Critical Care Nurse, 11,* 50–58.

Kilbride, S.S. (1994). Cardiac tamponade. In J. Gross & B.L. Johnson (Eds.), *Handbook of oncology nursing* (2nd ed., pp. 658–673). Boston: Jones & Bartlett.

Kohnoe, S., Maehara, Y., Takahashi, I., Saito, A., Okada, Y., & Sugimachi, K. (1994). Intrapericardial mitomycin C for the management of malignant pericardial effusion secondary to gastric cancer: Case report and review. *Chemotherapy, 40*(1), 57–60.

Laham, R.J., Cohen, D.J., Kuntz, R.E., Baim, D.S., Lorell, B.H., & Simons, M. (1996). Pericardial effusion in patients with cancer: Outcome with contemporary management strategies. *Heart, 75*(1), 67–71.

Mangan, C.M. (1992). Malignant pericardial effusions: Pathophysiology and clinical outcomes. *Oncology Nursing Forum, 19,* 1215–1223.

Martel, M.K., Sahijdak, W.M., Haken, R.K.T., Kessler, M.L., & Turrisi, A.T. (1998). Fraction size and dose parameters related to the incidence of pericardial effusions. *Journal of Radiation Oncology, Biology, and Physics, 40,* 155–161.

Mueller, X.M., Tevaearai, H.T., Hurni, M., Ruchat, P., Fischer, A.P., Stumpe, F., & von Segesser, L.K. (1997). Long-term results of surgical subxiphoid pericardial drainage. *Thoracic Cardiovascular Surgery, 45*(2), 65–69.

Okamoto, H., Shinkai, T., Yamakido, M., & Saijo, N. (1993). Cardiac tamponade caused by primary lung cancer and the management of pericardial effusion. *Cancer, 71,* 93–98.

Shuey, K.M. (1994). Heart, lung and endocrine complications of solid tumors. *Seminars in Oncology Nursing, 10*(3), 177–188.

Tomkowski, W., Szturmoxicz, M., Fijalkowska, A., Filipecki, S., & Figura-Chojak, E. (1994). Intrapericardial cisplatin for the management of patients with large malignant pericardial effusion. *Journal of Cancer Research and Clinical Oncology, 120*(7), 434–436.

Vaitkus, P.T., Hermann, H.C., & LeWinter, M.M. (1994). Treatment of malignant pericardial effusion. *Journal of the American Medical Association, 272*(1), 59–64.

Wang, N., Feikes, J.R., Mogensen, T., Vymeister, E.E., & Bailey, L.L. (1994). Pericardioperitoneal shunt: An alternative treatment for malignant pericardial effusion. *Annals of Thoracic Surgery, 57*(2), 289–292.

49. Peripheral Vascular Disease

Mary Ann Winokur, CRNP, MSN

I. Definition
  A. Peripheral vascular disease (PVD) is any disturbance in blood flow in the arterial and venous systems that disrupts the delivery of oxygen and nutrients and the elimination of waste products.
  B. Claudication is the ischemic pain associated with chronic arterial insufficiency that occurs with exercise and is relieved with rest.

II. Physiology/Pathophysiology
  A. Normal: The peripheral vascular system includes the arterial and venous systems that carry oxygenated blood from the heart and return it to the right atrium.
  B. Pathophysiology
    1. Any decrease in the perfusion within the arterial or venous system promotes activation of compensatory mechanisms.
    2. These mechanisms are
      a) Vasodilatation
      b) Development of collateral circulation
      c) Anaerobic metabolism with local mediating factors.
    3. Ischemia develops if these compensatory mechanisms insufficiently meet oxygen demands by the tissues; tissue death will result if the ischemia continues.

III. Clinical features
  A. Risk factors
    1. Nonmodifiable risk factors
      a) Familial hyperlipidemia
      b) Positive family history of cardiovascular diseases
      c) Diabetes mellitus
      d) Advancing age
      e) Gender: Men present with symptoms of the disease approximately 30 years earlier than women.
      f) Recent operative procedure with resultant immobility of extremities
    2. Modifiable risk factors
      a) Cigarette smoking

   b) High-fat diet

   c) Sedentary lifestyle

 B. Etiology

  1. Atherosclerosis: The major underlying factor contributing to PVD

   a) Arteriosclerotic plaques producing stenosis or occlusion of the arterial lumen often are segmentally distributed, with a predilection for arterial bifurcationes. Femoral and popliteal arteries are the most commonly affected.

   b) Other sites include the infrarenal abdominal aorta, aortic bifurcation, and iliac bifurcation artery

   c) Pressure and blood flow are not significantly diminished until at least 75% of the vein is occluded by the disease.

  2. Atherosclerosis obliterans (AO)

   a) Most prevalent vascular disorder

   b) Patients have an increased incidence of coronary artery disease (CAD) because of shared risk factors associated with an increased incidence of myocardial infarction (MI).

   c) Femoral and popliteal arteries are most commonly affected.

 C. History

  1. History of cancer and cancer treatment

  2. Current medications: Prescribed and over-the-counter

  3. History of presenting symptom(s): Precipitating factors, onset, location, and duration. Associated symptoms are leg pain at rest or with activity, dangling legs over side of bed relieve discomfort, hair loss on lower extremities, and inability to have an erection

  4. Changes in activities of daily living

  5. Recent surgeries

 D. Signs and symptoms

  1. Pain

   a) Mild muscular pain when exercising to severe pain when resting, which is relieved with dependency of the extremity

   b) Pain, generally in the muscle group distal to the occluded area

  2. Unilateral or bilateral cramping in calf, hip, thigh, or buttocks when walking

  3. Impotence

  4. Hair loss, thickened nails, smooth and shiny skin

 E. Physical exam

  1. Vital signs: Hypertension

  2. Integument exam

   a) Skin atrophy: Indicates loss of arterial perfusion

   b) Pallor or dependent rubor: Indicates poor venous return

   c) Cyanotic discoloration of digits, ulceration, necrosis, or gangrene: Indicates poor arterial flow

   d) Skin temperature: May be cool to the touch

  3. Cardiac exam

   a) Palpate all peripheral pulses (i.e., femoral, dorsalis pedis, posterior tibial).

    (1) Patients with intermittent claudication usually have normal or diminished pulses at rest, which reduce with exercise.

         (2) Patients with pain at rest will have loss of pulses distal to the stenotic area.

      b) Bruits: Assess for abdominal, femoral, and carotid bruits.

   4. Extremities exam: Limbs with severe insufficiency or obstruction will blanch when raised above the level of the heart while the patient is in a supine position.

     a) Pallor beyond 60 seconds is an ominous sign.

     b) A suddenly cold extremity is a sign of acute arterial occlusion.

IV. Diagnostic tests

  A. Laboratory: Both laboratory tests are used to evaluate the patient's cardiac risk factor profile.

    1. Serum cholesterol level

    2. Fasting blood sugar

  B. Radiology

    1. Noninvasive testing

     a) Ankle-arm index (AAI): Performed by using Doppler stethoscope

       (1) The ankle pressure is divided by the brachial systolic pressure; ankle pressure normally is equal to or greater than the brachial systolic pressure.

       (2) Normal AAI is > 0.9 or 90%; an AAI < 0.9 suggests arterial obstruction in the lower extremity.

     b) Segmental doppler studies: Measure leg pressures in segments.

     c) Duplex scan: Combines ultrasonography with Doppler flow studies to evaluate the quality of the arterial and venous flow and to look for any evidence of obstruction.

    2. Invasive testing: Arteriography provides both physiologic and anatomic information (e.g., ulcerating plaques, hemorrhage, degree of stenosis or obstruction).

V. Differential diagnosis

  A. Acute arterial occlusion

  B. Raynaud's phenomenon

  C. Radiation-induced fibrosis

  D. Antiphospholipid antibody (APA) syndrome

VI. Treatment

  A. Goals

    1. Modify risk factors

    2. Optimize blood flow

    3. Implement foot care

  B. Exercise: Can improve blood flow

    1. Progressive walking increases collateral circulation.

    2. Instruct patient to walk to the point of claudication, rest, and then resume walking until pain reappears.

    3. Walking should be done at least twice daily and, preferably, four times/day for at least 20 minutes.

  C. Risk factor modification

    1. Smoking cessation

      2. Weight loss or control

      3. Reduced fat intake

      4. Medication compliance

  D. Foot care

      1. Keep feet clean, dry, and free from trauma and local heat.

      2. Always wear shoes.

      3. Avoid tight restrictive socks or hose.

      4. Clip toenails straight across.

  E. Pharmacotherapy

      1. Hemorrheologic agents (Trental and aspirin): May enhance blood flow.

         a) Trental® (pentoxifylline, Hoechst Marion Roussel, Kansas City, KS): 400 mg tid; affects microcirculation by improving blood cell flexibility, reducing blood viscosity, and decreasing platelet aggregation.

         b) Aspirin and dipyridamole (Persantine®, Boehringer Ingelheim, Ridgefield, CT): Prevent platelet aggregation at the site of the occlusion. Most patients presenting with symptoms of PVD have coexisting ischemic coronary disease and already should be using aspirin therapy as part of the standard of care.

      2. Lipid-lowering medications: For patients presenting with hyperlipidemia (see Chapter 42)

  F. Invasive/surgical therapy

      1. Indications

         a) Claudication that affects normal activities of daily living

         b) Nonhealing ulcers

         c) Ischemic pain at rest

         d) Impending gangrene

      2. Angioplasty: Three-year patency rates are approximately 70%–80%, which is comparable to bypass surgery.

      3. Stent placement: Indications for stent are acute dissections and restenosis in native or bypassed grafts after angioplasty (e.g., iliac and femoropopliteal lesions).

      4. Surgical bypass grafting: Involves bypassing the occluded segment or segments; effective treatment for complex aortoiliac occlusive disease.

VII. Follow-Up

  A. Monthly to evaluate patient's response to therapy

  B. Continued encouragement: To maintain or initiate lifestyle modifications

  C. Revise program as needed: Every six months for mild PVD (mild symptoms not interfering with lifestyle), every three months for moderate PVD (symptoms begin to interfere with lifestyle), and monthly for severe PVD (symptoms occur at rest).

VIII. Referrals

  A. Vascular specialist: Patients requiring surgical intervention

  B. Cardiologist: Patients with cardiac risk factors or symptoms of coronary artery disease, poorly controlled hypertension, and CHF

  C. Endocrinologist: Patients with diabetes mellitus

References

Cookingham, A. (1995). Peripheral vascular disease: Educational concerns for patients with a chronic disease in a changing health care environment. *AACN Clinical Issues, 6*(4), 670–676.

Krenzer, M.E. (1995). Peripheral vascular assessment: Finding your way through arteries and veins. *AACN Clinical Issues, 6*(4), 631–644.

McDermott, M.M., & McCarthy, W. (1995). Intermittent claudication. The natural history. *Surgical Clinics of North America, 75*(4), 581–591.

Santilli, J.D., Rodnick, J.E., & Santilli, S.M. (1996). Claudication: Diagnosis and treatment. *American Family Physician, 53*(4), 1245–1253.

Welch, H.J. (1997). Chronic lower extremity ischemia. *Comprehensive Therapy, 23,* 534–538.

Wheeler, E., & Brenner, Z. (1995). Peripheral vascular anatomy, physiology, and pathophysiology. *AACN Clinical Issues, 6*(4), 505–515.

Section VI. Gastrointestinal

Symptoms

Medical Diagnosis

Chapter

50. Abdominal Pain
George Bryant, ND, APN

I. Definition: Pain originating from the abdomen
   A. Chronic: Pain is a slow, progressive process that persists over a long period of time.
   B. Acute: Pain is characterized by sudden onset and severe intensity and is incapacitating to the patient.
   C. Acute surgical abdomen: A type of hyperacute pain that requires immediate surgical or medical intervention

II. Pathophysiology
   A. Visceral pain: Results from spasm, contraction, or distention of the muscle wall
   B. Parietal pain: Associated with inflammation of the linings that cover the viscera
   C. Referred pain: Can be visceral or parietal in origin; in either case, a remote site shares nerve pathways with the organ of origin or the linings of the viscera.
   D. Neurogenic pain: Also referred as causalgia; the result of nerve injury from encroachment or irritation along the nerve pathway
   E. Psychogenic pain: Elicited by certain psychologic stressors that lead to a physiological response not associated with organ dysfunction

III. Clinical features: Pain is caused by three processes—ischemia, inflammation, or muscle contraction or distention.
   A. Etiology
      1. Pain location is important in determining the cause for the symptom. Abdominal pain can be divided into three forms.
         a) Pain involving the digestive system
         b) Pain as a result of metabolic disease
         c) Pain from a psychogenic origin
      2. Generally, the abdomen is divided into geographic regions with specific identifiable structures. Possible causes of pain are listed.
         a) Generalized/diffuse: Bowel obstruction, constipation, metabolic disturbances, peritonitis, gastroenteritis, mesenteric ischemia, and psychogenic pain
         b) Right upper quadrant: Cholecystitis, hepatitis, peptic ulcer disease (PUD), colitis, diverticulitis, pancreatitis, pulmonary embolism, nephrolithiasis, and cancer of the colon, esophagus, stomach, and pancreas

   c) Epigastric: Aortic aneurysm; gastroenteritis; myocardial infarction; early appendicitis; colitis; pancreatitis; cancer of the colon, liver, esophagus, stomach, or pancreas; cholecystitis; and inflammatory bowel disease

   d) Left upper quadrant: Splenic enlargement, colitis, PUD, pyelonephritis, pancreatitis, pneumonia, gastritis, urinary tract infection, and colon cancer

   e) Umbilical: Appendicitis, aortic aneurysm, gastroenteritis, hernia, mesenteric ischemia, bowel obstruction, inflammatory bowel disease, and pancreatitis

   f) Right lower quadrant (with flank pain): Ectopic pregnancy, menstrual cramps, endometriosis, pelvic inflammatory disease (PID), ovarian cyst, testicular torsion, psoas abscess, penetrating or perforating ulcer, inflammatory bowel disease, hernia, diverticulitis, appendicitis, colon or ovarian cancer, salpingitis, and kidney stones

   g) Left lower quadrant (with flank pain): Ectopic pregnancy, menstrual cramps, PID, endometriosis, ovarian cyst, testicular torsion, kidney stones, psoas abscess, penetrating or perforating ulcer, inflammatory bowel disease, diverticulitis, appendicitis, colon or ovarian cancer, hernia, salpingitis, and kidney stones

   h) Hypogastrium: Bowel obstruction, cystitis, prostatitis, ectopic pregnancy, hernia, ovarian cyst/torsion, diverticulitis, enteritis, aortic aneurysm, inflammatory bowel disease, colon cancer, and cecal volvulus

   i) Subxiphoid or substernal: Esophageal reflux, esophageal carcinoma, peptic ulcer, penetrating ulcer, myocardial infarction, and angina

 B. History

  1. History of cancer and cancer treatment

  2. Current medications: Prescribed and over-the-counter

  3. History of presenting symptom(s): precipitating factors, onset, location, and duration. Associated symptoms are nausea, emesis, diarrhea, bloating, anorexia, constipation, lightheadedness, syncope, weight loss, or fever with chills.

  4. Duration of pain

   a) Chronic: Usually involves periods of symptom exacerbation and clinical remission

   b) Acute: Multiple signs and symptoms are associated with the pain and usually precede the initial onset of pain.

  5. Changes in activities of daily living

  6. Medical history: Abdominal surgery, sexually transmitted diseases (STD)

  7. For women

   a) History of menstrual cycle

   b) Medical history: Abnormal vaginal bleeding or discharge, ectopic pregnancy

  8. Social history: Alcohol intake, sexual history

 C. Signs and symptoms

  1. Nausea/vomiting

  2. Diarrhea or constipation

  3. Hematemesis

  4. Melena: Maroon or bright-red blood in stool

  5. Syncope

    6. Dysuria, urgency, frequency, or hematuria

    7. Rectal pain

    8. Abnormal/missed menses (women)

    9. Abnormal vaginal bleeding (women)

   10. Jaundice

   11. Abdominal distention

   12. Anorexia

   13. Fevers and chills

D. Physical exam

    1. Vital signs

      a) Blood pressure: Orthostatic, tachycardia, or hypotension

        (1) Postural changes secondary to obstruction, peritonitis, bowel infarction

        (2) Hypertension secondary to pain

        (3) Hypotension secondary to dehydration

      b) Pulse: Tachycardia (> 100 bpm) or bradycardia (< 50 bpm)

      c) Respiration: Tachypnea (> 20)

      d) Temperature: Fever (> 38.3 °C; 101 °F) may indicate infection, but lack of fever does not rule out etiology.

    2. General appearance

      a) Level of distress

      b) Positioning

        (1) Patient avoids movement; peritoneal irritation

        (2) Patient is very restless; may indicate obstruction

    3. Integument exam

      a) Jaundice and other stigmata of chronic liver disease

      b) Sclerae: Icterus suggests liver disease.

      c) Rashes or lesions: Macules, papules, petechiae (vesicles are pattern of distribution)

      d) Signs of trauma

      e) Poor skin turgor: Indicates dehydration

      f) Ecchymotic areas: Disseminated intravascular coagulation (DIC), liver disease

    4. Cardiovascular exam

      a) Murmurs/abnormal heart sounds: Ectopic beats with mesenteric ischemia

      b) Bruit: Abdominal aortic aneurysm

      c) Jugular vein distention (JVD): Hepatomegaly associated with congestive heart failure (CHF)

      d) Splinting: Indicates inflammation

    5. Pulmonary exam

      a) Breath sounds

        (1) Diminished with CHF

        (2) Absent with consolidation

        (3) Grating sound with pleural friction rub

      b) Respirations: Increase in frequency with pain

    6. Abdominal exam

       a) Local tenderness, rebound tenderness, guarding tenderness located over affected digestive system in visceral pain

       b) Rigidity: Suggests peritoneal irritation

       c) Bowel sounds: High-pitched tinkling, bruits, or absent

       d) Distention: Obstruction, appendicitis, ascites

       e) Hepatosplenomegaly: Venous congestion associated with CHF, visible abdominal venous pattern indicates portal hypertension

       f) Pulsatile/nonpulsatile masses: Aortic aneurysm

       g) Flank tenderness: Pyelonephritis

7. Rectal exam (includes prostate exam in men)

       a) Masses

          (1) Heme-positive stools: PUD or upper GI bleed

          (2) Prostate is enlarged or with nodules

       b) Tenderness: Thrombosed hemorrhoids

       c) Gross rectal bleeding: Lower GI bleed (e.g., colon cancer)

8. Pelvic exam: To rule out PID, STD, cancer

       a) Vaginal or cervical discharge

       b) Cervical motion tenderness

       c) Adnexal masses or tenderness

9. Male genitourinary exam

       a) Testicular swelling, masses, or tenderness

       b) Scrotal masses or swelling

       c) Perineal edema

10. Special tests (see Appendix 13)

       a) Peritoneal irritation

          (1) Obturator sign: Have patient sit in supine position and flex knee to 90°, examiner immobilizes the ankle while performing internal/external rotation of the knee; pain with rotation is positive.

          (2) Iliopsoas sign: Have patient sit in supine position and extend knee, attempting to flex thigh against resistance; pain during maneuver is positive.

       b) Cholecystitis sign (i.e., Murphy's sign)

          (1) Have patient breathe in while palpating the edge of the liver.

          (2) Positive sign is when patient stops breathing suddenly during inspiration because of pain.

11. Surgical abdomen exam

       a) General overview: Extreme pallor, jaundice, restlessness, writhing with pain, rigidity, immobility may be present.

       b) Vital signs: High fever, tachypnea, irregular/thready pulse, orthostatic changes

       c) Abdominal exam: Absent or high-pitched bowel sounds, distended abdomen, severe localized tenderness, mass

IV. Diagnostic tests

  A. Laboratory studies

    1. CBC: To rule out infection, anemia

       a) Elevated WBC: Indicates inflammatory or infectious process

       b) Differential: Left shift indicates infection

   c) Low hematocrit and hemoglobin with bleeding
  2. BUN/creatinine, electrolytes, and glucose: To rule out dehydration or imbalances
  3. Stool for occult or gross blood: To rule out associated GI bleed
  4. Amylase/lipase: Elevated level may indicate pancreatitis, perforation, intestinal obstruction
  5. Urinalysis: Presence of hematuria or pyuria indicates urinary tract infection/pyelonephritis
  6. Quantitative urine pregnancy test: For women of childbearing age to rule out ectopic pregnancy
  7. Liver function studies: May indicate hepatitis, cirrhosis, or hepatotoxicity with elevated values
 B. Radiology
  1. Plain and upright films of the abdomen: To evaluate for obstructive processes, perforation (free air under diaphragm), ascites, or abnormal gas pattern
  2. Upper GI series: To rule out ulcer, cancer, small bowel obstruction
  3. Barium enema: If patient is bleeding to rule out cancer, inflammatory bowel
  4. Ultrasound: To rule out gallstones, biliary obstruction, ureteral obstruction, uterine or ovarian mass
  5. IV pyelogram: To rule out renal obstruction, mass, and stones

V. Differential diagnosis
 A. GI disorders
  1. Pancreatitis (see Chapter 72)
  2. Appendicitis
  3. Cholecystitis/choledocholithiasis
  4. Small bowel obstruction (see Chapter 63)
  5. Large bowel obstruction (see Chapter 63)
  6. Crohn's disease
  7. Ulcerative colitis
  8. Irritable bowel syndrome (see Chapter 71)
  9. Peptic ulcer disease (see Chapter 73)
  10. Intestinal infarct or ischemia
  11. Diverticulitis
  12. Hepatitis (see Chapter 69)
  13. Gastroenteritis/gastritis (see Chapter 67)
  14. Colon/liver/gastric/pancreatic cancers
  15. Splenomegaly (see Chapter 61)
  16. Abdominal hernia
  17. Hepatomegaly (see Chapter 56)
  18. Constipation (see Chapter 52)
 B. Genitourinary disorders
  1. Women
   a) PID
   b) Ectopic pregnancy

        c) Endometriosis

        d) Uterine fibroids

        e) Salpingitis

        f) Menstrual cramps/PMS

        g) Ovarian cyst/torsion/cancer

    2. Men

        a) Prostatitis (see Chapter 92)

        b) Testicular torsion/ cancer

        c) Prostate cancer

        d) Seminal vesiculitis

    3. Women and men

        a) Urinary tract infection (see Chapter 91)

        b) Pyelonephritis (see Chapter 93)

        c) Ureteral calculi

        d) Nephrolithiasis

C. Metabolic disorders

    1. Addison's disease

    2. Hyperparathyroidism

    3. Diabetic ketoacidosis

    4. Acute intermittent porphyria

D. Cardiovascular disorders

    1. Myocardial infarction/ischemia/angina pectoris (see Chapter 47)

    2. Aortic aneurysm

    3. Sickle cell anemia (see Chapter 118)

E. Pulmonary disorders

    1. Pulmonary embolism (see Chapter 33)

    2. Pneumonia (see Chapter 30)

F. Neurogenic disorders: Herpes zoster (see Chapter 20)

G. Drug-induced disorders

    1. Vinca alkaloids: Ileus, constipation

    2. Opioids: Ileus, constipation

    3. NSAIDs: Peptic ulcer disease, esophagitis

    4. Alcohol: Gastritis, esophagitis, cirrhosis

    5. Selective serotonin reuptake inhibitors (SSRIs): Gastritis

VI. Treatment

A. The degree of pain and number of associated symptoms correlates with the degree of intervention (i.e., great degree of pain and associated symptoms requires referral to emergency department/surgeon to rule out acute abdomen).

B. Narcotics generally are contraindicated for pain control and should not be given until a source for the pain has been identified. Narcotics generally decrease bowel motility as well as mask pain. Meperidine is usually the drug of choice because it does not decrease the GI motility.

C. Admission criteria for acute abdomen

    1. GI bleeding

2. Signs of infection (impending sepsis)
3. Significant intravascular volume depletion
4. Fever
5. Bowel obstruction with nausea and vomiting
6. Worsening of pain or tenderness during serial abdominal exam
7. Biliary tree obstruction
8. Presence of adnexal mass
9. General appearance of clinical toxicity

D. Introduce dietary measures depending on the diagnosis, which can include nothing by mouth (npo) status, clear liquids, or low-fat/low-residue diet until the problem has resolved or has been diagnosed.

VII. Follow-up
A. Short-term: Patients with nonacute abdomen; depending on the diagnosis, some disease states (e.g., reflux) require only dietary measures, while others (e.g., PUD) may require medical management
B. Long-term: Patients requiring intensive measures (e.g., surgical intervention beginning with the postoperative or recovery period)
C. Patients experiencing chronic symptoms (i.e., pancreatitis, reflux) need regular follow-up to monitor disease exacerbation and to determine if aggressive therapy should be initiated.

VIII. Referrals
A. General surgeon/emergency room: Immediately refer patients with acute abdomen or possible bowel obstruction.
B. Obstetrician/gynecologist: Immediately refer women presenting with adnexal masses or who are pregnant.
C. Gastroenterologist: Refer patients with GI bleeding for guidance in evaluation or if the diagnosis is uncertain.
D. Urologist: Refer patients with severe urinary tract infection or with urolithiasis.

References

American College of Emergency Physicians. (1994). Clinical policy for the initial approach to patients presenting with a chief complaint of nontraumatic acute abdominal pain. *Annals of Emergency Medicine, 23,* 906–922.

Blackington, E. (1998). Acute abdominal pain. *Advance for Nurse Practitioners, 6*(8), 46–50, 52, 90.

DeBanto, J.R., Varilek, G.W., & Yaas, L. (1999). What could be causing chronic abdominal pain? Anything from common peptic ulcers to uncommon pancreatic trauma. *Postgraduate Medicine, 106*(3), 141–146.

Klinkman, M.S. (1996). Episodes of care for abdominal pain in a primary care practice. *Archives of Family Medicine, 5*(5), 279–285.

Schuster, M.M. (1995). Abdominal pain. In L.R. Barker, J.R. Burton, & P.D. Zieve (Eds.), *Principles of ambulatory medicine* (4th ed.) (pp. 447–456). Baltimore: Williams & Wilkins.

Stone, R. (1996). Primary care diagnosis of acute abdominal pain. *Nurse Practitioner, 21*(12), 19–39.

Trott, A.L., Trunkey, D.D., & Wilson, S.R. (1995). Acute abdominal pain: A guide to crisis management. *Patient Care, 29*(13), 104–133.

Zuccaro, G. (1997). Treatment and referral guidelines in gastroenterology. *Gastroenterology Clinics of North America, 26,* 845–857.

Chapter

51. Ascites

Gail Egan Sansivero, MS, ANP, AOCN®

I. Definition: Accumulation of excessive fluid within the peritoneal cavity

II. Physiology/Pathophysiology
   A. Normal
      1. The peritoneal surface is a semipermeable membrane through which passive diffusion of water and solutes and exchanges between the abdominal cavity and the subperitoneal vascular and lymphatic channels occur.
      2. Fluid crosses the membrane at a rate of approximately 30–35 cc/hour.
   B. Pathophysiology: Ascites results when changes occur in the formation and absorption of this fluid.
      1. Inflammation causes protein to leak into the ascites fluid, resulting in exudate from damage to capillaries and disruption of lymphatics.
      2. Transudate: Pathophysiology mechanisms are uncertain. Various mechanisms proposed include a combination of increased portal pressure, increased capillary pressure, increased lymph production, decreased osmotic pressure, and impaired renal excretion of sodium and water.

III. Clinical features: Ascites is classified as exudate or transudate. Malignant and nonmalignant ascites are associated with a poor prognosis.
   A. Etiology
      1. Ascites occurs most frequently because of decompensation of previously existing liver disease (e.g., cirrhosis).
      2. Malignant ascites accounts for 10% of all cases of ascites and is a manifestation of advanced disease.
      3. Exudate: Etiologies include tumor, infection, or trauma.
      4. Transudate: Etiologies include congestive heart failure, cirrhosis, or nephrotic syndrome.
   B. History
      1. History of cancer and cancer treatment
      2. Current medications: Prescribed and over-the-counter
      3. History of presenting system(s): Precipitating factors, onset, location, and duration. Associated symptoms are shortness of breath, weight gain, change in abdomen size, edema of ankles or legs, and change in appetite.

    4. Changes in activities of daily living

    5. Social history: Alcohol intake

    6. Past medical history: Liver disease

C. Signs and symptoms

    1. Abdominal pain

    2. Abdominal fullness or pressure

    3. Abdominal distention

    4. Shortness of breath

    5. Nausea

    6. Anorexia

    7. Early satiety

    8. Weight gain

    9. Flank pain

    10. Penile and scrotal edema

    11. Orthopnea

    12. Peripheral edema

    13. Altered bowel habits

D. Physical exam: Not very sensitive for early ascites; at least several hundred milliliters of fluid must be present to detect by physical exam.

    1. Vital signs: Assess weight and compare to baseline.

    2. Pulmonary: Auscultate and percuss for dullness and decreased or absent breath sounds, indicating pulmonary effusions, or rales, indicating congestion.

    3. Abdominal exam: To confirm presence of fluid

        a) Fluid wave, in the presence of ascites, will be positive.

        b) Assess for shifting dullness to ascertain for ascites; dullness at the dependent side indicates ascites.

        c) Bulging flank indicates ascites.

        d) Increased venous distention occurs with abdominal distention.

        e) Monitoring abdominal girth is an unreliable gauge of fluid loss because of GI tract influences.

    4. Assess for edema: May be present in the extremities, sacrum, penis, scrotum, and other areas, indicating ascites

IV. Diagnostic tests

A. Laboratory

    1. CBC: To evaluate for an infection

    2. Liver function tests: Elevations may indicate liver damage or failure.

    3. Prothrombin time: Prolongation suggests advanced liver disease.

    4. Amylase is elevated in pancreatic disorders.

    5. Diagnostic paracentesis

        a) Test fluid for cell count and total protein; determine the albumin gradient, culture and sensitivity, cytology, and amylase.

        b) Transudate fluid is clear or straw-colored with low protein content ($<$ 25 g/l), low specific gravity ($<$ 1.016), low cell count, and a high gradient difference in the albumin concentration between the serum and ascitic fluid.

      c) Exudate fluid has a low gradient difference in the albumin concentration and high protein (> 25 g/l). Serum-ascitic albumin gradient (SAAG)

         (1) The gradient is calculated by subtracting the albumin concentration of the ascitic fluid from the serum albumin concentration collected on the same day. Traditionally, the total protein concentration of ascitic fluid and lactic dehydrogenase (LDH) have been used to classify ascitic fluid as transudate or exudate, but this is not as accurate as SAAG.

         (2) Patients with a high gradient (> 1.1 g/dl) are likely to have cirrhosis, alcoholic hepatitis, cardiac failure, hepatic failure, or portal vein thrombosis.

         (3) Patients with a lower gradient are more likely to have malignant ascites, pancreatic or biliary ascites, peritoneal tuberculosis (TB), nephrotic syndrome, bowel obstruction, or infarction.

      d) RBCs suggest hemorrhagic ascites, usually from malignancy, TB, or trauma.

      e) Amylase elevation suggests pancreatic disorders.

      f) Elevation of mononuclear cells (i.e., WBCs) suggests TB or fungal infection.

      g) Elevation of polymorphonuclear cells suggests bacterial infection.

      h) pH < 7 suggests bacterial infection.

      i) Cytology: May be positive in malignancy; only 60% of malignant aspirates are cytologically positive.

    6. Tumor markers may be indicated (see Appendix 16).

    7. Electrolytes: To assess for azotemia, indicating renal failure

    8. Ammonia level: If encephalopathy suspected

  B. Radiology

    1. Abdominal ultrasound: To confirm presence of ascites and rule out veno-occlusive disease

    2. Abdominal CT or laparotomy: May be indicated to identify source

V. Differential diagnosis

  A. Alcohol-induced hepatitis or cirrhosis (see Chapters 64 and 69)

  B. Cardiomyopathy (see Chapter 39)

  C. Peritoneal disease

  D. Portal hypertension

  E. Malignancy-related disorder

    1. Adenocarcinoma of the peritoneum

    2. Primary mesothelioma

    3. Ovarian cancer

    4. Chronic lymphocytic leukemia

    5. Peritoneal and abdominal metastasis

  F. Liver disease

    1. Acute liver disease

    2. Hepatic vein occlusion (i.e., Budd-Chiari syndrome)

    3. Bile ascites

  G. Mesenteric inflammatory disease

  H. Constrictive pericarditis (see Chapter 48)

  I. Hemochromatosis

   J. Amyloidosis
   K. Mucinous spur cell hemolytic anemia
   L. TB peritonitis
   M. Inferior vena cava obstruction
   N. Hypoalbuminemia
      1. Nephrotic syndrome
      2. Protein-losing enteropathy
      3. Malnutrition
   O. Myxedema
   P. Pancreatitis (see Chapter 72)
   Q. Chylous ascites
   R. Ovarian overstimulation syndrome

VI. Treatment: Under optimal conditions, the capacity to reabsorb ascitic fluid is no more than 700–900 ml/day; therefore, diuresis should proceed gradually.
   A. Monitor weights daily or every other day.
   B. Attempt dietary restriction of sodium to 2 g/day in patients with nonmalignant ascites (e.g., portal hypertension).
      1. Noncompliance with dietary restriction sometimes is overlooked as a cause of refractory ascites.
      2. In the absence of encephalopathy, a protein intake of 50 g/day is recommended.
      3. Excessive free water intake (> 1,500 ml/day) should be avoided, especially if serum sodium is < 130.
   C. The goal of diuretic therapy should be a daily weight loss of 0.5–1.0 kg with edema and 0.25 kg without edema if diuresis has not occurred with dietary restriction of sodium.
      1. Spironolactone: 100 mg/day with furosemide 40 mg/day po is most effective for rapid diminution of ascites.
      2. Doses of both drugs are increased if there is no decrease in body weight or increase in urinary sodium excretion after two to three days.
      3. Maximum daily doses should be 400–500 mg spironolactone and 160 mg furosemide.
   D. In patients with malignant ascites, systemic or intraperitoneal chemotherapy is aimed at the primary tumor. When the primary site is unknown, median survival is rarely affected by empiric therapy.
   E. Therapeutic paracentesis is performed for symptomatic relief in patients with pain, shortness of breath, and cardiac dysfunction.
      1. Paracentesis of up to one liter/day may provide relief of acute respiratory symptoms; in portal hypertension, three to four liters can safely be removed.
      2. Care must be taken to preserve intravascular volume.
      3. In larger volume paracentesis, replacement of albumin 10 g IV for each liter of ascitic fluid removed may prevent reduction in plasma volume; however, this is rarely necessary.
      4. Other volume expanders (e.g., dextran) may be used, although their effect on morbidity and mortality is uncertain. Dextran may precipitate variceal hemorrhage in patients with portal hypertension.

F. Peritoneovenous shunts (e.g., LeVeen, Denver) are used for patients who are fractory to all medical interventions and with disabling symptoms.
   1. Restrict use of shunts for patients with normal hepatic function.
   2. Shunts have poor outcomes and often fail early after placement, therefore, they usually are not indicated for malignant ascites.
G. Transjugular intrahepatic portosystemic shunt (TIPS) is a nonsurgical technique to decompress the portal circulation.
   1. Survival after TIPS is related to severity of liver function impairment.
   2. Occlusions occur frequently and can lead to hepatic (i.e., portosystemic) encephalopathy.
H. Supportive measures to provide symptomatic relief (e.g., positioning, lower extremity elevation, immersion in pool or jacuzzi, use of pillows to support abdomen) may be beneficial.

VII. Follow-up: Depends upon disease state
   A. Patient will need regular healthcare provider visits to monitor laboratory values (BUN, creatinine, electrolytes, ammonia) and nutritional status and for physical exam.
   B. Shunt patency must be monitored with abdominal ultrasound at least every six months in patients who have undergone a TIPS procedure.
   C. Patients with peritoneovenous shunts need frequent monitoring of shunt function.

VIII. Referrals
   A. Dietitian: For dietary modification/counseling
   B. Gastroenterologist: If endoscopy is indicated for diagnostic purposes
   C. Surgeon: If biopsy is indicated or for shunt placement
   D. Oncologist/hematologist: If malignancy is suspected or confirmed
   E. Internist: For newly diagnosed ascites, worsening encephalopathy, unexplained fever, increasing azotemia, and GI bleeding
   F. Hospice: Consider for patients receiving palliative treatment to manage ascites.

References

Parsons, S.L., Watson, S.A., & Steele, J.C. (1996). Malignant ascites. *British Journal of Surgery, 83,* 6–14.

Ringenberg, Q.S., Doll, D.C., Loy, T.S., & Yarbro, J.W. (1989). Malignant ascites of unknown origin. *Cancer, 64,* 753–755.

Runyon, B.A. (1994). Care of the patient with ascites. *New England Journal of Medicine, 330,* 337–342.

Runyon, B.A. (1997). Patient selection is important in studying the impact of large-volume paracentesis on intravascular volume. *American Journal of Gastroenterology, 92,* 371–373.

Runyon, B.A., Montano, A.A., Akriviadis, E.A., Antillon, M.R., Irving, M.A., & McHutchison, J.G. (1992). The serum-ascites albumin gradient is superior to the exudate-transudate concept in the differential diagnosis of ascites. *Annals of Internal Medicine, 117,* 215–220.

Williams, J.W., & Simel, D.L. (1992). Does this patient have ascites? How to divine fluid in the abdomen. *JAMA, 267,* 2645–2648.

Chapter

52. Constipation
Rebecca A. Hawkins, RN, MSN, ANP, AOCN®

I. Definition: Passage of excessively hard stool or the infrequent passage of stool

II. Physiology/Pathophysiology
   A. Normal: Elimination of fecal waste requires two processes.
      1. Filling of the rectum by colonic transport
      2. Defecation or reflex of stool
   B. Pathophysiology: Decreased colonic motility as a result of metabolic and endocrine disturbances or decreased storage capacity of the proximal colon

III. Clinical features: Normal frequency of bowel movements varies greatly, from two or three movements daily to one movement every three to five days. A change or decrease in the patient's normal frequency is significant.
   A. History
      1. History of cancer and cancer treatment
      2. Current medications: Prescribed and over-the-counter
      3. History of presenting symptom(s): Precipitating factors, onset, location, and duration
      4. Changes in activities of daily living
      5. History of normal bowel habits
   B. Signs and symptoms
      1. Increased hardness of the stool or difficulty in moving bowels
      2. Decreased frequency of defecation
      3. Abdominal distention
      4. Abdominal pain
      5. Anal pain or tenderness
      6. Nausea and vomiting
   C. Physical exam
      1. Abdominal exam
         a) Normal or hypoactive bowel sounds
         b) No hyperactive rushes or tinkles: Hyperactive rushes suggest obstruction.
         c) No abdominal tenderness but distention may be present
         d) Palpable stool in lower quadrants
      2. Rectal exam
         a) Note stool for color and consistency, and test for occult blood.
         b) Inspect and palpate for masses, fissures, inflammation, and hard stool.

      c) Note sphincter control.

      d) Observe for external or prolapsed hemorrhoids.

IV. Diagnostic tests

    A. Laboratory

       1. Stool specimen: For occult blood

       2. Potassium level: To rule out hypokalemia

       3. Thyroid-stimulating hormone: To rule out hypothyroidism after other causes have been ruled out

       4. Calcium level: To rule out hypercalcemia

       5. BUN and creatinine levels: To evaluate hydration status

    B. Radiology: Not indicated unless obstruction or ileus are being considered

V. Differential diagnosis

    A. Medication-induced disorders

       1. Opioids: Narcotic bowel syndrome

       2. Anticholinergic agents

       3. Antidepressants

       4. Antiserotonin antiemetics

       5. Chronic laxative use

       6. Vinca alkaloids and taxanes

       7. Iron preparations

       8. Calcium- or aluminum-containing antacids

       9. Diuretics

    B. Colonic tumors

    C. Hypothyroidism (see Chapter 150)

    D. Irritable bowel syndrome (see Chapter 71)

    E. Diabetes mellitus (see Chapter 143)

    F. Cushing's syndrome

    G. Diverticulitis

    H. Radiographic barium impaction

    I. Dehydration (see Chapter 147)

    J. Immobility

    K. Neurologic disorders

       1. Spinal cord compression (see Chapter 138)

       2. Neuropathy

    L. Electrolyte imbalances (e.g., hypercalcemia, hypokalemia) (see Chapter 144–148)

    M. Emotional difficulties

VI. Treatment: Anticipate and prevent constipation.

    A. Diet modification

       1. Encourage a high-fiber diet and increased fluid intake.

       2. Changing diet may not be sufficient to treat constipation, especially in patients with terminal illness.

       3. Diet will not affect constipation caused by opioids.

    B. Encourage activity and exercise, if appropriate.

Table 52-1. Pharmacologic Therapy for Constipation

Therapy	Action	Onset	Examples	Comments
Bulk laxatives	Increase peristalsis by increasing size and weight of stool	Twelve hours to several days	Calcium polycarbophil (Fiber Con[a]) Two caplets qd to qid po Psyllium (Metamucil[b]): one teaspoon qd to tid po	Works best with increased amounts of fluids and may not be feasible in patients with cancer
Lubricants	Coat the stool and reduce friction	Eight hours	Mineral oil: 10–30 cc/day po	Excessive doses can lead to seepage and can lead to malabsorption of fat-soluble vitamins.
Saline laxatives	Increase gastric, pancreatic, and small intestinal secretion and increases motor activity of the small and large bowel	1–12 hours	Magnesium hydroxide (milk of magnesia), 30–60 cc po; magnesium citrate, 200 cc po; sodium phosphate (Fleet® Phospho-Soda[c]), 30 cc po, Fleet enema	Avoid in patients with renal dysfunction; may be problematic in patients with cardiac or renal disease.
Osmotic laxatives	Nonabsorbable sugars that exert an osmotic effect in both the small and large intestine	30 minutes to several hours	Lactulose (5 grains/15 ml), 15–30 ml qd up to 60 ml/day; sorbitol, 30–60 cc po qd; glycerin suppository; Golytely[®d], 8–16 oz/day po	Watch for signs of dehydration.
Detergent laxatives	Reduce surface tension and allow penetration of water and fats into the stool	Several hours	Docusate sodium, 50–500 mg po qd; castor oil, 15 cc qd po	—
Large bowel stimulants	Stimulate colonic motility	Several hours to days	Senna (Senokot® or Senokot-S[®e]), one to six tablets/day po; bisacodyl (Dulcolax[®f], 10–15 mg/day po; phenolphthalein (Ex-Lax[®f] or Correctal[®f]), one or two tablets q hs po; casanthranol plus docusate sodium (Peri-Colace[®g]), one or two capsules qd or tid po	—

[a] American Cyanamid Company, Wagner, NJ; [b] Procter & Gamble Pharmaceuticals, Cincinnati, OH; [c] C.B. Fleet Co., Inc., Lynchberg, VA; [d] Braintree Laboratories, Inc., Braintree, MA; [e] The Purdue Frederick Company; Norwalk, CT; [f] Novartis Pharmaceuticals, East Hanover, NJ; [g] Roberts Laboratories, Eatontown, NJ

C. Set up a bowel regimen; must be simple and used for prevention in patients receiving opioids (see Table 52-1).
 1. Chronic constipation, such as with the use of opioids, requires a stool softener and a laxative.
 2. If bowel program does not work within two days of initiating, change medications or classes of drugs.

VII. Follow-up
 A. Short-term: Patients should be called to see if bowel program is working within 24–48 hours of starting the medications.
 B. Long-term: Patients with cancer, especially those on opioids, need constant follow-up regarding constipation and the effectiveness of their bowel program.

VIII. Referrals
 A. Dietitian: To make diet and hydration recommendations when appropriate
 B. Internist: If unable to relieve constipation effectively
 C. Oncologist: If patient needs to be admitted for narcotic bowel syndrome

References

Abrahm, J.L. (1998). Promoting symptom control in palliative care. *Seminars in Oncology Nursing, 14,* 95–109.

Bisanz, A. (1997). Managing bowel elimination problems in patients with cancer. *Oncology Nursing Forum, 24,* 679–686.

Canty, S.L. (1994). Constipation as a side effect of opioids. *Oncology Nursing Forum, 21,* 739–745.

Levy, M.H. (1991). Constipation and diarrhea in cancer patients. *Cancer Bulletin, 43,* 412–422.

Wright, P.S., & Thomas, S.L. (1995). Constipation and diarrhea: The neglected symptom. *Seminars in Oncology Nursing, 11,* 289–297.

53. Diarrhea

Jeanne Held-Warmkessel, MSN, RN, CS, AOCN®

I. Definition: Abnormal increase in frequency, volume, and/or liquid content of stool
   A. Pseudodiarrhea: Increased frequency of defecation without change in stool consistency
   B. Fecal incontinence: Inability to control stool evacuation

II. Physiology/Pathophysiology
   A. Normal
      1. Food is passed through the stomach to the bowel, where nutrients and water are absorbed.
      2. The majority of liquid is removed from the stool as it transits the bowel so that only 200 ml of water usually is present in a formed stool as it is evacuated.
      3. Peristaltic waves are responsible for the movement of stool through the bowel.
   B. Pathophysiology
      1. Osmotic diarrhea: Results from consumption of substances (food or drug) that create an increased amount of osmotic activity in the intestine. This increases the amount of water drawn into the colon and, thus, in the stool.
      2. Secretory diarrhea: Results from disruption in normal colonic epithelial cell transport of ions with increased intestinal mucosal secretion of fluid and electrolytes.
      3. Motility abnormalities: Slow colon transit times allow bacterial overgrowth, which may cause diarrhea. Increased motility may cause reduced absorption.
      4. Exudative diarrhea: Alteration in the integrity of colonic mucosa from ulcers, inflammatory process, or radiation therapy.
      5. Malabsorptive diarrhea: Results from a combination of altered mucosal contiguity, altered bowel structure, or enzyme changes.
      6. Chemotherapy-induced diarrhea: Results from a combination of intestinal inflammation, changes in villi, malabsorption, and secretory changes.
      7. Radiation to abdomen and pelvis causes loss of villi and bile malabsorption.

III. Clinical features: Classified as acute or chronic; acute diarrhea lasts for no more than two to three weeks, and chronic diarrhea lasts four weeks or longer. Diarrhea is subjective in its definition.
   A. Etiologies: See Figure 53-1
   B. History

Figure 53-1. Partial List of Etiologies for Acute and Chronic Diarrhea

Acute	Chronic
Food/diet, sorbitol	Food/diet
Bacteria, virus, protozoal fungus, food poisoning	HIV-induced diarrhea, chronic infections
Fecal impaction	Fecal impaction, fecal incontinence
Radiation injury	Chronic radiation-induced enteritis
Partial bowel obstruction	Post-GI tract surgical changes
Premenstrual syndrome, dysmenorrhea	Colon cancer, hormone-producing malignancies
Dihydropyrimidine dehydrogenase deficiency	Fistula
Medications	Chronic graft-versus-host disease
Acute graft-versus-host disease	Inflammatory bowel diseases (e.g., ulcerative colitis, Crohn's disease), diverticular disease, irritable bowel syndrome
	Malabsorption
	Alcoholism
	Collagen vascular diseases
	Endocrine disorders

1. History of cancer and cancer treatment
2. Current medications: Prescribed and over-the-counter
3. History of presenting symptom(s): Precipitating factors, onset, duration, and frequency. Associated symptoms are abdominal pain, fever, weight loss, stool incontinence, and cramps.
4. Changes in activities of daily living
5. History of bowel habits
   a) Liquid versus formed stool
   b) Color, odor, presence of undigested food or fat
   c) Presence of blood or mucus
6. Diet history: Food intolerance, aversions, allergies
7. Social history: Recent travel abroad, exposure to farm animals or animal feces, or consumption of well water, unpasteurized milk or its products, or raw seafood
8. Past medical history: Bowel disease, bowel surgery
C. Signs and symptoms
   1. Cramping
   2. Abdominal pain
   3. Rectal urgency, tenesmus
   4. Fever combined with dizziness, bloody diarrhea, or abdominal pain suggests severe infection.
   5. Dry mucous membranes
   6. Loose, watery, frequent stools

D. Physical exam
   1. Vital signs
      a) Orthostatic BP and pulse: To assess hydration status
      b) Weight
      c) Temperature: To assess for signs of infection or inflammation
   2. Integument exam: Poor skin turgor, dry mucous membranes, indicating dehydration
   3. Abdominal exam
      a) Tenderness, suggesting inflammation
      b) Organomegaly
      c) Distention, indicating flatus
      d) Hyperactive or hypoactive bowel sounds
      e) Tympany, indicating flatus
      f) Guarding, indicating infection or peritoneum irritation
      g) Rebound tenderness, indicating inflammation
   4. Rectal exam
      a) Assess for impaction, if suspected
      b) Irritated perirectal or peristomal skin
      c) Occult blood in stool
      d) Sphincter tone
      e) Tenderness

IV. Diagnostic tests
   A. Laboratory
      1. CBC: Increased WBC count present with infection
      2. BUN/creatinine ratio: Increased ratio present with dehydration
      3. Serum electrolytes: Decreased potassium and magnesium and increased or
         decreased sodium present with diarrhea
      4. Consider measuring dihydropyrimidine dehydrogenase deficiency (DPD) enzyme
         level if patient is receiving 5-fluorouracil (5-FU) and diarrhea occurs with acute onset
         (i.e., 24–48 hours after initiating chemotherapy). DPD tests are not routinely
         available at most cancer centers.
      5. Consider obtaining blood cultures if patient is febrile.
      6. Stool specimens
         a) *Clostridium difficile (C. difficile)* toxin stool specimen: If patient has postantibiotic
            diarrhea or has been exposed to another person with *C. difficile*
         b) Spot stool sample: For WBCs, ova and parasites, fat, and occult blood
         c) Stool culture and sensitivity: If infection other than *C. difficile* is suspected
            (1) Used to isolate diarrhea of unknown cause; often not positive and is
                expensive
            (2) May be used if patient is febrile or has bloody diarrhea, abdominal pain, or
                dizziness
         d) Stool for fecal fat: For chronic diarrhea; presence of fat suggests malabsorption
            or pancreatic insufficiency. A 48–72-hour stool collection can be measured for
            fat content; patient must be on a diet including 50–150 g of fat daily for three
            days.

    e) For chronic diarrhea, send 48–72-hour stool collection for quantitative analysis of volume to evaluate for malabsorption or pancreatic insufficiency.

    f) Blood and mucus visible in stool from exudative diarrhea

B. Radiology

1. Plain abdominal film and obstruction series if partial bowel obstruction is suspected: Dilated bowel loops or U-shaped bowel loops will be demonstrated in the presence of obstruction.

2. Barium studies: For chronic diarrhea, used to evaluate causes from colon abnormalities (e.g., tumors, colitis). First administer barium enema (BE), then upper GI series with small bowel follow-through if BE does not reveal cause. Note: Always administer BE first if both BE and upper GI are needed because barium from an upper GI obscures colon for several days, making a BE impossible.

C. Other

1. Volume of stool: Measure to assess fluid and protein loss.

2. Sigmoidoscopy/colonoscopy: Useful if antibiotic-induced pseudomembranous colitis is suspected; for chronic diarrhea, to take biopsies and cultures.

3. Upper endoscopy: To take biopsies and cultures for chronic diarrhea.

V. Differential diagnosis

A. Diet-induced

1. Fat substitute used in high-fat foods (e.g., olestra)

2. Enteral tube feedings: Initiation or change in formula or rate of infusion

3. Lactose intolerance

4. Food allergy

B. Infection

1. Bacteria: *C. difficile*, food poisoning

2. Protozoa

3. Parasites

4. Viruses, including HIV/AIDS, viral gastroenteritis

C. Drug-induced

1. Antibiotics

2. Chemotherapy: 5-FU, irinotecan, interleukin-2

3. Laxatives

4. Diuretics

5. Antihypertensives

6. Antiemetics and prokinetic agents: Metoclopramide, cisapride, 5-HT$_3$ antagonists)

7. H$_2$ blockers: Cimetidine, famotidine, ranitidine, nizatidine

8. Sorbitol-based liquid medications (e.g., Kayexalate®, Sanofi Pharmaceuticals, New York, NY)

9. Erythropoietin

10. Magnesium-based antacids

11. NSAIDs: Ibuprofen, oxaprozin

12. Caffeine, alcohol

D. Pelvic radiation therapy

E. Surgery that interrupts or alters intestinal continuity or function

    1. Small or large bowel resection
    2. Ileostomy, colostomy, ileoanal anastomosis
    3. Billroth I or II, gastrectomy
    4. Pancreatectomy
    5. Biliary surgery
    6. Vagotomy
    7. Cholecystectomy
F. Diseases of bowel
    1. Malignancies that produce hormones: VIPomas, carcinoid
    2. Inflammatory bowel diseases: Crohn's disease, ulcerative colitis
    3. Irritable bowel syndrome (see Chapter 71)
    4. Partial bowel obstruction (see Chapter 63)
    5. Diverticulosis
    6. Enterocoelic fistula
    7. Villous adenoma
    8. Diabetes mellitus and other endocrine diseases (see Chapter 143)
    9. Collagen vascular diseases
   10. Malabsorption: Fatty acid, bile salt, carbohydrate
   11. Sprue
   12. Hyperthyroidism (see Chapter 149), hypoparathyroidism
G. Psychiatric disorders: Anxiety, nervousness, narcotic withdrawal in addicts
H. Fecal impaction with continuous oozing of liquid stool
I. Graft-versus-host disease

VI. Treatment
A. Severe, profuse, watery diarrhea is a life-threatening emergency requiring hospitalization for hydration and electrolyte replacement.
B. Diet
    1. Alterations in diet used alone may insufficiently control cancer treatment-induced diarrhea.
    2. Eliminate offending food item(s).
    3. Use fiber-based formula tube feeding. Change rate of infusion of tube feeding, concentration, or type of formula.
    4. Initiate BRATT diet (i.e., bananas, rice, applesauce, white toast, decaffeinated tea) for maximum of one week.
    5. Recommend low-residue diet (i.e., small, frequent bland foods high in potassium, three liters of fluid/day).
    6. Suggest isotonic oral diet supplements (e.g., Isocal®, Mead Johnson & Co., Evansville, IN) with added flavoring. Avoid hypertonic supplements and high-glucose foods, which increase diarrhea.
C. Infection
    1. Enteric precautions
    2. For positive *C. difficile* toxin, start appropriate antibiotic therapy and stop causative agent, or replace with other antibiotic if treatment still required.
      a) Action: Eliminate bacteria, *C. difficile*

   b) Onset: Not known
   c) Examples
      (1) Metronidazole: Preferred choice; 250 mg po tid for 7–14 days or 500 mg IV q six hours if patient cannot take po
      (2) Vancomycin: 125 mg po qid for 7–14 days (may promote vancomycin-resistant enterococcus [VRE] colonization)
      (3) Bacitracin: 25,000 units po qid for 7–14 days
   d) Comments: Do not use antidiarrheal agents for *C. difficile* diarrhea.
   3. For patients with fever and orthostatic symptoms, bloody stool, or severe abdominal pain, begin antibiotic therapy with an oral quinolone (e.g., ciprofloxacin) (see Appendix 1).
D. Replace fluid volume and electrolytes and correct acid-base derangement.
E. Secretory diarrhea
   1. Action: Somatostatin analogue inhibits serotonin, VIP, gastrin, and other hormones; onset is 30 minutes.
   2. Example: Octreotide sq 100–200 mcg q eight hours; titrate dose as needed to control diarrhea.
F. Antidiarrheal: Antiperistalsis
   1. Loperamide (Imodium®, Johnson & Johnson, New Brunswick, NJ): 4 mg po (first dose), followed by 2 mg after each loose stool, up to 16 mg/day. More aggressive dosing is required for irinotecan-induced diarrhea; 4 mg at first evidence of diarrhea and then 2 mg q two hours (4 mg q four hours during night) until diarrhea-free for 12 hours.
   2. Diphenoxylate and atropine (Lomotil®, G.D. Searle & Co., Chicago, IL): Caution: Not for use in patients with advanced liver disease because it can cause hepatic coma. Recommended dose is two tablets po qid, titrate dose as needed; stop if no response after two days.
   3. Opium tincture: Improves GI tract muscle tone; 0.3–1 ml po qid, not to exceed 6 ml/day
   4. Psyllium (Metamucil®, Procter & Gamble, Cincinnati, OH): 1 teaspoon in 2 oz water po; titrate dose up to amount required to produce formed stool.
G. Rectal skin care: Cleanse skin after each stool with a mild soap and water or aloe-based baby wipe and apply a soothing topical agent (e.g., A & D® Ointment, Schering-Plough Healthcare Products, Inc., Memphis, TN).
H. Patient education
   1. Balance fiber consumption with the amount of stool produced.
   2. Consume minimum of two to three liters of fluid per day.
   3. Implement oral electrolyte replacement with sports drinks or Pedialyte® (Abbott Laboratories, Abbott Park, IL).
   4. Eliminate diarrhea-producing foods (e.g., milk products, carbonated drinks, caffeinated drinks, gas-producing foods, spicy foods).
   5. Add soluble fiber (e.g., oatmeal, apples, bananas) to diet to absorb fluid from bowel or use absorptive pharmacotherapy cholestyramine 4 mg po tid (Questran®, Bristol-Myers Squibb Co., Princeton, NJ).

    6. Institute low-fiber diet with initiation of abdominal/pelvic radiation therapy; continue throughout treatment and for approximately two weeks after treatment is completed or until diarrhea stops.

  I. Disimpact stool if impacted and start daily laxative regimen.

  J. If patient has DPD deficiency, consider IV thymidine given at least 12 hours after last dose of 5-FU (5-FU dose must be decreased or eliminated from treatment plan).

VII. Follow-up

  A. For patients with *C. difficile*, improvement often is seen four to five days after initiating metronidazole, but may take up to 13 days.

  B. For patients treated for positive *C. difficile* toxin, repeat test after antibiotic treatment is completed.

    1. If diarrhea persists, consider retreating with metronidazole and referring patient to gastroenterologist.

    2. Relapses range up to 50%, and symptoms will return in 3–10 days after antibiotic therapy is stopped in patients in whom the bacteria has not been cleared.

  C. Diarrhea lasting longer than four weeks is classified as chronic diarrhea and requires workup to determine the etiology so effective treatment can be instituted.

VIII. Referrals

  A. Dietitian: For dietary education

  B. Gastroenterologist: For sigmoidoscopy or colonoscopy

  C. Enterostomal therapist: For patients with ostomies

  D. Social worker: To assist patients with chronic diarrhea with coping and medication expenses

  E. Internist: For hospitalization of patients with dehydration or electrolyte/acid-base imbalance

References

Bartlett, J.G. (1998). Pseudomembranous enterocolitis and antibiotic-associated colitis. In M. Feldman, B.F. Scharschmidt, & M.H. Sleisenger (Eds.), *Sleisenger & Fordtran's gastrointestinal and liver disease: Pathophysiology, management* (pp. 1633–1647). Philadelphia: Saunders.

Bisanz, A. (1997). Managing bowel elimination problems in patients with cancer. *Oncology Nursing Forum, 24,* 679–686.

Briggs, J.M., & Beazlie, L.H. (1996). Nursing management of symptoms influenced by HIV infection of the endocrine system. *Nursing Clinics of North America, 31,* 845–865.

Cerda, J.J., Drossman, D.A., & Scherl, R.J. (1996, January 15). Effective, compassionate, management of IBS. *Patient Care,* pp. 131–144.

Finek, D. (1998). Diarrhea. In M. Feldman, B.F. Scharschmidt, & M.H. Sleisenger (Eds.), *Sleisenger & Fordtran's gastrointestinal and liver disease: Pathophysiology, management* (pp. 128–152). Philadelphia: Saunders

Harris, A.G., O'Dorisio, T.M., Woltering, E.A., Anthony, L.B., Burton, F.R., Geller, R.B., Grendell, J.H., Levin, B., & Redfern, J.S. (1995). Consensus statement: Octreotide dose titration in secretory diarrhea. *Digestive Diseases and Sciences, 40,* 1464–1473.

Hogan, C.M. (1998). The nurse's role in diarrhea management. *Oncology Nursing Forum, 25,* 879–886.

Meriney, D.K. (1996). Pathophysiology and management of VIPoma: A case study. *Oncology Nursing Forum, 23,* 941–948.

Morrison, G.B., Bastian, A., Dela Rosa, T.B., Diasio, R., & Takimoto, C.H. (1997). Dihydropyrimidine dehydrogenase deficiency: A pharmacogenetic defect causing severe adverse reactions to 5-fluorouracil-based chemotherapy. *Oncology Nursing Forum, 24,* 83–88.

Reese, J.L., Means, M.E., Hanrahan, K., Clearman, B., Colwill, M., & Dawson, C. (1996). Diarrhea associated with nasogastric feedings. *Oncology Nursing Forum, 23,* 59–66.

Rutledge, D.N., & Engelking, C. (1998). Cancer-related diarrhea: Selected findings of a national survey of oncology nurse experiences. *Oncology Nursing Forum, 25,* 861–873.

Takimoto, C.H., Zhi-Hong Lu, Zhang, R., Liang, M.D., Larson, L.V., Cantilena, R., Jr., Grem, J.L., Allegra, C.J., Diasio, R.B., & Chu, E. (1996). Severe neurotoxicity following 5-fluorouracil based chemotherapy in a patient with dihydropyrimidine dehydrogenase deficiency. *Clinical Cancer Research, 2,* 477–481.

Wright, P.S., & Thomas, S.L. (1995). Constipation and diarrhea: The neglected symptoms. *Seminars in Oncology Nursing, 11,* 289–297.

54. Heartburn/Indigestion/Dyspepsia

Gail Egan Sansivero, MS, ANP, AOCN®

I. Definition
   A. Heartburn: Retrosternal burning that radiates upward
   B. Indigestion: Incomplete or imperfect digestion
   C. Dyspepsia: Vague abdominal discomfort associated with indigestion

II. Physiology/Pathophysiology
   A. Normal
      1. The lower esophageal sphincter (LES) maintains a pressure barrier between the esophagus and the stomach.
      2. The hormone gastrin, alpha-adrenergic stimulation, and the vagus nerve promote relaxation of the smooth muscle of the LES.
   B. Pathophysiology: Heartburn is the symptom produced by increased reflux at the esophago-gastric junction and decreased clearance of stomach acid by gravity or esophageal peristalsis.

III. Clinical features
   A. Etiology
      1. Pharmacologic agents that decrease LES tone
         a) Antibiotics
         b) NSAIDs
         c) Iron preparations
         d) Xanthines
         e) Beta-adrenergic antagonists
         f) Anticholinergics
         g) Calcium channel blockers
         h) Theophylline
         i) Digoxin
         j) Oral steroids
      2. Tobacco
      3. Chocolate
      4. Ethanol
      5. High-fat foods

      6. Increased abdominal pressure such as obesity, ascites
      7. Delayed gastric emptying
      8. Alteration in esophageal mucosa

  B. History
      1. History of cancer and cancer treatment
      2. Current medications: Prescribed and over-the-counter
      3. History of presenting symptom(s): Precipitating factors, onset, location, and duration. Associated symptoms are dysphagia, nausea, vomiting, pain with swallowing, and hoarseness.
      4. Changes in activities of daily living
      5. Diet history: Food intolerances, carbohydrate intolerances
      6. Past medical history: Trauma to the abdomen, throat, or esophagus; hiatal hernia, ingestion of caustic materials, ulcers, irritable bowel syndrome, gallstones
      7. Social history: Tobacco and alcohol use

  C. Signs and symptoms
      1. Retrosternal burning that radiates upward
      2. Dull substernal discomfort or ache
      3. Feelings of abdominal distention
      4. Nausea, vomiting
      5. Sensation of reflux of gastric contents
      6. Worsening symptoms with certain foods
      7. Worsening symptoms with food ingestion just prior to sleep
      8. Dyspnea
      9. Pyrosis (sour or burning taste in mouth)

  D. Physical exam
      1. Vital signs: Assess weight; unexplained weight loss could indicate malignancy.
      2. HEENT/oral cavity exam: Assess for ulcers and thrush.
      3. Abdominal exam
          a) Epigastric tenderness on light or deep palpation
          b) Normal bowel sounds
          c) Masses and organomegaly
          d) Murphy's sign (if positive), indicative of gallbladder disease (see Appendix 13)
          e) Abdominal distention
      4. Lymph node exam: Assess cervical supraclavicular lymph nodes for enlargement indicative of malignancy.
      5. Rectal exam: Test stool for occult blood.

IV. Diagnostic tests
  A. Laboratory
      1. *Helicobacter pylori* (*H. pylori*) serology: Rule out infection with *H. pylori* if a gastric or duodenal ulcer is present.
      2. 24-hour esophageal pH monitoring: Use in selected cases when dietary and behavioral modification, as well as medical therapy, have failed.
  B. Radiology: Upper GI series—include esophagram; evaluate for hiatal hernia, confirm gastroesophageal reflux.

    C. Other: Endoscopy—evaluate for esophagitis and hiatal hernia; allows direct visualization and biopsy.

V. Differential diagnosis
    A. Esophageal diseases
        1. Motility disorders (e.g., achalasia, scleroderma, diabetic neuropathy, amyloidosis)
        2. Gastroesophageal reflux disease (see Chapter 66)
        3. Esophagitis
    B. Ulcers: Esophageal, gastric, or duodenal (see Chapter 73)
    C. Gastritis (see Chapter 67)
    D. Cholelithiasis
    E. Pancreatitis (see Chapter 72)
    F. Myocardial infarction (see Chapter 47)
    G. Psychiatric disorders
        1. Anxiety disorders (see Chapter 152)
        2. Depression (see Chapter 154)

VI. Treatment
    A. Lifestyle alterations
        1. Discuss dietary modification: Eliminate foods that initiate or aggravate symptoms (e.g., chocolate, alcohol, oils, peppermint, garlic, onion, fatty foods).
        2. Eliminate alcohol intake (especially white wines).
        3. Encourage smoking cessation.
        4. Avoid eating for at least two hours before bedtime.
        5. Drink fluids after eating to clear the esophagus.
        6. Elevate the head of the bed six inches for sleeping, or use a pillow wedge.
        7. Eliminate or modify the dose of medications that reduce lower esophageal sphincter tone, if possible.
        8. Eliminate medications that irritate esophageal mucosa, if possible.
        9. Lose weight, if necessary.
    B. Pharmacologic
        1. Begin trial of over-the-counter antacids before meals and HS (see Table 54-1).
        2. Begin trial of H_2 blockers (see Table 54-1).
        3. Begin proton pump inhibitors (see Table 54-1).
        4. Institute *H. pylori* treatment if patient is seropositive (see Chapter 73).
        5. Treat infectious causes (e.g., *Candida* esophagitis, cytomegalovirus, herpes simplex).
    C. Other procedures
        1. Endoscopy with dilatation: Patients with dysphagia
        2. Antireflux surgery: Consider if symptoms incapacitating.

VII. Follow-up
    A. Short-term
        1. Patients should be re-evaluated within one month of instituting dietary modification or medications.

Table 54-1. Medications Used to Treat Heartburn

Medication	Action	Examples	Comments
Antacids	Neutralize gastric acid (raising the pH), inhibiting proteolytic activity of pepsin	• Mylanta[a], Maalox[b]: 15–30 cc po after meals and at bedtime • Sodium bicarbonate: Two tablets in six ounces of water po every four hours prn • Calcium carbonate: Two tablets po every four hours prn • Dihydroxyaluminum sodium carbonate (Rolaids[c]): One or two tablets po every hour, not to exceed 14/day • Magnesium trisilicate and sodium bicarbonate (Gaviscon[d]): Two to four tablets po after meals and at bedtime	Should be taken after meals and at bedtime. May alter absorption of some medications. May cause constipation (aluminum hydroxide) or diarrhea (magnesium hydroxide).
H₂ blockers	Reduce volume and acidity of gastric parietal cell secretions	• Cimetidine (Tagamet[e]): 200–400 mg bid–tid or 800 mg HS • Ranitidine (Zantac[f]): 150 mg bid or 300 mg po at bedtime • Famotidine (Pepcid[g]): 20 mg bid or 40 mg po at bedtime • Nizatidine (Axid[h]): 150 mg bid or 300 mg po at bedtime	In milder cases, once-a-day dosing may be adequate. Patient may have tried over-the-counter doses prior to seeking medical evaluation.
Gastric proton pump inhibitors	Suppress gastric acid production	• Omeprazole (Prilosec[i]): 20–40 mg po qd • Lansoprazole (Prevacid[j]): 15–30 mg po qd	Appropriate for patients with severe symptoms or patients unable to follow dietary modification and other drug therapy.
Dopamine receptor antagonist therapy (prokinetic drugs)	Augments gastric emptying, raises lower esophageal sphincter (LES) tone, improves peristalsis	• Metoclopramide (Reglan[k]): 5–15 mg po before meals and at bedtime • Cisapride (Propulsid[l]): 10–20 mg po 15 minutes before meals and at bedtime	May induce diarrhea. Contraindicated when stimulation of GI motility may be dangerous (i.e., in the presence of mechanical obstruction or perforation). Many drug interactions have been identified.
Cholinergic agents	Raise LES pressure, improve acid clearance by esophagus	• Bethanechol (Urecholine[m]): 5–15 mg po tid–qid	Contraindicated in patients with asthma and other conditions exacerbated by anticholinergic therapy.

[a]Johnson & Johnson-Merck Consumer Pharmaceutical Co., Ft. Washington, PA; [b]Rhone-Poulec Rorer Pharmaceuticals, Inc., Collegeville, PA; [c]Warner Lambert Co., Morris Plains, NJ; [d]SmithKline Beecham Consumer Healthcare, LP, Pittsburgh, PA; [e]SmithKline Beecham Pharmaceutical Co., Philadelphia, PA; [f]Glaxo-Wellcome, Inc., Research Triangle Park, NC; [g]Merck & Co., Inc., West Point, PA; [h]Eli Lilly and Co., Indianapolis, IN; [i]Astra Merck, Inc., Wayne, PA; [j]Tap Pharmaceuticals, Inc., Deerfield, IL; [k]A.H. Robins Company, Richmond, VA; [l]Janssen Pharmaceuticals, Inc., Titusville, NJ; [m]Merck & Co., Inc., Research Triangle Park, NC

2. Evaluation should include nutritional status, effect of modification on symptoms, and assessment of need for further diagnostic testing or intervention.

B. Long-term patients with chronic or recurrent symptoms should be followed regularly.
   1. These patients are at risk for development of severe esophagitis, strictures, and esophageal malignancy.
   2. Patients with Barrett's esophagus are at increased risk for development of esophageal adenocarcinoma. Some practitioners advise periodic endoscopy for surveillance monitoring of patients with Barrett's esophagus.

VIII. Referrals
   A. Dietitian: For assistance with dietary modification, if appropriate
   B. Gastroenterologist: For further evaluation if symptoms remain refractory after eight weeks of therapy or if endoscopy is indicated

References

Bouchier, I.A. (1996). Indigestion. In I.A. Bouchier, H. Ellis, & P.R. Fleming (Eds.), *French's index of differential diagnosis* (13th ed) (pp. 307–310). Oxford, England: Butterworth-Heinemann.

DeVault, K.R., & Castell, D.O. (1994). Current diagnosis and treatment of gastroesophageal reflux disease. *Mayo Clinic Proceedings, 69,* 867–876.

Drugs for treatment of peptic ulcers. (1997). *Medical Letter on Drugs and Therapeutics, 39*(991), 1–4.

Horwitz, B.J., & Fisher, R.S. (1995). Intervening in GERD: The phases of management. *Hospital Practice, 30*(9), 43–52.

Kahrilas, P.J. (1996). Gastroesophageal reflux disease. *JAMA, 276,* 983–988.

Middlemiss, C. (1997). Gastroesophageal reflux disease: A common condition in the elderly. *Nurse Practitioner, 22*(11), 51–59.

Richter, J.M. (1995). Approach to the patient with heartburn and reflux. In A.H. Goroll, L.A. May, & A.G. Mulley (Eds.), *Primary care medicine: Office evaluation and management of the adult patient* (3rd ed.) (pp. 344–347). Philadelphia: Lippincott.

Robinson, M. (1995). Prokinetic therapy for gastroesophageal reflux disease. *American Family Physician, 52,* 957–962.

Rodriguez, S., Miner, P., Robinson, M., Greenwood, B., Maton, P.N., & Pappa, K. (1998). Meal type affects heartburn severity. *Digestive Diseases and Sciences, 43,* 485–490.

Sullivan, C.A., & Samuelson, W.M. (1996). Gastroesophageal reflux: A common exacerbating factor in adult asthma. *Nurse Practitioner, 21*(11), 82–96.

Wright, R.A., Sagatellan, M.A., Simons, M.E., McClave, S.A., & Roy, T.M. (1996). Exercise-induced asthma: Is gastroesophageal reflux a factor? *Digestive Diseases and Sciences, 41,* 921–925.

55. Hematemesis

Jeanne Held-Warmkessel, MSN, RN, CS, AOCN®

I. Definition: Vomiting blood from stomach, duodenum, or proximal jejunum

II. Pathophysiology
   A. Bleeding from the GI mucosa from irritation, ulceration, or trauma results in stimulation to the GI pathways, initiating emesis.
   B. Bleeding source is above the ligament of Treitz in the upper GI tract; the bleeding source is rarely more distal.

III. Clinical features: Overt bleeding is potentially a life-threatening emergency. Bleeding may be described as coffee-ground emesis (signifying contact with gastric secretions) or bright-red. Occult blood in the emesis may not be readily apparent and can be identified only by testing. In many cases, the bleeding stops spontaneously.
   A. History
      1. History of cancer and cancer treatment
      2. Current medications: Prescribed and over-the-counter
      3. History of presenting symptom(s): Precipitating factors, onset, and duration. Associated symptoms are change in bowel habits, nose bleeds, and mouth bleeds.
      4. Changes in activities of daily living
      5. Social history: Alcohol and tobacco use
      6. Past medical history: Pancreatic disease, renal disease, ulcer, liver disease
   B. Signs and symptoms
      1. Retching and nausea
      2. Vomiting: Blood may or may not be visible.
      3. Pallor
      4. Decreased level of consciousness
      5. Dizziness
      6. Weakness
      7. Abdominal pain
   C. Physical exam
      1. Vital signs: Check for hypotension, tachycardia, and other signs of hypovolemia or shock.
         a) Loss of < 500 ml blood: Few signs occur except in patients with preexisting anemia and in the elderly.

        b) Loss of 1,000 ml blood (20% of blood volume): Tachycardia and/or orthostatic hypotension (fall of 10 mm Hg) alone or with lightheadedness, nausea, thirst, and diaphoresis may be present.

        c) Loss of 1,500 ml blood (30% of blood volume): Orthostatic hypotension develops, and previously listed signs and symptoms are present.

        d) Loss of 2,500 ml blood (40% of blood volume): Supine hypotension, pallor, and cool skin are present.

        e) Assess for weight loss.

  2. HEENT exam

        a) Oral cavity: Assess for dry mucous membranes, indicating poor hydration status, and for bleeding.

        b) Tooth enamel: Assess for acid damage caused by decalcification from gastric acid.

        c) Nose: Assess for bleeding.

  3. Integument exam: Assess for pallor, temperature, petechiae, ecchymosis, telangiectasis, jaundice, and spider angioma, indicating bleeding.

  4. Lymph node exam: Assess regional lymph nodes for enlargement (e.g., left supraclavicular enlargement [Virchow's node]), suggestive of intra-abdominal malignancy.

  5. Abdominal exam: Assess for ascites, pain (epigastric with peptic ulcer disease [PUD]), masses, tenderness, and distention.

        a) Assess for hyperactive bowel sounds.

        b) Assess for rigidity and guarding, indicating possibility of peritonitis.

  6. Rectal exam: Test stool for occult blood.

IV. Diagnostic tests

  A. Laboratory

    1. CBC: Evaluate for anemia—low hemoglobin and hematocrit

        a) MCV: Low with chronic blood loss

        b) Low platelet count: Indicates thrombocytopenia, which may contribute to bleeding

        c) Hemoglobin and hematocrit: May not reflect extent of acute blood loss

    2. Prothrombin time/partial thromboplastin time: To assess for bleeding disorders or prolonged clotting time

    3. Type and cross match: If transfusion considered

    4. BUN: May be increased from hypovolemia and blood degradation from upper GI tract

    5. Liver function tests: Abnormal values present with liver disorders, which may promote upper GI bleeding.

  B. Radiology: Indicated with active bleeding when source has not been found during esophagogastroduodenoscopy (EGD)

  C. Other

    1. Nasogastric tube: Insert and aspirate for gross blood; occult blood tests can be compromised by mucosal-induced bleeding from tube placement.

    2. EGD: To evaluate for bleeding source and to obtain biopsies of abnormal areas or suspected malignancy; EGD is preferred over barium study of upper GI tract, as barium may interfere with usefulness of other tests.

    3. Emesis: Visually inspect for blood, food, liquids, drugs, or other contents and test for occult blood.

   4. Selective arteriography: May be diagnostic and/or therapeutic
   5. Technetium-99 scan: May be useful
   6. Assess for oxygen saturation.

V. Differential diagnosis
   A. Esophageal
      1. Esophageal rupture
      2. Esophageal varices
      3. GERD (see Chapter 66)
   B. Gastric
      1. PUD (see Chapter 73)
      2. Mucosal erosion
      3. Gastritis (see Chapter 67)
      4. Gastric varices
      5. Hiatal hernia
      6. Dieulafoy's lesion: Large artery in GI tract mucosa that erodes through mucosa and bleeds
      7. Mallory-Weiss tear at esophageal gastric junction
   C. Duodenal
      1. Erosive duodenitis
      2. Duodenal ulcers
   D. Cancer
      1. Esophageal: Squamous or adenocarcinoma
      2. Gastric: Adenocarcinoma, lymphoma
   E. Connective tissue diseases that cause bleeding disorders (e.g., pseudoxanthoma elasticum)
   F. Fistulas between large blood vessels and GI tract (e.g., aorta-duodenal fistula)
   G. Arteriovenous malformations (AVMs), angiodysplasia (dilated arteriole-venule-capillary network complex)
   H. Bleeding secondary to lung etiology
   I. Trauma or surgery of nose or mouth

VI. Treatment: May require emergency management depending on patient's vital signs and hemodynamic stability. Transfer unstable patients to hospital/emergency room by ambulance, then to intensive care unit, if necessary.
   A. Insert two large-gauge IV cannulas, and rapidly replace lost fluid volume with isotonic (normal saline [NS]) fluids, intake and output, frequent vital signs.
   B. Replace/correct anemia with RBC transfusions; maintain hematocrit around 30%, particularly for active bleeding.
   C. Supplemental oxygen if pulse oximetry is < 90%.
   D. Correct bleeding abnormalities; transfuse appropriate blood products.
      1. Vitamin K: 2.5–10 mg po, sq, or IM may be repeated to correct warfarin (Coumadin®, Dupont Pharma, Wilmington, DE) overanticoagulation or vitamin K deficiency.
      2. Transfuse fresh frozen plasma: To replace all clotting factors
      3. Transfuse platelets: If < 20,000
      4. Other clotting factors (e.g., factor VIII): As needed

    E. Patient should be npo.

    F. Insert nasogaotric (NG) tube for assessment of gastric contents and for irrigation.

       1. Connect NG tube to low intermittent suction; consider room-temperature tap water lavage to remove blood.

       2. Flush as needed to keep tube patent and assess blood loss.

    G. Insert indwelling urinary catheter to monitor renal function and monitor patient for oliguria, which often is present with hypovolemia.

    H. Recommend bed rest; elevate head of bed to 30°–45° to reduce risk of aspiration.

    I. Place airway-suction equipment at bedside in case of aspiration.

    J. Upper endoscopy performed after initial stabilization to treat bleeding thermally (e.g., laser cautery or heater probe) or injection of saline and epinephrine; thermal treatment and injection often are used in combination.

    K. Start IV H_2-receptor blockers (e.g., famotidine 20 mg IV q 12 hours); convert to po when patient takes oral fluids and medications or an oral proton pump inhibitor (e.g., omeprazole, lansoprazole) to reduce gastric acid production.

    L. Implement arteriography with vasopressin infusion or embolization if EGD is unsuccessful in managing or locating source of bleeding.

    M. Eliminate drug causes.

    N. Administer oral iron supplements after patient is stable.

VII. Follow-up: Monitor for further bleeding episodes and relapse of identified etiology.

VIII. Referrals

    A. Gastroenterologist: To perform EGD and control bleeding

    B. Medical internist: For hospital admission

    C. Surgeon: For surgery to correct bleeding etiology if other measures fail or are not appropriate

References

Eastwood, G.L. (1998). Gastrointestinal bleeding. In J.H. Stein (Ed.), *Internal medicine* (pp. 2008–2014). St. Louis: Mosby.

Fisher, R.L., Pipkin, G.A., & Wood, J.R. (1995). Stress-related mucosal disease: Pathophysiology, prevention and treatment. *Critical Care Clinics, 11,* 323–345.

Fred, H.L., & Hariharan, R. (1995). Hematemesis in a woman with skin, eye, and heart abnormalities. *Hospital Practice, 30*(9), 28R, 28U.

Kankaria, A.G., & Fleischer, D.E. (1995). The critical care management of nonvariceal upper gastrointestinal bleeding. *Critical Care Clinics, 11,* 347–368.

Labovich, T.M. (1994). Selected complications in patients with cancer: Spinal cord compression, malignant bowel obstruction, malignant ascites and gastrointestinal bleeding. *Seminars in Oncology Nursing, 10,* 189–197.

Longstreth, G.F. (1995). Epidemiology of hospitalization for acute upper gastrointestinal hemorrhage: A population-based study. *American Journal of Gastroenterology, 90,* 206–210.

Shapiro, M.J. (1994). The role of the radiologist in the management of gastrointestinal bleeding. *Gastroenterology Clinics of North America, 23,* 123–181.

Chapter

56. Hepatomegaly

Dawn Camp-Sorrell, RN, MSN, FNP, AOCN®

I. Definition: Enlargement of the liver

II. Physiology/Pathophysiology
   A. Normal
      1. The liver span is approximately 6–12 cm, and it lies in the right upper quadrant of the abdomen, just below the diaphragm.
      2. Inferior surface lies close to the gallbladder, stomach, duodenum, and hepatic flexure of the colon.
      3. Each lobule is made up of liver cells (hepatocytes) radiating around a central vein from branches of the portal vein, hepatic artery, and bile duct.
      4. Bile is secreted by the hepatocytes into bile canaliculi then to the hepatic duct, which joins the cystic duct from the gallbladder to form the common bile duct. This duct empties through the ampulla of Vater, which empties into the duodenum.
      5. The liver is a highly vascularized organ.
         a) The hepatic artery transports blood to the liver directly from the aorta, and the portal vein carries blood from the digestive tract and spleen to the liver.
         b) Three hepatic veins carry blood from the liver and empty into the inferior vena cava.
      6. Functions of the liver
         a) Metabolizes carbohydrates, fats, and proteins
         b) Converts glucose and stores it as glycogen; when stimulated, reconverts glycogen to glucose for secretion
         c) Uses cholesterol to form bile salts
         d) Metabolizes proteins to amino acids and converts their waste products to urea for excretion
         e) Stores several vitamins and iron
         f) Detoxifies potentially harmful substances
         g) Produces prothrombin, fibrinogen, and other substances for blood coagulation
         h) Conjugates and excretes steroid hormones
   B. Pathophysiology
      1. Hepatomegaly can result from destruction of the liver parenchyma, resulting in scarring and fat formation.

2. In diabetes mellitus, hepatocellular glycogen accumulation can occur.
    a) During periods of hyperglycemia, glucose freely enters the hepatocytes, stimulating glycogen synthesis.
    b) Accumulation of excessive amounts of glycogen in the hepatocytes is a function of intermittent episodes of hyperglycemia and hypoglycemia and the use of excessive insulin.

III. Clinical features
  A. Etiology
    1. Destruction of the liver by toxins, viruses, or bacteria
    2. Tumor involvement, primary or metastatic
    3. Alterations in hepatic venous outflow (i.e., from CHF, Budd-Chiari syndrome)
    4. Extra medullary hematopoiesis
  B. History
    1. History of cancer and cancer treatment
    2. Current medications: Prescribed and over-the-counter (e.g., acetaminophen, oral contraceptives, androgenic steroids)
    3. History of presenting symptoms(s): Precipitating factors, onset, location, and duration. Associated symptoms are abdominal pain, fatigue, jaundice, color changes of stool or urine, and somnolence.
    4. Changes in activities of daily living
    5. Social history: Alcohol intake, illicit drug use
    6. Past medical history: Liver disease, hepatitis, cirrhosis
    7. Family history: Liver disease
  C. Signs and symptoms
    1. Jaundice
    2. Confusion (end stage)
    3. Right upper quadrant pain and fullness
    4. Nausea and vomiting
    5. Malaise
    6. Fatigue, somnolence
    7. Ascites
    8. Light-colored stools
    9. Dark urine
    10. Anorexia
    11. Weight loss
    12. Pruritus
  D. Physical exam
    1. Integument exam
        a) Inspect the palmar surfaces for erythema, suggesting chronic hepatitis.
        b) Assess for signs of excoriation.
        c) Spider angioma can be seen on the head, neck, chest, arms, and upper abdomen almost exclusively in the drainage of the superior vena cava, suggesting chronic hepatitis.
    2. HEENT/eye exam: Assess for icteric sclerae.

3. Cardiac exam: Auscultate the heart for murmurs, extra heart sounds, or rubs that suggest CHF or tricuspid regurgitation.
4. Abdominal exam
  a) Auscultate for bruit, venous hum, or hepatic rub.
    (1) Friction rubs are high-pitched and heard in association with respiration.
    (2) Venous hum is soft, low-pitched, and continuous, which occurs with increased collateral circulation between portal and systemic venous systems.
    (3) Scratch test is useful when the abdomen is distended (see Appendix 13).
  b) Palpate the liver for contour and texture. Left lobe may be palpable in epigastrium.
    (1) Focal enlargement or rock-like consistency suggests tumor.
    (2) Tenderness suggests inflammation.
    (3) Rapid enlargement suggests heart failure.
    (4) Firm and nodular suggests cirrhosis; nodules often are difficult to palpate.
    (5) Scarred cirrhotic liver may be small and not palpable.
  c) Percuss the liver margins to ascertain the size; normal vertical span is 6–12 cm, normal midsternal span is 4–8 cm.
    (1) Normally, dullness is heard at the right costal margin or slightly below it.
    (2) Lower liver border that is more than 2–3 cm below the right costal margin suggests enlargement or downward displacement of the diaphragm secondary to pulmonary disease.
    (3) Upper liver border usually begins at the fifth to seventh intercostal space.
      (a) Upper border below this may indicate downward displacement or liver atrophy.
      (b) Dullness extending above suggests upward displacement from ascites or masses.
  d) Assess wave fluid for ascites.

IV. Diagnostic tests: Tests are nonspecific in end-stage cirrhosis and may be normal even in extensive metastatic disease.
  A. Laboratory
    1. LFTs: Enzymes may be elevated or normal.
      a) Serum glutamic-oxaloacetic transaminase (SGOT) or aspartate aminotransferase (AST): Increased or normal
      b) Alkaline phosphatase: Increased or normal
    2. Serum albumin: Usually decreased
    3. Globulin levels: Often increased
    4. Bilirubin values: Usually elevated in obstructed diseases, acute and chronic hepatitis, end-stage liver disease, and drug toxicity
    5. Carcinoembryonic antigen (CEA) value or alpha-fetoprotein levels: If hepatic metastasis or primary hepatic carcinoma is suspected (see Appendix 16)
  B. Radiology
    1. Ultrasound: Best technique to assess the liver size
    2. CT scan: To evaluate the liver size, masses, and extrahepatic disease
  C. Other: Biopsy of the liver may be necessary to confirm diagnosis

V. Differential diagnosis
  A. Pulmonary etiology
    1. Lung hyperinflation
    2. Chronic obstructive pulmonary disease (see Chapter 28)
  B. Vascular congestion
    1. CHF (see Chapter 40)
    2. Tricuspid valve regurgitation
    3. Budd-Chiari syndrome
  C. Inflammatory disorders
    1. Hepatitis (see Chapter 69)
    2. Hepatotoxicity (see Chapter 70)
    3. Cirrhosis (see Chapter 64)
  D. Malignancy
    1. Hepatocellular carcinoma
    2. Metastatic cancer
  E. Infiltrative disorders
    1. Diabetes mellitus (see Chapter 143)
    2. Extramedullary hematopoiesis
    3. Amyloidosis
    4. Infection (e.g., TB [see Chapter 34], sarcoidosis, cytomegalovirus [CMV])
  F. Other
    1. Polycythemia vera (see Chapter 122)
    2. Alcoholism
    3. Hemolytic uremic syndrome
    4. Vitamin A toxicity
    5. HIV (see Chapter 156)
    6. Thalassemia
    7. Cysts, adenomas

VI. Treatment: Depends on underlying cause
  A. Avoid hepatotoxic medications.
  B. Place on a low-protein diet if in liver failure.
  C. May need a low-sodium diet if ascites is present.

VII. Follow-up: Depends on underlying cause

VIII. Referrals: Depend on underlying cause
  A. Infectious disease consult: To develop treatment plan for infections
  B. Oncologist: For evaluation and treatment of cancer
  C. Surgeon or interventional radiologist: For liver biopsy

References

Chatila, R., & West, A.B. (1996). Hepatomegaly and abnormal liver tests due to glycogenosis in adults with diabetes. *Medicine, 75,* 327–333.

Mainenti, P.P., Petrelli, B., Lamanda, R., Amalfi, G., & Castigione, F. (1997). Primary systemic amyloidosis with giant hepatomegaly and a swiftly progressive course. *Journal of Clinical Gastroenterology, 24,* 173–175.

Rose, A.A., Iseri, O., Fishbein, G., & Knodell, R.G. (1991). Nodular regenerative hyperplasia. A cause of ascites and hepatomegaly after chemotherapy for leukemia. *American Journal of Gastroenterology, 86,* 86–88.

Tucher, W.N., Saab., S., Rickman, L.S., & Mathews, W.C. (1997). The scratch test is unreliable for detecting the liver edge. *Journal of Clinical Gastroenterology, 25,* 410–414.

Zoli, M., Magalotti, D., Grimaldi, M., Gueli, C., Marchesini, G., & Pisi, E. (1995). Physical examination of the liver: Is it still worth it? *American Journal of Gastroenterology, 90,* 1428–1432.

Chapter

57. Jaundice

Cindy Jo Horrell, MS, CRNP, AOCN®

I. Definition: Condition in which the skin, sclerae, and mucous membranes acquire a yellowish discoloration

II. Physiology/Pathophysiology
   A. Normal: Bilirubin is the end product of heme degradation, with 70%–80% coming from hemoglobin.
      1. The remaining 20%–30% comes from breakdown of nonhemoglobin hemoproteins in the liver (e.g., catalase, cytochrome oxidase).
      2. Unconjugated bilirubin (water-insoluble) is transported in plasma tightly bound to albumin.
      3. Elimination of bilirubin requires conversion to water-soluble conjugates by the liver and secretion into bile.
      4. Bilirubin is deconjugated by bacterial enzymes in the terminal ileum and colon, converted to urobilinogen and other porphyrins, and excreted mostly in stool (minimally in urine).
   B. Pathophysiology: Jaundice occurs as a result of elevated concentrations of serum bilirubin.
      1. Serum bilirubin levels must reach 2–2.5 mg/100 ml for jaundice to occur.
      2. Bilirubin is readily bound to elastic tissue, which accounts for skin, ocular sclerae, and blood vessel color changes.

III. Clinical features (see Table 57-1)
   A. Risk factors
      1. Blood transfusions
      2. IV drug abuse
      3. Tuberculin testing
      4. Dental treatment
      5. Tattooing
      6. Sexual practices
   B. Etiology (see Table 57-1)
      1. Excess bilirubin production
      2. Decreased hepatic uptake of bilirubin

Table 57-1. Clinical Features of Jaundice

Etiology	Onset	Signs/Symptoms	Laboratory	Physical Findings
Excess bilirubin production	Usually sudden	Pale yellow skin Dark stool	Increase reticulocyte count Increase indirect bilirubin Increase urine urobilinogen Decrease HGB/HCT (hemolysis)	Splenomegaly
Impaired bilirubin uptake in the liver	Episodic, self-limiting	Mild jaundice	Increase indirect bilirubin	None
Impaired bilirubin conjugation	Neonatal type: First week of life, transient Hereditary type	Jaundice Intermittent jaundice	Increase indirect bilirubin	Kernicterus
Intrahepatic cholestasis	Gradual	Anorexia, malaise, myalgias; mild to deep orange-yellow skin; dark urine; pale stool	Increase alkaline phosphatase Increase direct/indirect bilirubin Increase urine bilirubin Increase prothrombin time Increase AST, SGOT	Ascites, abdominal veins, spider angioma, ecchymosis, hepatosplenomegaly, encephalopathy
Extrahepatic obstruction	Gradual	Jaundice; persistent pruritis; mild to deep yellow-green skin; dark urine; clay-colored stool; fever; pain	Increase alkaline phosphatase Increase direct/indirect bilirubin Increase urine bilirubin If prothrombin time is increased, will normalize with vitamin K administration Increase transaminase	Abdominal tenderness may be present Palpable abdominal mass

      3. Impaired bilirubin conjugation

      4. Intrahepatic cholestasis

      5. Extrahepatic obstruction

      6. Hepatocellular injury

  C. History

      1. History of cancer and cancer treatment

      2. Current medications: Prescribed and over-the-counter

      3. History of presenting symptom(s): Precipitating factors, onset, location, and duration. Associated symptoms are anorexia, dyspepsia, morning nausea, diarrhea, low-grade fever, pruritus, weight loss, and pain in right upper abdominal quadrant.

      4. Changes in activities of daily living

      5. History of recent contact with a person with jaundice or viral hepatitis, recent foreign travel, recent consumption of raw shellfish or oysters

      6. Family history: Liver disease or anemia

      7. Social history: Alcohol intake, illicit drug use

      9. Past medical history: Blood or plasma transfusions, fat intolerance, biliary colic, surgical procedures

  D. Signs and symptoms (see Table 57-1)

  E. Physical exam (see Table 57-1)

      1. Vital signs: Assess for weight loss.

      2. Integument exam

        a) Bruising: May indicate clotting defect

        b) Purpuric spots on forearms, axillae, or shins; vascular spiders; palmar erythema: May indicate cirrhosis

        c) Ecchymoses: May indicate obstructive or hepatocellular disease

        d) Scratch marks (from itching); melanin pigmentation; finger clubbing; xanthomas on eyelids, extensor surfaces, and palmar creases; and hyperkeratosis in chronic cholestasis

      3. Abdominal exam

        a) Dilated periumbilical veins: Indicate portal collateral circulation and cirrhosis

        b) Ascites: Indicates cirrhosis or metastatic disease

        c) Hepatomegaly: Indicates liver disease

        d) Splenomegaly: Indicates cirrhosis

        e) Palpable gallbladder: May indicate obstruction of common bile duct; usually malignant

IV. Diagnostic tests

  A. Laboratory (see Table 57-1)

      1. Initial test

        a) CBC and reticulocyte: Initial test to evaluate for hemolysis

        b) Bilirubin: Increase in direct and indirect indicates liver disease severity.

        c) Transaminase (AST, SGOT): Increase indicates hepatocellular disease.

        d) Alkaline phosphatase, SGPT: Levels three times the normal indicate obstruction (intrahepatic and extrahepatic) and prolonged cholestasis; more sensitive in liver injury than SGOT.

    e) Albumin: Decreased indicates hepatocellular disease.
   2. Secondary tests
    a) Urine: Bilirubin provides a measure of bilirubin excretion; increased values indicate cholestasis, obstruction, or hepatocellular injury.
    b) Prothrombin time: Prolonged suggests cholestasis and obstruction; if not reversible with vitamin K administration, suggests hepatocellular disease.
    c) Hepatitis A and B titers: To assess for hepatitis virus
  B. Radiology
   1. Abdominal ultrasound: Determines size of extrahepatic biliary trees; reveals intra- or extrahepatic lesions and/or gallstones (may not be useful in obese patients or patients with overlying bowel gas)
   2. CT scan of abdomen: To assess liver size, structure, and associated abnormalities (e.g., tumor)
   3. Percutaneous transhepatic cholangiography: Indicated when ultrasound and CT scan are positive to evaluate obstruction

 V. Differential diagnosis
  A. Conditions that increase bilirubin formation
   1. Hemolysis: Hemolytic anemia
   2. Ineffective erythropoiesis (rare): Megaloblastic anemia (rare)
  B. Conditions in which hepatic clearance is decreased
   1. Hereditary disorders of bilirubin metabolism (e.g., Gilbert's syndrome)
   2. Drug-induced (e.g., rifampin)
  C. Liver disease
   1. Acute or chronic dysfunction
    a) Viral hepatitis (see Chapter 69)
    b) Wilson's disease (rare), hemachromatosis, hepatotoxin (e.g., alcohol, medications, poison)
   2. Diffuse infiltrative disorders (e.g., sarcoidosis, lymphoma, amyloidosis)
   3. Inflammation of intrahepatic bile ducts and/or portal tracts
    a) Graft-versus-host disease
    b) Primary biliary cirrhosis
   4. Malignancy
    a) Metastatic cancer
    b) Primary liver cancer (hepatoma)
    c) Pancreatic cancer
    d) Ampullary cancer
    e) Cholangiosarcoma
    f) Gallbladder carcinoma
  D. Obstruction of bile ducts
   1. Gallstones
   2. Inflammation/infection (e.g., AIDS, hepatic arterial chemotherapy, postoperative strictures, primary sclerosing cholangitis)
   3. Extrinsic compression of biliary tree (e.g., pancreatitis [see Chapter 72], cancer)

VI. Treatment
    A. Obstructed bile ducts: Mechanical relief of obstruction via surgery
        1. Removal of obstruction
        2. Stent placement
        3. Internal or external drain placement
    B. Cholestatic liver disease
        1. Cessation of alcohol
        2. Discontinuation of offending drug
    C. Management of pruritus
        1. Antihistamines: Rarely provide significant relief apart from drowsiness
            a) Diphenhydramine: 25–50 mg po qid
            b) Hydroxyzine: 25 mg po tid
        2. Cholestyramine: 4–6 g po 30 minutes before meals (absorbs bile acids). Adverse effects include fat malabsorption, decreased absorption of other medications, constipation
        3. Emollients, mild fragrance-free soaps, less frequent bathing, light clothing, short fingernails

VII. Follow-up: Depends on etiology and stage of disease

VIII. Referrals
    A. Gastroenterologist: For endoscopic retrograde cholangiopancreatography (ERCP)
    B. Hematologist: For hemolytic anemia
    C. Surgeon: For gallstones and other surgically amenable conditions

References

Cohen, S.A., & Siegel, J.H. (1995). Biliary tract emergencies. *Critical Care Clinics, 11,* 279–285.

Fred, H.L., Hariharan, R., Doucet, J., & Mehta, N. (1996). Jaundice and extreme hypercholesterolemia after a stroke. *Hospital Practice, 31*(9), 33–37.

Lidofsky, S., & Scharschmidt, B.F. (1997). Jaundice. In M. Feldman, B.F. Scharschmidt, & M.H. Sleisinger (Eds.), *Gastrointestinal and liver disease: Pathophysiology/diagnosis/management* (6th ed.) (pp. 220–231). Philadelphia: Saunders.

Mankarious, R., Zaafran, S., McDonald, G., & Moody, F. (1995). Jaundice and massive abdominal lymphadenopathy. *Hospital Practice, 30*(6), 31–32.

Sherlock, S., & Dooley, J. (1996). *Diseases of the liver and biliary system* (10th ed.) (pp. 201–241). England: Blackwell.

Stewart, J.A., Gunn, M.C., Rathbone, B.J., & Robertson, G.S. (1997). Shortness of breath and jaundice. *Postgraduate Medical Journal, 73,* 759–760.

Chapter

58. Melena

Jeanne Held-Warmkessel, MSN, RN, CS, AOCN®

I. Definition: Foul-smelling, black, tarry stool associated with an upper GI source

II. Pathophysiology
  A. Blood is lost proximal to the ileocecal valve where hemoglobin is converted into hematin, which gives it a tarry appearance.
  B. Blood usually originates from the upper GI tract above the ligament of Treitz and is degraded as it passes through the small and large bowel.
  C. Right colonic bleeding may cause melena when transit is slow.

III. Clinical features (see Table 58-1)
  A. History
    1. History of cancer and cancer treatment
    2. Current medications: Prescribed and over-the-counter
    3. History of presenting symptom(s): Precipitating factors, onset, and duration. Associated symptoms are black tarry stools, bleeding, abdominal pain, back pain, vomiting, retching, dysphagia, indigestion, altered bowel habits, and weight loss
    4. Changes in activities of daily living
    5. Past medical history: Ulcers, abdominal surgery
    6. Social history: Alcohol intake
    7. Family history: Bowel disorders (e.g., Crohn's disease, colitis, polyps)
  B. Signs and symptoms (secondary)
    1. Black, tarry stool

Table 58-1. Clinical Features of Upper Gastrointestinal Bleed

Blood Loss	Clinical Manifestation
60–200 ml	Black, tarry stools (larger volumes may cause maroon stools)
< 500 ml	No associated hemodynamic instability
> 500 ml	Signs of hemodynamic instability
> 20% blood loss	Orthostatic blood pressure falls >10 mm Hg or pulse rises > 10/minute

   2. Pallor
   3. Diaphoresis
   4. Dizziness
   5. Syncope
   6. Nausea and vomiting
   7. Thirst
   8. Bruising, hematuria, abnormal vaginal bleeding (suggestive of coagulopathy)
 C. Physical exam
   1. Vital signs: Assess hemodynamic instability.
      a) Orthostatic hypotension
      b) Tachycardia
   2. Integument exam: Assess for pallor, ecchymosis, petechiae, and temperature.
   3. HEENT exam: Assess nose and mouth for bleeding, oral telangiectasis.
   4. Abdominal exam
      a) Distention
      b) Hyperactive bowel sounds (upper GI source)
      c) Tenderness
      d) Masses
   5. Rectal exam
      a) Test stool for occult blood.
      b) Assess for rectal mass, tenderness, and fecal impaction.

IV. Diagnostic tests: Perform concurrently with treatment.
 A. Laboratory
   1. CBC
      a) Indicating signs of anemia
         (1) Low mean corpuscular volume (MCV): With chronic blood loss
         (2) Fall in hemoglobin and hematocrit: May not reflect volume of blood loss for 24–72 hours
      b) Platelets, indicating thrombocytopenia
   2. Prothrombin time (PT), partial thromboplastin time (PTT): To assess for prolonged values, which facilitate bleeding
   3. Liver function tests: To assess for abnormal values, indicating liver disorders
   4. BUN: Increased with hypovolemia; if ratio above 25:1, consider upper GI bleed. Digested blood protein increases BUN and creatinine.
   5. Type and crossmatch: If transfusion is considered
   6. Albumin: Low in liver dysfunction
 B. Radiology
   1. Selective celiac and or mesenteric angiogram/arteriogram (depending on suspected site of bleed)
      a) If endoscopy does not identify bleeding source
      b) If massive bleeding precludes adequate endoscopic visualization
      c) If patient is unstable and cannot have adequate precolonoscope bowel preparation
      d) Lesion must bleed at rate of 0.5 ml/minute or greater for angiograph to be diagnostic.

      2.   Upper GI/barium enema: Not useful in active bleeding

      3. Small bowel series: If other tests are negative

      4. CT scan of abdomen: To assess for masses, hematoma formation

      5. Tc-99m labeled RBC scintigraphy: Useful when colonoscopy is not diagnostic; performed before angiogram

  C. Other

      1. Upper endoscopy (EGD): Preferred test used to assess upper GI tract as source of bleeding; perform even if NG aspirate is negative for blood (bleeding source identified in 90% of cases). If ulcer or erosion, obtain biopsy for *H. pylori*.

      2. NG aspirate: To assess for upper GI source

      3. Colonoscopy: Used when scintigraphy is negative or suggests a colonic source of bleeding or upper endoscopy not diagnostic

          a) Can be done emergently, if deemed appropriate, to identify bleeding site and institute treatment.

          b) Should be done within 24 hours of bleeding episode if upper GI evaluation is unrevealing.

      4. Pulse oximetry: To assess oxygen saturation in massive GI bleed

V. Differential diagnoses

  A. Medications

      1. NSAIDs/acetylsalicylic acid (ASA): Most common etiology in elderly

      2. Corticosteroids

  B. Peptic ulcer disease with or without associated *H. pylori* infection (see Chapter 73)

  C. Gastritis (see Chapter 67)

  D. Mallory-Weiss tears

  E. Erosive gastritis

  F. Gastroesophageal reflux disease (see Chapter 66)

  G. Duodenal ulcer

  H. Portal hypertensive gastropathy or colopathy

  I. Cancer

      1. Esophageal

      2. Gastric

      3. Small bowel

      4. Colorectal

  J. Gastric polyps

  K. Esophageal varices

  L. Infection: CMV enteritis

  M. Aortoenteric fistula: After repair of abdominal aortic aneurysm

  N. Mesenteric vascular occlusion secondary to clot

  O. Graft-versus-host disease

  P. Pseudomelena: From iron, bismuth, licorice, beets, blueberries, charcoal

  Q. Any cause of lower GI bleeding

      1. Crohn's disease

      2. Infectious colitis

      3. Chronic inflammatory bowel disease

VI. Treatment: Concurrently with diagnosis
  A. Specific treatment may not be indicated if bleeding stops spontaneously.
  B. Insert two large-gauge IV cannulas and infuse IV isotonic (NS) fluids; monitor continuously for hemodynamic stability.
  C. Transfuse appropriate blood products.
     1. Administer, as appropriate, packed RBCs (PRBCs) to restore blood volume.
     2. Correct bleeding abnormalities (e.g., prolonged PT) with transfusions of fresh frozen plasma; one unit often is administered after four units of PRBC transfusions.
     3. Platelets: To correct bleeding caused by thrombocytopenia
     4. Coagulation factors: To correct identified deficiencies
  D. Administer vitamin K 2.5–10 mg po, SQ, or IM to correct bleeding abnormalities from warfarin over-anticoagulation or vitamin K deficiency.
  E. If npo
     1. Insert NG tube to aspirate for blood.
     2. If aspirate is positive for blood, leave NG tube in place to decompress stomach, approximate blood loss, and remove blood and lavage to prepare patient for endoscopy. Flush as needed to keep tube patent.
  F. Administer oxygen if pulse oximetry is low or patient is unable to tolerate hypoxia because of cardiopulmonary disease; oxygen saturation > 90% is desirable
  G. Upper endoscopy
  H. Bedrest: To prevent syncope if hypotensive and to conserve energy
  I. Start IV H_2 blockers (e.g., famotidine 20 mg IV q 12 hours or rantidine 50 mg IV q 8 hours); convert to PO when patient is stable and taking oral fluids.
  J. Arteriography with embolization, injection of vasopressin during procedure: Indicated when continued or recurrent bleeding occurs and guided by results of nuclear GI bleed scan
  K. Oral iron (ferrous sulfate 250–325 mg po tid): After patient is stable (see Chapters 111–116)

VII. Follow-up: Monitor patient for further bleeding after discharge and relapse of identified etiology.
  A. Inform patient to report blood in stool.
  B. Perform rectal exam at next office visit and test stool for blood.
  C. Repeat rectal exam based on patient's reports of blood in stool and at least annually if no further reports of bleeding (or more often based on assessment).

VIII. Referrals
  A. Gastroenterologist: Consult for diagnostic evaluation, including endoscopy.
  B. Medical internist: For admission
  C. Surgeon: For surgery if patient does not respond to endoscopic therapy

References

Catalano, M.F., & Grace, N.D. (1996). Getting to the cause of rectal bleeding. *Patient Care, 30*(16), 32–59.

Labovich, T.M. (1994). Selected complications in the patient with cancer: Spinal cord compression, malignant bowel obstruction, malignant ascites and gastrointestinal bleeding. *Seminars in Oncology Nursing, 10,* 189–197.

Laine, L. (1998). Acute and chronic gastrointestinal bleeding. In M. Feldman, B.F. Scharschmidt, M.H. Sleisenger (Eds.), *Sleisenger & Fordtran's gastrointestinal and liver disease: Pathophysiology, management* (pp. 198–219). Philadelphia: Saunders.

Nankhonya, J.M., Datta-Chaudhuri, M.L., & Bhan, G.L. (1997). Acute upper gastrointestinal hemorrhage in older people: A prospective study in two neighboring districts. *Journal of American Geriatric Society, 45,* 752–754.

Roberts, S.K., & Dudley, F.J. (1997). Management of haematemesis and melena. *Medical Journal of Australia, 166,* 549–553.

Vella, A., & Farrugia, G. (1996). 90-year-old man with fever and melena. *Mayo Clinic Proceedings, 71,* 1205–1208.

Chapter

59. Nausea and Vomiting

Kathleen Murphy-Ende, RN, PhD, CFNP

I. Definition
   A. Nausea: A nebulous, unpleasant sensation described as the need to vomit, motion sickness, or queasiness that may occur before, with, or without vomiting
   B. Vomiting: The expulsion of gastric contents through the mouth
      1. Incoercible vomiting: Uncontrollable vomiting
      2. Projectile vomiting: Ejection of vomitus with great force
      3. Stercoraceous vomiting: Expulsion of fecal matter
   C. Retching: Spasmodic respiratory and abdominal muscle movement; may or may not accompany nausea and vomiting

II. Pathophysiology
   A. Neural structures in the fourth ventricle and brain stem, multiple afferent nerve fibers, and several neurotransmitters are involved in the nausea and vomiting reflex.
   B. Vomiting center (VC)
      1. Located in the medullary reticular formation of the brain
      2. Stimulated by neurotransmitters, the chemoreceptor trigger zone (CTZ), vestibular apparatus, and vagus nerve receive stimulation from the viscera or higher brain centers.
         a) Once stimulated, impulses are sent to the autonomic nervous system, causing nausea, and to the somatic and visceral system to produce vomiting.
         b) Nausea
            (1) The stomach relaxes, and gastric acid secretion is inhibited.
            (2) A single, retrograde, giant contraction of the small intestine causes the alkaline contents of the small bowel to be propelled into the stomach.
         c) Vomiting
            (1) The abdominal muscles contract, and the periesophageal diaphragm relaxes.
            (2) Compression of the stomach causes reflux of the contents through the esophagus and mouth.
   C. Neural connection between the higher cortical centers in the cortex and the VC may be responsible for anticipatory nausea.
      1. Vagus nerve terminates in the proximal gut wall.
         a) Mechanical changes in the GI tract (i.e., from chemotherapy and radiation) cause the enterochromaffin cells in the gut wall to release serotonin ($5\text{-}HT_3$), which

binds to the chemoreceptors of the afferent vagus nerve in the stomach and proximal small intestine.

b) Stimulation of the afferent vagus sends an impulse to the VC and CTZ.

D. The CTZ, located on the floor of the fourth ventricle, is linked to the vomiting center by the fasciculus solitarius.

1. Neurotransmitters and hormones in the cerebrospinal fluid and blood bind with the chemoreceptors, transmitting an impulse to the VC to cause nausea and vomiting.

2. These neurotransmitters and hormones include serotonin, noradrenaline, somatostatin, substance P, enkephalin, acetylcholine, aminobutyric acid, vasopressin (antidiuretic hormone), and cortisol.

3. Metabolic chemicals resulting from paraneoplastic syndromes (see Appendix 12) such as hypercalcemia, hyponatremia, and uremia, or metabolites from tumor proliferation may stimulate the CTZ and VC.

a) The accumulation of morphine metabolites can stimulate the vestibular apparatus, resulting in chronic nausea.

b) The products of cellular breakdown after chemotherapy administration also may contribute to nausea.

c) Opioids directly stimulate the CTZ's serotonin and dopaminergic receptor sites.

E. Visceral alteration from gastric irritation, intestinal obstruction, or gastric, liver, or splenic distention may stimulate the vagal nerve. The vagal efferent fibers directly stimulate the vomiting center by their release of histaminergic, serotoninergic, and cholinergic neurotransmitters.

F. Vestibular apparatus located in the inner ear is stimulated by histaminergic and muscarinic cholinergic receptors, which communicate with the VC.

G. Psychological factors (e.g., anxiety) stimulate the sympathetic nervous system, mediating the release of hormones from the pituitary and adrenal glands.

H. In the CNS, an increase in intracranial pressure stimulates the histaminergic receptors in the vomiting center.

III. Clinical features: Nausea and vomiting are common symptoms found in patients with cancer related to the treatment or to the disease process. The cause of these symptoms spans a wide variety of factors and often is multifactorial.

A. Etiology: Nausea and vomiting may be structural (e.g., CNS, visceral, vestibular), psychological, chemical, metabolic, or a combination.

B. History

1. History of cancer and cancer treatment

2. Current medications: Prescribed and over-the-counter

3. History of presenting symtom(s): Precipitating factors, onset, and duration. Associated symptoms are increased salivation, diaphoresis, tachycardia, diarrhea, retching, dysphagia, and thirst.

4. Changes in activities of daily living

C. Signs and symptoms (depend on etiology): Nausea, vomiting, and anorexia with poor or absent oral intake

1. Decreased urine output secondary to dehydration

2. Weight loss

       3. Constipation
       4. Pain: Abdominal, chest, head, or ear
       5. Manifestations of hypokalemia: Malaise, fatigue, weakness, palpitations, paresthesias, cramps, and restless leg syndrome
       6. Manifestations of metabolic alkalosis: Impaired mentation, hypotension, and hypoventilation
       7. Viral symptoms: Malaise, myalgia, arthralgia, rhinorrhea, headache, stiff neck, vertigo, tinnitus, anorexia, chest pain, cough, fever (also consider household members with similar symptoms)
       8. Neurologic symptoms: Headache, projectile vomiting, incoordination with altered vision, personality change, paralysis, convulsion, seizure
       9. Vestibular symptoms: Tinnitus, nausea worse with head motion, decreased hearing, skull tenderness

  D. Physical exam
       1. Vital signs
          a) Temperature decreased with dehydration, increased with infection
          b) Increased respirations in acidosis, respiratory abnormalities with increased intracranial pressure (ICP)
          c) Orthostatic hypotension and tachycardia with dehydration; hypertension with bradycardia could indicate increased ICP, hypertension with increased ICP, slow pulse with ICP
          d) Weight loss
       2. Neurologic exam
          a) Diagnostic signs of meningitis: Neck rigidity, Kernig and Brudzinski signs, disconjugate ocular movements, pupillary abnormalities
          b) CNS involvement: Usually associated with abnormal neurologic function
       3. HEENT/oral cavity exam: Assess for dry mucous membranes, indicating dehydration, *Candida* lesions (may exacerbate nausea)
       4. Integument exam: Tenting skin turgor
       5. Cardiac exam: Assess for regularity of rhythm to evaluate for dysrhythmia.
       6. Abdominal exam: Assess for hepatosplenomegaly, masses, ascites, rigidity, hyper/hypoactive bowel sounds or tenderness.
       7. Rectal exam: Evaluate for fecal impaction.

IV. Diagnostic tests
  A. Laboratory
       1. Electrolytes: Potassium and chloride may be low in dehydration, and sodium may be elevated or low
       2. BUN and creatinine: Ratio above 10:1 in fluid volume deficit (FVD)
       3. Carbon dioxide: High in alkalosis
       4. Urinalysis: Specific gravity and osmolality increase in fluid volume deficit or dehydration; chloride is decreased in metabolic alkalosis.
       5. Liver function tests: Abnormal with liver metastases
       6. Elevated amylase in pancreatic disease
       7. Serum levels of drug toxicity (e.g., digoxin, theophylline)
       8. Serum beta-human chorionic gonadotropin (B-HCG): Suspect pregnancy

B. Radiology
1. Abdominal flat plate and upright: Free intraperitoneal air if perforation or dilated loops of small bowel in mechanical small bowel obstruction
2. Scintigraphic study: Delayed gastric emptying indicates gastroparesis if obstruction has been excluded.
3. Barium upper GI study: May show evidence of gastric outlet obstruction
4. Upper endoscopy: May show evidence of gastric outlet obstruction, ulceration, tumor, gastritis, or esophagitis
5. Abdominal ultrasound: May show blockage in the GI tract; a biliary obstruction can be noted but not bowel obstruction
6. Abdominal CT: May show bowel obstruction or a mass causing direct pressure on the bowel
7. Brain CT or MRI: May show CNS involvement, such as brain metastasis
C. Other
1. Saline load test: More than 400 ml residual 30 minutes after instillation of 750 ml of NS indicates obstruction or gastroparesis.
2. EKG: Prominent U-waves and QRS widening in hypokalemia; dysrhythmia
3. Lumbar puncture (LP): To evaluate ICP and for meningitis

V. Differential diagnosis
A. Treatment-related causes
1. Chemotherapy
2. Radiation therapy to the GI tract
3. Surgery
4. Drug-induced
a) Opioids
b) Hormonal agents
c) Antidepressants
d) Antibiotics
e) NSAIDs
B. Malignancy-related causes
1. Hepatomegaly (see Chapter 56)
2. Splenomegaly (see Chapter 61)
3. CNS metastasis
4. Vestibular neuroma
5. Carcinoid tumor
6. Paraneoplastic syndrome (see Appendix 12)
C. Gastrointestinal
1. Upper GI
a) Gastroenteritis
b) Peptic ulcer disease (see Chapter 73)
c) Gastroparesis
2. Lower GI
a) Appendicitis

       b) Constipation (see Chapter 52)

       c) Diverticulosis

   3. Hepatobiliary

       a) Biliary tract disease (cholecystitis)

       b) Hepatitis (see Chapter 69)

   4. Other

       a) Adhesions

       b) Bowel obstruction (see Chapter 63)

       c) Food poisoning

       d) Organ distention

       e) Pancreatitis (see Chapter 72)

       f) Peritonitis

       g) Superior mesenteric artery syndrome

       h) Zollinger-Ellison syndrome

D. Endocrine

   1. Adrenal insufficiency

   2. Diabetic ketoacidosis (see Chapter 143)

   3. Hyperparathyroidism

   4. Pregnancy

   5. Thyroid disease (see Chapters 149 and 150)

   6. Hypercalcemia (see Chapter 144)

E. CNS

   1. Increased intracranial pressure

   2. Labyrinthitis

   3. Menière's disease

   4. Meningitis (see Chapter 136)

   5. Migraine headaches (see Chapter 135)

F. Cardiac disease

   1. Glycoside treatment (digoxin)

   2. Myocardial infarction (see Chapter 47)

   3. CHF (see Chapter 40)

G. Psychological

   1. Anxiety (see Chapter 152)

   2. Cyclical vomiting

   3. Depression (see Chapter 154)

   4. Eating disorders

H. Renal

   1. Urinary tract infections (see Chapter 91)

   2. Uremia

I. Vestibular

   1. Primary vestibular disorder

   2. Acoustic neuroma

   3. Brain tumors or carcinomatous meningitis

J. Miscellaneous

       1. Drug withdrawal

       2. Binge drinking

VI. Treatment: Direct the treatment of nausea and vomiting to the underlying disorder, and consider individual characteristics before initiating a treatment plan.

    A. Antiemetics (see Appendix 3)

    B. Nonpharmacologic treatment

       1. Relaxation

       2. Hypnosis

       3. Imagery

       4. Diversion or attention distraction

       5. Systematic desensitization

       6. Dietary modification

    C. Nasogastric tube placement: Placed for relief of symptoms; aspiration of more than 200 ml of fluid in a fasting patient may indicate obstruction or gastroparesis.

VII. Follow-up

    A. Regularly assess the effectiveness of a treatment plan.

       1. If nausea or vomiting persists after 24 hours of antiemetic treatment, further evaluation warranted.

       2. Monitor the patient for side effects; modify drugs and doses accordingly.

    B. Self-care strategies and patient education should focus on the treatment plan, preventive measures, and appropriate follow-up medical/nursing consultation.

VIII. Referrals

    A. Surgeon: Promptly refer patients who have evidence of an acute dysfunction that may require surgical intervention.

    B. Oncologist/internist: Notify regarding progressive metastatic process or uncontrollable nausea and vomiting.

References

Cunningham, R. (1997). 5-HT$_3$ receptor antagonists: A review of pharmacology and clinical efficacy. *Oncology Nursing Forum, 24*(Suppl.7), 33–40.

Doherty, K.M. (1999). Closing the gap in prophylactic antiemetic therapy: Patient factors in calculating emetogenic potential of chemotherapy. *Clinical Journal of Oncology Nursing, 3,* 113–119.

Fessele, K. (1996). Managing the multiple causes of nausea and vomiting in the patient with cancer. *Oncology Nursing Forum, 23,* 1409–1415.

Goodman, M. (1997). Risk factors and antiemetic management of chemotherapy-induced nausea and vomiting. *Oncology Nursing Forum, 24*(Suppl. 7), 20–32.

Gralla, R., Osoba, D., Kris, M., Kirkbride, P., Hesketh, P., Chinnery, L., Clark-Snow, R., Gill, D., Groshen, S., Grunberg, S., Koller, J., Morrow, G., Preaze, E., Silber, J., & Pfister, D. (1999). Recommendations for the use of antiemetics: Evidence-based clinical practice guidelines. *Journal of Clinical Oncology, 17,* 2971–2994

Hogan, C.M., & Grant, M. (1997). Physiologic mechanisms of nausea and vomiting in patients with cancer. *Oncology Nursing Forum, 24*(Suppl. 7), 8–12.

Lichter, I. (1996). Nausea and vomiting in patients with cancer. *Pain and Palliative Care, 10*(1), 207–220.

Chapter

60. Rectal Bleeding (Hematochezia)

Jeanne Held-Warmkessel, MSN, RN, CS, AOCN®

I. Definition: Bright-red to maroon blood from rectum associated more often with lower GI tract

II. Pathophysiology
   A. Bleeding of GI mucosa from irritation, ulceration, or trauma
   B. Bleeding often originates in the left colon or anorectal region, although very brisk movement of blood from the right colon, small bowel, or stomach can lead to similar presentation.

III. Clinical features: Bleeding may be pure or mixed with stool, clots, or diarrhea. Blood may be obvious or occult and may range from a life-threatening event to spontaneous cessation. The colon will continue to eliminate blood even after active bleeding stops because of its storage capability.
   A. History
      1. History of cancer and cancer treatment
      2. Current medications: Prescribed and over-the-counter
      3. History of presenting symptom(s): Precipitating factors, onset, and duration. Associated symptoms are weight loss, change in bowel habits, abdominal pain, dyspepsia, nausea, and vomiting.
      4. Changes in activities of daily living
      5. Past medical history: Rectal or colon disease, hemorrhoids, anal fissure
      6. Social history: Alcohol intake
   B. Signs and symptoms
      1. Visible blood at the rectum or passing of blood through rectum
      2. Vomiting
      3. Lightheadedness
      4. Pallor
      5. Weakness
      6. Diaphoresis
      7. Pain (abdominal cramps occur with diverticular bleeding)
   C. Physical exam
      1. Vital signs: Assess for hemodynamic instability.

        a) Orthostatic hypotension

        b) Tachycardia

    2. Integument exam

        a) Lesions: Many GI disorders are associated with skin changes (e.g., telangiectasis).

        b) Pallor

        c) Temperature

    3. Abdominal exam

        a) Masses

        b) Ascites

        c) Tenderness

        d) Distention

        e) Spider veins (angionoma)

        f) Hyperactive bowel sounds

    4. Digital rectal exam: Assess for masses, tenderness, and stool impaction.

IV. Diagnostic tests (see Figure 60-1)

  A. Laboratory tests

    1. CBC

        a) Indicating signs of anemia

           (1) Low MCV with chronic blood loss; no change with acute loss

           (2) Fall in hemoglobin and hematocrit; may not reflect volume of blood loss for 24–72 hours

        b) Platelets, indicating thrombocytopenia

    2. PT/PTT: To assess for anticoagulation/coagulopathy, which increase the risk of bleeding

    3. Liver function tests (LFTs): Abnormal values may indicate liver dysfunction.

    4. BUN/creatinine: If ratio is above 25:1, consider upper GI bleed; digested blood protein increases BUN value, as well as volume depletion.

    5. Type and cross match if transfusion is considered.

  B. Radiology

    1. Selective visceral arteriography/angiography

        a) Useful with massive bleeding; embolization of a bleeding vessel or infusion of vasopressin can be done during procedure (0.2–0.4 units/minute).

        b) Done if proctosigmoidoscopy or colonoscopy is not diagnostic or if patient is too unstable for endoscopy.

        c) Procedure of choice if nuclear technetium (Tc) scan is positive and if bleeding is rapid.

        d) Lesion must be bleeding at time of test for it to be useful in identifying bleeding site.

        e) Blood loss as slow as 0.5–2 ml/minute can be detected.

    2. Barium enema: Not useful in active bleeding situations

    3. Small bowel series: Used after other tests are unsuccessful in revealing source of blood loss

    4. Scintigraphy Tc 99m-labeled RBCs

        a) Useful for lesions that bleed on intermittent basis.

        b) Labeled RBCs enter bowel at bleeding site.

Figure 60-1. Diagnostic Approach to the Patient With Gastrointestinal Hemorrhage

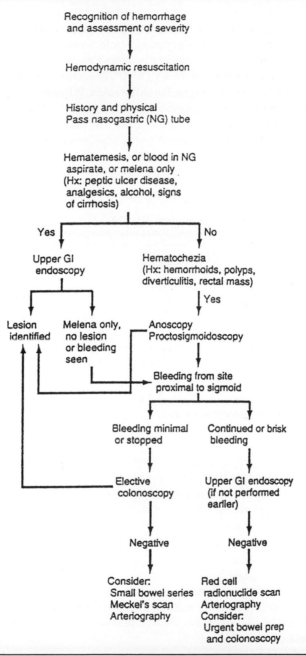

Note. From *Cecil Essentials of Medicine* (4th ed.) (p. 260), by T. Andreoli, J. Bennett, C. Carpenter, and F. Plum, 1997, Philadelphia: W.B. Saunders Company. Copyright 1997 by W.B. Saunders Company. Reprinted with permission.

        c) Lesion must be bleeding at time of test for it to be useful in identifying bleeding site.

        d) Done if NG aspirate and rectal exam do not reveal bleeding source.

  C. Other

    1. NG aspirate: To assess for upper GI source/upper endoscopy

    2. Test stool for occult blood and possible infectious causes to identify bleeding source.

    3. Proctosigmoidoscopy/anoscopy to identify bleed

    4. Colonoscopy: Oral prep (GoLYTELY®, Braintree Laboratories, Braintree, MA, or CoLyte®, Schwartz Pharma, Inc., Milwaukee, WI) required unless massive bleeding is present or patient is unstable.

        a) If colon is full of blood or stool, test may not identify source of bleeding.

        b) Useful after scintigraphy if test is negative or if patient is stable and bleeding source is identified in the colon.

    5. Test oxygen saturation with pulse oximetry.

V. Differential diagnosis

  A. Vascular abnormalities: Abnormal colon blood vessel structure with capillary dilation

    1. Vasculitis

    2. Vascular anomalies

    3. Mesenteric ischemia

    4. Ischemic colitis

  B. Diverticular disease

  C. Cancers

    1. Colorectal

    2. Small bowel

  D. Polyps

  E. Hemorrhoids (internal) (see Chapter 68)

  F. Rectal ulcer

  G. Small bowel or colorectal varices

  H. Lacerations, rectal trauma

  I. Fistula

  J. Anal fissure

  K. Drugs such as NSAIDs/ASA

  L. Thrombocytopenia, altered coagulation (see Chapter 123)

  M. Inflammatory bowel diseases

    1. Ulcerative colitis

    2. Crohn's disease

    3. Ischemic colitis

    4. Infectious colitis

  N. Aortoenteric fistula (after abdominal aortic aneurysm repair)

  O. Radiation colitis, proctitis: more than six months postradiation therapy

VI. Treatment for lower GI bleed

  A. Insert large-gauge IV cannulas (two) and rapidly infuse isotonic (NS) fluids to achieve hemodynamic stability.

  B. Monitor urine output, as oliguria may develop with hypovolemia.

C. Check vital signs frequently for hemodynamic instability.

D. Replace/correct anemia with RBC transfusion to correct hematocrit to approximately 30%.

E. Provide supplemental oxygen as needed if patient is unable to tolerate low oxygen saturation or has a history of cardiac disease.

F. Correct bleeding problems.

   1. Administer vitamin K 2.5–10 mg po, SC, or IM if overanticoagulated from warfarin or from vitamin K deficiency.

   2. Administer platelets if platelet count is low.

   3. Use fresh frozen plasma to replace all clotting factors if coagulopathy is present.

G. Bedrest: To conserve energy and prevent syncope

H. Colonoscopy: To perform cautery, laser, polypectomy, or other methods to stop bleeding

I. Radiation proctitis: Topical or systemic corticosteroids or other anti-inflammatory medications, sucralfate, oral sulfasalazine, laser, or other coagulation method during colonoscopy

J. Iron supplements: When patient is stable, ferrous sulfate 250–325 mg po tid (see Chapter 116)

VII. Follow-up: Monitor patient for further bleeding or for relapse from previously identified bleeding source.

VIII. Referrals

A. Gastroenterologist: For endoscopy

B. Medical internist: For admission

C. Surgeon: For surgery

References

Billingham, R.P. (1997). The conundrum of lower gastrointestinal bleeding. *Surgical Clinics of North America, 77,* 241–252.

Ellis, D.J., & Reinus, J.F. (1995). Lower intestinal hemorrhage. *Critical Care Clinics, 11,* 369–389.

Labovich, T.M. (1994). Selected complications in the patient with cancer: Spinal cord compression, malignant bowel obstruction, malignant ascites, and gastrointestinal bleeding. *Seminars in Oncology Nursing, 10,* 189–197.

Miller, L.S., Barbarevech, C., & Friedman, L.S. (1994). Less frequent causes of lower gastrointestinal bleeding. *Gastroenterology Clinics of North America, 23,* 21–52.

Reinus, J.F., & Brandt, L.J. (1994). Vascular ectasias and diverticulosis: Common causes of lower intestinal bleeding. *Gastroenterology Clinics of North America, 23,* 1–20.

Richter, J.M. (1994). Occult gastrointestinal bleeding. *Gastrointestinal Clinics of North America, 23,* 53–66.

Shapiro, M.J. (1994). The role of the radiologist in the management of gastrointestinal bleeding. *Gastroenterology Clinics of North America, 23,* 123–181.

61. Splenomegaly

Gail Egan Sansivero, MS, ANP, AOCN®

I. Definition: Enlargement of the spleen

II. Physiology/Pathophysiology
   A. Normal
      1. The normal spleen is shaped like a curved wedge and follows the course of the left tenth rib, lying entirely within the rib cage; thus, it normally is not palpable.
      2. It is located in the left upper quadrant lying above the left kidney and below the diaphragm.
      3. It receives blood flow of approximately 300 ml/minute.
      4. Normal splenic size includes a length of 12 cm, a width of 7 cm, and a volume of 250 cm; however, splenic size does vary.
      5. The normal spleen is the body's largest lymphoid organ and is involved in the production and maintenance of RBCs, certain circulating WBCs, and platelets.
         a) Plays a major role in the cellular and humoral immune response to infection and inflammation
         b) Primary filter for circulating senescent (i.e., damaged) cells, antigens, and microorganisms
      6. The spleen is divided into white pulp (i.e., lymphoid tissue) and red pulp.
         a) The white pulp functions as part of the reticuloendothelial system to filter blood and to manufacture lymphocytes and monocytes. It also serves as a major source of immunoglobulin M (IgM) production.
         b) The red pulp contains a capillary network and venous sinus system, allowing for the storage and release of blood. New reticulocytes are conditioned in this environment.
      7. The spleen serves as a reservoir for platelets, housing up to a third of the body's total platelet mass sequestered in a freely exchangeable pool.
   B. Pathophysiology
      1. Hypersplenism results in exaggerated splenic function with enhanced filtration and phagocytosis of cellular components of blood, resulting in cytopenia.
      2. Hematopoiesis in the adult spleen occurs only as a result of pathologic conditions.
      3. Splenomegaly that occurs in hepatic cirrhosis complicated by portal hypertension may result from reticuloendothelial hyperplasia and the hemodynamic changes associated with portal hypertension.

III. Clinical features
  A. Etiology: Splenic enlargement is caused by the following general mechanisms.
      1. Reactive proliferation of lymphoid cells
      2. Infiltration by neoplastic cells
      3. Extramedullary hematopoiesis
      4. Proliferation of phagocytic cells
      5. Vascular congestion
  B. History
      1. History of cancer and cancer treatment
      2. Current medications: Prescribed and over-the-counter
      3. History of presenting symptom(s): Precipitating factors, onset, location, and duration. Associated symptoms are abdominal discomfort, bruising, and bleeding.
      4. Changes in activities of daily living
      5. Past medical history: Recent abdominal injuries, immune disorders, blood disorders, recent infections or illnesses
      6. History of recent travel to tropical climates
  C. Signs and symptoms
      1. Petechiae, ecchymoses
      2. Fatigue
      3. Malaise
      4. Feeling of abdominal fullness, especially in left upper quadrant
      5. Early satiety, anorexia
  D. Physical exam
      1. HEENT/oral cavity
          a) Assess for petechiae, indicating thrombocytopenia
          b) Assess for exudate and erythema, indicating infection
      2. Integument exam
          a) Petechiae and ecchymoses of skin, indicating thrombocytopenia
          b) Exudate and erythema of skin indicating signs of infection
      3. Lymph node exam: Palpate for adenopathy, indicating signs of infection or malignancy
      4. Abdominal exam
          a) Physical exam techniques have a low sensitivity for detecting splenomegaly unless it is massive.
          b) When the spleen is enlarged, the lower edge moves down and to the right of the midclavicular line.
          c) Splenomegaly may present with upper quadrant fullness or bulging from beneath the left costal margin. Fullness should descend on inspiration.
          d) Percussion is used to identify the size and density of the spleen; dullness suggests spleen enlargement.

IV. Diagnostic tests
  A. Laboratory tests
      1. CBC with differential: To evaluate for pancytopenia (may be present with mild enlargement)

    2. Chemistry profile including LFTs: To rule out liver failure

    3. Monospot: To rule out mononucleosis

    4. HIV testing: If patient has known risk factors

    5. Bone marrow aspiration and biopsy: To evaluate for hyperplastic marrow

  B. Radiology

    1. Ultrasound of the spleen: To confirm splenomegaly and provide dimensions more useful than flat plate of abdomen

    2. Liver/spleen scan (with isotopes): To confirm splenomegaly and to detect diffuse parenchymal disease in liver, which may cause portal hypertension

    3. CT scan of abdomen: To delineate size and location of spleen, assess for presence of malignancy, and identify enlarged mesenteric or retroperitoneal lymph nodes

V. Differential diagnosis

  A. Polycythemia vera (see Chapter 122)

  B. Congenital syphilis

  C. AIDS (see Chapter 156)

  D. Infection (lymphoid hyperplasia)

    1. Mononucleosis (Epstein-Barr virus)

    2. Cytomegalovirus infections (CMV)

    3. Toxoplasmosis

    4. Chronic viral hepatitis (see Chapter 69)

    5. Influenza

    6. Malaria

    7. Rickettsial infection (Rocky Mountain spotted fever)

  E. Inflammation (lymphoid hyperplasia)

    1. Sarcoidosis

    2. Rheumatoid arthritis (see Chapter 108)

    3. Systemic lupus erythematosus

    4. Renal dialysis (occurs in 10% of uremic patients)

  F. Neoplasms (infiltrative or myeloproliferative)

    1. Leukemia (acute and chronic)

    2. Lymphoma

    3. Metastatic tumors (rare)

    4. Primary tumors (rare)

  G. Hemolytic disease (phagocytic hyperplasia)

    1. Spherocytosis

    2. Thalassemia major

    3. Pyruvate kinase deficiency

    4. Idiopathic thrombocytopenic purpura (see Chapter 120)

  H. Infiltration

    1. Gaucher's disease

    2. Niemann-Pick disease

    3. Amyloidosis

    4. Extramedullary hematopoiesis

  I. Splenic vein hypertension (vascular congestion)

   1. Cirrhosis (see Chapter 64)
   2. Splenic or portal vein thrombosis
   3. Chronic congestive hepatopathy (with or without cardiac cirrhosis)
J. Endocrine
   1. Grave's disease (see Chapter 144)
   2. Hashimoto's thyroiditis (see Chapter 150)
K. Hemophilia
L. Chronic congestive splenomegaly (Banti's syndrome)

VI. Treatment: Directed at underlying cause of splenomegaly
   A. Patients with polycythemia vera
      1. Smoking cessation
      2. Phlebotomy (when HCT rises above approximately 50)
      3. Oxygen therapy
      4. Myelosuppressive therapy
   B. Patients with leukemia or lymphoma: Treatment with chemotherapy and/or radiation therapy as indicated, depending on type and stage of disease.
   C. Patients with sarcoidosis: Treatment is aimed at relieving symptoms and active pulmonary disease, primarily using oral corticosteroids. This therapy is most effective if begun before pulmonary fibrosis occurs.
   D. Patients with congestive splenomegaly or secondary hypersplenism
      1. Splenectomy
      2. Irradiation
      3. Transjugular intrahepatic portosystemic shunt (TIPS)
      4. Splenic embolization
   E. Patients with limited splenomegaly and correctable coagulopathy
      1. Laparoscopic splenectomy may be a surgical option
      2. The major operative risk for splenectomy is intra- and postprocedure bleeding.
      3. Pneumovax® (Merck & Co., Inc., West Point, PA), *Haemophilus influenzae*, and meningococcal vaccines should be given prior to surgery whenever possible or immediately afterwards.
   F. Patient education
      1. Instruct patients with splenomegaly to avoid activities that place them at risk for splenic injury/rupture (e.g., contact sports).
      2. Post-splenectomy patients are at increased risk for sepsis with encapsulated organisms (e.g., *Streptococcus pneumoniae, Haemophilus influenzae, Neisseria meningitis*).
         a) Signs and symptoms of infection should be reported immediately.
         b) A viral infection may predispose a patient to fulminant bacterial infection.
         c) Aggressive empiric therapy should be initiated in the patient with sepsis of unknown origin.

VII. Follow-up: Laboratory tests and healthcare provider visits will be dictated by the patient's underlying disease process.

VIII. Referrals
    A. Internist: For patients with newly discovered splenomegaly, consult for workup plan and diagnosis.
    B. Infectious disease/AIDS specialist: For patients with newly diagnosed HIV infection, consult for treatment planning.
    C. Hematologist/oncologist: For patients with newly diagnosed hematologic malignancy, consult for treatment planning.
    D. Hematologist: For patients with newly diagnosed polycythemia vera, consult for treatment planning.
    E. Pulmonologist: For patients with newly diagnosed sarcoidosis, refer depending on stage and sites involved.
    F. Consider social work referral for patients with newly diagnosed malignancy or HIV infection.

References

Barkun, A.N., Camus, M., Green, L., Meagher, T., Coupal, L., DeStempel, J., & Grover, S.A. (1991). The bedside assessment of splenic enlargement. *American Journal of Medicine, 91,* 512–518.

Farid, H., & O'Connell, T.X. (1996). Surgical management of massive splenomegaly. *The American Surgeon, 62,* 803–805.

Flowers, J.L., Lefor, A.T., Steers, J., Heyman, M., Graham, S.M., & Imbembo, A.L. (1996). Laparoscopic splenectomy in patients with hematologic diseases. *Annals of Surgery, 224,* 19–28.

Grover, S.A., Barkun, A.N., & Sackett, D.L. (1993). Does this patient have splenomegaly? *JAMA, 270,* 2218 2221.

Kcnawi, M.M., El-Ghamrawi, K.A., Mohammad, A.A., Kenawi, A., & El-Sadek, A.Z. (1997). Splenic irradiation for the treatment of hypersplenism from congestive splenomegaly. *British Journal of Surgery, 84,* 860–861.

Orozco, H., Mercado, H.A., Martinez, R., Tielve, M., Chan, C., Vasquez, M., Zenteno-Guichard, G., & Pantoja, J.P. (1998). Is splenectomy necessary in devascularization procedures for treatment of bleeding portal hypertension? *Archives of Surgery, 133,* 36–38.

Pursnani, K.G., Sillin, L.F., & Kaplan, D.S. (1997). Effect of transjugular intrahepatic portosystemic shunt on secondary hypersplenism. *American Journal of Surgery, 173,* 169–173.

Shah, S.H., Hayes, P.C., Allan, P.L., Nicoll, J., & Finlayson, N.D. (1996). Measurement of spleen size and its relation to hypersplenism and portal hemodynamics in portal hypertension due to hepatic cirrhosis. *American Journal of Gastroenterology, 91,* 2580–2583.

Wilhelm, M.C., Jones, R.E., McGehee, R., Mitchener, J.S., Sandusky, W.R., & Hess, C.E. (1988). Splenectomy in hematologic disorders. *Annals of Surgery, 207,* 581–589.

62. Anorexia/Cachexia

Margaret Q. Rosenzweig, CRNP-C, MSN, AOCN®

I. Definition
   A. Anorexia is the aversion to food.
   B. Cachexia is a general lack of nutrition and wasting occurring in the course of a chronic disease or emotional disturbance.
   C. Anorexia-cachexia is a syndrome of profound weight loss—a decrease in baseline weight by 10% or more in six months or 5% in one month.

II. Pathophysiology
   A. Cachexia is the outcome of net negative energy balance.
      1. In cachexia, the patient appears to overproduce glucose, despite relative insulin resistance or diminished insulin levels.
      2. In chronic disease states, the employment of the relatively energy-inefficient pathway of anaerobic gluconeogenesis results in high lactate levels.
      3. An imbalance is noted in the host energy needs and glucose production through the Cori cycle, a phenomenon labeled futile cycling.
   B. Because of inefficient glucose usage from the breakdown of skeletal muscle protein into its component amino acids, wasting occurs.
      1. In patients with cancer, protein mobilization is an early source of calories, rather than the use of carbohydrate and fat deposits during starvation.
      2. As a result of protein usage, hypoalbuminemia occurs from the increased breakdown of albumin and, in part, to hemodilution. Other effects include
         a) Decrease in protein mass
         b) Atrophy of skin and skeletal muscle mass.
   C. Abnormal depletion of lipid stores occurs from reduced lipogenesis or increased lipolysis or a combination of both. Consequently, the patient often will have increased serum triglycerides and glycerol and decreased high-density lipoproteins and cholesterol.
   D. While the exact etiology is not yet fully understood, cancer cachexia is considered to be a complex paraneoplastic syndrome of anorexia, weight loss, and wasting mediated, at least in part, through cytokines.
   E. One of the most significant cytokines in anorexia and cachexia is the macrophage-derived protein cachectin (i.e., tumor necrosis factor), which is capable of inducing muscle wasting and mediating adverse metabolic changes.

III. Clinical features: Cancer cachexia may occur in up to 80% of all patients with cancer. When the daily physiologic demands exceed the patient's dietary consumption, the body reserves are used to meet energy and protein needs.

    A. Etiology: Cancer cachexia appears to be multifactorial (e.g., social, psychological, physiological) rather than caused by poor dietary intake.

        1. Inadequate intake

            a) Changes in taste or smell of foods

            b) Fear of provoking nausea, vomiting, or abdominal cramping

            c) Disinterest in food

        2. Associated symptoms of food aversion

            a) Depression

            b) Anxiety

            c) Uncontrolled pain

            d) Xerostomia

        3. Malfunction of GI tract

            a) Malabsorption

            b) Mucosa damage

            c) Obstruction

        4. Paraneoplastic syndrome

    B. History: A complete history regarding weight patterns, gain and loss cycles, and nutritional intake patterns are essential to the diagnosis of the etiology and management of this symptom. Conduct complete nutritional assessment at the time of diagnosis and periodically throughout therapy.

        1. History of cancer and cancer treatment

        2. Current medications: Prescribed and over-the-counter

        3. History of presenting symptom(s): Precipitating factors, onset, and duration. Associated symptoms are difficulty chewing and swallowing, sore throat, xerostomia, caries, and altered taste.

        4. Changes in activities of daily living

        5. Diet: History of typical 24-hour diet prior to cancer diagnosis and current 24-hour diet; use of nutritional supplements, vitamins, and minerals

    C. Signs and symptoms

        1. Significant decreased weight over the last six months

        2. Loss of appetite

        3. Nausea/vomiting

        4. Fatigue/weakness

        5. Amenorrhea

        6. Polyuria

        7. Cold intolerance

    D. Physical exam

        1. Vital signs

            a) Height and weight, including anthropometric measurements

            b) Blood pressure: Usually orthostatic

            c) Tachycardia

        d) Tachypnea
    2. Integument exam
        a) Dry skin with poor turgor
        b) Dry brittle hair and/or nails
    3. HEENT exam: Poor dentition, stomatitis, lesions, dry membranes
    4. Cardiovascular exam: Irregular heart rate may indicate dysrhythmia.
    5. Musculoskeletal exam: Loss of muscle mass, poor muscle tone, temporal wasting
    6. Abdominal exam: Protuberant, distended abdomen in late stage from ascites

IV. Diagnostic tests
  A. Laboratory
    1. Hemoglobin and hematocrit: May be decreased secondary to nutritional depletion
    2. Chemistry profile: Electrolytes may be altered
        a) Sodium: May be decreased with weight loss, anorexia
        b) Potassium: May be decreased with weight loss, anorexia
    3. Serum albumin/serum protein: Will be decreased even though these values are considered to be nonspecific indicators of nutrition
        a) Prealbumin: Will be depressed in malnutrition
        b) Prealbumin is the precursor of albumin and is a sensitive measure of nutritional status
    4. Glucose: Will be decreased; however, is considered to be a nonspecific indicator of generalized nutrition
    5. BUN/creatinine ratio: Helps to differentiate between dehydration and renal disease; will be increased with cancer cachexia or volume depletion
    6. Iron status
        a) Folate: Will be decreased in malnutrition
        b) Serum transferrin: Indicates visceral protein and may be depressed with extended periods of malnutrition
        c) Iron and iron saturation: Not specific in nutritional assessment
  B. Radiology
    1. Upper GI series or barium swallow: To rule out obstructive process if symptoms warrant
    2. Other radiographic studies: CT, MRI, ultrasound, chest x-ray to rule out progressive disease

V. Differential diagnosis
  A. Dementia
  B. Congestive heart failure (see Chapter 40)
  C. Malignancy: Primary or metastatic
  D. Alcoholism
  E. Electrolyte imbalance (see Chapters 144–148)
  F. Drug-induced disorder (e.g., from amphetamines, chemotherapy)
  G. Depression (see Chapter 154)
  H. Anxiety (see Chapter 152)
   I. Fatigue (see Chapter 155)

J. Pain
K. Constipation (see Chapter 52)
L. Impaired absorption
 1. Cholestasis
 2. Postgastrectomy
 3. Small bowel or pancreatic disease
 4. Parasitic infection (e.g., giardiasis)
 5. AIDS (see Chapter 156)
 6. Mechanical obstruction (see Chapter 63)
M. Increased nutrient loss
 1. Diabetes mellitus (see Chapter 143)
 2. Chronic diarrhea (see Chapter 53)
 3. Chronic nausea and vomiting (see Chapter 59)
 4. Hyperthyroidism (see Chapter 149)
 5. Fever (see Chapter 140)

VI. Treatment
 A. Specific interventions for a specific etiology of weight loss and malnutrition can be implemented.
  1. No evidence exists to show that the paraneoplastic process of cancer cachexia can be reversed.
  2. No evidence exists to support or discourage dietary intervention with end-stage disease.
  3. Evidence supports the benefit of early nutritional intervention.
  4. Severely malnourished patients or patients with GI toxicity interfering with intake for greater than one week will benefit from enteral or parenteral supplements.
 B. Patient education to stimulate appetite
  1. Discuss diet and encourage intake of high-calorie, high-protein foods frequently throughout the day.
  2. Encourage activity, as tolerated, for appetite stimulation.
 C. For associated symptoms, prescribe appropriate medications.
  1. Nausea and/or vomiting (see Chapter 59)
  2. Constipation (see Chapter 52)
  3. Diarrhea (see Chapter 53)
  4. Dysphagia (see Chapter 65)
  5. Irritable bowel syndrome (see Chapter 71)
 D. Anticipatory guidance: Continue to help patients to view their weight loss as a symptom with an expected pattern specific to their disease/treatment. Use every patient encounter as an opportunity for anticipatory guidance.
 E. Consider the following medications for appetite stimulation/increased well being.
  1. Megestrol acetate: 800 mg po qd (available in suspension); low dose of 320 mg/day is effective for patients with advanced-stage cancer.
  2. Glucocorticoid/dexamethasone: 4 mg po qd; significant side effect profile with long-term usage

3. Metoclopramide: 10 mg po 30 minutes before each meal and at bedtime for two to eight weeks or cisapride 10–20 mg po qd; increases gastric emptying in the treatment of early satiety and postprandial fullness
4. Dronabinol (Marinol®, Roxane Laboratories, Inc., Columbus, OH): 2.5 mg po twice daily before lunch and dinner; a derivative of cannabinoid, increases hunger to increase weight

VII. Follow-up: Short-term: Patients should be followed frequently to monitor weight and to determine the effectiveness of dietary interventions.

VIII. Referrals
   A. Surgeon: If extent of disease is not certain, surgery may be needed for evaluative process or curative or palliative treatment.
   B. Dietitian: For assessment of dietary intake and suggestions for nutritional supplements and elimination of mechanical barriers
   C. Psychologist/counselor: If depression or other emotional disturbances appear to be a contributing factor to weight loss, refer for suggestions on appropriate behavioral counseling, medication, and follow-up.

References

Ahlbrecht, J.T., & Canada, T.W. (1996). Cachexia and anorexia in malignancy. *Hematology-Oncology Clinics of North America, 10,* 791–800.

Cangiano, C., Laviano, A., Muscaritoli, M., Meguid, M., Cascino, A., & Fanelli, F.R. (1996). Cancer anorexia: New pathogenic and therapeutic insights. *Nutrition, 12*(Suppl. 1), S48–S51.

Chernecky, C., & Berger, B. (1998). *Laboratory tests and diagnostic procedures* (2nd ed.). Philadelphia: Saunders.

DeConno, R., Marini, C., Zecca, E., Balzerini, A., Venturino, P., Groff, L., & Carneni, A. (1998). Megestrol acetate for anorexia in patients with far advanced cancer: A double blind controlled clinical trial. *European Journal of Cancer 34,* 1705–1709.

Glynn-Tucker, E. (1998). Malnutrition/cachexia. In C. Chernecky & B. Berger (Eds.), *Advanced and critical care oncology nursing* (pp. 461–475). Philadelphia: Saunders.

King, C. (1997). Nonpharmacologic management of chemotherapy-induced nausea and vomiting. *Oncology Nursing Forum, 24*(Suppl. 7), 41–48.

Laviano, A., Meguid, M., Yang, Z., Gleason, J.R., Cangiano, C., & Fanelli, F.R. (1996). Cracking the riddle of cancer anorexia. *Nutrition, 12,* 706–710.

Ottery, F. (1994). Rethinking nutritional support of the cancer patient: The new field of nutritional oncology. *Seminars in Oncology, 21,* 770–778.

Plata-Salaman, C.R. (1996). Anorexia during acute and chronic disease. *Nutrition, 12*(2), 69–78.

Rivadeneira, D., Evoy, D., Fahey, T., Leibermon, M., & Dray, J. (1998). Nutritional support of the cancer patient. *CA: A Cancer Journal for Clinicians, 48*(2), 69–80.

Chapter

63. Bowel Obstruction and Ileus
Jeanne Held-Warmkessel, MSN, RN, CS, AOCN®

I. Definition: Failure of intestinal materials to move forward in the normal manner

II. Physiology/Pathophysiology
   A. Normal GI fluid secretion totals seven to eight liters per day, which is mostly reabsorbed as it transits the length of the bowel.
   B. Pathophysiology
      1. Altered bowel motility
         a) Bowel becomes hyperactive above the obstruction, attempting to force bowel contents beyond the obstruction.
         b) After time, the bowel tires and stops its attempts to move the contents beyond the obstruction
         c) Bowel below the obstruction continues to function and produce stool until the bowel is emptied below the obstruction.
         d) Swallowed air accounts for much of the trapped gas in bowel obstruction.
      2. Loss of normal absorption capacity and the continued influx of fluids and electrolytes into the bowel causes bowel distention and depletes the intravascular volume.
      3. Bacterial overgrowth (aerobic and anaerobic)
         a) Overgrowth increases bowel gas, interferes with bowel absorption, and injures the bowel mucosa.
         b) Bacteria migrate through the bowel wall into the lymph nodes and blood stream.
         c) Bacterial endotoxins enter the peritoneal cavity, allowing more bacteria to migrate through the bowel wall.
      4. Damage to intestinal mucosa develops quickly when blood supply is impaired by increased intestinal intraluminal pressure from fluid accumulation. Fluids leak into the bowel and the mucosa may slough and bleed.
      5. Distant organ responses occur from release of systemic inflammatory substances.
      6. Pseudo-obstruction has no known cause but may be caused by autonomic nervous system dysfunction. The bowel functions as if obstructed, though no mechanical blockage is present.

III. Clinical features: Obstruction may be acute in onset, chronic, or recurrent. Ninety percent of bowel obstructions involve the small bowel.

A. History
    1. History of cancer and cancer treatment
    2. Current medications: Prescribed and over-the-counter
    3. History of presenting symptom(s): Precipitating factors, onset, and duration. Associated symptoms are vomiting, bowel changes, pain, flatus, and decreased urine output
    4. Changes in activities of daily living
    5. Past medical history: Abdominal surgery, Crohn's disease, irritable bowel syndrome, diverticulitis

B. Signs and symptoms
    1. Abdominal pain
        a) Spasmodic, colicky, crampy mid- to upper-abdominal pain
        b) May be diffuse or localized
    2. Abdominal distention: The more distal the obstruction, the worse the distention
    3. Reduced amount, reduced caliber, or absence of stool; as the distal bowel evacuates the remaining contents, stool will be eliminated, and obstipation occurs.
    4. Fever, chills: Suggest strangulation
    5. Retching and vomiting: May be feculent with small bowel obstruction. The more proximal the blockage, the worse the vomiting; the more distal the blockage, the longer it takes for vomiting to start.
    6. No flatus occurs if the obstruction is complete.

C. Physical exam
    1. Vital signs: Check for orthostatic hypotension; tachycardia, tachypnea, and hypotension occur from hypovolemia, fever.
    2. Neurological exam: Assess for change in mental status from hypovolemia, electrolyte imbalances.
    3. Integument exam: Assess for inguinal, femoral, or ventral hernia; radiation markings, abdominal mass(es), scars for possible causes of obstruction (e.g., adhesions). Assess skin and mucous membranes for dehydration.
    4. Pulmonary exam: Increased respiratory rate and decreased respiratory depth occur from pressure on the diaphragm secondary to obstruction.
    5. Abdominal exam
        a) Tenderness: Diffuse or at site of blockage; guarding could represent bowel strangulation or ischemia. Rebound tenderness indicates bowel ischemia.
        b) Distention: Measure baseline abdominal girth and monitor size to assess response to treatment.
        c) Bowel sounds: Usually hyperactive, high-pitched sounds (i.e., borborygmus) with periods of absence; as bowel tires, sounds stop.
        d) Ileus: No bowel sounds occur.
    6. Rectal exam: Assess for impaction; test for occult blood.

IV. Diagnostic tests
    A. Laboratory
        1. Electrolytes
            a) Decreased potassium, chloride, and bicarbonate levels with bowel obstruction
            b) Increased phosphorus and potassium with bowel strangulation

2. BUN/creatinine: Increased ratio from intravascular volume depletion from vomiting and bowel sequestration of fluid

3. CBC: Increased WBC with inflammation, ischemia, or perforation

4. Amylase and lipase: If strangulation is suspected, levels are increased, but the tests are not a reliable indicator.

5. Blood pH

   a) Metabolic alkalosis: With high intestinal obstruction

   b) Metabolic acidosis: With lower intestinal obstruction and bowel infarction, bowel gangrene, intravascular volume depletion

B. Radiology

1. Plain abdominal film and obstruction series (see Figure 63-1)

   a) In presence of complete bowel obstruction, x-rays show dilated bowel above obstruction, U-shaped bowel loops, minimal or no gas in large bowel, and air-fluid levels in multiple areas of bowel.

   b) With a partial small bowel obstruction, gas is present in the large bowel.

2. CT scan: For acute bowel obstruction, dilated bowel, or bowel filled with air above obstruction; may show etiology of obstruction (e.g., mass)

3. Barium sulfate contrast study: Contrast given orally (small bowel series); used if plain films are nondiagnostic and clinical findings identify obstruction and area of

---

Figure 63-1. Algorithm for Diagnostic Triage of Patients With Suspected Intestinal Obstruction

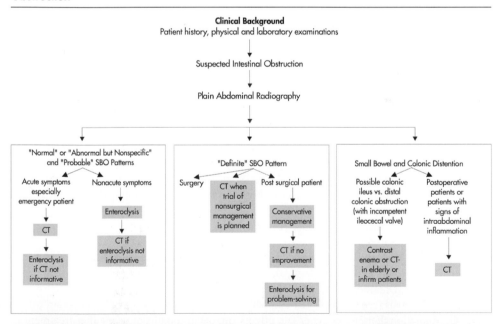

Note. From "The Role of Radiology in the Diagnosis of Small-Bowel Obstruction," by D.D. Maglinte, E.S. Balthzar, F.M. Kelvin, and A.J. Megibow, 1997, *American Journal of Roentgenology, 168,* p. 1178. Copyright 1997 by the American Roentgen Ray Society. Reprinted with permission.

blockage (water-soluble contrast agents [e.g., Gastrografin®, Olin Mathieson Chemical Corp., New York, NY] are diluted and fail to reveal blockage). Note: small bowel enema or enteroclysis require placement of a nasojejunal tube, through which barium and ethylcellulose are injected.

    4. Water-soluble contrast enema: Only used for large bowel obstruction to demonstrate area of blockage

C. Other: Endoscopic

    1. Proctosigmoidoscopy: To evaluate for large bowel obstruction

    2. Colonoscopy: Used to diagnose cancer or other obstructing lesions; has limited utility because oral preparation cannot be taken in presence of bowel obstruction

V. Differential diagnosis

A. Mechanical

    1. Small bowel

        a) Adhesions: From prior abdominal surgery, intra-abdominal infection

        b) Hernia: Inguinal, ventral, femoral

        c) Malignancy

        d) Inflammatory stenosis: From Crohn's disease

    2. Large bowel (most are sigmoid)

        a) Malignancy originating intraluminal (e.g., colon cancer), extrinsical (e.g., ovarian cancer), or metastatic

        b) Diverticular disease

        c) Volvulus: Bowel twisted on itself 180°

        d) Fecal impaction

B. Nonmechanical: Paralytic ileus secondary to

    1. Postoperative surgical complication

    2. Electrolyte abnormalities (e.g., hypokalemia) (see Chapter 144–148)

    3. Abdominal cavity inflammatory process: From infection, pancreatitis (see Chapter 72), peritonitis, inflammatory bowel disease

    4. Bowel blood vessel embolus or thrombus

    5. Fracture of spine, ribs, or pelvis: Possibly from reflex inhibition (see Chapter 104)

    6. Myocardial infarction: From impaired blood flow to bowel (see Chapter 47)

    7. Respiratory disorder: Pneumonia (see Chapter 30), pulmonary embolus (see Chapter 33)

    8. Retroperitoneal bleeding or inflammation: Ruptured abdominal aortic aneurysm, pyelonephritis

    9. Drug-/medication-induced disorder from

        a) Narcotics

        b) Plant alkaloids from neurotoxicity (e.g., vinblastine, vincristine)

        c) Anticholinergics (e.g., dicyclomine, hyoscyamine)

        d) Diuretics, causing hypokalemia

   10. Sepsis (see Chapters 121 and 140)

C. Radiation therapy: Acute or late effects can occur months or years after treatment is completed.

    1. Early: Ulceration may cause contraction of the wall with resultant obstruction.

    2. Late: Scarring over a period of months to years may cause strictures.

D. Strangulated (bowel dies quickly) versus nonstrangulated
E. Fecal impaction
F. Perforation versus nonperforation
G. Closed loop (two blockages) versus open loop (one blockage)
H. Porphyria: A heme biosynthesis metabolic disorder causing an attack that can be confused with a bowel obstruction.

VI. Treatment
A. Complete bowel obstruction or the presence of strangulation (i.e., loss of blood supply) indicates the need for emergency surgery after stabilizing the patient.
B. Partial bowel obstruction may be managed conservatively.
   1. Failure to improve in 48 hours indicates need for surgical intervention.
   2. Medically managed patients require frequent assessment and monitoring so surgery can be performed promptly if normal bowel function is not restored.
   3. Large bowel obstruction is managed similarly, but, usually, only 24 hours should lapse before surgery is performed.
C. Relieve distention and vomiting by decompressing bowel.
   1. Insert nasogastric (NG) tube and connect to low intermittent suction.
   2. Flush NG tube prn to maintain patency.
   3. Patient should have nothing by mouth.
   4. Monitor abdominal girth to assess response to bowel decompression. NG tube insertion and drainage should result in decreased abdominal girth.
D. Replace fluids and electrolytes.
   1. Start IV fluids; aggressive isotonic (NS) fluid replacement may be needed.
   2. Replace electrolytes as needed based on serum electrolyte results.
   3. Insert indwelling urinary catheter to monitor urine output with hypovolemia; oliguria often accompanies dehydration.
   4. Correct metabolic acidosis with sodium bicarbonate in IV fluids (alkalosis occurs with proximal small bowel obstruction) to return pH to normal range.
   5. Monitor intake and output closely.
E. Relieve pain
   1. Pain should decrease with NG tube decompression.
   2. Administer parenteral narcotics (usually meperidine) as needed to keep patient comfortable.
F. Monitor for signs and symptoms of ongoing complications (e.g., fever, nausea and vomiting, tachypnea, abdominal tenderness, guarding, blood pressure changes, change in mental status, oliguria), indicating possible
   1. Strangulation
   2. Perforation
   3. Peritonitis
   4. Sepsis
   5. Respiratory compromise
G. Surgical intervention (e.g., laparotomy) is required for most patients with complete small and large bowel obstruction, perforation, or ischemia to resect affected bowel or lyse adhesions.

H. Management of advanced or recurrent abdominal malignancy causing bowel obstruction
   1. Percutaneous endoscopic gastrostomy: For continuous drainage of chronic obstruction if it cannot be corrected surgically or with medication
   2. Long intestinal tube (e.g., Miller-Abbott tube) will accomplish same objective (rarely used).
   3. Placement of stent (endoprosthesis), or use of laser, dilation, or tube decompression: To prepare bowel for resection of malignant obstruction
I. Parenteral nutrition: If npo for at least seven days
J. Activity: Ambulate with ileus to promote bowel function.

VII. Follow-up
   A. Monitor for recurrence of obstruction after discharge.
      1. Patients with abdominal metastases may reobstruct if not resected.
      2. Some patients may not be surgical candidates because of extensive carcinomatosis and are at risk for reobstruction.
   B. Educate patient to call healthcare provider at first onset of symptoms so prompt treatment can be instituted.

VIII. Referrals
   A. Surgeon: To evaluate patient for acute abdomen
   B. Gastroenterologist: For diagnostic evaluation and endoscopy
   C. Oncologist: If malignancy-induced or malignancy suspected

References

Labovich, T.M. (1994). Selected complications in the patient with cancer: Spinal cord compression, malignant bowel obstruction, malignant ascites, and gastrointestinal bleeding. *Seminars in Oncology Nursing, 10,* 189–197.

Lopez-Kostner, F., Hool, G.R., & Lavery, I.C. (1997). Management and causes of large-bowel obstruction. *Surgical Clinics of North America, 77,* 1265–1290.

Maglinte, D.T., Balthazar, E.J., Kelvin, F.M., & Megibow, A.J. (1997). The role of radiology in the diagnosis of small-bowel obstruction. *American Journal of Radiology, 168,* 1171–1180.

Saclarides, T.J. (1997). Radiation injuries of the gastrointestinal tract. *Surgical Clinics of North America, 77,* 261–268.

Saida, Y., Sumiyama, Y., Nagao, J., & Takase, M. (1996). Stent endoprosthesis for obstructing colorectal cancers. *Diseases of the Colon and Rectum, 39,* 552–555.

Sagar, P.M., MacFie, J., Sedman, P., May, J., Mancey-Jones, B., & Johnstone, D. (1995). Intestinal obstruction promotes gut translocation of bacteria. *Diseases of the Colon and Rectum, 38,* 640–644.

Stone, R. (1996). Primary care diagnosis of acute abdominal pain. *Nurse Practitioner, 21,* 19–39.

Turnage, R.H., & Bergen, P.C. (1998). Intestinal obstruction and ileus. In M. Feldman, B.F. Scharschmidt, & M.H. Sleisenger (Eds.), *Sleisenger & Fordtran's gastrointestinal and liver disease: Pathophysiology, management* (pp. 1799–1810). Philadelphia: Saunders.

Chapter

64. Cirrhosis

Cindy Jo Horrell, MS, CRNP, AOCN®

I. Definition: Widespread fibrosis that surrounds regenerative nodules of the liver

II. Pathophysiology
   A. Hepatic lobules collapse from exposure to toxins, bacteria, and viruses.
      1. Injury occurs, ranging from limited necrosis of liver cells to destruction of entire lobules with collapse of reticulin framework within the area.
      2. Repair process involves production of connective tissue (collagen) to bridge gaps within the liver structure and regeneration or hypertrophy results of hepatocytes.
   B. Anatomic distortions, because of underlying collagen replacement, change the liver's structure.
      1. Regenerated lobules are perfused by the hepatic artery and may not have a draining central vein.
      2. Reduction in blood flow increases the resistance within the portal system, resulting in portal hypertension.

III. Clinical features: Liver failure appears when numerous functioning hepatocytes decrease or when resistance to portal venous flow results in symptomatic portal hypertension.
   A. History
      1. History of cancer and cancer treatment
      2. Current medications: Prescribed and over-the-counter
      3. History of presenting symptom(s): Precipitating factors, onset, location, and duration
      4. Changes in activities of daily living
      5. Past medical history: Hepatitis, alcohol abuse, hereditary liver disorders (e.g., hemachromatosis, Wilson's disease)
   B. Signs and symptoms
      1. Hepatocellular dysfunction
         a) Spider angioma
         b) Gynecomastia
         c) Palmar erythema
         d) Jaundice
         e) Testicular atrophy

    f) Impotence
    g) Weight loss
    h) Malnutrition
    i) Fatigue
    j) Pruritus
    k) Steatorrhea (late sign)
    l) Bleeding problems (late sign)
    m) Changes in mental function (late sign)
   2. Portal hypertension
    a) Bleeding
    b) Ascites
    c) Abdominal vein distention
  C. Physical exam
   1. Integument exam
    a) Presence of jaundice
    b) Hyperpigmentation
    c) Purpura
    d) Vascular spiders, spider angiomas
    e) Palmar erythema
   2. Thorax exam: Assess for gynecomastia, loss of axillary hair.
   3. Abdominal exam
    a) Presence of ascites
    b) Prominent abdominal wall veins
    c) Hepatosplenomegaly
    d) Firm liver edge: Indicates portal hypertension
    e) Presence of varicose veins radiating from the umbilicus (i.e., caput medusae)
   4. Extremities exam
    a) Peripheral edema
    b) Clubbing of fingers
   5. Neurologic exam: Mental status change, tremor, stupor, indicating encephalopathy
   6. Genitourinary exam
    a) Testicular exam: Atrophy
    b) Loss of pubic hair
    c) Rectal exam: Hemorrhoids

IV. Diagnostic tests
  A. Laboratory
   1. Bilirubin
    a) Total bilirubin is increased with hepatocellular damage.
    b) Direct and indirect bilirubin are increased with hepatocellular necrosis and cirrhosis.
   2. Transaminase
    a) AST: May be elevated or normal
    b) ALT: May be elevated or normal
   3. Alkaline phosphatase: Increased
   4. Albumin and immunoglobulins

        a) Albumin: Decreased

        b) IgA: May be elevated with alcoholic cirrhosis

        c) Total globulin level: Usually increased

    5. Prothrombin time: Prolonged

    6. Clotting factors: Decreased

    7. Blood ammonia: Increases with worsening of disease

    8. Electrolytes: Hyponatremia, hypokalemia

  B. Radiology

    1. Barium swallow: To evaluate varices in portal hypertension

    2. Ultrasound: To assess liver size and visualize nodular surface; to rule out veno-occlusive disease or obstruction

    3. Abdominal CT scan: If ultrasound is inconclusive

V. Differential diagnosis

  A. Alcoholic cirrhosis

  B. Primary biliary obstruction or cirrhosis

  C. Hepatitis (see Chapter 69)

  D. Hereditary liver disease

  E. Right-sided heart failure

  F. Tricuspid insufficiency

  G. Syphilis (see Chapter 95)

VI. Treatment

  A. Lifestyle changes

    1. Eat a well-balanced diet.

        a) Limit protein load.

        b) Administer branched-chain-enriched amino acid supplement to improve protein tolerance.

    2. Take a multivitamin daily.

    3. Cease alcohol intake.

    4. Restrict sodium to 1–2 g/day and diuretics in patients with edema and ascites.

    5. Caution against the use of hepatotoxic drugs (e.g., acetaminophen, aspirin).

  B. Pharmacologic treatment of cirrhosis (see Table 64-1)

    1. With known varices, administer H₂ blockers to decrease chance of bleeding; however, no scientific basis supports this practice.

    2. Spironolactone (Aldactone®, G.D. Searle & Co., Chicago, IL) is the first choice because it inhibits the hyperaldosteronism of portal hypertension.

        a) 100 mg po qd; maximum 400 mg/day

        b) If unable to tolerate because of tender gynecomastia, amiloride hydrochloride or triamterene is alternative (Midamor®, Merck & Co., Inc., West Point, PA)

  C. Pharmacologic treatment of portal hypertension (Maxzide®, Bertek Pharmeceuticals, Inc., Sugarland, TX)

    1. Prevent initial hemorrhage to lower portal venous pressure.

        a) Propranolol (Inderal®, American Home Products Corp., Madison, NJ): Start 10–20 mg po bid; titrate weekly to maximum of 160 mg per day, maintaining heart rate at 55 beats/minute or greater.

Table 64-1. Pharmacologic Management of Cirrhosis

Drug	Indication	Dose	Comments
Spironolactone	Edema/ascites	100 mg po qd in divided doses Maximum dose = 400 mg qd	Inhibits hyperaldosteronism of portal hypertension; can cause tender gynecomastia, hyperkalemia.
Furosemide	Given with spironolactone for persistent edema/ascites	20–40 mg po qd Maximum dose = 80 mg bid	Check weight, serum electrolytes, renal function frequently.
Propranolol	Lower portal venous pressure	10–20 mg po qd; titrate weekly to maximum dose 160 mg po qd	Maintain heart rate at ≥ 55 beats/minute.
Isosorbide dinitrate	Lower portal venous pressure	10–20 mg po qd; titrate according to blood pressure response	
Vasopressin (use with nitroglycerin)	Manage acute bleeding	20μ IV over 15–20 minutes, then 0.1 to 0.4μ/minute	Use with care in patients with coronary artery disease.
Nitroglycerin (use with vasopressin)	Manage acute bleeding	0.3 mg sublingual q hour or 0.2 mg/minute IV	Same as vasopressin
Vitamin K	Correct clotting abnormalities	10 mg sq qd x three days	
Octreotide	Mange acute bleeding	50 mg IV bolus, then 50 mg/hour IV up to five days	
Lactulose	Hepatic encephalopathy	15–45 ml po qd	Adjust to produce two to four stools/day.
Neomycin sulfate	Hepatic encephalopathy	1 g po bid–qid	
Metronidazole	Hepatic encephalopathy	500 mg po tid	
H₂ blockers	Reduce gastric acidity/reflux esophagitis in patients with varices	Cimetidine: 300–400 mg po bid Ranitidine: 150 mg po bid Famotidine: 20–40 mg po at bedtime	

       b) Isosorbide dinitrate (Isordil®, Ives-Cameron Company, New York, NY): 10–20 mg po per day; titrate according to blood pressure response.

  2. Management of acute bleeding

       a) Administer fresh frozen plasma to replace clotting factors.

       b) Vasopressin (Pitressin®, Warner-Lambert Co., Morris Plains, NJ): 20 units IV over 15–20 minutes, then 0.1 to 0.4 units/minute, *plus* nitroglycerin 0.3 mg every hour sublingual or 0.2 µg/minute IV. Use with care in patients with coronary artery disease or alcoholic cardiomyopathy.

       c) Octreotide (Sandostatin®, Novartis, East Hanover, NJ): 50 µg IV bolus, then 50 µg/hour IV up to five days

D. Bacterial peritonitis

  1. Patients with total serum protein of < 1g/dl have a 20% risk of developing bacterial peritonitis the first year after diagnosis. Ascitic fluid with a neutrophil count > 250 cells/mm^3 even if culture negative is diagnostic.

  2. Prevalent organisms include *Escherichia coli*, *Streptococcus pneumoniae*, and *Klebsiella pneumoniae*.

  3. Appropriate antibiotics include a five-day course of third-generation cephalosporins followed by quinolone therapy (see Appendix 1).

E. Peritoneovenous (LeVeen) shunting: Placed between abdominal cavity and internal jugular vein to manage ascites

F. Management of encephalopathy

  1. Lactulose: 15–45 ml po q four to six hours

  2. Monitor ammonia levels.

  3. If condition worsens, try neomycin sulfate 1 g po bid–qid/day, metronidazole 500 mg orally three times/day, or vancomycin 500 mg orally four times/day.

G. Nonpharmacologic management of variceal hemorrhage

  1. Transjugular intrahepatic portacaval shunts (TIPS): To lower portal vein pressure in patients with Child's C cirrhosis, Budd-Chiari syndrome, or diuretic refractory ascites

  2. Endoscopic injection: Sclerotherapy to achieve hemostasis by inducing thrombosis of bleeding vessel

  3. Variceal obturation: Injection of tissue adhesives into variceal lumen, causing nearly immediate occlusion

  4. Endoscopic banding ligation: Placement of rubber O rings on variceal columns, causing hemostasis through physical constriction of the varix

  5. Short-term control (less than 24 hours): Producing tamponade by the Sengstaken-Blakemore, Minnesota, or Linton-Nachlas tubes; use is restricted to situations in which pharmacotherapy or endoscopic therapy is ineffective

  6. Liver transplantation

VII. Follow-up: Depends on etiology

VIII. Referrals

A. Gastroenterologist: For management of varices

B. Hematologist: For anemia and coagulopathies
C. Alcohol/drug counselor: Refer if appropriate
D. Dietitian: For assistance with protein-calorie malnutrition
E. Surgeon: For placement of portacaval shunt, liver transplantation or resection

References

Brown, J.J., Naylor, M.J., & Yagan, N. (1997). Imaging of hepatic cirrhosis. *Radiology, 202,* 1–16.

Chung, R.T., Jaffe, D.L., & Friedman, L.S. (1995). Complications of chronic liver disease. *Critical Care Clinics, 11,* 431–441.

Gershwin, M.E., & Mackay, I.R. (1995). New knowledge in primary biliary cirrhosis. *Hospital Practice, 30*(8), 29–36, 79, 81.

McGuire, B.M., & Bloomer, J.R. (1998). Complications of cirrhosis. *Postgraduate Medicine, 103*(2), 209, 212, 217–218, 223–225.

Schiff, R.R., Sorrell, M.F., & Maddrey, W.C. (1998). *Schiff's diseases of the liver* (8th ed.). Philadelphia: Lippincott-Raven.

Trevillyan, J., & Carroll, P.J. (1997). Management of portal hypertension and esophageal varices in alcoholic cirrhosis. *American Family Physician, 55,* 1851–1858.

Chapter

65. Dysphagia

Gail Egan Sansivero, MS, ANP, AOCN®

I. Definition
   A. Dysphagia: Sensation of difficulty swallowing
   B. Odynophagia: Painful swallowing
   C. Achalasia: Progressive loss of motility

II. Pathophysiology
   A. Transfer dysphagia (also called oropharyngeal dysphagia) is a consequence of neuro-logic or neuromuscular disease, such as cerebral vascular accident, CNS tumor, or degenerative disease.
   B. Aging is associated with reduced upper esophageal sphincter (UES) pressures and delayed UES relaxation, which may contribute to an increased incidence of dysphagia.

III. Clinical features: The esophageal lumen generally is narrowed at least 40% before an individual exhibits dysphagia as a result of stenosis. Intermittent dysphagia suggests a motility disorder, while progressive, unremitting dysphagia is more likely related to an obstructive process.
   A. Etiologies: Dysphagia can occur as a result of
      1. Failure of the lower esophageal sphincter (LES) to relax
      2. Dysmotility (e.g., diffuse esophageal spasm)
      3. Esophageal stricture from cancer or benign reflux
      4. Extrinsic compression of the esophagus (e.g., lung cancer)
      5. Inflammatory processes related to infection or radiation reaction also may be present with dysphagia and may or may not cause fever.
      6. Age-related changes that may contribute to dysphagia include increase in fatty and connective tissue in the tongue, atrophy of alveolar bone, decreased esophageal muscle tone, and decreased salivary gland production.
   B. History: A tentative diagnosis can be made on the basis of thorough history.
      1. History of cancer and cancer treatment
      2. Current medications: Prescribed and over-the-counter
      3. History of presenting symptom(s): Precipitating factors, onset, and duration. Asso-ciated symptoms are choking, cough, weight loss, nausea, vomiting, and tremors.
      4. Changes in activities of daily living

      5. Diet history: Solids versus liquids, change in appetite
      6. Past medical history: Stroke, reflux disease, esophageal infections, Barrett's esophagus, immunosuppressive therapy, or immunodeficiency
      7. Social history: Smoking and alcohol intake

C. Signs and symptoms
    1. Subjective sensation of difficulty swallowing
    2. Pain with swallowing
    3. Sensation of heartburn or reflux
    4. Substernal chest pain
    5. Aspiration or regurgitation of fluid into the nose
    6. Halitosis (i.e., bad breath)
    7. Hiccups
    8. Sensation of a substernal lump
    9. Fatigue
   10. Weight loss
   11. Hoarseness (late sign, indicating laryngeal involvement)

D. Physical exam
    1. Vital signs: Assess weight
    2. Integument exam: Observe for hyperkeratosis on the palms and soles (a rare sign of esophageal carcinoma).
    3. HEENT exam
      a) Examine oropharynx for masses and inflammatory lesions.
      b) Examine dentures for fit and any signs of irritation.
    4. Neck exam
      a) Palpate lymph nodes for lymphadenopathy, suggesting malignancy or infection.
      b) Examine thyroid for masses or enlargement that may impinge on the esophagus.
    5. Pulmonary exam: Decreased breath sounds, crackles, and consolidation to rule out aspiration pneumonia
    6. Abdominal exam: For masses, tenderness, hepatosplenomegaly
    7. Rectal exam with stool testing: For occult blood
    8. Neurologic exam: Presence/absence of tremors, rigidity, and cranial nerve function (e.g., gag reflex, palatal movement, tongue movement)

IV. Diagnostic tests
A. Laboratory: Not indicated
B. Radiology: Barium swallow generally is the first step in the diagnostic process; provides a fluoroscopic record of swallowing difficulty and motor dysfunction.
    1. Sensitivity is excellent in determining the location and severity of an obstructing mass or lesion.
    2. Lacks sensitivity in identifying the nature of the lesion.
    3. Patient must be able to tolerate the supine position.
C. Other: Upper GI endoscopy is performed when a lesion is discovered and requires biopsy or if barium swallow is nondiagnostic.
    1. Allows dilatation to be performed at the same time as the diagnostic study if stricture is the problem
    2. Does not assess motor function.

V. Differential diagnosis
    A. Motor causes
        1. Transfer dysphagia
            a) Pseudobulbar palsy
            b) Myasthenia gravis
            c) Multiple sclerosis
            d) Amyotrophic lateral sclerosis
            e) Parkinson's disease
            f) Stroke
        2. Achalasia
        3. Scleroderma (progressive systemic sclerosis)
        4. Diffuse esophageal spasm
        5. Diabetic neuropathy (see Chapter 143)
        6. Hypertensive lower esophageal sphincter
        7. Metabolic myopathy (hypothyroidism, hyperthyroidism) (see Chapters 149 and 150)
    B. Obstructing lesions
        1. Esophageal cancer
        2. Benign esophageal strictures (e.g., reflux strictures or Schatzki rings)
        3. Zenker's diverticulum (weakness of the posterior hypopharyngeal wall)
        4. Plummer-Vinson syndrome (symptomatic hypopharyngeal webs occurring in women with iron deficiency)
        5. Lymphadenopathy (see Chapter 109)
        6. Mediastinal tumor
        7. Aortic aneurysm
        8. Food impaction
        9. Goiter (see Chapter 149)
        10. Postsurgical complications (e.g., laryngectomy)
        11. Foreign body

IV. Treatment
    A. Patients with reflux disease should be treated with antireflux therapy, consisting of behavioral recommendations, promotility drugs, acid-relieving medication, or a combination.
        1. Therapy may consist of a promotility agent.
            a) Cisapride (Propulsid®, Johnson & Johnson, New Brunswick, NJ): 10–20 mg po before meals (ac) and at bedtime (hs), which has action on both upper and lower sphincters. Avoid concomitant use of systemic oral antifungal and cisapride.
            b) Metoclopramide (Reglan®, A.H. Robins Company, Inc., Richmond, VA): 5–15 mg po ac and hs, which acts primarily on the lower esophageal sphincter LES. Extrapyramidal reactions are a common side effect.
            c) Diarrhea is a common side effect of these agents.
    B. Acid-reducing medications (see Chapter 66): Cimetidine, ranitidine, famotidine, antacids
    C. Behavioral modification
        1. Stop smoking.

  2. Stop or decrease alcohol intake.

  3. Decrease intake of spicy, irritating foods.

  4. Elevate head of bed for sleep.

  5. Avoid food ingestion two hours prior to sleeping.

  6. Decrease caffeine intake.

 D. When possible, give medications in liquid form.

 E. Treat patients with xerostomia with artificial saliva or systemic medication.

  1. For systemic dosing, pilocarpine hydrochloride (Salagen®, MGI Pharma, Inc., East Minnesota, MN) 5 mg po tid, with total doses of 15–30 mg/day, may be helpful. It may take up to 12 weeks to achieve maximal response from this therapy.

  2. For short-term relief of xerostomia, artificial saliva used prn may prove to be helpful.

 F. In patients with mild, nonspecific motor disease, symptomatic therapy may suffice.

  1. Advise patients to drink small quantities at a time, eat and swallow slowly, and thoroughly chew all foods.

  2. Avoid cold foods if they are particularly problematic.

  3. The goal is adequate nutritional intake with minimal discomfort.

 G. Antidepressants, antianxiety medications, and behavioral therapy may be helpful in patients with stress-related symptoms (see Appendix 2 and Chapter 152).

 H. Antifungal therapy is indicated in the treatment of patients with *Candida* esophagitis.

  1. Fluconazole (Diflucan®, Pfizer, Inc., New York, NY): 200 mg po initially, followed by 100 mg po for 3–14 days, depending upon severity

  2. Clotrimazole troches (Mycelex®, Bayer Corporation, Pharmaceutical Division, West Haven, CT): 10 mg dissolved in mouth (five/day) for 7–14 days

  3. Nystatin: 100,000 u/ml 5 ml swish and swallow qid for 7–14 days

 I. Esophageal pneumatic dilatation or surgical myotomy is indicated in patients with achalasia for whom more conservative measures provide no relief. Endoscopic injection of botulism toxin (Botox®, Allergan, Inc., Irvine, CA) also can be used in some patients.

 J. Patients with esophageal carcinoma may require multimodality therapy.

  1. Endoscopic laser ablation and esophageal endoprosthesis or stents

  2. Radiation therapy and/or chemotherapy or combination

 K. Benign strictures usually are best managed with endoscopic dilatation.

V. Follow-up

 A. Consistent follow-up with a dietitian to assess nutritional status is important.

 B. Intermittent assessment of albumin levels (approximately twice a year) may be helpful in evaluating nutritional status.

 C. Regular follow-up with an ear, nose, throat physician and a medical and/or surgical oncologist for patients with head and neck or esophageal carcinoma is indicated.

VI. Referrals

 A. Dietitian: For dietary modification; patients who aspirate during barium boluses may require a nonoral feeding program.

 B. Speech pathologist: For training and compensatory techniques that may treat oropharyngeal dysphagia

   C. Dentist: If ill-fitting dentures or poor dentition are problems

   D. Gastroenterologist: Patients with an obstructive lesion require referral for endoscopy, biopsy, and, often, for symptomatic management, including dilatation and stenting.

   E. Surgeon, medical oncologist, and/or radiation oncologist: For treatment following initial biopsy if malignant

References

Ali, G.N., Wallace, K.L., Schwartz, R., DeCarle, D.J., Zagami, A.S., & Cook, I.J. (1996). Mechanisms of oral-pharyngeal dysphagia in patients with Parkinson's disease. *Gastroenterology, 110,* 383–392.

Fulp, S.R., Dalton, C.B., Castell, J.A., & Castell, D.O. (1990). Aging-related alterations in human upper esophageal sphincter function. *American Journal of Gastroenterology, 85,* 1569–1572.

Logemann, J.A. (1990). Effects of aging on the swallowing mechanism. *Otolaryngologic Clinics of North America, 23,* 1045–1056.

Paterson, W.G. (1996). Dysphagia in the elderly. *Canadian Family Physician, 42,* 925–932.

Parkman, H.P., Maurer, A.H., Caroline, D.F., Miller, D.L., Krevsky, B., & Fisher, R.S. (1996). Optimal evaluation of patients with nonobstructive esophageal dysphagia: Manometry, scintigraphy, or videoesophagography? *Digestive Diseases and Sciences, 41,* 1355–1368.

Shaker, R., Ren, J., Zamir, Z., Sarna, A., Liu, J., & Sui, Z. (1994). Effect of aging, position, and temperature on the threshold volume triggering pharyngeal swallows. *Gastroenterology, 107,* 396–402.

Shaker, R., Ren, J., Podvrsan, B., Dodds, W., Hogan, W., Kern, M., Hoffman, R., & Hintz, J. (1993). Effect of aging and bolus variables on pharyngeal and upper esophageal sphincter motor function. *American Journal of Physicians, 264,* G427–G432.

Chapter

66. Gastroesophageal Reflux Disease
Diane G. Cope, PhD, ARNP-CS, AOCN®

I. Definition: Regurgitation of GI contents into the esophagus with or without manifestations of esophageal, laryngeal, or pulmonary injury

II. Physiology/Pathophysiology
    A. Normal
        1. The lower esophageal sphincter (LES) maintains a pressure barrier between the esophagus and the stomach.
        2. The hormone gastrin, alpha-adrenergic stimulation, and the vagus nerve promote relaxation of the smooth muscle of the LES.
    B. Pathophysiology
        1. Absence of the high-pressure barrier between the stomach and the esophagus increases reflux
        2. Intermittent relaxation of the LES as a result of inhibitory reflexes triggered by gastric distention increases reflux
        3. Inflammation of the esophageal mucosa that delays peristalsis, increasing the time gastric reflux remains in the esophagus; salivation and neutralization of gastric secretions are decreased.
        4. Reduced gastric storage capacity and increased postprandial intragastric pressure from conditions such as partial gastric resection can increase reflux.

III. Clinical features
    A. Etiology
        1. Abnormalities of the LES
            a) Incompetent LES
                (1) Drug-induced: Hormones, anticholinergics, calcium antagonists, theophylline, meperidine
                (2) Nicotine
                (3) Alcohol
                (4) Foods: High-fat, chocolate, peppermint
            b) Decreased LES tone: Gastric distention from obesity or ascites
        2. Impaired esophageal peristalsis
            a) Sleeping, which ceases swallowing

        b) Lying in a horizontal position, which increases time of gastric reflux contact with the esophageal mucosa

    3. Gastric emptying abnormalities

  B. History

    1. History of cancer and cancer treatment

    2. Current medications: Prescribed and over-the-counter

    3. History of presenting symptom(s): Precipitating factors, onset, and duration. Associated symptoms are voice changes and respiratory problems.

    4. Changes in activities of daily living

    5. History of diet

    6. Social history: Tobacco and alcohol use

  C. Signs and symptoms

    1. Heartburn: More common symptom

        a) Presents as substernal burning

        b) Usually occurs after meals

        c) Aggravated by position change

    2. Acid regurgitation: Most common symptom

    3. If reflux becomes severe, esophageal, laryngeal, or pulmonary injury may occur exhibiting the following symptoms.

        a) Chest pain

        b) Sore throat

        c) Dyspepsia

        d) Vomiting

        e) Belching

        f) Chronic cough

        g) Hoarseness

        h) Wheezing

    4. Dental erosions

    5. Hematemesis

    6. Weight loss

    7. Dysphagia

  D. Physical exam

    1. Vital signs: Assess weight; unexplained weight loss could indicate malignancy.

    2. Integument exam: Observe for signs of compromised nutritional status (e.g., poor skin turgor, loss of subcutaneous fat).

    3. HEENT: Observe for erythematous oropharynx, halitosis, and acid corrosion of teeth.

    4. Abdominal exam

        a) Abdominal appearance is usually normal but slight distention may be present.

        b) Mild pain may be elicited upon palpation of the epigastric area.

        c) Listen for normal bowel sounds.

    5. Rectal exam: Evaluate for occult blood, bright red blood, or melena.

IV. Diagnostic tests

  A. Laboratory: *Helicobacter pylori* serology to rule out infection

B. Radiology: Barium upper GI radiographic exam detects sequelae of gastroesophageal reflux disease (GERD) (e.g., ulceration, obstruction, stricture)

C. Other: Endoscopy detects sequelae of GERD (e.g., esophagitis, ulceration, stricture, Barrett's esophagus)

V. Differential diagnosis
   A. Cardiac disease
   B. Lower respiratory infections
   C. Gastric or duodenal ulcer disease (see Chapter 73)
   D. Cholelithiasis
   E. Esophageal infections (e.g., *Candida*)
   F. Barrett's esophagus

VI. Treatment
   A. Postural measures
      1. Place head of bed on four- to six-inch blocks.
      2. Avoid recumbent position for at least two hours after eating.
   B. Dietary measures
      1. Reduce meal size, and avoid late or large evening meals.
      2. Diet should be low in fat, avoiding spices, sweets, acidic foods, caffeine, alcohol, peppermint, spearmint, and chocolate.
      3. Limit chewing gum, sucking on hard candy, and drinking carbonated beverages.
   C. Lifestyle modifications
      1. Smoking cessation
      2. Weight reduction
   D. Pharmacologic interventions
      1. Modify or discontinue medications that decrease LES pressure (e.g., theophylline, anticholinergics, calcium antagonists, hormones).
      2. Antisecretory drugs: For erosive esophagitis
         a) H$_2$ blockers
            (1) Cimetidine (Tagamet®, SmithKline Beecham Consumer Healthcare, LP, Pittsburgh, PA): 400 mg po bid or 800 mg hs
            (2) Famotidine (Pepcid®, Merck & Co., Inc., West Point, PA): 20 mg po bid or 40 mg hs
            (3) Ranitidine (Zantac®, Glaxo Wellcome, Inc., Research Triangle Park, NC): 150 mg po bid or 300 mg hs
            (4) Nizatidine (Axid®, Eli Lilly and Co., Indianapolis, IN): 150 mg bid
         b) Proton pump inhibitors: For severe esophagitis or if refractory to antisecretory treatment for three months
            (1) Omeprazole (Prilosec®, AstraZeneca LP, Wayne, PA): 20–40 mg po qd
            (2) Lansoprazole (Prevacid®, Tap Pharmaceuticals, Deerfield, IL): 15–30 mg po qd
      3. Gastrokinetic drugs: Increase LES pressure and enhance gastric emptying
         a) Metoclopramide (Reglan®, A.H. Robins Co., Inc., Richmond, VA): 5–15 mg ac and hs

       b) Cisapride (Propulsid®, Janssen Pharmaceutica Inc., Titusville, NJ): 10–20 mg po ac and hs

       c) Bethanechol (Urecholine®, Merck & Co., Inc., West Point, PA): 25 mg po qid

    4. Cytoprotectant drugs: Sucralfate (Carafate®, Hoechst Marion Roussel, Kansas City, MO): 1 g po qid ac and hs

    5. Antacids

       a) Sodium bicarbonate (Alka-Seltzer®, Bayer Corp., Elkhart, IN): Two tablets dissolved in six ounces of water every four hours po prn not to exceed eight/day

       b) Calcium carbonate (Tums®, SmithKline Beecham, Philadelphia, PA): Two tablets po every four hours prn

       c) Dihydroxyaluminum sodium carbonate (Rolaids®, Warner Lambert Co., Morris Plains, NJ): One to two tablets po every hour prn not to exceed 14/day

       d) Sodium citrate and sodium bicarbonate (Di-Gel®, Plough, Inc., Memphis, TN)

       e) Magnesium trisilicate and sodium bicarbonate (Gaviscon®, SmithKline Beecham Consumer Healthcare, LP, Pittsburgh, PA): 80 mg tablets, two to four po pc and hs; liquid, 15–30 ml po one hour pc and hs

       f) Magnesium and aluminum hydroxides (Mylanta®, Johnson & Johnson-Merck Consumer Pharmaceutical Co., Ft. Washington, PA): 10–20 ml po one hour pc and hs

       g) Magnesium and aluminum hydroxides and simethicone (Mylanta II): 10–20 ml po one hour pc and hs

       h) Magaldrate (Riopan®, Altana, Inc., Melville, NY): 5–10 ml po one hour pc and hs

VII. Follow-up

    A. Short-term: Symptoms should improve in four weeks with H_2 receptor antagonist, antacids, and lifestyle modifications. If no improvement, patient may use proton pump inhibitor for four to eight weeks of therapy. If no improvement after eight weeks, refer to gastroenterologist.

    B. Long-term

      1. Encourage continued lifestyle modifications.

      2. Consider maintenance therapy after response with H_2 receptor antagonists.

VIII. Referrals

    A. Dietitian: To assist with dietary modifications

    B. Cardiologist: If suspect chest pain as cardiac origin

    C. Gastroenterologist: For further evaluation if symptoms remain refractory after eight weeks of therapy

References

Castell, D.O., & Johnston, B.T. (1996). Gastroesophageal reflux disease. Current strategies for patient management. *Archives of Family Medicine, 5,* 221–227.

Chiba, N., DeGara, C.J., Wilkinson, J.M., & Hunt, R.H. (1997). Speed of healing and symptom relief in Grade II to IV gastroesophageal reflux disease: A meta-analysis. *Gastroenterology, 112,* 1798–1810.

Isolauri, J., Luostarinen, M., Isolauri, E., Reinikainen, P., Viljakka, M., & Keyrilainen, O. (1997). Natural course of GERD: 17–22 year follow-up of 60 patients. *American Journal of Gastroenterology, 92*(1), 37–41.

Lagergren, J., Bergstrom, R., Lindgren, A., & Nyren, O. (1999). Symptomatic gastroesophageal reflux as a risk factor for esophageal adenocarcinoma. *New England Journal of Medicine, 340,* 825–831.

Locke, G.R., Talley, N.J., Fett, S.L., Zinsmeister, A.R., & Melton, L.J. (1999). Risk factors associated with symptoms of gastroesophageal reflux. *American Journal of Medicine, 106,* 642–649.

Middlemiss, C. (1997). Gastroesophageal reflux disease: A common condition in the elderly. *Nurse Practitioner, 22*(11), 51–61.

Parks, S.M. (1997). Omeprazole maintenance therapy for GERD. *Journal of Family Practice, 45,* 292–293.

Salzberg, S.A., & Newton, W.P. (1999). Omeprazole or ranitidine for intermittent treatment of GERD. *Journal of Family Practice, 48,* 332–333.

Scott, M., & Gelhot, A.R. (1999). Gastroesophageal reflux disease: Diagnosis and management. *American Family Physician, 59,* 1161–1169, 1199.

Sullivan, C.A., & Samuelson, W.M. (1996). Gastroesophageal reflux: A common exacerbating factor in adult asthma. *The Nurse Practitioner, 21*(11), 82–84, 93–94, 96.

Szarka, L.A., & Locke, G.R. (1999). Practical pointers for grappling with GERD. *Postgraduate Medicine, 105*(7), 88–90, 95–98, 103–106.

Chapter

67. Gastritis

Kristine Turner Story, RN, MSN, ARNP

I. Definition: Inflammation of the stomach (may be acute or chronic)

II. Pathophysiology
   A. Endoscopically, gastritis is gross mucosal changes of the gastric lining characterized by erythema, subepithelial hemorrhage, and erosions.
   B. *Helicobacter pylori* (*H. pylori*) gastritis is erosive and hemorrhagic or nonerosive and nonspecific.
      1. Erosive/hemorrhagic gastritis: Endoscopic findings include subepithelial hemorrhage, petechiae, and erosions that are superficial and patchy, local, or diffuse.
      2. There is no inflammation on pathology.
   C. Nonspecific gastritis: Findings seen on endoscopy range from normal to erythema to erosions to areas of gross ulceration. The diagnosis may require biopsy.
      1. Type A (atrophy) involves the proximal acid-secreting portion of the stomach.
      2. Type B (idiopathic) involves mainly the antrum but may involve the entire stomach.
         a) *H. pylori* is a spiral gram-negative rod that resides under the gastric mucosal layer next to epithelial cells.
         b) Initial infection by *H. pylori* causes an acute gastritis, followed by chronic mucosal inflammation.

III. Clinical features: May be asymptomatic to symptomatic with symptoms poorly correlated with endoscopic changes; characterized as acute or chronic
   A. Risk factors: See Figure 67-1
   B. Etiology: Gastritis is classified as erosive (hemorrhagic) or nonerosive (nonspecific)
      1. Erosive/hemorrhagic gastritis
         a) The most common cause is the use of NSAIDs, which cause mucosal erosion and gastric mucosal prostaglandin inhibition.
         b) Other causes are alcohol ingestion, aspirin use, stress during severe illness, and portal hypertension.
         c) In immunocompromised patients, erosive gastritis may be caused by bacterial infection, cytomegalovirus, or fungal infections of the stomach lining.
      2. Nonerosive/nonspecific gastritis

a) Type A: Relatively uncommon
  (1) The major cause is pernicious anemia, an autoimmune gastritis of the fundic gland caused by vitamin B_{12} deficiency, which causes mucosal atrophy (atrophic gastritis) and achlorhydria.
  (2) Three to five percent of patients with pernicious anemia develop gastric carcinoid tumors.
  (3) There is a small increase in the risk of adenocarcinoma of the stomach.
b) Type B: More common
  (1) The primary cause is *H. pylori* infection.
  (2) *H. pylori* is present in 30%–50% of the population.
  (3) Exact mechanism of spread of *H. pylori* is unknown; some evidence supports fecal-oral and oral-oral spread.
c) Most patients infected with *H. pylori* remain asymptomatic, and only a minority develop peptic ulcer disease (PUD).
  (1) The reasons are unclear but may be a combination of virulence of the strain of *H. pylori* and differences in host defense mechanisms.
  (2) Early age of developing the infection and smoking may increase the risk of PUD development.
d) Chronic *H. pylori* gastritis has the potential to induce metaplasia and dysplasia, causing an increased risk of gastric adenocarcinoma and non-Hodgkin's lymphoma of mucosa-associated lymphoid tissue (MALT-oma).

C. History
  1. History of cancer and cancer treatment
  2. Current medications: Prescribed and over-the-counter
  3. History of presenting symptom(s): Precipitating factors, onset, and duration. Associated symptoms are weight loss, nausea, vomiting, bloody stools, and bloody vomitus.
  4. Changes in activities of daily living
  5. Social history: Tobacco, alcohol, and caffeine use
D. Symptoms/signs
  1. Erosive
    a) Often asymptomatic
    b) Symptoms correlate poorly with endoscopic changes.
    c) The most common clinical manifestation is upper GI bleed.
      (1) Coffee-ground emesis

Figure 67-1. Risk Factors for Erosive Gastritis With NSAIDs

Medication-Related
- Concomitant steroid use
- High NSAID dose
- Concomitant NSAID use
- Type of NSAID (long-acting create a greater risk of gastritis than short-acting agents)
- Usage longer than three months

Past Medical History
- Prior history of peptic ulcer disease
- Smoking
- Alcohol use
- Coexisting systemic disease

Demographics
- Age ≥ 60 years
- Gender female

---

      (2)   Blood in nasogastric aspirate

      (3)   Melena

    d) Ulcer-like dyspepsia: Gnawing or burning sensation in the epigastric region that is relieved by food, antacids, or antisecretory drugs (less common)

    e) Dysmotility-like dyspepsia: Indigestion with bloating, belching, and fullness

    f) Nausea and/or vomiting, often postprandial

    g) Anorexia

  2. Nonerosive

    a) May have a transient clinical illness with acute infection characterized by nausea and abdominal pain for several days

    b) Chronic infections usually are asymptomatic unless there is PUD.

E. Physical exam

  1. Abdominal exam

    a) May have epigastric tenderness to deep palpation

    b) Normal bowel sounds

    c) No masses palpable

    d) No organomegaly

  2. Rectal exam

    a) No rectal masses

    b) Test stool for occult blood.

IV. Diagnostic tests

A. Laboratory

  1. CBC: To rule out anemia

  2. Chemistry profile: To rule out liver toxicity

  3. Serum IgG and IgA antibodies for *H. pylori*: IgG more sensitive and preferred; results reported as positive or negative

    a) Quantitative testing using enzyme-linked immunosorbent assays (ELISA)

    b) Qualitative in-office testing available for *H. pylori* test; results available in 10 minutes

    c) Antibodies will not differentiate acute from chronic infection and are not useful for determining eradication of active infection, as they will remain positive after successful treatment. They are most valuable in determining the likelihood that someone with upper GI symptoms may have active *H. pylori* infection.

B. Radiology: Upper GI series (least sensitive test for gastritis and will not allow biopsy)

C. Other

  1. Endoscopy with biopsy and use of rapid urease test: To detect production of ammonia by *H. pylori*

  2. Urea breath test: Detects production of *H. pylori* urease; more expensive than serum testing but less expensive than endoscopy.

  3. Recent treatment for *H. pylori* may result in false negative results on the above tests.

V. Differential diagnosis

A. PUD (see Chapter 73)

B. Gastroesophageal reflux disease (see Chapter 66)

  C. Gastric carcinoma and gastric lymphoma
  D. Biliary tract disease
  E. Food poisoning
  F. Viral gastroenteritis
  G. Nonulcer dyspepsia (see Chapter 54)
  H. Patients with severe pain at presentation
    1. Perforating or penetrating ulcer
    2. Pancreatic disease (see Chapter 72)
    3. Esophageal rupture
    4. Ruptured aortic aneurysm
    5. Ureteral colic
    6. Myocardial infarction (see Chapter 47)
  I. Patients with GI bleeding at presentation
    1. Esophageal varices or severe esophagitis
    2. Mallory-Weiss tear
    3. Arteriovenous malformation

VI. Treatment
  A. Erosive gastritis
    1. Eliminate the cause, if possible.
      a) Discontinue the use of all NSAIDs.
      b) Encourage smoking cessation.
      c) Encourage decreased alcohol and caffeine intake.
      d) Dietary modification plays no specific role.
    2. If NSAID use is necessary
      a) Use lowest effective dose possible.
      b) Switch to nonacetylated salicylate (Disalcid®, Riker Laboratories, Inc., St. Paul, MN) 500–3,000 mg/day po in divided doses or a nonacidic NSAID (nabumetone [Relafen®, SmithKline Beecham Inc., Philadelphia, PA]) 1 g/day po
      c) Coadminister a proton pump inhibitor with the NSAID.
      d) Coadminister mucosal protective agent.
    3. Treatment options for erosive gastritis
      a) Antacids: Administer one and three hours after meals
      b) Histamine receptor blockers: Generally given for six to eight weeks
        (1) Cimetidine (Tagamet®, SmithKline Beecham Consumer Healthcare, LP, Pittsburgh, PA): 800 mg po q hs or 400 mg bid
        (2) Famotidine (Pepcid®, Merck & Co., Inc., West Point, PA): 40 mg po q hs or 20 mg bid
        (3) Nizatidine (Axid®, Eli Lilly and Co., Indianapolis, IN): 300 mg po q hs or 150 mg po bid
        (4) Ranitidine (Zantac®, Glaxo Wellcome, Inc., Research Triangle Park, NC): 300 mg po q hs or 150 mg bid
      c) Proton pump inhibitors: Generally given for four to eight weeks
        (1) Omeprazole (Prilosec®, AstraZeneca LP, Wayne, PA): 20 mg po qd
        (2) Lansoprazole (Prevacid®, TAP Pharmaceuticals Inc., Deerfield, IL): 15–30 mg po qd

(3) Rabeprazole (AcipHex®, Eisai, Inc., Teaneck, NJ): 20 mg po qd
d) Mucosal protective agents
(1) Sucralfate (Carafate®, Hoechst Marion Roussel, Kansas City, MO): 1 g po qid for six to eight weeks
(2) Consider misoprostol (Cytotec®, G.D. Searle & Co., Chicago, IL): 100 mg po bid; titrate weekly up to 200 mg qid.
B. Nonerosive gastritis
1. The appropriate treatment for nonerosive gastritis is controversial.
2. Some authors recommend treating patients with nonulcer dyspepsia empirically with histamine receptor blockers or proton pump inhibitors for six to eight weeks before performing endoscopy.
3. Other authors suggest treating *H. pylori*-seropositive patients with dyspepsia with antibiotics without need for endoscopy.
4. Data do not currently support treatment of *H. pylori* infection for nonulcer dyspepsia or for the prevention of gastric cancer, although whether certain individuals or populations may benefit from such treatment remains uncertain.
5. Treatment options for *H. pylori* gastritis (see Chapter 73) are rapidly changing; consult the most recent literature or experts in the field of *H. pylori* for recommendations. At the time of publication, the following regimens are examples of treatment.
   a) Triple therapy for 14 days: Greater than 90% eradication rate
      (1) BTM: Bismuth 600 mg (two tablets) po qid, tetracycline 500 mg po qid, metronidazole (Flagyl®, G.D. Searle & Co., Chicago, IL) 250 mg po qid
         (a) Available pre-packaged under the trade name Helidac® (Procter & Gamble Pharmaceuticals Inc., Cincinnati, OH) and is the least expensive
         (b) Generally given with two to four weeks of a histamine receptor blocker
      (2) BTC: Bismuth, tetracycline, clarithromycin 500 mg po tid
      (3) RCA: Ranitidine bismuth subcitrate (Tritek®, Glaxo Wellcome, Inc., Research Triangle Park, NC) 400 mg po bid, clarithromycin 500 mg po bid, amoxicillin 1,000 mg po bid
      (4) RCM: Ranitidine bismuth subcitrate 400 mg po bid, clarithromycin 500 mg po bid, metronidazole 500 mg po bid

VII. Follow-up
A. Short-term
1. Patients should be seen two to four weeks after initiating therapy for symptom evaluation and to confirm compliance with medication.
2. Urea breath test is useful to determine eradication of *H. pylori* post-treatment, especially if symptoms have not resolved entirely.
B. Long-term
1. One-third of patients with bleeding ulcers re-bleed in one to two years; these patients require close follow-up (every two to three months).
2. Preventive treatment for patients with erosive gastritis is unclear.
   a) Long-term acid blockers at half dose is suggested.
   b) Some authors recommend full-dose long-term acid blockers.

VIII. Referrals
   A. Gastroenterologist: For endoscopy, acute GI bleed, evaluation of severe pain, and acute symptomatology
   B. Surgeon: For evaluation in acute GI bleed, severe pain, and acute symptomatology

References

Ament, P.W., & Childers, R.S. (1997). Prophylaxis and treatment of NSAID-induced gastropathy. *American Family Physician, 55,* 1323–1332.

Anand, B.S., & Graham, D.Y. (1999). Ulcer and gastritis. *Endoscopy, 31,* 215–225.

Cave, D.R. (1996). Transmission and epidemiology of *Helicobacter pylori. American Journal of Medicine, 100*(5A), 12S–18S.

Dattilo, M., & Figura, N. (1998). *Helicobacter pylori* infection, chronic gastritis, and proton pump inhibitors. *Journal of Clinical Gastroenterology, 27*(Suppl. 1). S163–S169.

Fay, M., & Jaffe, P.E. (1996). Diagnostic and treatment guidelines for *Helicobacter pylori. Nurse Practitioner, 21*(7), 28–38.

Fisher, R.S., & Parkman, H.P. (1998). Management of nonulcer dyspepsia. *New England Journal of Medicine, 339,* 1376–1381.

Forbes, G.M. (1997). Review: *Helicobacter pylori.* Current issues and new directions. *Journal of Gastroenterology and Hepatology, 12,* 419–424.

Hayat, M., Arora, D.S., Dixon, M.F., Clark, B., & O'Mahony, S. (1999). Effects of *Helicobacter pylori* eradication on the natural history of lymphocytic gastritis. *Gut, 45,* 495–498.

Huang, J.Q., & Hunt, R.H. (1997). Review: Eradication of *Helicobacter pylori.* Problems and recommendations. *Journal of Gastroenterology and Hepatology, 12,* 590–598.

Maton, P.N., & Burton, M.E. (1999). Antacids revisited: A review of their clinical pharmacology and recommended therapeutic use. *Drugs, 57,* 855–870.

McFarlane, G.A., & Munro, A. (1997). *Helicobacter pylori* and gastric cancer. *British Journal of Surgery, 84,* 1190–1199.

Ofman, J.J., Etchason, J., Fullerton, S., Kahn, K.L., & Soll, A.H. (1997). Management strategies for *Helicobacter pylori*-seropositive patients with dyspepsia: Clinical and economic consequences. *Annals of Internal Medicine, 126,* 280–291.

Peek, R.M., & Blaser, M.J. (1997). Pathophysiology of *Helicobacter pylori*-induced gastritis and peptic ulcer disease. *American Journal of Medicine, 102,* 200–207.

Chapter

68. Hemorrhoids

George Bryant, ND, APN

I. Definition: Dilatation of the arteriovenous complexes arising from the rectal mucosa

II. Pathophysiology
   A. External hemorrhoidal tag is fibrotic tissue that no longer has a dilated vein but can still become inflamed. It protrudes from the rectum, arising at the anal verge and extending down from the pectinate line.
   B. Thrombosed hemorrhoid is an internal hemorrhoid that has clotted.
   C. Internal hemorrhoids occur when the surrounding anovascular cushion prolapses into the anal canal arising above the pectinate line and can protrude through the anal canal. This causes the cushion to become entrapped and engorged by the internal anal sphincter.

III. Clinical features: External hemorrhoids are more likely to cause a burning sensation. Internal hemorrhoids do not cause pain and become symptomatic when prolapse and excessive engorgement occur, causing painless rectal bleeding noted after defecation. They are classified by location and position superior or inferior to the dentate (pectinate) line. This border area is a zone of transition between the rectum and anal canal mucosa.
   A. Etiology: Hemorrhoids can be related to
      1. Certain types of medications
      2. Lifestyle changes
      3. Medical conditions
      4. Carcinomas
      5. Increased portal/systemic venous pressure
      6. Liver disease
      7. Congestive heart failure
      8. A result of a shearing force, such as in moderate to severe constipation, causing prolapse
      9. Increased straining accompanied by Valsalva maneuver
      10. Constipation and diarrhea (contribute to hemorrhoidal development secondary to irritation)
   B. History
      1. History of cancer and cancer treatment

    2. Current medications: Prescribed and over-the-counter

    3. History of presenting symptom(s): Precipitating factors, onset, and duration. Associated symptoms are pain, itching, or burning during or after a bowel movement, and blood in stool or on the toilet paper.

    4. Changes in activities of daily living

    5. Past medical history

    6. Bowel pattern, diet recall

C. Signs and symptoms

    1. Anal itching (i.e., pruritus ani)

    2. Anal pain during defecation or between bowel movements

    3. Abdominal pain

    4. Bleeding

    5. Constipation/diarrhea

    6. Burning sensation (external)

    7. Difficulty sitting for prolonged periods

D. Physical exam

    1. Abdominal exam

        a) Normal bowel sounds

        b) Usually no abdominal tenderness

    2. Rectal exam

        a) External: Visible, palpable masses on exam; protuberant purplish nodules covered by mucosa are prolapsed internal hemorrhoids.

        b) Digital rectal exam (DRE): Usually no palpable masses unless external; then, a firm mass on the anal surface may be palpated.

            (1) Not tender unless thrombosed (a rope-like mass is felt)

            (2) Rectal vault is usually smooth; internal hemorrhoid usually cannot be palpated.

            (3) Assess for a rectal mass as a source of bleeding.

E. Internal hemorrhoids are graded on a scale of I–IV.

    1. Grade I: Not prolapsed

    2. Grade II: Prolapse upon straining but reduce spontaneously

    3. Grade III: Prolapse upon straining but require manual reduction

    4. Grade IV: Always prolapsed, not reducible

IV. Diagnostic tests

A. Laboratory: Hemoccult stool

    1. Will be positive if any blood is present

    2. Not reliable as first-line diagnosis

B. Radiology: When a definitive diagnosis cannot be made

    1. Barium enema: To rule out colon cancer or polyps; not as sensitive or specific in diagnosing rectal bleeding

    2. Air-contrast barium enema: To rule out carcinoma and inflammatory patterns

C. Other: Sigmoidoscopy is performed with flexible fiberoptic sigmoidoscope to verify diagnosis and assess hemorrhoid.

V. Differential diagnosis
   A. Anal fissure
   B. Prolapse of rectal mucosa (more common in the elderly)
   C. Protruding tumors (e.g., rectal polyp, carcinoma)
   D. Perianal abscess and fistula
   E. Condylomata acuminate
   F. Pruritus ani
   G. Anorectal Crohn's disease/ulcerative colitis
   H. Anal skin tags
   I. Hypertrophied anal papilla

VI. Treatment
   A. Nonsurgical methods: Aimed at conservative measures, alleviating symptoms, and promoting spontaneous healing
      1. Avoidance of direct pressure (i.e., sitting on a doughnut-type pillow) especially with thrombosed external hemorrhoids
      2. Sitz baths two to three times daily using warm water
      3. High-fiber diet with increased water intake
      4. Stool softeners/stimulant laxatives
         a) Docusate sodium (Colace®, Roberts Pharmaceutical Corporation, Eatontown, NJ): 100 mg po bid to start, then qd
         b) Casanthrol plus docusate sodium (Peri-Colace®, Roberts Pharmaceutical Corporation, Eatontown, NJ): One tablet (30/100 mg) po at hs
      5. Bulk laxatives: Patient must be able to increase fluid intake; Psyllium (Metamucil®, Procter & Gamble, Cincinnati, OH; Citrucel®, Merrell Pharmaceuticals, Inc., Cincinnati, OH; Fiberall®, Ciba-Geigy Corporation, New York, NY): One teaspoon po mixed in water as directed at hs
      6. Lubricants: Mineral oil: 10–30 cc po/day
      7. Topical preparations: To alleviate the pain and itching associated with hemorrhoids
         a) Hydrocortisone acetate 25 mg (Anusol® HC cream, Monarch Pharmaceuticals, Bristol, TN): Apply rectally bid.
         b) Praxomine 1%/hydrocortisone acetate1% (Proctofoam®-HC aerosol, Schwartz Pharma, Inc., Milwaukee, WI): Apply rectally bid.
         c) Witch hazel (Tucks®, Warner-Lambert Consumer Healthcare, Morris Plains, NJ): Use after each bowel movement.
      8. Analgesic topical rectal preparations: To help to alleviate pain
         a) Nupercainal-anesthetic: Use tid or qid.
         b) Anusol-anesthetic + emollient + protectant: Use three to four times/day.
         c) Live yeast cell derivative with 3% shark oil and polymercuric nitrate (antiseptic) (Preparation-H™, American Home Products Corporation, New York, NY): Use twice/day.
         d) Lidocaine 2.5% cream: Use twice/day.
      9. Systemic analgesics: Used in treating thrombosed hemorrhoids or in postsurgical thrombectomy.
         a) Acetaminophen: 650 mg po every four to six hours prn

      b) Oxycodone 5 mg/acetaminophen 650 mg (Tylox®, Ortho-McNeil Pharmaceutical, Raritan, NJ): One capsule po every six hours prn

B. Surgery
1. Endoscopy: If conservative measures are unsuccessful after one to two weeks and hemorrhoids are at least grade III or IV
2. Endoscopy: If thrombosis occurs, causing severe pain and evidence of strangulation or ulceration
3. Partial internal sphincterotomy: To relieve obstruction
4. Laser therapy/infrared coagulation (grades I, II, and III)
5. Hemorrhoidectomy (grades III and IV)
6. Electrocoagulation: For thrombosed and bleeding higher-grade hemorrhoids

C. Less frequent measures
1. Rubber band ligation: Grade I, II, or III
2. Injection with sclerosing agent (seldom used): Grade I or II
   a) Quinine and urea hydrochloride
   b) 5% phenol in almond oil
3. Manual dilatation of the anus (not standard therapy): To alleviate pressure from obstruction of the anal canal from thrombosed internal hemorrhoids

VII. Follow-up
A. Conservative therapy requires no follow-up if symptoms have spontaneously resolved using a nonsurgical treatment, especially for nonthrombosed external hemorrhoids or for grades I and II internal hemorrhoids.
B. Higher-grade hemorrhoids usually require closer follow-up after a procedure is performed; follow-up is generally one to two weeks postprocedure.

VIII. Referrals
A. Gastroenterologist/surgeon: Refer patients who do not respond to conservative measures for further evaluation.
B. Surgeon: Immediately refer patients with thrombosed hemorrhoids that cause severe pain and bleeding, resulting in strangulation and ulceration.

References

Mazier, P.W. (1994). Hemorrhoids, fissures, and pruritus ani. *Surgical Clinics of North America, 74,* 1277–1292.

Metcalf, A. (1995). Anorectal disorders; five common causes of pain, itching, and bleeding. *Postgraduate Medicine, 98*(5), 81–94.

Nagle, D., & Rolandelli, R. (1996). The primary care office management of perianal and anal disease. *Primary Care Clinics, 23,* 609–620.

Orkin, B.A., Schwartz, A.M., & Orkin, M. (1999). Hemorrhoids: What the dermatologist should know. *Journal of American Academy of Dermatology, 41*(3, Part 1), 449–456.

Pfenninger, J.L., & Surell, J.S. (1995). Nonsurgical treatment options for internal hemorrhoids. *American Family Physician, 52,* 821–834.

Polglase, A.L. (1997). Hemorrhoids: A clinical update. *Medical Journal of Australia, 167*(21), 85–88.

Schuster, M.M. (1995). Abdominal pain. In L.R. Barker, J.R. Burton, & P.D. Zieve (Eds.), *Principles of ambulatory medicine* (4th ed.) (pp. 447–456). Baltimore: Williams & Wilkins.

Trowers, E.A., Ganga, U., Rizk, R., Ojo, R., & Hodges, D. (1998). Endoscopic hemorrhoidal ligation: Preliminary clinical experience. *Gastrointestinal Endoscopy, 48*(1), 49–52.

Yussain, J.N. (1999). Hemorrhoids. *Primary Care Clinics, 26*(1), 35–51.

Chapter

69. Hepatitis

Gena Schottmuller, RN, BA, CIC, and

Nancy C. Grandt, RN, CNP, MS, AOCN®

I. Definition: An inflammation of the liver caused by a virus or toxic substance

II. Pathophysiology
   A. The hepatic inflammatory process includes lymphocytes and other nonmononuclear cells, as well as cell necrosis.
      1. Microscopic findings include hepatocellular necrosis, inflammatory infiltrates, and liver cell regeneration.
      2. The histologic pattern in the variety of hepatitis diseases cannot be clearly recognized nor used as a predictor of illness severity. Variability in the lesions may account for the differences in the damage to the liver.
   B. Typical morphologic changes include the portal, periportal, and lobular areas or may involve the entire liver.
   C. Types of viruses
      1. Hepatitis A: A RNA enterovirus; belongs to one serotype
      2. Hepatitis B: A DNA virus; produces an excess of hepatitis B surface antigen (HbsAg), which can be detected in the serum and associated with polyarteritis nodosa. This is a multisystem condition caused by inflammation and damage to small-sized arteries.
      3. Hepatitis C: A single-strand RNA virus with no unusual histopathologic finding
      4. Hepatitis D: A RNA virus; requires hepatitis B to be present and is able to replicate only in the presence of HBV
      5. Glomerulonephritis and cryoglobulinemia related to chronic hepatitis C are thought to be caused by immune complex deposition of viral antigen and/or antibody within the glomerular membrane.

III. Clinical features: Hepatitis may present without symptoms, as a subclinical illness, or as fulminate hepatic failure. Four clinical stages are easily identified: incubation period, preicteric phase, icteric phase, and convalescent phase. Not all individuals experience each phase.
   A. Etiology (see Table 69-1)
      1. Hepatitis A
         a) Contaminated food and water

Table 69-1. Characteristics of Hepatitis A Through Hepatitis E

Characteristics	Hepatitis A (HAV)	Hepatitis B (HBV)	Hepatitis C (HCV)	Hepatitis D (HDV)	Hepatitis E (HEV)
Epidemiology	• Worldwide, sporadic, and epidemic • Daycare-related exposures • Foodborne outbreaks • Most common among school-aged children and young adults	• Worldwide • Higher prevalence: Africa, Asia, and South America; seen in infancy and childhood • Lower prevalence: United States; most common in young adults (200,000–300,000 cases annually in United States) • 35% of cases of hepatitis	• Worldwide 20%–40% of cases of acute hepatitis • Major cause of non-epidemic hepatitis • Estimated 30,000 new acute infections annually in United States; 25%–30% are diagnosed • 1.5%–4.4% of general population have positive HCV antibodies • Leading reason for liver transplant	• Worldwide • Associated with HBV coinfection or super-infection • Self-limited or chronic progression	• Not endemic to United States • Epidemic in Asia, North and West Africa • Waterborne outbreaks • Common in young adults • Uncommon in children and elderly
Incubation period	• Two to six weeks; average three to four weeks	• Two to six months; average two to three months	• Two to 24 weeks; average six to nine weeks	• One to 24 weeks; average two to eight weeks	• Two to nine weeks; average four to six weeks
Transmission	• Fecal/oral route; person to person • Common source outbreaks: Contaminated water and food, poor hygiene, poor sanitation • Rarely: Blood transfusions, sexual contact • Greatest infectivity two weeks before jaundice	• Percutaneous and permucosal exposure: Blood, saliva, semen, vaginal fluids • Sexual contact • Perinatal • Illicit drug use • Needlestick, accidental • Tattooing and acupuncture	• Percutaneous blood exposure • Transfusion • Illicit drug use • Needlestick, accidental (rate is approximately 3%–10% following a needlestick) • Less frequently: Sexual contact • Perinatal	• Blood and serous body fluids • Parenteral exposure (common in drug-injecting population and hemophiliacs) • Sexual contact	• Fecal/oral route, person to person • Contaminated water

(Continued on next page)

Table 69-1. Characteristics of Hepatitis A Through Hepatitis E *(Continued)*

Characteristics	Hepatitis A (HAV)	Hepatitis B (HBV)	Hepatitis C (HCV)	Hepatitis D (HDV)	Hepatitis E (HEV)
Clinical signs and symptoms	• Malaise, anorexia, nausea, vomiting, fever, abdominal pain, jaundice, dark urine, lymphadenopathy, hepatomegaly • Can be asymptomatic	• Malaise, abdominal pain, diarrhea, anorexia, nausea, vomiting, fever, muscle and joint pain, jaundice, rash • Can be asymptomatic	• Malaise, anorexia, nausea, vomiting, abdominal pa n, jaundice • Commonly c symptomatic	• Resemble those of HBV; always associated with coexistent HBV infection; super-infection with HBV more severe than coinfection	• Similar to HAV
Onset	• Abrupt, severity related to age .	• Insidious	• Insidious	• Abrupt	• Abrupt
Specific tests	• Anti-HAV • Anti-HAV/IgM • Liver function tests	• HBsAg • Anti-HBc/IgM • Anti-HBs • HBeAg • Liver function tests	• Anti-HCV (if negative during acute phase, repeat in six months) • RIBA • HCV RNA • Liver function tests	• Anti-HDV (anti-delta)	• Anti-HEV not commercially available (test available at CDC) Exclusion of other hepatitis • Liver function tests
Vaccine	• Havrix®[a] • Vaqta®[b]	• Recombivax[b] HB • Engerix[a] B	• None	• Hepatitis B vaccine will prevent HDV infection	• None
Treatment	• None	• Alpha interferon and ribavirin may help chronic carriers	• Alpha interferon may help	• None	• None

[a] SmithKline Beecham Pharmaceuticals, Philadelphia, PA; [b] Merck & Co., Inc., West Point, PA

        b) Poor hygiene

        c) Poor sanitation

    2. Hepatitis B

        a) Blood contamination

        b) Saliva

        c) Body fluids

        d) Illicit drug use

        e) Accidental needle sticks or contaminated needles

    3. Hepatitis C

        a) Transfusions

        b) IV drug use

        c) Needle sticks

        d) Sexually transmitted disease

    4. Hepatitis D

        a) Blood and serous fluid

        b) Transfusion

        c) Sexual contact

    5. Hepatitis E: Fecal/oral route

B. Classification of hepatitis (see Table 69-1)

    1. Hepatitis A virus (HAV)

    2. Hepatitis B virus (HBV)

    3. Hepatitis C virus (HCV, formerly identified as non-A non-B)

    4. Hepatitis virus (HDV)

    5. Hepatitis E virus (HEV)

    6. Hepatitis F virus (isolated in human stool)

    7. Hepatitis G virus (seen in liver transplant patients and caused by chronic liver disease)

C. History

    1. History of cancer and cancer treatment

    2. Current medications: Prescribed and over-the-counter

    3. History of presenting symptom(s): Precipitating factors, onset, location, and duration

    4. Changes in activities of daily living

    5. Social history: Recent foreign travel, alcohol use, illicit drug use, tattoos, sexual orientation

    6. Past medical history: Exposure to blood or body fluids, blood transfusions

D. Signs and symptoms: Some individuals (especially children) may be asymptomatic (see Table 69-1).

    1. Incubation period: From exposure to symptoms

    2. Preicteric phase: From symptoms to jaundice; symptoms may include fever, malaise, anorexia, nausea, vomiting, and abdominal pain. Rash (typically pruritic hives, macular-papular lesions, or patches of erythema), myalgia, and arthralgia are often seen in HBV.

    3. Icteric phase: Jaundice, abdominal tenderness, dark urine, gray-colored stools, and pruritus may be present.

    4. Convalescent phase: Jaundice is gone. General fatigue and malaise may continue.

E. Physical exam
   1. Integument exam
      a) Vascular spiders may be found on light-colored skin on chest, arms, and hands.
      b) Skin excoriation from severe pruritus
      c) Rash common HBV-macular-papular, hives, erythema
   2. Abdominal exam
      a) Slightly enlarged and/or tender liver with smooth, regular border indicates acute hepatitis.
      b) Enlarged firm nodular liver indicates chronic hepatitis.
      c) Splenomegaly may be present.
   3. Neurologic exam: Assess for fulminant (late-stage) hepatitis; evaluate for lethargy, confusion, somnolence, forgetfulness, stupor, and coma.

IV. Diagnostic tests
  A. Laboratory
    1. Specific serologic assays (see Table 69-1)
      a) To rule out/confirm hepatitis
      b) Hepatitis Be antigen (HBeAg) is positive in early course of infection and persists in chronic disease; potential for more liver damage occurs.
      c) HBV DNA testing by molecular methods is useful in monitoring therapeutic responsiveness in chronically infected patients.
      d) To confirm positive anti-HCV, a follow-up HCV RNA test is performed.
    2. Liver function tests (LFTs)
      a) Aspartate aminotransferase (AST): 1.5–15 times normal
      b) Alanine aminotransferase (ALT): 1.5–15 times normal
      c) In chronic HCV, an increase in ALT and AST ranges from 1–20 times the upper limits.
    3. Bilirubin level: Variably elevated during the icteric phase
    4. Prothrombin time (PT): Typically normal in acute hepatitis and prolonged when more severe liver necrosis and fulminant hepatic failure are suspected
  B. Radiology: Ultrasound to rule out obstruction
  C. Other: Liver biopsy generally is not necessary but is indicated in the following situations.
    1. When diagnosis is not clear in spite of clinical and serologic data
    2. If more than one explanation of acute hepatitis is considered

V. Differential diagnosis (includes infectious as well as noninfectious hepatitis)
  A. Bacterial infections (pneumococcal pneumonia)
  B. Viral infections
    1. Hepatitis A–G
    2. CMV
    3. Epstein-Barr virus
    4. Herpes simplex (see Chapter 89)
    5. Varicella zoster
    6. Rubella
    7. Rubeola

8. Coxsackie
9. Adenovirus yellow fever
C. Drug- or toxin-induced
   1. Acetaminophen
   2. Chlorpromazine
   3. Halothane
   4. Methotrexate
   5. Isoniazid (INH)
   6. Phenytoin
   7. Methyldopa
   8. Inhaled anesthetics
   9. Phenothiazine
D. Autoimmune hepatitis
E. Cancer of the liver or metastasis
F. Radiation hepatitis with doses > 2,500 cGy to the liver

VI. Prevention
   A. Vaccine recommendations
      1. Hepatitis A vaccine: Havrix® (SmithKline Beecham Pharmaceuticals, Philadelphia, PA) 1 ml IM and Vaqta® (Merck & Co., Inc., West Point, PA) 1 ml IM
         a) Typically administered in two doses
         b) Effective four weeks after receiving vaccine
         c) Booster given 6–12 months later
         d) Individuals to immunize
            (1) Travelers to or workers in areas where HAV is endemic, excluding Australia, Canada, Japan, New Zealand, Western Europe, and Scandinavia
            (2) Sexually active homosexuals or bisexuals
            (3) IV drug users
            (4) Patients with chronic liver disease (include chronic HCV) who may be at higher risk for severe or fulminant HAV
            (5) Others possibly at increased risk (e.g., childcare workers, food handlers)
            (6) People in the general public who wish to achieve immunity
      2. HBV vaccine: Recombivax® IIB 1 ml (Merck & Co., Inc., West Point, PA) and Engerix® B 1 ml (SmithKline Beecham Pharmaceuticals, Philadelphia, PA) (see Table 69-2)
         a) Typically three doses: Initially, one month later, and six months later
         b) Given IM into the arm
         c) Individuals to immunize
            (1) All infants and adolescents not yet vaccinated
            (2) IV drug users
             (3) Sexually active homosexual and bisexual men
            (4) Household and sexual partners of HBV carriers
            (5) Patients in hemodialysis units
            (6) Recipients of clotting factor concentrate
            (7) Healthcare workers, and public safety workers who are exposed to blood and bloody body fluids

Table 69-2. Interpretation of the Hepatitis B Profile Recommendations for Hepatitis B Vaccination

Tests	Results	Interpretation	Recommendation
HBsAg	Negative	Susceptible	Vaccinate
Anti-HBc	Negative		
Anti-HBs	Negative		
HBsAg	Negative	Immune	Vaccination not needed
Anti-HBc	Negative or positive		
Anti-HBs	Positive		
HBsAg	Positive	Acutely infected	Do not vaccinate
Anti-HBc	Positive		
IgM anti-HBc	Positive		
Anti-HBs	Negative		
HBsAg	Positive	Chronically infected	Do not vaccinate
Anti-HBc	Positive		
IgM anti-HBc	Negative		
Anti-HBs	Negative		
HBsAg	Negative	Four interpretations	Vaccinate if clinical
Anti-HBc	Positive	possible*	situation warrants
Anti-HBs	Negative		

1. May be recovering from acute HBV infection.
2. May be distantly immune and test not sensitive enough to detect very low level of anti-HBs in serum.
3. May be susceptible with a false positive anti-HBc.
4. May be undetectable level of HBsAg present in the serum and the person is actually a carrier.

Note. Table adapted from Immunization Action Coalition (www.immunize.org/genr.d/quesfreq.htm).

        (8) Clients and staff working with institutionalized, developmentally disabled individuals
        (9) Inmates of long-term correctional facilities
      (10) Patients with chronic HCV infection
      (11) Pregnant women who are chronic carriers
      (12) Infants born to HBsAg-positive mothers
      (13) Travelers to countries with high HBV rate (e.g., Africa, Asia, South America)

B. Management of close contacts of HAV
    1. Immune globulin (IG) given IM, 0.02 mg/kg of body weight, as soon as possible after direct contact exposure (within 48 hours of exposure) may be protective up to two weeks after contact.
    2. HAV vaccine 1 ml IM (Havrix® or Vaqta®) may be considered for postexposure prophylaxis and administered concurrently with IG at a separate anatomic injection site.

C. Management of individuals exposed to HBV (see Table 69-3)
    1. Immediate: Wash with soap and water, apply disinfectant to puncture wounds and cutaneous injuries, and flush exposed mucous membrane with copious amounts of water/saline.

Table 69-3. Recommended Postexposure Prophylaxis for Percutaneous or Permucosal Exposure to Hepatitis B Virus

Vaccination and antibody response status of exposed person	Treatment when source is		
	HBsAg[a]-Positive	HBsAg-Negative	Source Not Tested or Status Unknown
Unvaccinated	HBIG[b] x 1: Initiate HB vaccine series[c]	Initiate HB vaccine series	Initiate HB vaccine series
Previously vaccinated, known responder[d]	No treatment	No treatment	No treatment
Known non-responder	HBIG x 2 or HBIG x 1 and initiate revaccination	No treatment	If known high-risk source, treat as if source were HBsAg-positive
Antibody response unknown	Test exposed person for anti-HBs[e] 1. If adequate[d], no treatment 2. In inadequate[d], HBIG x 1 and vaccine booster	No treatment	Test exposed person for anti-HBs 1. If adequate[d], no treatment 2. If inadequate[d], initiate revaccination

[a]Hepatitis B surface antigen; [b]Hepatitis B immune globulin: Dose 0.06 ml/kg IM; [c]Hepatitis B vaccine; [d]Responder is defined as a person with adequate levels of serum antibody to hepatitis B surface antigen (i.e., anti-HBs $\geq$ 10 mIU/ml); inadequate response to vaccination defined as serum anti-HBs < 10 mIU/ml.; [e]Antibody to hepatitis B surface antigen

Note. From "Immunization of Health-Care Workers. Recommendations of the Advisory Committee on Immunization Practices (ACIP) and the Hospital Infection Control Practices Advisory Committee (HICPAC)," by Centers for Disease Control and Prevention, 1997, *MMWR, 46*(No. RR-18), pp. 1–42.

2. Draw blood to determine HBV antibody status if unknown. It is not necessary to do further testing on individuals who have had a positive antibody response following a series of three doses of vaccine.
3. Hepatitis B immune globulin (HBIG) should be given for prophylactic treatment to exposed susceptible individuals.
    a) Give a single dose, 0.06 ml/kg or 5 ml for adults, IM as soon as possible, within 24 hours of a high-risk exposure.
    b) Initiate HBV vaccine series.
4. HBV vaccine: Typically administered in three doses (initially, one month later, and six months later) given IM into the arm.

VII. Treatment
    A. No specific therapies are well-accepted for acute viral hepatitis.
    B. Interferon alfa-2b has been effective for chronic HBV and HCV to slow down progressive destruction and to decrease viral load. No beneficial effect has been shown in treating fulminant HBV.

1. Chronic HCV: Treat with alpha interferon dose of three million units three times/week subcutaneously for 6–12 months. Patients who do not normalize the ALT after 16 weeks of therapy rarely achieve a sustained response with extension of treatment.
2. Specific criteria must be met (persistent elevated ALT for six months and a positive HCV RNA). Liver bioposy may be performed to demonstrate portal fibrosis, inflammation, and necrosis.
3. Ribavirin is indicated in combination with alpha interferon for the treatment of chronic HCV in patients with compensated liver disease previously untreated with interferon or who have relapsed following alpha interferon therapy. Doses are as follows (administered as aerosol using SPAG-2 aerosol generator).
   a) Body weight less than 75 kg: 400 mg every am and 600 mg every pm
   b) Body weight greater than 75 kg: 600 mg q 12 hours.
4. Chronic HBV: Treat with alpha interferon five million units SC daily or 10 million units subcutaneously three times/week for 16 weeks.
C. Corticosteroids have not been shown to shorten the course or to help the healing process.
D. Evaluate all of patient's current medications; limit those metabolized in the liver.

VIII. Follow-up
A. Short-term
   1. Monitor LFTs during acute phase regularly and specifically for three to six months.
   2. Monitor ALT, AST, alkaline phosphatase, bilirubin levels, and PT one or two times weekly and every one to two weeks until normal.
   3. Provide education for prevention of transmission and good health maintenance.
      a) Refrain from donating blood, organs, tissues, or semen.
      b) Practice safe sex.
      c) Refrain from sharing razors and toothbrushes.
   4. Monitor CBC and ALT monthly while on interferon and/or ribavirin.
B. Long-term
   1. HAV: Typically a self-limiting disease; monitor older patients for acute liver failure.
   2. HBV
      a) If HBsAg is positive, repeat every one to two months until it is undetectable.
      b) HBeAg requested when HBsAg is positive; indicates a high likelihood of infectivity.
      c) The presence of HBsAg and HBeAg four to six months after acute disease indicates chronic carrier state.
   3. HCV
      a) When serology for HCV is negative initially, recheck antibodies in six months. If positive, conduct further follow-up to rule out chronic HCV.
      b) To confirm a positive anti-HCV, conduct a follow-up HCV RNA.
      c) HAV and HBV vaccination is recommended for all HCV-positive patients.

IX. Referrals: Upon positive serology and/or persistent abnormal LFTs
A. Infectious disease specialist to develop treatment plan
B. Gastroenterologist/hepatologist to perform liver biopsy

C. Public health departments (reportable disease)
D. Resource: Advisory Committee on Immunization Practices (ACIP): Phone number is 800-232-2522.

References

Baker, D.A. (1996). Viral hepatitis. In R.N. Olmstead (Ed.), *APIC infection control and applied epidemiology: Principles and practice* (II, B, pp. 1–9) St. Louis: Mosby.

Benenson, A.S. (Ed.). (1995). *Control of communicable diseases manual* (16th ed.). New York: American Public Health Association.

Centers for Disease Control and Prevention. (1996). Prevention of hepatitis A through active or passive immunization. Recommendations of the Advisory Committee on Immunization Practices (ACIP). *MMWR, 45*(No. RR-15), 1–30.

Centers for Disease Control and Prevention. (1997). Immunization of health-care workers. Recommendations of the Advisory Committee on Immunization Practices (ACIP) and the Hospital Infection Control Practices Advisory Committee (HICPAC). *MMWR, 46*(No. RR-18), 1–42.

Hoofnagle, J.H., & DiBisceglie, A.M. (1997). The treatment of chronic viral hepatitis. *New England Journal of Medicine, 336,* 347–356.

Johnson, R.J., Gretch, D.R., Yamabe, H., Hart, J., Bacchi, C.E., Hartwell, P., Couser, W.G., Corey, L., Weller, M.H., Alpers, C.E., & Willson, R. (1993). Membranoproliferative glomerulonephritis associated with hepatitis C virus infection. *New England Journal of Medicine, 328,* 465–470.

Lee, W.A. (1997). Hepatitis B virus infection. *New England Journal of Medicine, 337,* 1733–1745.

Marcus, E.L., & Tur-Kaspa, R. (1997). Viral hepatitis in older adults. *Journal of the American Geriatrics Society, 45,* 755–763.

Minnesota Department of Health. (1998). Viral hepatitis prevention: What providers can do. *Disease Control Newsletter, 26*(3), 21–28.

Najm, W. (1997). Viral hepatitis: How to manage type C and D infection. *Geriatrics, 52*(5), 28–37.

National Institutes of Health. (1997). Management of hepatitis C. *NIH Consensus Statement, 15*(3), 1–41.

Schiff, E.R., Sorrell, M.F., & Maddrey, W.C. (1999). *Schiff's diseases of the liver* (8th ed.). Philadelphia: Lippincott-Raven.

Weiss, R. (1999). Hepatitis B virus: DNA quantitation (viral load). In ARUP Laboratories, Inc. (Ed.), *ARUP's guide to clinical laboratory testing* (p. 271). Salt Lake City: ARUP Laboratories Inc.

Zimmerman, R.K., Ruben, F.L., & Ahwesh, E.R. (1997). Hepatitis B virus infection, HBV and HBIG. *Journal of Family Practice, 45,* 295–309.

70. Hepatotoxicity

Cindy Jo Horrell, MS, CRNP, AOCN®

I. Definition: Damage to the liver caused by disturbances in portal and hepatic circulation, hepatobiliary tract disorders, and/or hepatocellular changes

II. Physiology/Pathophysiology
   A. Normal
      1. Metabolic functions of the liver
         a) Carbohydrate metabolism
            (1) Maintains blood glucose levels
            (2) Provides energy for cells
            (3) Stores excess carbohydrates as glycogen and fat
         b) Fat metabolism
            (1) Synthesizes and degrades fats to fatty acids
            (2) Synthesizes and degrades triglycerides, cholesterol, phospholipids, and lipoproteins
            (3) Forms bile salts through metabolism of cholesterol
         c) Protein metabolism
            (1) Synthesizes and releases plasma proteins and enzymes
            (2) Deaminates amino acids
            (3) Converts ammonia to urea
            (4) Synthesizes blood clotting factors (I, II, V, VII, IX, X)
         d) Transforms drugs into active metabolites or harmless substances for excretion
      2. Normal filtration functions: Kupffer's cells remove bacteria, antigens, and by-products of coagulation, as well as other harmful substances from the blood.
      3. Normal storage functions
         a) Sinusoids hold blood for shunting into general circulation.
         b) Stores fat-soluble vitamins (A, D, E, K) as well as the water-soluble vitamin B_{12}
         c) Stores copper and iron minerals
      4. Normal excretion of bilirubin
         a) After formation in reticuloendothelial cells, bilirubin is bound to albumin and transported to liver, conjugated, and excreted into the bile.
         b) From there, bilirubin is excreted via biliary tree into small intestine.

    c) Intestinal bacteria reduce conjugated bilirubin into urobilinogen, which is excreted in stool or urine or reabsorbed into portal blood.

  B. Pathophysiology

   1. Pathologic changes of the liver are broadly categorized as neoplastic, inflammatory, or fibrotic.

   2. Damage to hepatocytes

    a) Leads to impaired metabolism and elimination of bilirubin

    b) Depresses synthesis of Factors I, II, V, VII, IX, and X

    c) Diminishes glucose synthesis

    d) Decreases lactate uptake or increases intracellular lactate generation caused by anaerobic glycolysis

    e) Triggers hepatocellular injury from direct toxin effects or as an idiosyncratic reaction

III. Clinical features

  A. Etiology: Mechanisms causing an elevated bilirubin

   1. Overproduction of bilirubin

   2. Reduction in its hepatic uptake or conjugation

   3. Decreased biliary excretion

    a) By cell mechanisms (e.g., intrahepatic cholestasis)

    b) By duct obstruction (e.g., extrahepatic cholestasis)

  B. History

   1. History of cancer and cancer treatment

   2. Current medications: Prescribed and over-the-counter

   3. History of presenting symptom(s): Precipitating factors, onset, location, and duration

   4. Changes in activities of daily living

   5. Social history: Alcohol intake, use of illicit drugs, recent foreign travel

   6. Past medical history: Organ transplant (e.g., liver, renal, bone marrow/peripheral blood stem cell), hepatitis or exposure to infected individuals

   7. Family history: Hereditary liver diseases

  C. Signs and symptoms

   1. Varying degrees of jaundice

   2. Varying color changes in urine and stool

   3. Pruritus

   4. Edema

   5. Ecchymosis

   6. Malaise, anorexia, headache, muscle and joint aches, and low-grade fever, suggesting hepatitis

  D. Physical exam

   1. Vital signs: Fever may suggest hepatitis.

   2. Integument exam

    a) Assess for jaundice.

    b) Assess for ecchymosis and petechia.

   3. HEENT exam: Assess for icteric sclera.

   4. Neurologic exam: Assess for altered behavior, level of orientation, and mental status.

   5. Cardiac and pulmonary exam: Assess for signs of congestive heart failure (e.g., peripheral edema, extra heart sound, rales)

      6. Abdominal exam
        a) Assess for ascites.
        b) Assess liver for hepatomegaly, contour, and texture.

IV. Diagnostic tests
  A. Laboratory
    1. Serum aminotransferase: Elevated levels indicate liver injury from either cell necrosis or increased cell permeability.
      a) ALT: Specific indicator of liver damage
      b) AST: Generally sensitive for liver disease; elevation of AST often greater than ALT in alcohol-related liver disease (an increase in AST can come from muscle breakdown, as well)
    2. Alkaline phosphatase (ALP): Released by disorders affecting the bile duct; markedly elevated levels reflect hepatotoxicity, prolonged cholestasis, and extrahepatic and intrahepatic obstruction.
    3. GGT: Sensitive but not specific; used in conjunction with alkaline phosphatase, can help to distinguish liver origin from bone
    4. Serum bilirubin
      a) Elevated indirect (unconjugated) bilirubin indicates liver damage and is seen in hemolytic anemia, congenital enzyme deficiencies, and severe chronic hepatic damage.
      b) Elevated direct (conjugated) bilirubin reflects excess amounts excreted into serum from obstruction of bile ducts and is seen in viral hepatitis, cirrhosis, and obstruction to bile flow (e.g., gallstones, cancer of the head of the pancreas or ampulla of Vater).
  B. Radiology: Percutaneous transhepatic cholangiography (PTC)
    1. Complements endoscopic retrograde cholangiopancreatography (ERCP)
    2. Useful when biliary obstruction is proximal to common hepatic duct or with altered anatomy or postsurgical alterations

V. Differential diagnosis
  A. Portal and hepatic circulation disturbances
    1. Portal hypertension
    2. Budd-Chiari syndrome (thrombosis of hepatic vein)
    3. Congestive heart failure (see Chapter 40)
    4. Veno-occlusive disease
  B. Hepatobiliary tract disorders
    1. Primary biliary cirrhosis
    2. Sclerosing cholangitis
    3. Wilson's disease (inherited disorder of metabolism creating copper overload)
    4. Malignancy
  C. Hepatocellular disturbances
    1. Hepatitis (see Chapter 69)
    2. Cirrhosis (see Chapter 64)
    3. $Alpha_1$-antitrypsin deficiency

    4. Hemochromatosis
    5. Hepatic failure
    6. Reye's syndrome
    7. Diabetes mellitus (see Chapter 143)
  D. Drug-induced: Any hepatotoxic drugs
    1. Acetaminophen
    2. Halothane
    3. Isoniazid
    4. Methyldopa
    5. Valproic acid
    6. Trimethoprim-sulfamethizole
    7. Erythromycin
    8. Chlorpromazine
    9. NSAIDs

  VI. Treatment: Depends on diagnosis (see related sections)

 VII. Follow-up: Depends on diagnosis (see related sections)

VIII. Referrals: Depend on diagnosis (see related sections)

References

Bach, N. (1994). A pragmatic approach to liver function tests. *Hospital Medicine, 30,* 45–46, 51–53, 73–75.

Ginsberg, A.L. (1996). Liver enzyme abnormalities: How to interpret the diagnostic implications. *Consultant, 36,* 575–378.

Gordon, R.D. (1997). Liver transplantation and venous disorders of the liver. *Liver Transplantation and Surgery, 3*(5, Suppl. 1), 541–551.

Herlong, H.F. (1994). Approach to the patient with abnormal liver enzymes. *Hospital Practice, 29*(11), 32–38.

Lidofsky, S.D. (1995). Fulminant hepatic failure. *Critical Care Clinics, 11,* 415–430.

Porth, C.M. (1994). *Pathophysiology: Concepts of altered health states* (4th ed.) (pp. 844–850). Philadelphia: Lippincott.

Scheig, R. (1996). Evaluation of tests used to screen patients with liver disorders. *Primary Care: Clinics in Office Practice, 23,* 551–560.

71. Irritable Bowel Syndrome

Kristine Turner Story, RN, MSN, ARNP

I. Definition
   A. A functional disorder or disturbance of intestinal motility and visceral perception strongly influenced by emotional factors
   B. By definition, no structural abnormalities or organic diseases should be identifiable for symptoms. Diagnosis of irritable bowel syndrome (IBS) is by exclusion.

II. Pathophysiology: Results from dysregulation of intestinal motor and sensory function as modulated by the central nervous system

III. Clinical features: Symptoms usually are intermittent, lasting days, weeks, or months with the same amount of symptom-free time. IBS usually presents in adolescence and young adulthood; onset after age 50 is unlikely. Women usually have a higher incidence of IBS, although the incidence in men and women actually may be similar, as men may be underdiagnosed. Many women with IBS have a history of sexual or verbal abuse.
   A. Etiology: Studies have identified a combination of factors that contribute to the syndrome.
      1. Abnormal gut motility: Characterized by increased motility and abnormal bowel contractions
      2. Enhanced visceral perception: Increased sensitivity of the bowel; may worsen after intestinal infection or surgery, suggesting inflammation may be an activating factor.
      3. Psychosocial factors: People with IBS have an increased effect of stress on the gut and tend to have more stress than people without IBS.
   B. History
      1. History of cancer and cancer treatment
      2. Current medications: Prescribed and over-the-counter
      3. History of presenting symptom(s): Precipitating factors, onset, and duration. Associated symptoms are weight loss, fever, night sweats, nausea, and vomiting.
      4. Changes in activities of daily living
      5. History of bowel habits, diet intake, current stress level
   C. Signs and symptoms: Symptoms will wax and wane or occur intermittently.
      1. The Rome Criteria (see Figure 71-1) provides a model for differentiating IBS from other conditions. Use of these criteria may save the patient from unnecessary and costly testing.

a) If symptoms other than these are present, more extensive testing is necessary to rule out other etiologies.

b) The hallmark of IBS is abdominal pain relieved by defecation or change in stool consistency.

2. IBS may be diarrhea-predominant, constipation-predominant, or a combination of both.

3. Abdominal pain

a) Poorly localized but often occurs in the left lower quadrant or lower abdomen

b) May be initiated by or worsen with meals

c) May be initiated or exacerbated by stress

d) Does not awaken the patient from sleep

e) May worsen with menses

4. Extraintestinal symptoms

a) Urinary frequency

b) Dyspareunia

c) Dysmenorrhea

d) Sexual dysfunction

e) Myalgia

D. Physical exam

1. Abdominal exam

a) Normal bowel sounds

b) Soft, nondistended abdomen

c) Normal to slightly tympanic to percussion

d) No tenderness or mild left lower quadrant tenderness to palpation

e) No abdominal masses; tender, cord-like sigmoid may be present in the left lower quadrant

2. Rectal exam

a) No rectal masses; may have increased sensitivity to rectal exam

b) Test stool for occult blood.

IV. Diagnostic tests: The goal of testing is to conduct enough testing early in the diagnostic process to rule out organic causes of disease and avoid repeat testing, which leads the patient to question the reliability of the diagnosis.

A. Laboratory

1. CBC: To rule out microcytic anemia

Figure 71-1. Rome Diagnostic Criteria for Irritable Bowel Syndrome

At least three months of continuous or recurrent symptoms

Abdominal pain or discomfort that is relieved with defecation

and/or

associated with a change in frequency of stool

and/or

associated with a change in consistency of stool

plus

Two or more of the following, on at least one-fourth of occasions or days

• Altered stool frequency

• Altered stool form (lumpy and hard or loose and watery)

• Altered stool passage (straining, urgency, or feeling of incomplete evacuation)

• Passage of mucous

• Bloating or feeling of abdominal distention

Note. From *Functional Gastrointestinal Disorders: Diagnosis, Pathophysiology, and Treatment: A Multinational Consensus* (pp. 120–121) by D.A. Drossman (Ed.), 1994, Boston: Little, Brown, and Co. Copyright 1994 by Little, Brown, and Co. Adapted with permission.

   2. Erythrocyte sedimentation rate: To rule out occult malignancy or inflammatory process
   3. Thyroid function testing: To rule out thyroid disease
   4. Electrolytes: To rule out metabolic complications of diarrhea; hypokalemia can cause decreased bowel contractility and produce an ileus.
   5. Stool for culture and sensitivity, ova and parasites, and 24-hour volume: If diarrhea is present
   6. Urinalysis: To rule out urinary tract infection
   B. Radiology
   1. Abdominal film: To rule out obstruction
   2. Barium enema, sigmoidoscopy, or colonoscopy: For patients older than age 50 if a mass or lesion is suspected or for persistent diarrhea or constipation to rule out cancer, inflammatory bowel disease, or colitis
   C. Other
   1. Hydrogen breath test or trial of lactose-free diet: If lactose intolerance is suspected
   2. Psychological assessment: To evaluate stress

V. Differential diagnosis
    A. Malabsorption
    1. Food intolerance
    2. Lactose intolerance
    B. Functional disorders: Nonulcer dyspepsia
    C. Organic disorders
    1. Gastroesophageal reflux disease (GERD) (see Chapter 66)
    2. Peptic ulcer disease (PUD) (see Chapter 73)
    3. Malignant lesions
    4. Inflammatory bowel disease
    5. Gallstones and biliary spasm
    6. Infectious diarrhea (see Chapter 53)
    7. Diverticulosis
    8. Bowel obstruction (see Chapter 63)
    9. Diabetic autonomic neuropathy
    10. Peripheral neuropathy (see Chapter 131)
    11. Thyroid dysfunction (see Chapters 149 and 150)
    D. Psychiatric disorders
    1. Anxiety (see Chapter 152)
    2. Depression (see Chapter 154)
    3. Somatization disorders

VI. Treatment: Treatment is primarily supportive with large placebo effect; no therapies have been clinically proven as beneficial in the treatment of IBS. Establishing a trusting, therapeutic relationship with the patient is essential.
    A. Reassurance as to the benign nature of the disease and the lack of progression to a more serious condition
    B. Use of a diary to identify symptom patterns, causative factors

C. Dietary modification
   1. Avoid offending agents: Dairy products (if lactose-intolerant), lentils, beans, peas, gas-forming vegetables (e.g., cabbage, broccoli, cauliflower, cucumbers, brussels sprouts, onions, leafy vegetables), fatty foods, alcohol, sorbitol-containing products (e.g., sugar-free candies), cola, caffeine; reintroduce slowly when symptoms are controlled
   2. High-fiber, low-fat foods
   3. Increase fluids
   4. Regular meal times
D. Use of bulk laxatives: Take with 8–16 oz of water
   1. Psyllium (Metamucil®, Procter & Gamble, Cincinnati, OH; Perdiem® Fiber Therapy, Novartis Consumer Health, Inc., Summit, NJ): One teaspoon to one tablespoon qd–tid
   2. Methylcellulose (Citrucel®, Merrell Dow Pharmaceuticals, Cincinnati, OH): One-half to one tablespoon qd–tid
   3. Calcium polycarbophil (Fibercon®, American Cyanamid Company, Wayne, NJ): One to two tablets qd–tid
E. Bowel training: Encourage patient to sit on toilet for 15–20 minutes after breakfast, which stimulates the gastrocolic reflex
F. Control of excess gas: Simethicone (Mylicon®, Merek & Co., Inc., West Point, PA): One to two tablets po with meals and at bedtime
G. Management of pain
   1. Antispasmodic agents
      a) Dicyclomine (Bentyl®, Merrell Pharmaceuticals, Cincinnati, OH): 10–20 mg po tid–qid
      b) Hyoscyamine sulfate (Levsin®, Schwartz Pharma Inc., Milwaukee, WI): One to two tablets sublingual q four hours prn or one tablet po bid of the sustained-release product (Levbid®, Schwartz Pharma Inc., Milwaukee, WI)
      c) Clidinium bromide and chlordiazepoxide (Librax®, Hoffman-La Roche, Inc., Nutley, NJ): One to two capsules po tid–qid
      d) Belladonna alkaloids (Donnatal®, A.H. Robins Co., Inc., Richmond, VA): One to two tablets po tid–qid
   2. Antidepressants (see Appendix 2)
      a) Amitriptyline (Elavil®, AstraZeneca, Wilmington, DE): 10–150 mg/day po in divided doses
      b) Doxepin (Sinequan®, Pfizer Inc., New York, NY): 10–100 mg/day po in divided doses
      c) Protriptyline (Vivactil®, Merck & Co., Inc., West Point, PA): 5–15 mg/day po in divided doses
      d) Nortriptyline (Pamelor®, Novartis Pharmaceutical Corp., East Hanover, NJ): 10–150 mg/day po in divided doses
      e) Trazodone (Desyrel®, Mead Johnson & Co., Evansville, IN): 50–150 mg/day po in divided doses
H. Management of diarrhea (see Chapter 53)
   1. Loperamide (Immodium®, McNeil Consumer Healthcare, Fort Washington, PA): 4 mg po initially, then 2 mg after each loose stool; maximum 16 mg/day

   2. Diphenoxylate with atropine sulfate (Lomotil®, G.D. Searle & Co., Chicago, IL): Two tablets po qid
   3. Cholestyramine (Questran®, Mead Johnson & Co., Evansville, IN): One scoop mixed in water or noncarbonated liquid po qd–qid
 I. Management of constipation (see Chapter 52)
   1. Osmotic agents
      a) Lactulose: 15–30 cc po qd
      b) Sorbitol: 15–30 cc po qd
      c) Magnesium hydroxide: 15–30 cc po qd
 J. Behavioral modification therapies as necessary
   1. Relaxation
   2. Hypnosis
   3. Biofeedback
   4. Cognitive-behavioral therapies
 K. Evolving potential therapies
   1. 5-HT$_3$ receptor antagonists (Zofran®, Glaxo Wellcome, Inc., Research Triangle Park, NJ; Kytril®, SmithKline Beecham Pharmaceuticals, Philadelphia, PA)
   2. Selective serotonin reuptake inhibitors (Prozac®, Dista Products Company, Indianapolis, IN; Paxil®, SmithKline Beecham Pharmaceuticals; Zoloft®, Pfizer Inc., New York, NY)
   3. Prokinetic agents (Propulsid®, Janssen Pharmaceutica, Inc., Titusville, NJ)
   4. Calcium channel blockers (verapamil [Calan®, C.D. Searle & Co., Chicago IL]) (diltiazem [Cardizem®, Hoechst Marion Roussel, Kansas City, MO])

VII. Follow-up
 A. Short-term: Important to establish a therapeutic relationship; see frequently at time of diagnosis, less often as control is achieved.
 B. Long-term
   1. Whenever necessary for new symptoms
   2. Annually for routine follow-up

VIII. Referrals
 A. Dietitian: For dietary interventions
 B. Gastroenterologist: For refractory or disabling symptoms
 C. Behavioral health specialist: For behavior modification techniques

References

Alderman, J. (1999). Managing irritable bowel syndrome. *Advance for Nurse Practitioners, 7,* 40–41, 45–46, 78.

Barsky, A.J., & Borus, J.F. (1999). Functional somatic syndromes. *Annals of Internal Medicine, 130,* 910–921.

Bonis, P.A.L., & Norton, R.A. (1996). The challenge of irritable bowel syndrome. *American Family Physician, 53,* 1229–1236.

Browning, S.M. (1999). Constipation, diarrhea, and irritable bowel syndrome. *Primary Care, 26,* 113–139.

Camilleri, M., Mayer, E.A., Drossman, D.A., Heath, A., Dukes, G.E., McSorley, D., Kong, S., Mange, A.W., & Northcutt, A.R. (1999). Improvement in pain and bowel function in female irritable bowel patients with alosetron, 5HT3 receptor antagonist. *Alimentary Pharmacology Therapeutics, 13,* 1149–1159.

Carlson, E. (1998). Irritable bowel syndrome. *Nurse Practitioner, 23,* 82–91.

Dalton, C.B., & Drossman, D.A. (1997). Diagnosis and treatment of irritable bowel syndrome. *American Family Physician, 55,* 875–880.

Drossman, D.A. (1995). Diagnosing and treating patients with refractory functional gastrointestinal disorders. *Annals of Internal Medicine, 123,* 688–697.

Hamm, L.R., Sorrells, S.C., Harding, J.P., Northcutt, A.R., Heath, A.T., Kapke, G.F., Hunt, C.M., & Mangel A.W. (1999). Additional investigations fail to alter the diagnosis of irritable bowel syndrome in subjects fulfilling the Rome criteria. *American Journal of Gastroenterology, 94,* 1279–1282.

Harris, M.W. (1997). Irritable bowel syndrome. A cost-effective approach for primary care physicians. *Postgraduate Medicine, 101,* 215–226.

Thompson, W.G., Longstreth, G.F., Drossman, D.A., Heaton, K.W., Irvine, E.J., & Mullerl-Lissner, S.A. (1999). Functional bowel disorders and functional abdominal pain. *Gut, 45*(Suppl. 2), 1143–1147.

Thompson, W.G., & Gick, M. (1996). Irritable bowel syndrome. *Seminars in Gastrointestinal Disease, 7*(4), 217–229.

Verne, M.N., & Cerda, J.J. (1997). Irritable bowel syndrome. Streamlining the diagnosis. *Postgraduate Medicine, 102,* 197–208.

Chapter

72. Pancreatitis

Cindy Jo Horrell, MS, CRNP, AOCN®

I. Definition: Inflammation of the pancreas

II. Pathophysiology
   A. Acute: Caused by premature activation of proteolytic enzymes triggering the autodigestion process; initial injury occurs within the acinar cell.
      1. Pancreatic enzymes leak into interstitium, causing edema, inflammation, and peripancreatic fat necrosis.
      2. Activated pancreatic enzymes are absorbed into systemic circulation, causing widespread toxicity and damage to specific organs, including the lungs.
      3. Intestinal permeability to bacteria is increased, and translocation of bacteria from colon to pancreas occurs.
      4. Response in the inflammatory state can dictate whether pancreatitis is a self-limiting process (e.g., gallstone) or more severe process (e.g., sepsis secondary to alcohol abuse), which can be unrelenting.
   B. Chronic: Pathophysiology of chronic pancreatitis remains unclear.
      1. Pancreatitis is a well-compensated process in which the pancreas, between insults, is able to regenerate itself.
      2. Process can result in a life-threatening condition if the cause is not identified and removed.
      3. It results in destruction of exocrine tissue, fibrosis, and, in some patients, loss of endocrine tissue.

III. Clinical features: Course may range from mild to fulminant based on the degree of pancreatic necrosis.
   A. History
      1. History of cancer and cancer treatment
      2. Current medications: Prescribed and over-the-counter
      3. History of presenting symptom(s): Precipitating factors, onset, location, and duration
      4. Changes in activities of daily living
      5. Social history: Alcohol intake, illicit drug use
      6. Past medical history: Gallstones

B. Signs and symptoms: Presenting symptoms can be vague and range from mild pain and low-grade fever to clinical signs of hypovolemic shock (see Figure 72-1).
1. Pain
2. Nausea/vomiting
3. Fever
4. Jaundice
5. Weight loss (seen in chronic pancreatitis, as well as diarrhea and fatty stools)

C. Physical exam
1. Vital signs
   a) Tachycardia
   b) Blood pressure: Normal or slightly increased from pain; hypotension will occur with severe pancreatitis
   c) Respirations: Shallow from pain or tachypnea with severe pancreatitis
   d) Low-grade fever
2. HEENT exam: Xanthoma and lipemia retinalis with pancreatitis secondary to hyperlipidemia
3. Pulmonary exam: May reveal basilar consolidation, decreased basilar breath sounds, indicating severe pancreatitis and minimal left-sided effusion
4. Abdominal exam
   a) Spider angioma and thickening of palmar sheaths: With alcohol-induced pancreatitis
   b) Rebound tenderness with voluntary and/or involuntary guarding
   c) Hypoactive/absent bowel sounds
   d) Flank or periumbilical ecchymosis: Suggests severe pancreatitis
   e) Distention

IV. Diagnostic tests
A. Laboratory
1. Serum amylase: > 250 u/dl; not diagnostic of pancreatitis
2. Serum lipase: > 110 u/l
3. Serum glucose: > 180 mg/dl if endocrine function compromised
4. Hematocrit (HCT): Increased with third spacing and hemoconcentration; decrease with GI bleed
5. Increased WBC with left shift: < 10,000/mm^3
6. Increased serum AST/ALT: If caused by alcohol or biliary tract obstruction
7. Increased total bilirubin: < 1 mg/dl if caused by alcohol or biliary tract obstruction

---

Figure 72-1. Acute Versus Chronic Pancreatitis: Signs/Symptoms

---

Acute
- Constant epigastric, periumbilical, or left/right upper abdominal pain
- Radiating pain to the back
- Persistent nausea/vomiting
- Elevated serum amylase, lipase, triglycerides
- Frequently elevated WBCs
- Elevated liver function tests (LFTs): Higher with biliary tract disease than with alcoholic pancreatitis

Chronic
- Mild to severe recurrent epigastric pain; frequently nocturnal
- Decreased pain with sitting up
- Nausea/vomiting after eating or drinking alcohol
- Usually normal serum amylase and lipase; elevated with blocked pancreatic duct, pseudocyst, or superimposed acute inflammation
- Possible abnormal LFTs with compression of intrapancreatic common bile duct (e.g., elevated alkaline phosphatase, occasional elevated bilirubin)
- Decreased calcium and albumin with significant weight loss and malnutrition
- Steatorrhea with complete blockage of pancreatic duct

---

8. Liver enzymes: May be elevated
9. Coagulation profile: Usually prolonged
B. Radiology
  1. Abdominal flat plate and upright: To detect nonpancreatic sources of pain
  2. Chest films: To rule out pneumonia and identify atelectasis, pleural effusion
  3. CT scan: Modality of choice to identify a mass
    a) Especially useful with rapid sequence scanning after IV contrast bolus
    b) Best way to differentiate edematous from necrotizing pancreatitis
  4. Ultrasound: To evaluate the biliary tract for stones and dilatation; reveals edema of pancreas (not useful in obese patients or those with excessive colonic gas)

V. Differential diagnosis
  A. Excessive ethanol intake
  B. Acute cholelithiasis
  C. Drug-induced
    1. Asparaginase
    2. Didanosine
    3. Estrogens
    4. Ethacrynic acid
    5. Furosemide
    6. Mercaptopurine
    7. Pentamidine
    8. Thiazide diuretics
    9. Glucocorticosteroids
    10. Azathioprine
    11. Sulfonamides
    12. Tetracycline
    13. Valproic acid
  D. Hypertriglyceridemia
  E. Trauma
  F. Vascular insufficiency
  G. Cancer of pancreas
  H. Duodenal disease (ulcer/obstruction/inflammatory)
  I. Hyperparathyroidism (associated with hypercalcemia)
  J. Infections (mumps, hepatitis B)

VI. Treatment: Initial treatment is aimed at hemodynamic stabilization and decreasing pancreatic inflammation.
  A. Identify precipitating factors (e.g., medications, previous history of gallstones, alcohol ingestion).
  B. Vigorous hydration with electrolyte replacement (e.g., calcium, potassium, magnesium) as indicated
  C. Lipid-restricted diet
  D. Respiratory support (monitor O_2 saturation)
  E. NPO: If more than three to five days, consider total parenteral nutrition (TPN) to prevent malnutrition (see Chapter 158)

    F. Nasogastric tube: If patient has nausea/vomiting or ileus

    G. Pain management

       1. Meperidine (Demerol®, Sanofi Pharmaceuticals, New York, NY): 50–100 mg IM q three to four hours for mild pancreatitis

       2. Ketorolac (Toradol®, Roche Laboratories, Nutley, NJ): 30 mg IM/IV q six hours

          a) Maximum daily dose: 120 mg

          b) Reduce dose 50% for age ≥ 65 years and renal impairment.

          c) Maximum use: Five days

       3. Hydromorphone (Dilaudid®, Knoll Laboratories, Mount Olive, NJ)

          a) Indicated for severe pain

          b) Dose: 3–4 mg po/IV q three to four hours; administer IV slowly

       4. Morphine

          a) Use is controversial, although recent research found it has minimal effects on Oddi's sphincter.

          b) Can be given via patient-controlled analgesia pump at 1 mg/ml/hour with breakthrough doses titrated to patient need.

    H. Discontinue alcohol intake.

    I. Monitor closely for infection and organ failure.

VII. Follow-up: Depends on etiology

VIII. Referrals

    A. Surgeon: Refer as appropriate (e.g., cholelithiasis, pseudocyst, fistula, abscess).

    B. Gastroenterologist: For management

    C. Counselor: For help with alcohol abuse

    D. Dietitian: For counseling for fat-restricted diet

References

Banks, P.A. (1997). Practice guidelines in acute pancreatitis. *American Journal of Gastroenterology, 92,* 377–386.

Banks, P. (1997). Acute and chronic pancreatitis. In M. Feldman, B.F. Scharschmidt, & M.H. Sleisenger (Eds.), *Gastrointestinal and liver disease: Pathophysiology/diagnosis/management* (6th ed.) (pp. 817–818, 840–841). Philadelphia: Saunders.

Forsmark, C.E., & Toskes, P.P. (1995). Acute pancreatitis: Medical management. *Critical Care Clinics, 11,* 295–309.

Gupta, P., & Al-Kawas, F.H. (1995) Acute pancreatitis: Diagnosis and management. *American Family Physician, 52,* 435–443.

Gupta, P., & Al-Kawas, F.H. (1997). Vinorelbine-induced pancreatitis. *Journal of the National Cancer Institute, 89,* 1631.

Krumberger, J.M. (1993) Acute pancreatitis. *Critical Care Nursing Clinics of North America, 5*(1), 185–202.

Steinberg, W.M. (1997). Diagnosis and management of acute pancreatitis. *Cleveland Clinical Journal of Medicine, 64*(4), 182–186.

Chapter

73. Peptic Ulcer Disease

Jeanne Held-Warmkessel, MSN, RN, CS, AOCN®

I. Definition: Disruption of integrity of gastric mucosal layer (muscularis mucosa) resulting from gastric secretions with extension into submucosa or muscularis propria

II. Physiology/Pathophysiology
   A. Normal: The epithelial cells of the stomach are protected from pepsin and hydrochloric acid, the major acids of the stomach that digest food, by
      1. Rapidly reproducing mucosal lining
      2. Secreting bicarbonate to neutralize acid
      3. Mucus production promoted by blood supply and prostaglandin release.
   B. Pathophysiology
      1. Process by which *Helicobacter pylori* (*H. pylori*) causes peptic ulcer disease (PUD) is not well-understood.
         a) Bacteria secrete an enzyme, urease, which allows the bacteria to attach firmly to the stomach mucosa and produce an inflammatory response causing tissue damage.
         b) *H. pylori* colonizes the gastric mucosa and causes chronic superficial gastritis.
      2. ASA/NSAIDs cause gastric ulcers by interfering with the protective effect of prostaglandins in the stomach.
      3. Duodenal ulcers may develop from elevated levels of acid secretion and enhanced gastric emptying, even in the absence of *H. pylori* or ASA/NSAIDs.

III. Clinical features: At one year post-treatment, ulcer relapse rate is 2%.
   A. Risk factors
      1. Smoking
      2. Alcohol abuse
      3. High caffeine use (e.g., cola, coffee)
      4. Stress (increases acid secretion)
      5. Radiation to the stomach, causing mucosal damage
   B. Etiology
      1. Bacterial
         a) *H. pylori*: Bacteria present in 95% of patients with duodenal ulcers and 70% of patients with gastric ulcers
         b) Mycobacterium avium complex (MAC)

        2. Viral (rarely causes ulcers)
           a) Herpes simplex virus-1
           b) CMV
        3. Drug-induced
           a) ASA/NSAIDs
           b) Chemotherapy: Hepatic artery floxuridine infusion
           c) Crack cocaine
           d) Steroids
           e) Theophylline
           f) Digitalis

   C. History
      1. History of cancer and cancer treatment
      2. Current medications: Prescribed and over-the-counter
      3. History of presenting symptom(s): Precipitating factors, onset, location, and duration
      4. Changes in activities of daily living
      5. Social history: Tobacco and alcohol use

   D. Signs and symptoms
      1. Gnawing or burning epigastric pain two to three hours after meals and at night (pain may also occur in right or left upper quadrants or radiate to the back)
      2. Some patients are asymptomatic. Ulcer may perforate or bleed before symptoms develop in patients taking ASA/NSAIDs or in the elderly.
      3. Anorexia, nausea, vomiting
      4. Weight loss
      5. Heartburn
      6. Dyspepsia, bloating, distention, fatty food intolerance
      7. If ulcer bleeds, hematemesis or melena may occur.

   E. Physical exam: Nonspecific
      1. Abdominal exam
          a) Pain may be elicited on palpation.
          b) Assess for masses and organomegaly.
          c) Assess for epigastric tenderness.
          d) Assess for guarding (voluntary and involuntary) with rigidity.
      2. Rectal exam: To test stool for occult blood

IV. Diagnostic tests
   A. Laboratory: Hemoglobin/hematocrit if bleeding is suspected
   B. Radiology: Upper GI-barium to assess for ulcer
   C. Other
      1. *H. pylori* testing
          a) Antiulcer drugs (e.g., bismuth compounds, omeprazole) and antibiotics taken up to four weeks before tests for *H. pylori* (except serology) will cause false-negative results.
          b) Other drugs (e.g., misoprostol, sucralfate) taken one week prior to the breath test will interfere with test accuracy.
          c) Famotidine, cimetidine, rantidine taken one day prior to the breath test will interfere with test accuracy.

  (1) Serology for immune globulin G (IgG) blood levels of *H. pylori* antibodies induced by the bacterial infection

  (2) 13-$_C$ or 14-$_C$ urea breath test: A six-hour pretest fast is required.

   (a) The patient drinks a labeled urea solution, which the bacteria metabolizes.

   (b) Twenty minutes later, a series of breath samples are taken and sent for analysis for the presence of labeled carbon dioxide, which is released only from bacterial metabolism of urea.

   (c) Human cells do not have the enzyme urease necessary to metabolize urea in the bacteria.

 2. Upper endoscopy: For biopsy to rule out malignancy or infection, take *H. pylori* specimens from two to three areas of the stomach, and test the biopsies for urease activity.

 3. Gastric analysis: To quantitatively assess acid secretions

V. Differential diagnosis

 A. Infection

 B. Medication-/drug-induced

 C. GI disorders

  1. Inflammatory disease (e.g., Crohn's disease)

  2. Zollinger-Ellison syndrome

  3. Gastritis, gastroduodenitis (see Chapter 67)

VI. Treatment: The following list is only a suggestion of potential drug options available at the time of publication. Do not begin drugs at different times when treating *H. pylori*. If patient relapses after initial treatment, reevaluate and retreat. Treatment is undergoing continuous evolution; consult the most recent literature and experts in the field of *H. pylori* management.

 A. Antibiotics: If positive for *H. pylori*, treat with combination therapy for 10–14 days with a proton pump inhibitor (PPI) and two antibiotics followed by two more weeks of PPI at reduced dose. Bismuth can alternatively be used in combination with antibiotics. H_2 blocker can be used instead of a PPI for 14 days to six weeks, depending on drug regimen selected. **DO NOT** use monodrug therapy; use a combination of drugs to yield a 90% or greater response rate.

  1. Treatment options

   a) Triple therapy for 14 days (greater than 90% eradication rate)

    (1) BTM: Bismuth 600 mg po (two tablets) qid, tetracycline 500 mg po qid, metronidazole (Flagyl®, G.D. Searle & Co., Chicago, IL) 250 mg po qid

     (a) Available prepackaged under the trade name Helidac® (Procter & Gamble Pharmaceuticals, Inc., Cincinnati, OH) and is the least expensive

     (b) Generally given with two to four weeks of a histamine receptor blocker

    (2) BTC: Bismuth, tetracycline, and clarithromycin 500 mg po tid

    (3) RCA: Ranitidine bismuth subcitrate (Tritek®, Glaxo Wellcome, Philadelphia, PA) 400 mg po bid, clarithromycin 500 mg po bid, and amoxicillin 1,000 mg po bid

(4) RCM: Ranitidine bismuth subcitrate, clarithromycin 500 mg po bid, and metronidazole 500 mg po bid

(5) RCT: Ranitidine bismuth subcitrate, clarithromycin 500 mg po tid, and tetracycline 500 mg po qid

(6) RMA: Ranitidine bismuth subcitrate, metronidazole, and amoxicillin

(7) RMT: Ranitidine bismuth subcitrate, metronidazole, and tetracycline

   b) Other potential therapies

(1) Quadruple therapy: Triple therapy with the addition of a PPI

(2) Triple therapy: Consists of a PPI (omeprazole 20 mg po bid) for four weeks, clarithromycin 500 mg po bid for two weeks, and either metronidazole or amoxicillin for two weeks

   c) Use caution with the use of metronidazole and alcohol, as it may cause an antabuse effect. Do not use metronidazole if patient has prior exposure to drug because of the likelihood of drug resistance.

   d) H_2 blocker doses may need to be reduced for hepatic and renal failure. Start after antibiotic treatment of *H. pylori* is completed and continue for four to six weeks.

   e) Antacids: Do not use aluminum- or magnesium-based antacids in renal failure. Do not use sodium-based antacids for patients with cardiac, hypertensive, or renal failure.

B. Patient education

1. Avoid smoking, especially before nighttime dose of H_2 blocker, because cigarette smoke blocks bicarbonate release in the stomach.

2. Diet

   a) Avoid coffee and caffeine-containing foods and liquids, which may increase acid secretion.

   b) Eat regular meals; no snacking between regular meals, as food stimulates acid production.

   c) Avoid alcohol.

3. Stress management: Stress causes increased acid secretion; implement relaxation and quiet diversion.

VII. Follow-up

A. Improvement should be noted after several weeks of treatment. Healing should occur in four to six weeks with treatment.

B. Repeat urea breath test no earlier than four weeks post-treatment to avoid false-negative results. Repeat breath test in six to eight weeks after treatment for patients with bleeding or complicated ulcer(s) if *H. pylori* was diagnosed.

C. Development of fatigue, tachycardia, pallor, coffee-ground emesis, hematemesis, or black stools indicates bleeding/hemorrhage and prompt medical intervention is required.

D. Perforation requires prompt emergency surgical intervention. Peritonitis develops quickly over the next 6–12 hours.

E. Serology may remain positive for eight months after successful treatment of *H. pylori*. Immune globulin blood levels decrease slowly after *H. pylori* treatment.

VIII. Referrals: Gastroenterologist for esophagogastroduodenoscopy (EGD)

References

Cave, D.R., & Hoffman, J.S. (1996). Management of *Helicobacter pylori* infection in ulcer disease. *Hospital Practice, 31*(1), 63, 64, 67–69, 73–75.

Cerda, J.J., Go, M.F., & Yamada, T. (1995). Peptic ulcer disease: Now you can cure. *Patient Care, 29*(Dec. 15), 100–117.

Fay, M., & Jaffe, P.E. (1996). Diagnostic and treatment guidelines for *Helicobacter pylori*. *Nurse Practitioner, 21*(7), 28, 30, 33, 34, 38.

NIH Consensus Development Panel on *Helicobacter pylori* in Peptic Ulcer Disease. (1994). *Helicobacter pylori* in peptic ulcer disease. *JAMA, 272,* 65–69.

Peterson, W.L., & Graham, D.Y. (1998). *Helicobacter pylori.* In M. Feldman, B.F. Sharschemidt, & M.H. Sleisenger (Eds.), *Sleisenger & Fordtran's gastrointestinal and liver disease: Pathophysiology, diagnosis, and management* (6th ed.) (pp. 604–619). Phildadelphia: Saunders.

Podolski, J.L. (1996). Recent advances in peptic ulcer disease: *Helicobacter pylori* infection and its treatment. *Gastroenterology Nursing, 19,* 128–136.

Smoot, D.T., Hinds, T., Ahsktorab, H., Jagtap, J., Kim, K.S., & Scott, V.F. (1999). Effectiveness of ranitidine bismuth citrate, clarithromycin, and metronidazole therapy for treating *Helicobacter pylori. American Journal of Gastroenterology, 94,* 955–958.

Vakil, N., & Cutter, A. (1999). Ten-day triple therapy with ranitidine bismuth citrate, amoxicillin, and clarithromycin in eradicating *Helicobacter pylori. American Journal of Gastroenterology, 94,* 1197–1199.

Section VII. Genitourinary

Symptoms

Medical Diagnosis

74. Amenorrhea

Aurelie C. Cormier, RN, MS, AOCN®

I. Definition
   A. Primary: Lack of menses by age 14 without secondary sex characteristic development or lack of menses by age 16 with secondary sex characteristics
   B. Secondary: Lack of menses for 6 months in a woman who was regularly menstruating or 12 months in a woman who had oligomenorrhea

II. Physiology/Pathophysiology
   A. Normal
      1. Menstruation requires a functional hypothalamus, pituitary gland, ovarian system, and uterus, as well as a patent cervix and vaginal canal.
      2. Physiologically, the hypothalamus releases gonadotrophin-releasing hormone (GnRH) to stimulate the anterior pituitary to release follicle-stimulating hormone (FSH) and luteinizing hormone (LH).
         a) These two hormones stimulate the development of the follicle to produce estrogen and release the egg (i.e., ovulation).
         b) If the egg is not fertilized, the uterus sheds its lining.
         c) Menstrual flow passes through the cervix and down through the vagina.
   B. Pathophysiology
      1. Amenorrhea can occur from any disturbance at any level of the regulatory cascade or feedback.
      2. Hypothalamic amenorrhea usually represents a functional disorder of GnRH release, leading to loss of LH and failure to ovulate.
      3. Pituitary tumors can cause hyperprolactinemia, which inhibits GnRH release and impairs gonadotropin production.
      4. Disease of the ovary can cause hypergonadotropic response, leading to marked serum elevations in LH and FSH and low levels of estrogen and progesterone (i.e., menopause).
      5. Some chemotherapeutic agents can directly cause fibrosis and destruction of follicles, leading to ovarian failure.
      6. Follicles of varying size and maturation status will have radioresistance or sensitivity to radiation. Intermediate follicles are the most radiosensitive; small follicles are the most radioresistant.

    7. Radiation to the pituitary gland can cause flattening of the gland and result in pituitary dysfunction.

III. Clinical features
  A. Etiology
    1. Hypothalamic dysfunction is caused by
      a) Stress
      b) Malnutrition
      c) Congenital malformation
      d) Excessive exercise.
    2. Pituitary tumors
    3. Ovarian disease may be caused by
      a) Normal menopause
      b) Cancer
      c) Surgery
      d) Chemotherapy.
        (1) Ovarian dysfunction is usually a delayed side effect of chemotherapy, beginning two to three months after treatment starts. Menses may become irregular or stop during treatment; menstruation may resume in some patients, usually after treatment ends.
        (2) Increasing age of the patient (i.e., > 35), higher doses, cumulative dose, and type of chemotherapy (e.g., alkylating agents) are factors most predictive for ovarian failure.
      e) Pelvic radiation
        (1) Ovarian function may resume when eggs in the small radioresistant follicles mature and resume functioning.
        (2) Increasing age of the patient (i.e., > 40) and increasing dose of radiation are most predictive for adverse effects on the ovaries.
  B. History
    1. History of cancer and cancer treatment
    2. Current medications: Prescribed and over-the-counter
    3. History of presenting symptom(s): Precipitating factors, onset, and duration. Associated symptoms are weight loss, depression, stress, and galactorrhea.
    4. Changes in activities of daily living
    5. History of menstrual cycle, pregnancies, and miscarriages/abortions
    6. Past medical history: Gynecologic procedures, hypothalamic disorders, pituitary disorders, ovarian disorders, endometriosis, pelvic inflammatory disease, infertility, hypothyroidism
    7. Family history: Menstrual problems, infertility, endocrine diseases, autoimmune diseases, congenital anomalies, tuberculosis
  C. Signs and symptoms of ovarian failure
    1. Absence of menses
      a) Six months in women who have been normally menstruating
      b) Twelve months in women who have had few menses
    2. Hot flashes

    3. Night sweats

    4. Insomnia

    5. Fatigue

    6. Emotional lability

       a) Anxiety

       b) Depression

       c) Irritability

    7. Headache

    8. Joint pains

    9. Stomach upset

  10. Decreased cognition

  11. Forgetfulness

  12. Urinary: Dysuria, frequency, urge incontinence

  13. Vaginal dryness, pruritus, dyspareunia

D. Physical exam

    1. Head, eyes, ears, nose, and throat (HEENT) exam

       a) Assess hair distribution for signs of androgen deficiency (e.g., male pattern baldness).

       b) Eye exam: Inspect fundus for signs of intracranial pressure, indicating tumor presence.

       c) Presence of acne suggests high androgen levels.

       d) Assess face for excess hair distribution, indicating high androgen levels.

    2. Neurologic exam: Assess cranial nerves for abnormalities, indicating tumor (see Appendix 5).

    3. Thyroid exam: Assess for enlargement or nodules, indicating thyroid disease.

    4. Breast exam

       a) Assess breasts for sexual development or changes associated with pregnancy.

       b) Assess for galactorrhea, indicating inappropriate prolactin release.

       c) Assess for masses, edema, abnormal dimpling, or drainage.

       d) Assess chest for excess hair distribution, indicating high androgen level.

    5. Abdominal exam

       a) Note any abdominal striae in a nulliparous woman, indicating hypercortisolism

       b) Note excess hair distribution, indicating high androgen levels.

       c) Obesity with fat concentration in the trunk may suggest high androgen levels.

       d) Assess for abdominal mass and organomegaly.

    6. Gynecologic exam

       a) Assess external genitalia and vagina for evidence of low estrogen levels.

         (1) Dry, atrophic mucosa

         (2) Minimal cervical mucus

       b) Assess clitoris for enlargement (> 1 cm), indicating high androgen levels.

       c) Assess vaginal canal for imperforate hymen or vaginal septum defect preventing menstrual flow. Assess for vaginal stenosis.

       d) Assess cervix for signs of stricture or blockage preventing menstrual flow.

       e) Assess uterus and ovaries for presence or signs of enlargement or mass.

       f) Assess for signs of pregnancy.

(1) Purplish color of cervix

(2) Enlarged, doughy, or elastic uterus

7. Assess thighs for excess hair distribution, indicating high androgen levels.

IV. Diagnostic tests

A. Laboratory

1. Quantitative beta HCG: Must be done first to rule out pregnancy; results reported as positive or negative

2. Step-wise workup

a) TSH levels: To rule out hypothyroidism (normal < 5µU/m)

b) Serum prolactin levels: To rule out hyperprolactinemia (normal is 10–25 ng/ml)

c) Progestational challenge (see Other, next page)

(1) If withdrawal bleeding occurs two to seven days after progesterone administration and TSH level and prolactin level are normal, anovulation is confirmed.

(2) If the patient does not have galactorrhea with progesterone, no further workup is required.

3. If withdrawal bleeding does not occur within two to seven days after progesterone therapy, or did occur but then stopped, initiate further workup.

a) Further workup starts with determination of normal uterine function and patent cervix and vagina.

b) Prescribe conjugated estrogen 1.25 mg po for 21 days and medroxyprogesterone acetate 10 mg po days 17–21 for one cycle.

c) If no withdrawal bleeding occurs, repeat the medications for another cycle.

d) If withdrawal bleeding occurs, do further workup to determine the etiology of inadequate estrogen production.

(1) Workup must be done at least two weeks or longer from the time of estrogen/progesterone therapy.

(2) Serum FSH, LH: To rule out menopause, hypothalamic, or pituitary dysfunction

(a) Normal levels: FSH 5–30 IU/l (mid-cycle levels will be twice the baseline level); LH 5–20 IU/l (midcycle levels will be three times the baseline level)

(b) Hypothalamic or pituitary dysfunction: FSH < 5 IU/l; LH < 5 IU/l

4. If exhibiting signs of hirsutism: Serum dehydroepiandrosterone sulfate, 17-hydroxyprogesterone level, free testosterone levels to rule out androgen excess

5. If elevated FSH (see levels above)

a) CBC, sedimentation rate, antinuclear antibody, rheumatoid factor, total protein, albumin/globulin ratio, am cortisol, phosphorus, and calcium to rule out autoimmune disorder

b) Tests for autoimmune disease are not necessary if symptoms are not present.

B. Radiology

1. CT scan of sella turcica: To rule out pituitary tumor in the patient who presents with galactorrhea

   2. MRI of anterior pituitary: If the prolactin level is > 100 ng/ml or patient has symptoms of increased intracranial pressure
C. Other
   1. Progesterone challenge: To determine normal estrogen activity with evidence of withdrawal bleeding administered as
      a) Medroxyprogesterone acetate: 10 mg po qd for five days
      b) Progesterone in oil: 200 mg IM if there is doubt that patient will follow through with po medication
   2. Endometrial biopsy: In selected patients to rule out endometrial hyperplasia, precancerous lesions, or cancerous lesions if it has been determined that the patient was anovulatory for a prolonged period of time
   3. Chromosomal karyotypic studies: For patients younger than age 30 with elevated FSH and LH to rule out presence of Y chromosome and increased risk of germ cell malignancies or absence of X chromosome

V. Differential diagnosis: Irregular menses and amenorrhea are common side effects of cancer treatment, especially if higher doses of chemotherapy are used or if radiation or surgical treatment occurs in the pelvic area. However, other etiologies may need to be explored.
   A. Malignancies
      1. Pituitary microadenoma/macroadenoma
      2. Glioma
      3. Craniopharyngioma
      4. Meningioma
      5. Chordoma
   B. Medication-induced amenorrhea
      1. Chemotherapy
      2. Digoxin
      3. Marijuana
      4. Oral contraceptives (OCs)
      5. Antihypertensives
      6. Antidepressants
      7. Antipsychotics
   C. Premature ovarian failure secondary to
      1. Chromosomal abnormalities
      2. Autoimmune disorders (e.g., myasthenia gravis, idiopathic thrombocytopenic purpura (see Chapter 120), rheumatoid arthritis (see Chapter 108), vitiligo, autoimmune hemolytic anemia)
      3. Infections affecting ovarian follicles (e.g., mumps oophoritis)
      4. Radiation therapy
      5. Chemotherapy
   D. Hypothalamic disorder resulting from stress, infection, severe weight loss, depression (see Chapter 154), anorexia nervosa, or strenuous exercise
   F. Medical conditions (e.g., hypothyroidism [see Chapter 150], intrauterine adhesions, Cushing's syndrome, polycystic ovary syndrome, ovarian tumors, adrenal tumors)
   G. Menopause (see Chapter 151)

VI. Treatment
   A. Cyclic progesterone: Administer if patient is amenorrheic and has normal estrogen levels.
      1. Medroxyprogesterone acetate: 10 mg/day po for 7–10 days/month
      2. If contraception is needed, a low-dose oral contraceptive may be used instead of progesterone alone (see Table 74-1).
         a) OCs are now designed as monophasic, biphasic, or triphasic.
         b) The triphasic variety are more widely used today because they more closely mimic the natural hormone milieu of the body.
         c) OCs are contraindicated in women with a history of breast cancer, endometrial cancer, hepatic cancer, hepatic adenomas, prior jaundice with OC use, abnormal vaginal bleeding of unknown etiology, cerebral vascular disease, coronary artery disease, or a present or past history of thrombophlebitis or thromboembolic disorders.
         d) Side effects may include vaginal bleeding, breast tenderness, fluid retention, irregular darkening of the skin (especially of the face), nausea, headache,

Table 74-1. Characteristics of Oral Contraceptives

Drug	Dose	Comments
Ortho Tri-Cyclen®[a]	1 tablet qd x 28	Ethinyl estradiol and norgestimate (35 mcg/0.18 mg, 35 mcg/0.215 mg, 35 mcg/0.25 mg); triphasic and has been found to have less risk of spotting or intermenstrual bleeding, acne, oily skin, sebaceous cysts, pilonidal cysts, or weight gain; patients have better lipid levels than with other OCs.
Ortho-Novum® 7/7/7	1 tablet qd x 28	Ethinyl estradiol and norethindrone (35 mcg/0.5 mg, 35 mcg/0.75 mg, 35 mcg/1mg); triphasic
Triphasil®[b]-28	1 tablet qd x 28	Ethinyl estradiol and levonorgestrel (30 mcg/0.05 mg, 40 mcg/0.075 mg, 30 mcg/0.125 mg)
Lo/Ovral®[b]-28	1 tablet qd x 28	Ethinyl estradiol and norgestrel (30 mcg/0.3 mg); monophasic and has been found to have less side effects of breast tenderness, headaches, nausea, or breakthrough bleeding
Desogen®[c]	1 tablet qd x 28	Ethinyl estradiol and desogestrel (30 mcg/0.15 mg); monophasic and has less side effects of breast tenderness, nausea, headaches, weight gain, breakthrough bleeding, acne, oily skin, sebaceous cysts, or pilonidal cysts
Loestrin Fe®[d] 1/20	1 tablet qd x 21	Ethinyl estradiol and norethindrone acetate (20 mcg/1 mg); monophasic and is useful in women at higher risk of thrombosis; pill is taken for 21 days and next cycle is started 7 days after last pill.

[a] Ortho-McNeil Pharmaceuticals, Raritan, NJ; [b] Wyeth-Ayerst Pharmaceuticals, Philadelphia, PA; [c] Organon, Inc., West Orange, NJ; [d] Parke-Davis, Morris Plains, NJ

elevated blood pressure, altered sensitivity to contact lenses, irritability, depression, vaginal infections, acne, diminished libido, or weight gain.

e) For packs containing 21 pills, the easiest method of establishing a cycle is to start the pill on Sunday and continue for 21 days, discontinue for 7 days, and resume next cycle on Sunday.

f) For 28-pill packs, pills taken on days 22–28 are placebos.

B. If amenorrhea and hypoestrogenic

1. Use estrogen therapy to prophylactically treat for reduction in risk of osteoporosis or cardiovascular disease.

2. Controversy exists as to whether estrogen/progesterone therapy or the oral contraceptive is appropriate for premenopausal women.

C. If patient has breast or endometrial cancer, estrogen and/or progesterone therapy is contraindicated. In some studies, drug-induced amenorrhea has shown a survival benefit for early-stage breast cancer. In rare exceptions, if patient has severe symptoms, is ER/PR negative, and is at an increased risk for cardiovascular disease, estrogen and progesterone therapy may be used with special monitoring.

VII. Follow-up

A. Short-term: Patients started on estrogen or progesterone therapy should be followed two to three months after starting therapy to assess for response or side effects.

B. Long-term: Patients should be seen in one year and then followed periodically to determine if amenorrhea is resolving or is occurring because of premature menopause.

VIII. Referrals

A. Gynecologist, reproductive endocrinologist, or endocrinologist: If patient does not have withdrawal bleeding to progesterone challenge or has low levels of FSH and LH indicating a hypothalamic or pituitary disorder

B. Internist: For evaluation of other medical conditions

C. Psychotherapist or psychiatrist: To treat women with eating or psychiatric disorders

References

Aloi, J. (1995). Evaluation of amenorrhea. *Comprehensive Therapy, 21,* 575–578.

Averette, H., Boike, G., & Jarrell, M. (1990). Effects of cancer chemotherapy on gonadal function and reproductive capacity. *CA: A Cancer Journal for Clinicians, 40,* 199–209.

Del Mastro, L., Venturini, M., Sertoli, M.R., & Rosso, R. (1997). Amenorrhea induced by adjuvant chemotherapy in early breast cancer patients: Prognostic role and clinical implications. *Breast Cancer Research and Treatment, 43,* 183–190.

Feldman, J. (1989). Ovarian failure and cancer treatment: Incidence and interventions for the premenopausal woman. *Oncology Nursing Forum, 16,* 651–657.

Hatcher, R., Trussell, J., Stewart, F., Stewart, G., Kowal, D., Guest, F., Cates, W., & Policar, M. (Eds.). (1994). *Contraceptive technology* (16th ed.). New York: Irvington Publishers, Inc.

Kiningham, R., Apgar, B., & Schwenk, T. (1996). Evaluation of amenorrhea. *American Family Physician, 53,* 1185–1194.

Marshall, L. (1994). Clinical evaluation of amenorrhea in active and athletic women. *Clinics in Sports Medicine, 13,* 371–387.

Putukian, M. (1994). The female triad: Eating disorders, amenorrhea and osteoporosis. *Medical Clinics of North America, 78,* 345–356.

Schachter, M., & Shoham, Z. (1994). Amenorrhea during the reproductive years—Is it safe? *Fertility and Sterility, 62*(1), 1–16.

Speroff, L., Glass, R., & Kase, N. (1994). *Clinical gynecologic endocrinology and infertility* (5th ed.). Baltimore: Williams & Wilkins.

Warren, M. (1996). Evaluation of secondary amenorrhea. *Journal of Clinical Endocrinology and Metabolism, 81,* 437–442.

75. Dysuria

Barbara St. Marie, RN, MA, CNP, ANP, GNP

I. Definition: The presence of burning or difficult urination

II. Pathophysiology: Pain caused by inflammation from organisms that ascend the urethra

III. Clinical features
  A. Risk factors
    1. In women, a shorter urethra increases risk for infection.
    2. In men, the longer urethra, the absence of colonization of bacteria near the meatus, and the antibacterial factor present in the prostatic fluid create a lower incidence of urinary tract infection (UTI).
    3. Urinary catheterization
    4. Vaginal atrophy
    5. Pelvic surgery
  B. Etiology
    1. Invasion of the urinary tract by bacteria (e.g., *Escherichia coli*, *Klebsiella pneumoniae*) that ascends the urethra
    2. Urothelial inflammation associated with bacillus Calmette-Guérin (BCG) intravesical therapy
  C. History
    1. History of cancer and cancer treatment
    2. Current medications: Prescribed and over-the-counter
    3. History of presenting symptom(s): Precipitating factors, onset, location, and duration. Associated symptoms are flank tenderness, back pain, hematuria, urination urgency, frequency, and hesitancy.
    4. Changes in activities of daily living
    5. Past medical history: Sexually transmitted diseases, diabetes mellitus, urinary stress incontinence, vaginal atrophy, traumatic vaginal or pelvic injury
  D. Signs and symptoms
    1. Burning (suggests urethral inflammation)
    2. Urgency
    3. Frequency
    4. Characteristics of urine: Cloudy, foul-smelling
    5. Hematuria

E. Physical exam
   1. Vital signs: Elevated temperature in infection; often absent in the elderly
   2. Abdominal exam: Suprapubic tenderness suggests cystitis; not always present
   3. Costovertebral angle tenderness: Consistent with renal inflammation; not always present
   4. Genitourinary male exam
      a) Urethral discharge and erythema may be present with sexually transmitted diseases or penile cancer.
      b) Conduct prostate exam to assess for an inflamed prostate that may cause urethral symptoms.
      c) Expressed prostatic secretions or voiding after prostatic massage may help with diagnosis by showing bacterial count.
   5. Gynecologic exam
      a) Assess external genitalia for discharge, odor, labial irritation, prolapsed bladder, or evidence of trauma.
      b) Assess cervical motion tenderness to evaluate for pelvic inflammatory disease.

IV. Diagnostic tests
   A. Laboratory
      1. Urinalysis
         a) Color usually dark yellow (concentrated) or amber (hematuria)
         b) Pyuria: > 2–5 WBCs per high-power field is indicative of UTI.
            (1) Absence of pyuria suggests a vaginal cause for dysuria.
            (2) Sterile pyuria suggests renal tuberculosis.
            (3) WBC casts suggest renal parenchymal infection.
         c) Presence of one organism on high-power field represents clinically significant bacteriuria (> 10^5 organisms per/ml).
      2. Urine culture
         a) A colony count > 10^5 organisms per ml provides high specificity but poor sensitivity.
         b) Most common organism causing UTI is *Escherichia coli*.
            (1) Gram-positive organism (e.g., enterococcus, *Staphylococcus aureus*, Group B streptococci) can be involved.
            (2) *Staphylococcus epidermis* or diphtheroid are skin flora and are considered contaminants.
            (3) Candida is seldom correlated with symptoms of UTI and is most likely related to vaginal secretions in the urine sample.
      3. Culture drainage
         a) Urethral discharge at the urinary meatus suggests sexually transmitted disease.
         b) Vaginal cultures also can determine bacterial vaginitis or Candida infections (see Chapters 97 and 98).
   B. Radiology: Renal ultrasound: To evaluate for obstruction or masses

V. Differential diagnosis
   A. Urinary tract infection: Cystitis (see Chapter 91)
   B. Urethritis: Reiter's syndrome
   C. Infection in the urinary tract: Sexually transmitted diseases, pyelonephritis, acute bacterial prostatitis (see Chapters 92 and 93)
   D. Urethral stricture: Urinary obstruction (e.g., calculus)
   E. Benign prostatic hypertrophy, Chronic bacterial prostatitis, nonbacterial prostatitis (see Chapters 85 and 92)
   F. Tumor: Prostate, bladder, cervix
   G. Gynecologic disorders: Postmenopausal atrophic vaginitis (see Chapter 97), prolapse of uterus, cystocele, rectocele, metritis, dysmenorrhea
   H. Pelvic peritonitis and abscess: Sexually transmitted diseases, vulvovaginitis
   I. Psychological abnormalities
   J. Mechanical or chemical irritation: Sexual abuse, incidental trauma

VI. Treatment
   A. Symptomatic treatment for dysuria
      1. Phenazopyridine (Pyridium®, Warner Chilcott Laboratories, Rockaway, NJ): 200 mg po tid for one to three days; provides relief of annoying symptoms within hours of the first dose but will turn the urine dark orange.
   B. Symptomatic treatment for bladder spasms
      1. Oxybutynin: 5 mg po bid to tid
   C. Treatment of dysuria with pyuria depends upon organism (see Appendix 1). Antibiotic alternatives include
      1. Bactrim™ DS (Roche Pharmaceutical Laboratories, Nutley, NJ) 1 mg po bid
      2. Cipro® (Bayer Corp., West Haven, CT) 500 mg po bid.

VII. Follow-up: If the patient remains asymptomatic after treatment for dysuria, there is no need for further follow-up.

VIII. Referrals
   A. Urologist: For workup of suspected urologic neoplasm and diagnosis and management of long-term bladder compromise from cancer treatment, refractory dysuria, and persistent symptoms after initial treatment

References

Conovan, D.A., & Kenneally-Nicholas, P. (1997). Prostatitis: Diagnosis and treatment in primary care, *Nurse Practitioner, 22*(4) 144–156.

Criste, G., Gray, D., & Gallo, B. (1994). Prostatitis: A review of diagnosis and management. *Nursing Practice. 19*(7), 32–38.

Karlowicz, K.A. (1997). Pharmacologic therapy for acute cystitis in adults: A review of treatment options. *Urological Nursing, 17*(3), 106–114.

Kurowski, K. (1998). The women with dysuria. *American Family Physician, 57,* 2155–2164, 2169–2170.

Lipsky, B.A. (1989). Urinary tract infections in men. *Annals of Internal Medicine, 110,* 138.

Sant, G.R. (1997). Interstitial cystitis. *Current Opinions in Obstetrics and Gynecology, 9,* 332–336.

76. Hematuria
Deborah McCaffrey Boyle, RN, MSN, AOCN®, FAAN

I. Definition: Presence of blood in the urine

II. Physiology/Pathophysiology
   A. Normally, less than 100 RBCs are excreted into the urine each minute.
   B. Pathophysiology
      1. If the rate of excretion rises to 3,000–4,000 RBCs per minute (two to three RBCs per high-power field), microscopic hematuria occurs.
      2. If the excretion rate exceeds one million RBCs per minute, gross hematuria occurs.
      3. Greater than eight RBCs per high-power field is considered to be indicative of potentially serious pathology.
      4. Cystitis, urethritis, and genitourinary stones can cause hematuria because of intrinsic kidney disease and traumatic injury to the kidney.
      5. Hemorrhagic cystitis results from damage to the epithelial lining of the bladder from exposure to metabolites of alkylating agents during urinary excretion. As a result, scarring and fibrotic changes occur, causing bladder contraction and chronic urinary distress (i.e., dysuria, frequency, incontinence, bleeding).

III. Clinical features: Gross hematuria is indicative of disease or injury within the urinary system.
   A. Etiology
      1. Bladder cancer
      2. Genitourinary stones
      3. Alkylating agents (e.g., cyclophosphamide, ifosfamide)
      4. Pelvic radiation
      5. Cystitis
      6. Intrinsic genitourinary lesion involving the kidneys, ureter, bladder, prostate, and urethra
      7. Pyelonephritis
   B. History: Evaluate urinary patterns (past and present) and associated symptoms.
      1. History of cancer and cancer treatment
      2. Current medications: Prescribed and over-the-counter
      3. History of presenting symptom(s): Precipitating factors, onset, location, and duration. Associated symptoms are nocturia, blood clots in the urine, dysuria, abdominal pain, and flank pain.

    4. Changes in activities of daily living

    5. Recent history: Pelvic injury or trauma

C. Signs and symptoms

    1. Urine: May be blood-tinged, grossly bloody, or smoky brown in color; determine at what point during urination bleeding occurs.

       a) Bright red blood at onset of urination: Urethral origin

       b) Blood at the end of urination: Site near the bladder neck

       c) Bleeding throughout voiding: Site above bladder neck; characterizes blood mixed with urine in the bladder prior to elimination

       d) Blood that has remained in the urinary tract long enough to deteriorate will give the urine a smoky, brownish color; also may indicate a site of bleeding above the bladder neck

    2. Urinary frequency

    3. Dysuria characterized as sharp and burning

    4. Urinary urgency

    5. Presence of suprapubic or flank pain

    6. Fever and/or chills

    7. Nocturia

    8. Foul-smelling urine

D. Physical exam

    1. Vital signs

       a) Fever suggests infection.

       b) Hypertension may be noted in glomerulonephritis.

    2. Integument exam: Assess for ecchymosis, which is suggestive of coagulopathy.

    3. Abdominal exam: Assess for lower abdominal/pelvic tenderness, suprapubic pressure.

    4. Lymph exam: Check inguinal area for masses and lymph node enlargement.

    5. Posterior thorax exam: Palpate dorsal costovertebral region for tenderness, pain, and mass.

    6. Genitourinary exam

       a) Examine urethral orifice and external genitalia for evidence of sexually transmitted disease (STD), ulceration, or stenosis.

       b) Palpate prostate to rule out hypertrophy, nodules, or pain.

IV. Diagnostic tests

A. Laboratory

    1. CBC: Assess for elevated WBCs (infection), anemia, and thrombocytopenia.

    2. Prothrombin time and partial thromboplastin time: Assess for prolonged values, suggesting coagulopathy.

    3. Prostate-specific antigen (PSA): Assess for prostatic abnormality suspicious for cancer or benign hypertrophy.

    4. Urine

       a) Dipstick: A quick, inexpensive test performed in the clinic to confirm blood in the urine

       b) Urinalysis: Check for WBCs and bacteria suggestive of an infection.

          (1) WBC casts indicate pyelonephritis or interstitial nephritis.

        (2) RBCs in specimen indicate urinary tract disease.

        (3) RBC casts represent glomerulonephritis.

        (4) Malignant cytology

      c) Urine culture: To identify the type of bacterial organism and the number of bacterial colonies.

        (1) Greater than 100,000 colonies represent infection.

        (2) The number can be less if the patient is symptomatic.

      d) 24-hour urine for creatinine and protein: To assess renal function; elevated protein suggests glomerular lesions.

  B. Radiology

    1. Renal sonogram: To detect presence and location of kidney masses, obstruction, and stones

    2. CT scan of abdomen: To detect presence of urinary tract abnormalities

    3. Intravenous pyelogram (IVP): To reveal abnormalities in urinary tract architecture and blood flow; particularly helpful in determining presence and location of obstruction but is not used as frequently as the above tests

  C. Other: Cystoscopy permits visualization of urethra, bladder, and urethral orifices; documents epithelial inflammation, erythema, ulceration, and necrosis; and facilitates biopsy.

V. Differential diagnosis

  A. Diseases

    1. Malignancies originating within the urinary tract

    2. Nonurological malignancies causing external compression on urinary structures with resultant hematuria

    3. Infection (see Chapters 121 and 140)

    4. Benign prostatic hypertrophy (see Chapter 85)

    5. Intrinsic kidney disease

  B. Medications

    1. Cyclophosphamide: Particularly high single dose (> 2 g)

    2. Ifosfamide

    3. Intravesical chemotherapy/immunotherapy (i.e., mitomycin, thiotepa, doxorubicin, bacillus Calmette-Guérin [BCG] instillation): For primary treatment of bladder tumors; symptoms rarely persist following treatment cessation.

  C. Radiation therapy

    1. External beam

      a) Pelvic field total dose is 65–70 Gy

      b) Concurrent cyclophosphamide or cisplatin with external radiation heightens risk for hemorrhagic cystitis, as does administration of these drugs following pelvic irradiation.

    2. Brachytherapy: With radioactive seeds implanted near the bladder (i.e., prostate seed implants) symptoms resolve usually within 12–18 months after treatment but may continue for years.

VI. Treatment: Depends on etiology of hematuria

  A. Infection

1. Antibiotic regimen depends on the organism isolated (see Appendix 1).
   a) Cipro® (Bayer Corp., West Haven, CT): 500 mg po bid
   b) Bactrim™ DS (Roche Pharmaceutical Laboratories, Nutley, NJ): 1 mg po bid
2. Symptom control: Pyridium: 200 mg po q8° prn; side effect is urine discoloration (e.g., reddish, brown, orange).
3. Encourage fluid intake (i.e., at least eight 8 oz glasses of fluids per day)

B. Drug-induced hemorrhagic cystitis
   1. Vigorous hydration before and during high-dose cyclophosphamide and ifosfamide therapy
      a) Parenteral route
      b) Encourage oral fluids.
   2. Use of uroprotectant, mesna
      a) Blocks damage to the bladder epithelium, which results from chemotherapy crystallization
      b) Mesna binds to acrolein, the metabolic byproduct produced by metabolism of alkylating agents.
      c) Dose: Depends on chemotherapy dose (usually 60%–80% of total dose of chemotherapy); administered prior to chemotherapy agent and repeated four and eight hours after chemotherapy infusion or as a continuous infusion
   3. Sodium bicarbonate: Dose depends on urinary pH and response; administered IV or po to maintain alkaline urine (pH > 7.0)

C. Bleeding
   1. Continuous bladder irrigation with normal saline
   2. Intravesical instillation of alum, silver nitrate, or formalin to stop the bleeding (dose ranges vary)
   3. Cystoscopy with fulguration of bleeding source(s)
   4. Cystectomy with urinary diversion

D. Malignancy: Appropriate management of underlying cancer

VII. Follow-up
   A. Short-term: Assess resolution of symptoms and efficacy of interventions within a few days to a week.
   B. Long-term: Monitor bone marrow transplant patients treated with high-dose cyclophosphamide for potential long-term bladder sequela.

VIII. Referrals
   A. Urologist: For workup of suspected urologic neoplasm and diagnosis and management of long-term bladder compromise from previous chemotherapy
   B. Ostomy nurse: If cystectomy is required

References

Belldegrun, A., & deKernion, J.B. (1998). Renal tumors. In P.C. Walsh, A.B. Retick, E.D. Vaughan, & A.J. Wein (Eds.), *Campbell's urology* (7th ed., vol. 3) (pp. 2283–2326). Philadelphia: Saunders.

Bramble, F.J. (1997). Drug-induced cystitis: The need for vigilance. *British Journal of Urology, 79*(1), 3–7.

Choudhury, D., & Ahmed, Z. (1997). Drug-induced nephrotoxicity. *Medical Clinics of North America, 81,* 705–717.

Meisenberg, B., Lassiter, M., Hussein, A., Ross, M., Vredenburgh, J.J., & Peters, W.P. (1994). Prevention of hemorrhagic cystitis after high-dose alkylating agent chemotherapy and autologous bone marrow support. *Bone Marrow Transplantation, 142,* 287–291.

Ross, R.K., Jones, P.A., & Yu, M.C. (1996). Bladder cancer epidemiology and pathogenesis. *Seminars in Oncology, 23,* 536–545.

West, N.J. (1997). Prevention and treatment of hemorrhagic cystitis. *Pharmacotherapy, 17,* 696–707.

Chapter

77. Oliguria/Anuria/Azotemia

● Barbara St. Marie, RN, MA, CNP, ANP, GNP

I. Definition
   A. Oliguria is the amount of urine output below which the normal load of metabolic waste products cannot be excreted (usually 400–500 cc/24 hours).
   B. Anuria, a rare occurrence, is a urine output less than 100 cc/day.
   C. Azotemia is the retention of nitrogenous waste normally cleared by the kidney with more than 50% reduction in glomerular filtration rate.

II. Pathophysiology: Oliguria, anuria, and azotemia can be caused by urinary tract obstruction, infection, and renal perfusion impairment.

III. Clinical features
   A. Etiology
      1. Obstruction in the urinary tract
      2. Renal parenchymal disease
      3. Renal arterial occlusion
      4. Cortical necrosis
      5. Crescentic glomerulonephritis
      6. Severe acute tubular necrosis
      7. Hypovolemia (e.g., diarrhea, diuresis, poor intake)
      8. "Third space" losses (e.g., as in peritonitis)
   B. History
      1. History of cancer and cancer treatment
      2. Current medications: Prescribed and over-the-counter
      3. History of presenting symptoms: Precipitating factors, onset, location, and duration
      4. Changes in activities of daily living
      5. Past medical history: Stomach or intestinal bleeding, congestive heart failure (CHF), cirrhosis, nephrotic syndrome, peritonitis, bowel obstruction, diabetes mellitus
      6. Recent history of receiving contrast dyes
   C. Signs and symptoms
      1. Hypovolemia and prerenal azotemia
         a) Poor tissue turgor
         b) Thirst

        c) Dizziness, lightheadedness

        d) Weight loss

    2. CHF or cirrhosis of the liver

        a) Edema

        b) Shortness of breath

  D. Physical exam

    1. Vital signs

        a) Orthostatic hypotension: May indicate hypovolemia or prerenal azotemia

        b) Tachycardia: May indicate hypovolemia or prerenal azotemia

        c) Weight loss or gain: May be present depending upon etiology

    2. Abdominal exam

        a) Hepatomegaly: May indicate cirrhosis or CHF

        b) Hepatojugular reflux in supine or semirecumbent position: May indicate cirrhosis

        c) Distended bladder and flank pain: May indicate postrenal obstructive acute renal failure (ARF)

        d) Pelvic mass

    3. Integument exam: Poor skin turgor

    4. Lower extremities: Pitting edema, indicating cirrhosis or CHF

    5. Pulmonary exam

        a) Rales: Indicate CHF

        b) Inability to lie flat without shortness of breath: Indicates CHF

    6. Cardiac exam

        a) Sinus tachycardia

        b) S_3 gallop sound

IV. Diagnostic tests

  A. Laboratory

    1. Urinalysis

        a) Prerenal: Normal

        b) Acute renal failure: Muddy brown casts

        c) Postrenal: Crystals, WBCs, RBCs, and bacteria

    2. Urinary sodium

        a) Prerenal: < 20

        b) Acute renal failure: > 40

        c) Postrenal: Variable

    3. Urinary osmolality

        a) Prerenal: > 500

        b) Acute renal failure: < 350

        c) Postrenal: Variable

    4. 24-hour urine collection

    5. Chemistries

        a) Blood urea nitrogen- (BUN-) creatinine ratio: 10–14:1 in renal parenchymal disease

        b) BUN-creatinine ratio: 20:1 in prerenal disease

        c) Hyperchloremic acidosis: Suggests tubular dysfunction and interstitial disease

  B. Radiology
    1. Technetium scanning: To distinguish vascular occlusion from obstructive uropathy and renal parenchymal disease
    2. CT scan or ultrasound: To rule out obstruction
    3. Retrograde pyelography: If questions of obstruction remain after the above procedures are done

V. Differential diagnosis
  A. Volume depletion: Shock and dehydration
  B. CHF (see Chapter 40)
  C. Cirrhosis (see Chapter 64)
  D. Nephrotic syndrome
  E. Peritonitis
  F. Obstructive uropathy
    1. Urethral obstruction
    2. Bilateral ureteral obstruction
  G. Vascular disease
    1. Acute renal arterial obstruction
    2. Renal vein obstruction
  H. Renal parenchymal disease
    1. Diffuse acute glomerular disease
      a) Acute glomerulonephritis
      b) Acute vasculitis
    2. Acute tubular necrosis
      a) Prolonged prerenal failure
      b) Nephrotoxic agents
      c) Sepsis
      d) Myoglobinuria
    3. Acute interstitial nephritis
      a) Hypersensitivity to methicillin, ampicillin, NSAIDs, cephalosporins
      b) Acute urate nephropathy
      c) Hypercalcemic nephropathy
    4. Postcontrast media in preexisting renal failure
      a) Multiple myeloma
      b) Diabetes mellitus (see Chapter 143)

VI. Treatment
  A. Relieve underlying process
    1. Relieve obstruction with surgical intervention or stent placement.
    2. Attempt to establish a urine output with volume challenge or diuretics, administration of fluids (contraindicated in CHF).
    3. Relieve vascular obstruction.
  B. Correct electrolyte imbalances (see Chapters 144–148).
  C. Measure strict intake and output and daily weights.
  D. Discontinue all nephrotoxic medications and avoid radiographic studies with IV contrast.

VII. Follow-up: Depends on underlying etiology; serial observations are necessary to measure serum creatinine.

VIII. Referrals
    A. Nephrologist: To collaborate for evaluation and initial management
    B. Nurse practitioner: For follow-up visits to monitor laboratory status and physical exam

References

Adler, S., & Fairley, K. (1995). The patient with hematuria or proteinuria, or both, and abnormal findings on urinary microscopy. In R.W. Schreier (Ed.), *Manual of nephrology* (4th ed.). Boston: Little, Brown & Co.

Barretti, P., & Soares, V.A. (1997). Acute renal failure: Clinical outcome and causes of death. *Renal Failure, 19,* 253–257.

DePriest, J. (1997). Reversing oliguria in critically ill patients. *Postgraduate Medicine, 102,* 245–246, 251–252, 258.

Lesko, J., & Johnston, J.P. (1997). Oliguria. *AACN Clinical Issues, 8,* 459–468.

78. Penile Discharge

Roberta A. Strohl, RN, BSN, MN, AOCN®

I. Definition: Abnormal discharge or secretions from the penis

II. Pathophysiology: Inflammation and/or infection in the urethra

III. Clinical features
  A. Etiology
    1. STDs
    2. Cancer of the urethra
    3. Cancer of the penis with obstruction of ureter: Most common histology is squamous cell carcinoma.
  B. History
    1. History of cancer and cancer treatment
    2. Current medications: Prescribed and over-the-counter
    3. History of presenting symptom(s): Precipitating factors, onset, location, and duration
    4. Changes in activities of daily living
    5. Past medical history: Urethritis, STDs, HIV, recent exposure to anyone with an STD, unprotected sexual intercourse
  C. Signs and symptoms
    1. Area of induration
    2. Erythema of glans
    3. Warty growth, nodule, or superficial ulceration with bleeding
    4. Swelling of groin
    5. Difficulty voiding
    6. Purulent or bloody urethral discharge
    7. Fever
    8. Perineal pain, urinary retention
    9. Tender epididymis or prostate
  D. Physical exam
    1. Genitourinary exam
      a) Assess penis for lesions (occur on glans penis in uncircumcised males); note discharge and ulceration.
      b) Examine external genitalia for warts, lesions, abrasions, erythema, edema.
      c) Palpate scrotum to evaluate for masses, pain, edema.

    2. Rectal exam

       a) Examine anus for abrasion, warts, trauma.

       b) Evaluate for masses and intact rectal vault.

       c) Palpate prostate for tenderness, contour, edema.

    3. Abdominal exam: Palpate for masses and organomegaly.

    4. Lymph exam: Inguinal nodes may be enlarged from infection or malignancy.

IV. Diagnostic tests

    A. Laboratory

       1. Biopsy of suspicious lesions

       2. Gram stain of penile drainage

         a) Polymorphonuclear leukocytes containing gram-negative diplococci indicates gonorrhea.

         b) Nongonococcal urethritis yields polymorphonuclear leukocytes without bacteria.

       3. Biopsy of urethra: To rule out urethral cancer

    B. Radiology: CT of abdomen and pelvis to evaluate lymph node enlargement if etiology uncertain

V. Differential diagnosis

    A. Malignancy

    B. Urethritis

    C. STD

       1. Gonorrhea (see Chapter 87)

       2. Chlamydia trichomoniasis (see Chapter 86)

    D. Group A beta-hemolytic streptococcus

    E. Reiter's syndrome

VI. Treatment

    A. Penile cancer

       1. Surgery: May be limited (circumcision) or radical (total penectomy)

       2. Radiation and chemotherapy: May be indicated depending upon extent of disease

    B. STDs

       1. Gonorrhea: Ceftriaxone 125 mg IM single dose or cefixime 400 mg po single dose (see Chapter 87)

       2. Chlamydia trichomoniasis: Metronidazole 2 g po as a single dose (see Chapter 86)

    C. Urethral cancers: In men, treated with partial or total penectomy and possibly bilateral inguinal node dissection if clinically palpable groin nodes are present

VII. Follow-up

    A. Monitor for disease recurrence with physical examination and pelvic CT scan.

    B. Counsel patients on risk for recurrence of STD and preventive measures.

VIII. Referrals

    A. STD clinic and/or social worker: To assist patients in ongoing treatment and preventive strategies

    B. Surgeon, urologist, or oncologist: For management of cancer

References

Lindegaard, J.C. (1996). A retrospective analysis of 82 cases of cancer of the penis. *British Journal of Urology, 77,* 883–890.

Magoha, G.A. (1996). Management of carcinoma of the penis: A review. *East African Medical Journal, 72,* 547–550.

Micali, G. (1995). Squamous cell carcinoma of the penis. *Journal of American Academy of Dermatology, 34,* 715–716.

Chapter

79. Proteinuria

Barbara St. Marie, RN, MA, CNP, ANP, GNP

I. Definition: An abnormal excretion of protein >150 mg/24 hours

II. Physiology/Pathophysiology
   A. Normal
      1. Urinary proteins normally are composed of filtered proteins from plasma (50%) and proteins that are secreted into the urine from urinary tract cells (50%).
      2. The normal average amount of protein excreted per day is approximately 40–50 mg.
   B. Pathophysiology
      1. Proteinuria is classified into three major categories.
         a) Overflow proteinuria: Occurs when the filtration of a large amount of serum protein exceeds the absorption capacity of normal tubules
         b) Tubular proteinuria: Occurs when there is injury to the renal tubules, causing the tubules to fail to completely reabsorb small molecular weight proteins filtered by the glomerulus
         c) Glomerular proteinuria: Occurs with injury to the glomerulus, causing an increase in the clearance of serum proteins or an increase in glomerular permeability
      2. Proteinuria can occur from an increased production of abnormal proteins small enough to pass freely through the glomerulus (e.g., Bence Jones protein) and is seen in multiple myeloma.

III. Clinical features
   A. Etiology
      1. Hypertension
      2. Primary renal disease
      3. Diabetes mellitus
      4. Transient proteinuria after contact sports
      5. Pelvic or lower abdominal trauma
   B. History
      1. History of cancer and cancer treatment
      2. Current medications: Prescribed and over-the-counter
      3. History of presenting symptom(s): Precipitating factors, onset, location, duration, and urinary pattern

    4. Changes in activities of daily living
    5. Past medical history: Diabetes mellitus, kidney disease, connective tissue disease, amyloidosis, CHF, typhus, hepatitis, UTIs
    6. Family history: Diabetes mellitus, kidney disease
- C. Signs and symptoms
    1. Changes in urinary pattern
    2. Flank pain
    3. Arthralgia
    4. Skin rash
    5. Dry eyes (i.e., Sjogrens syndrome)
- D. Physical exam
    1. Vital signs: Hypertension
    2. Integument exam: Erythematous rash, suggestive of connective tissue disease
    3. Ophthalmologic exam: Diabetic retinopathy
    4. Evidence of CHF
        a) Lower extremity edema
        b) S_3
        c) Jugular vein distention
        d) Rales
        e) Bilateral lower extremity edema
    5. Abdominal exam
        a) Distended bladder, flank pain: Suggests acute postrenal obstructive renal failure
        b) Enlarged kidneys: Suggests polycystic disease
    6. Prostatic exam: Enlargement suggests postrenal obstructive acute renal failure.

IV. Diagnostic tests
- A. Laboratory
    1. Urinalysis (see Figure 79-1)
    2. 24-hour urinary protein collection: To analyze total protein and composition of urinary protein
        a) The test may not be necessary if urinalysis reveals trace or 1+ protein and no other evidence of renal disease.
        b) Patients with minimal to moderate proteinuria should be checked for postural or orthostatic proteinuria.
            (1) Orthostatic proteinuria can be differentiated from other etiologies by evaluating a urine sample collected upon arising and another after staying continuously upright for two hours.

Figure 79-1. Urinalysis Diagnostic Results

Nephrotic Syndrome	Glomerulonephritis	Diabetes mellitus
Fatty casts	Red cell casts	Glycosuria
Oval fat bodies	Hematuria Proteinuria	
Double refractile fat globules		

        (2) For patients with postural orthostatic proteinuria, the total urinary protein excretion exceeds 150 mg and < 1 g during urine collection; protein excreted during recumbency should not exceed 75 mg.

        (3) Procedure: Patient rests for two hours and voids prior to retiring in the evening to ensure an empty bladder while recumbent. Patient is recumbent for eight hours and, upon arising, voids in container labeled "recumbent urine." The patient stays up and performs nonvigorous activity, and all subsequent urine is collected over the next eight hours into a container labeled "ambulatory urine."

   3. 24-hour collection of urine (see Figure 79-2)

      a) Quantify the degree of proteinuria.

      b) Urinary albumin

      c) Urine creatinine: Depending on the muscle tone, the total 24-hour creatinine should be 15–24 mg/kg.

   4. Serum studies to determine etiology

      a) CBC: To evaluate for anemia that results from renal insufficiency and myeloma

      b) Serum creatinine: Clearance can be determined in conjunction with the urine creatinine.

      c) BUN: To follow renal function; less sensitive than creatinine clearance

      d) Glucose: To evaluate for diabetes mellitus

      e) Serum albumin: Inversely correlates with the severity of proteinuria

      f) Serum protein electrophoresis: Monoclonal gammopathy or multiple myeloma

  B. Radiology: Renal ultrasound to evaluate for

   1. Polycystic kidney disease

   2. Renal stones

   3. Obstruction

   4. Kidney size (small in chronic renal failure).

  C. Other: Renal biopsy to rule out glomerular disease

Figure 79-2. 24-Hour Collection of Urine

1. Empty the bladder and discard the first urine on the morning of collection.
2. Collect all subsequent urine for the next 24 hours.
3. The final urine at the end of the 24-hour period is kept as part of the collection.

Prerenal Acute Renal Failure	Intrarenal Acute Renal Failure	Chronic Renal Failure
1. Urine osmolality >500	1. Urine osmolality approximately 300	1. Glomerular filtration tests > 30 ml/min
2. Specific gravity > 1.020	2. Specific gravity approximately 1.010	2. Normal urine osmolality
3. Hyaline casts	3. Tubular casts	3. Normal specific gravity
	4. Tubular cells	
	5. Brownish muddy appearance due to brown granular casts	

V. Differential diagnosis
   A. Hypertension (see Chapter 45)
   B. Medication-induced
      1. Gold salts (oral or parenteral): Can cause nephropathy
      2. Penicillamine
      3. NSAIDs
   C. Prerenal diseases: Renal artery stenosis
   D. Renal parenchymal diseases
      1. Glomerular diseases
         a) Membranous glomerulonephritis
         b) HIV nephropathy
         c) Immunoglobulin A (IgA) nephropathy
         d) Diabetic glomerulosclerosis
      2. Tubulointerstitial diseases
         a) Drug-induced interstitial nephritis
         b) Chronic pyelonephritis with reflux (see Chapter 93)
         c) Analgesic nephropathy
         d) Radiation nephritis
         e) Polycystic kidney disease
         f) Sickle cell nephropathy (see Chapter 118)
      3. Vascular diseases
         a) Thrombotic thrombocytopenic purpura
         b) Hypertensive nephropathy
         c) Vasculitis
   E. Postrenal diseases
      1. Ureteral obstruction
      2. Bladder outlet obstruction
   F. Transient proteinuria induced by
      1. CHF (see Chapter 40)
      2. Fever (see Chapter 140)
      3. Heavy exercise
   G. Overflow proteinuria
      1. Multiple myeloma
      2. Amyloidosis
      3. Lymphoproliferative disorder

VI. Treatment
   A. When proteinuria is caused by acute renal failure (see Chapter 83), remove the nephrotoxin, if involved.
   B. When proteinuria is caused by chronic renal failure
      1. Control hypertension (see Chapter 45).
      2. In glomerular disease, the reduction of urinary protein excretion protects renal function.
         a) Dietary protein restriction

       b) Angiotensin-converting enzyme inhibitors are used to protect the kidney by improving blood flow.

   3. Correct fluid and electrolyte imbalance (see Chapters 144–148).

       a) Hypocalcemia from impaired vitamin D synthesis

       b) Serum phosphorous levels as the excretion of phosphorous is decreased

       c) Correct hyperphosphatemia with oral phosphate if present.

   4 Anemia results from the inability of the kidney to produce erythropoietin. When the hematocrit falls below 30%, as in end-stage renal disease, erythropoietin can be administered (see Chapter 112).

   5. Monitor for glucose intolerance, hypertriglyceridemia, and elevated uric acid.

VII. Follow-up: Depends on etiology

VIII. Referrals: To nephrologist if further evaluation is warranted, if autoimmune process is suspected, if etiology for proteinuria unknown, or if renal biopsy is necessary

References

Burton, C., & Harris, K.P. (1996). The role of proteinuria in the progression of chronic renal failure. *American Journal of Kidney Disease, 27,* 765–775.

Keane, W.F., & Eknoyan, G. (1999). Proteinuria, albuminuria, risk, assessment, detection, elimination (PARADE): A position paper of the National Kidney Foundation. *American Journal of Kidney Disease, 33,* 1104–1010.

Keilani, T., Schlueter, W., & Battle, D. (1995). Selected aspects of ACE inhibitor therapy for patients with renal disease: Impact on proteinuria, lipids and potassium. *Journal of Clinical Pharmacology, 35*(1), 87–97.

Pedersen, L.M., & Milman, N. (1996). Prevalence and prognostic significance of proteinuria in patients with lung cancer. *Acta Oncologica, 35,* 691–695.

Chapter

80. Urinary Incontinence

Deborah McCaffrey Boyle, RN, MSN, AOCN®, FAAN

I. Definition: An involuntary, uncontrolled loss of urine that produces a social and hygienic problem, as perceived by the patient, family, or caregivers

II. Physiology/Pathophysiology
   A. Normal
      1. The detrusor muscle of the bladder normally is under simultaneous sympathetic and parasympathetic control.
         a) During the filling phase, sympathetic tone predominates, whereas parasympathetic tone is inhibited.
         b) During voluntary emptying, parasympathetic stimulation produces detrusor contraction and sympathetic tone decreases.
            (1) External sphincter of pelvic floor relaxes and abdominal muscles tighten.
            (2) Urethra facilitates continence.
         c) A reflex arc between the detrusor and the brain stem initiates and amplifies bladder contraction by parasympathetic stimulation. Arc is under cortical inhibition.
      2. Continence depends on three factors.
         a) Detrusor stability
         b) Sphincter or pelvic competence
         c) Central autonomic nervous system function
   B. Pathophysiology
      1. Excessive and inappropriate bladder detrusor muscle contraction can reduce bladder volume capacity, causing frequent and incomplete voiding. Mechanism involves decreased or loss of cortical inhibition of detrusor contraction.
      2. Detrusor overactivity occurs from bladder irritation.
      3. Sphincter or pelvic incompetence occurs from pelvic floor laxity that develops from partial denervation, which reduces sphincter tone.
      4. Interference with sensation and coordination of the detrusor and sphincter activity above the sacral area of the spinal cord leads to detrusor spasticity and outlet obstruction.
      5. Detrusor hypotonia results from longstanding outlet obstruction, detrusor insufficiency, or impaired sensation.

          a) Outlet obstruction causes the detrusor to be constantly overstretched and eventually unable to generate enough pressure to empty the bladder.

          b) Detrusor insufficiency usually results from lower motor neuron damage.

    6. Frontal lobe dysfunction caused by cortical compromise results in the inability to void independently, despite having an intact urinary system.

III. Clinical features

  A. Etiology

    1. Detrusor impairment

      a) Bladder infection

      b) Chronic cystitis

      c) Dementia

      d) Radiation

      e) Detrusor hyperreflexia

      f) Detrusor hypertrophy

    2. Stress incontinence: Involuntary loss of urine in response to pelvic pressure in the absence of detrusor contraction

      a) Occurs during coughing, sneezing, laughing, or other physical activity

      b) Most commonly caused by pelvic descent associated with changes in circulating estrogens or multiple vaginal deliveries

      c) Autonomic neuropathy

      d) Perineal injury

      e) Urologic surgery

    3. Urge incontinence: Involuntary loss of urine caused by detrusor instability associated with an abrupt and strong desire to void (i.e., urgency)

      a) Enlarged prostate

      b) Infection

      c) Cystocele

      d) Stroke

      e) Multiple sclerosis

      f) Irritable bladder disorders (e.g., postinterstitial bladder chemotherapy)

      g) Primary urothelial tumors

    4. Overflow incontinence: Involuntary loss of urine associated with overdistention of the bladder

      a) Diabetes mellitus

      h) Medications with anticholinergic effects

      c) Peripheral neuropathy

      d) Disc herniation

      e) Sacral cord lesion

      f) Vitamin B_{12} deficiency

      g) Bladder outlet obstruction

    5. Functional incontinence: Related to alterations in mobility, dexterity, and/or cognition that interfere with the patient's ability to reach the bathroom

      a) Psychiatric disease

      b) Functional impairment

B. History: History-taking is enhanced by acknowledging embarrassment about symptoms and exercising sensitivity during the interview.
   1. History of cancer and cancer treatment
   2. Current medications: Prescribed and over-the-counter (see Table 80-1)
   3. History of presenting symptom(s): Precipitating factors, onset, location, and duration. Associated symptoms are polydipsia, fever, weight gain/loss, and change in bowel habits or sexual function.
   4. Changes in activities of daily living

C. Signs and symptoms: Symptoms of urinary incontinence may characterize a simple mechanical disorder of the urinary system or may be the direct or indirect result of a serious underlying illness (e.g., malignancy).
   1. Nocturia
   2. Dysuria
   3. Hesitancy
   4. Straining
   5. Interrupted stream
   6. Hematuria
   7. Pain
   8. Frequency
   9. Urgency
   10. Increased leakage
   11. Changes in bowel habits or sexual function
   12. Dribbling
   13. Weak stream

D. Physical exam
   1. Abdominal exam
      a) Palpate for masses and areas of fullness or tenderness.
      b) Palpate the bladder after patient voids for masses and distention.
   2. Genital exam (men)
      a) Assess for abnormalities of foreskin, glans penis, and perineal skin.
      b) Palpate prostate for enlargement.
   3. Pelvic exam (women)
      a) Assess for vaginal atrophy, bladder prolapse, perineal skin condition, tenderness, and muscle tone.
      b) Test continence by asking patient to cough or perform Valsalva maneuver. No urine should be noted if continence intact.
   4. Rectal exam: Test for rectal sensation, tone, fecal impaction, and masses.
   5. Neurologic exam: Assess nerve roots S2–S4 to determine deficits above, within, or distal to the autonomic reflex arc.
      a) Assess bulbocavernosus reflex by squeezing the clitoris or glans penis, which will normally cause the anal sphincter to contract.
      b) Anal tone is similar to the bladder sphincter tone; if the patient can contract anal sphincter voluntarily, the patient has an intact autonomic reflex arc.

Table 80-1. Characteristics of Drugs That Affect Continence

Medication	Potential Effects	Comments
Alcohol	Urinary frequency	Can cloud sensorium, impair mobility, and induce diuresis, resulting in incontinence
Anticholinergics	Urinary retention	Side effects of drugs with anticholinergic properties include urinary retention with associated urinary frequency and overflow incontinence. NOTE: Many over-the-counter medications (commonly taken for insomnia, coryza, pruritus, and vertigo) have anticholinergic effects.
Antihypertensives	Bladder outlet relaxation	Sphincter tone in the proximal urethra can be decreased by alpha-2 agonists, causing urinary retention.
Antipsychotics	Urinary retention	Have anticholinergic properties
Antidepressants	Urinary retention	Have anticholinergic properties
Calcium channel blockers	Urinary retention, frequency	Reduce smooth muscle contractility in the bladder and occasionally can cause urinary retention and overflow incontinence
Diuretics	Urinary frequency, urgency	A brisk diuresis induced by loop diuretics (e.g., furosemide, ethacrynic acid, bumetanide) can overwhelm bladder capacity and lead to polyuria, frequency, and urgency, thereby precipitating incontinence in a frail older person.
Narcotics	Urinary retention	Have anticholinergic properties
Sedatives/hypnotics	Urinary sphincter relaxation	Benzodiazepines, especially long-acting agents (e.g., fluazepam, diazepam), may accumulate in the elderly and cause confusion and secondary incontinence.

Note. Based on information from Agency for Health Care Policy and Research Urinary Incontinence Guidelines Panel, 1992.

IV. Diagnostic tests
  A. Laboratory
    1. Urinalysis: Helpful to rule out hematuria, pyuria, bacteriuria, glycosuria, and proteinuria
    2. CBC: To determine elevated WBC count and PSA level.
    3. Urine cytology to evaluate presence of infection
    4. Renal panel to evaluate for renal failure
  B. Radiology
    1. Voiding cystourethrogram: To determine lower urinary tract anatomy
    2. Pelvic ultrasound: To assess postvoid residual and prostate size
  C. Other
    1. Postvoid straight catheterization: To determine urine residual

2. Provocative stress testing: Another mechanism to measure the presence of residual urine

3. Cystoscopy: To evaluate presence of bladder lesions or urinary obstructive process

V. Differential diagnosis
   A. Infection (see Chapters 91, 92, and 93)
   B. Renal stones
   C. Spinal cord injury (see Chapter 138)
   D. Malignancy
   E. Benign prostrate hypertrophy (see Chapter 85)
   F. Drug-induced (see Table 80-1)

VI. Treatment: Within the realm of four intervention options
   A. Behavioral: Used only following completion of a basic incontinence evaluation and if overflow incontinence is ruled out
      1. Bladder training for urge and stress incontinence
      2. Habit training for urge incontinence
      3. Prompted toileting in frail or cognitively impaired patients
      4. Pelvic muscle exercises for urge and stress incontinence
      5. Restriction of fluid, coffee, tea, and alcohol
      6. Use of an absorbent pad and frequent changes to prevent skin irritation
      7. Elimination or decrease in dose of anticholinergic medication to determine if it is the cause
      8. Intermittent catheterization to manage overflow incontinence
   B. Pharmacologic
      1. Drugs for incontinence caused by detrusor overactivity
         a) Anticholinergic/antispasmodic agents, which relax the bladder and increase bladder capacity; contraindicated in patients with narrow-angle glaucoma
         b) Medications
            (1) Propantheline: 15 mg po q 8 hours
            (2) Oxybutynin: 5 mg po q 8 hours
            (3) Tofranil® (Novartis Pharmaceutical Corp., East Hanover, NJ): 25 mg po at bedtime or q 12°
            (4) Hyoscyamine: 0.375 mg po bid
            (5) Detrol™ (Pharmacia & Upjohn, Peapack, NJ): 2 mg po bid
            (6) Vitamin B12: If deficiency (see Chapter 114)
      2. Drugs for incontinence related to urethral sphincter insufficiency
         a) Alpha-adrenergic agonist agents decrease detrusor activity and increase internal sphincter tone.
         b) These drugs should be used with caution in patients with hypertension, hyperthyroidism, cardiac dysrhythmia, and angina.
         c) Medications
            (1) Phenylpropanolamine (PPA): 75 mg po bid

(2) Imipramine hydrochloride: 10–25 mg po qd to qid

(3) Estrogen cream: qd initially, then two or three times/week

3. Drugs for detrusor atony and reflex incontinence

   a) These drugs increase the detrusor tone.

   b) Examples include the following.

   (1) Bethanechol chloride: 5–25 mg po bid–qid

   (2) Prazosin hydrochloride: 1–5 mg po bid–qid

   (3) Terazosin hydrochloride: 1–2 mg po qd

C. Surgical

   1. Management of stress incontinence

      a) Retropubic suspension

      b) Needle endoscopic suspension

      c) Sling (primarily female)

      d) Artificial sphincter

      e) Urethral bulking

      f) Cystocele repair

   2. Management of urge incontinence

      a) Augmentation cystoplasty

      b) Removal of inflammatory or obstructive lesion

   3. Management of overflow incontinence: Surgical interventions to relieve obstruction.

D. Supportive: Required after or in conjunction with initial attempts to ablate incontinent episode by containing or collecting incontinent urine; methods include use of external catheters (e.g., condom, Texas catheter with leg bag), indwelling urinary catheters, external pads, or diapers.

VII. Follow-up

   A. Short-term

      1. Depends on the nature/etiology of incontinence

      2. Ongoing need for education and reinforcement of self-care techniques

      3. Need for follow-up associated with cancer-related cause of incontinence

   B. Long-term: Assess for long-term adaptation to urinary incontinence.

VIII. Referrals

   A. Urologist: For

      1. Uncertain diagnosis or inability to develop a reasonable management plan based on the diagnostic evaluation

      2. Failure to respond to a therapeutic trial of medications

      3. Incontinence associated with recurrent symptomatic urinary tract infections

      4. Hematuria without infection (also consider consultation to medical oncologist)

      5. Presence of known or suspected prostate nodule, bladder primary tumor, pelvic mass, or lymph node enlargement causing bladder outlet obstruction.

   B. Continence nurse or specialty service: If self-care skills concerning urinary care are required

References

Agency for Health Care Policy and Research Urinary Incontinence Guidelines Panel. (1992). *Urinary incontinence in adults: Clinical practice guideline* (AHCPR Publication No. 92-0038). Rockville, MD: U.S. Department of Health and Human Services.

Davila, G.W. (1994). Urinary incontinence in women. *Postgraduate Medicine, 96*(2), 103–110.

Fainsinger, R.L. (1996). Integrating medical and surgical treatments in gastrointestinal, genitourinary and biliary obstruction in patients with cancer. *Hematology/Oncology Clinics of North America, 10,* 173–188.

Pearson, B.D., & Kelber, S. (1996). Urinary incontinence: Treatments, interventions and outcomes. *Clinical Nurse Specialist, 10*(4), 177–182.

81. Vaginal Discharge

Roberta A. Strohl, RN, BSN, MN, AOCN®

I. Definition: Abnormal discharge or secretions from the vagina

II. Physiology/Pathophysiology
   A. Normal
      1. Physiologic changes in vaginal secretions are normal. Increase in secretions may occur up to the time of ovulation with a subsequent decrease until menses. Pregnancy, stress, and sexual excitement can alter the amount and/or quality of secretions.
      2. Normal vaginal secretions are colorless and odorless with a pH of 3.8–4.2. The predominant normal flora is gram-positive anaerobic *Doderlein bacillus*.
   B. Pathophysiology
      1. Abnormal vaginal discharge may be the result of a change in pH, which provides a favorable environment for the growth of other bacteria.
      2. Systemic antibiotics change the normal bacterial flora, which can promote other bacterial or fungal growth.
      3. Tumors or vaginal fistulas that disrupt the vaginal integrity or that drain into the vagina may result in vaginal discharge and/or bleeding.

III. Clinical features
   A. Etiology
      1. Carcinoma of proximal urethra tumors can invade the bladder and vagina, resulting in discharge and/or bleeding.
      2. Advanced pelvic tumors may invade the vaginal wall.
      3. Vaginal cancer can cause dysfunctional bleeding and discharge, initially presenting with postcoital bleeding.
      4. Cervical cancer can result in chronic cervicitis, which causes vaginal discharge.
      5. Candida
         a) Most commonly related to systemic antibiotics
         b) Occurs in women with diabetes mellitus and pregnant women because the increased glycogen content of vaginal fluid results in intense pruritus
      6. STDs
   B. History: Note normal vaginal secretions and any recent changes.

1. History of cancer and cancer treatment
2. Current medications: Prescribed and over-the-counter
3. History of presenting symptom(s): Precipitating factors, onset, and duration
4. Changes in activities of daily living
5. Past medical history: STDs, HIV

C. Signs and symptoms
   1. Increase in secretions
   2. White, yellow, green, or gray secretions
   3. Thick or bubbly secretions
   4. Bleeding
   5. Foul-smelling discharge
   6. Fever
   7. Burning/pain on urination
   8. Pelvic pain
   9. Burning or itching of introitus

D. Physical exam
   1. Pelvic exam: Note discharge (see Table 81-1) to determine etiology.
      a) Thin, gray discharge with fishy odor indicates bacterial infection.
      b) Thin, yellow, bubbly, frothy, malodorous discharge indicates trichomonas vaginitis.
      c) Thick, white, curd-like discharge indicates Candida (yeast) infection.
      d) Serosanguineous or yellow discharge indicates cervical cancer.
      e) Cervix, vagina, and labia may be painful and swollen.
      f) Ulceration and exophytic cervical lesions indicate malignancy.
      g) Thin vaginal epithelium occurs from low estrogen levels.
   2. If patient is hemorrhaging, pelvic exam may be contraindicated until bleeding can be controlled.

Table 81-1. Types, Symptoms, and Treatment of Vaginal Discharge

Type	Symptoms	Treatment
Trichomonas	Thin, yellow, bubbly, frothy discharge; burning and itching of introitus	Metronidazole: 250 mg po tid x 10 days; must also treat sexual partner
Candida	Thick, white discharge; curd-like appearance; intense pruritus	Nystatin: One applicator intravaginally; clotrimazole: 1 applicator daily for 3–7 days; daily consumption of eight ounces of yogurt; fluconazole: 100–150 mg po x 1 day
Bacterial vaginosis	Thin, gray discharge; persistent discharge; less itching	Metronidazole gel: 5 g vaginally bid x 5 days; clindamycin cream 2%: intravaginally qd x 7 days
Atrophic vaginitis	Clear discharge, soreness, pruritus	Estrogen vaginal cream: ½ to 2 g daily
Neisseria gonorrhea	Pus; red and swollen vaginal canal	Cefixime: 400 mg po x 1 day or ceftriaxone 125 mg IM

IV. Diagnostic tests
   A. Laboratory
      1. Microscopic examination of vaginal secretions: May identify *Trichomonas vaginalis* and *Candida albicans*
      2. CBC: To evaluate for infection or neutropenia
      3. Pregnancy test
      4. Urinalysis: To rule out infection
      5. HIV test
   B. Radiology: Not indicated

V. Differential diagnosis
   A. Malignancy
      1. Carcinoma of urethra proximal tumors
      2. Advanced pelvic tumors
      3. Cancer of the vulva
      4. Vaginal cancer
      5. Cervical cancer
   B. STDs (see Chapters 86, 87, 89, 95, 96, and 98)
   C. Bacterial vaginosis (see Chapter 97)
   D. Atrophic vaginitis (see Chapter 151)
   E. Foreign body: A forgotten tampon is the most common source of discharge from foreign objects.

VI. Treatment (see Table 81-1)
   A. Gynecologic cancers: Treatment of the primary cancer may involve a combined modality approach, usually with surgery and radiation therapy.
   B. Trichomonas vaginalitis is treated with oral metronidazole (Flagyl®, G.D. Searle & Co., Chicago, IL) 250 mg tid/10 days or a single 2 g dose.
   C. Candida
      1. Topical antifungal: Initial cure rate 90%
         a) Nystatin: One applicator intravaginally/seven nights
         b) Miconazole
            (1) Monistat 3® (Ortho Dermatological, Skillman, NJ): 200 mg suppository intravaginally at bedtime for three nights
            (2) Monistat-Derm® (Ortho Dermatological) or Gyne-Lotrimin™ (Schering Corp., Kenilworth, NJ) vaginal cream: One applicator intravaginally at bedtime for seven nights
            (3) 100 mg vaginal tablet intravaginally at bedtime for seven nights
         c) Butoconazole (Femstat™, Syntex [USA] Inc., Palo Alto, CA): 2% cream, one applicator full vaginally at bed time for three nights
         d) Tioconazole: 65 mg, one pre-filled syringe intravaginally at bedtime
      2. Persistent or recurrent cases: May require treatment on days 5–11 of four consecutive menstrual cycles; Fluconazole: 100–150 mg po for one dose
      3. Prophylaxis

          a) Clotrimazole (Mycelex™-G, Bayer Corp., West Haven, CT): 500 mg vaginal tablet once a month

          b) Daily consumption of eight ounces of yogurt containing *lactobacillus acidophilus*

  D. Bacterial vaginosis (see Chapter 97)

    1. Metronidazole gel: 5 g vaginally bid for five days

    2. Clindamycin: 2% cream 5 g intravaginally at bedtime for three or seven consecutive days

  E. Atrophic vaginitis: Estrogen vaginal cream ½ to 2 g daily, depending on the severity of infection (see Chapter 151)

  F. *Neisseria gonorrheae*: Ceftriaxone 125 mg IM in a single dose or cefixime 400 mg orally in a single dose (see Chapter 87)

  G. Foreign body: Remove object.

VII. Follow-up

  A. Follow response to treatment by assessing symptomatic relief and decrease in discharge.

  B. Follow patients on broad-spectrum antibiotic therapy for the development of vaginal infections.

  C. Surgical consult may be needed to remove foreign object.

VIII. Referrals

  A. Gynecologist: To manage persistent problems

  B. HIV/AIDS specialist: For management of problems related to HIV/AIDS diagnosis

References

Daily, R.H. (1996). Vaginal discharge in the adult: A practice guideline. *Journal of Emergency Medicine, 14*(2), 227–232.

Fox, K.K. (1998). Vaginal discharge: How to pinpoint the cause. *Postgraduate Medicine, 3*, 87–90, 93–96, 101.

Fruchter, R.G., Maiman, M., & Sillman, F. (1994). Characteristics of cervical intraepithelial neoplasia in women infected with human immunodeficiency virus. *American Journal of Obstetrics and Gynecology, 171*, 531–537.

McKay, M. (1996). Disorders of the female genitalia. *Western Journal of Medicine, 164*(6), 5–20.

Wathne, B. (1994) Vaginal discharge: A comparison of clinical, laboratory and microbiology findings. *Acta Obstetricaet Gynecologica Scandanavica, 73*, 802–808.

Chapter

82. Vaginal Stenosis

Jennifer S. Jockel, RN, BSN, OCN®

I. Definition: A narrowing and stricture of the vaginal canal

II. Pathophysiology
   A. Stenosis occurs as a result of scarring of the vaginal mucosa, resulting in loss of its pliability and narrowing of the vaginal introitus.
   B. A decrease in blood supply causes the vaginal tissue to become dry and tender and to lose elastic tissue, resulting in fibrous and tough tissue.
   C. Lack of estrogen production causes decreased vaginal lubrication, pruritus, and dyspareunia.

III. Clinical features
   A. Etiology
      1. Pelvic radiation (external and internal) causes a decrease in blood supply to the radiated area.
      2. Surgery that results in shortening the vagina
         a) Radical hysterectomy
         b) Radical vulvectomy
         c) Partial vaginectomy
         d) Pelvic exenteration
      3. Menopause
         a) Natural onset
         b) Medically induced: Chemotherapy
         c) Surgically induced: Bilateral oophorectomy
         d) Radiation-induced: To the lower abdomen or pelvis
   B. History
      1. History of cancer and cancer treatment
      2. Current medications: Prescribed and over-the-counter
      3. History of presenting symptom(s): Precipitating factors, onset, and duration
      4. Changes in activities of daily living
      5. Past medical history: Gynecologic surgery, menopausal state
   C. Signs and symptoms
      1. Dyspareunia

517

      2. Vaginal dryness

      3. Inability to have sexual intercourse

      4. Ulceration

      5. Peeling

   D. Physical exam: Pelvic exam reveals

      1. Shortened vagina

      2. Atrophy of the vaginal walls; thin, friable vaginal mucosa

      3. Narrowed introitus: Can cause difficulty when passing the speculum; use a narrow or pediatric speculum lubricated with water.

      4. Labial agglutination: Clumping together of labia/vaginal tissue usually caused by excessive dryness and lack of vaginal dilation; adhesions can be manually broken and then treated aggressively for dryness.

      5. Scarred vaginal tissue; possible ulceration

      6. Excessive dryness

IV. Diagnostic tests: Noncontributory

V. Differential diagnosis

   A. Disease-related

      1. Vaginal ulcers

      2. Vaginismus: A psychophysiologic genital reaction in women characterized by contraction of the perineal and paravaginal muscles, tightly closing the vaginal introitus

      3. STD (see Chapters 86, 90, and 95)

      4. Vaginitis (see Chapter 97)

      5. Menopause (see Chapter 151)

VI. Treatment

   A. Sexual intercourse

      1. Sexually active patients should be encouraged to engage in sexual intercourse at least three times/week to maintain pliability of the vaginal tissue.

      2. Application of water-soluble lubrication before intercourse is recommended (see Figure 82-1).

   B. Dilator (see Figure 82-2)

      1. Vaginal dilators should be used regularly (i.e., at least three times/week) in patients who are not sexually active or in conjunction with sexual activity; maintains pliability of vaginal tissue and patency of the vaginal vault.

         a) Postoperative use should begin four weeks after surgery or after complete healing of vaginal wall.

Figure 82-1. Recommended Lubrication

1. Replens® (Columbia Laboratories, Coconut Grove, FL)

2. K-Y Jelly® (Johnson & Johnson, Brunswick, NJ)

3. Astroglide® (Astro-Lube Inc., North Hollywood, CA)

4. Estrogen vaginal cream: Usual dosage is ½–2 g daily, depending on the severity (contraindicated in estrogen-dependent tumors).

Figure 82-2. Instructions on Using a Vaginal Dilator

---

1. Wash your hands and the dilator with soap and water.

2. Liberally lubricate the dilator with water-soluble lubricant.

3. Lie on your back, bend your knees, and open your legs.

4. Insert the vaginal dilator slowly, as far as it will go without hurting.

5. Close your knees, and straighten your legs.

6. Maintain this position for at least 10 minutes.

7. Bend your knees, open your legs, and slowly remove the dilator.

8. Wash dilator with soap and water and dry.

Note. Dilators come in small, medium, and large sizes. The patient should start with a dilator she is able to partially insert into her vagina. Remember, using a vaginal dilator for prevention or treatment can be uncomfortable and frustrating. It is important to stay relaxed and be persistent to experience positive results.

      b) After radiation to the vaginal area, use should begin approximately four weeks after completion of radiation or after vaginal discomfort has dissipated.

    2. Water-soluble lubrication is recommended to facilitate dilator use to prevent trauma and pain; do not use oil-based lubricants (e.g., petroleum jelly).

  C. Surgery: Neovaginal reconstruction

  D. Prevention of vaginal dryness

    1. Insert one vitamin E capsule, 400 U, intravaginally, three times/week at bedtime.

    2. Alternate vitamin E with a vaginal lubricant (see Figure 82-1) three times/week at bedtime.

    3. Use liberal application of lubricant with sexual intercourse or with vaginal dilator.

    4. Unless contraindicated by the presence of an estrogen-dependent tumor, prescribe an estrogen cream, patch, or tablets to relieve vaginal dryness. Estrogen vaginal cream has a usual dosage of ½–2 g daily, depending on the severity (contraindicated in hormonally related tumors).

VII. Follow-up

  A. Short-term: For complications related to stenosis (e.g., fistula)

  B. Long-term: After surgery or radiation, the patient is seen every three to six months for two to three years, then annually.

  C. Patients with menopausal-induced stenosis should be seen annually for pelvic exams.

VIII. Referrals

  A. Gynecologist or gynecologic oncologist: For frequent exams for recurrence and long-term complications (e.g., fistula, vaginal necrosis)

  B. Plastic surgeon: For vaginal reconstruction

  C. Sex therapist: To assist with sexual dysfunction and to discuss alternatives to sexual expression (i.e., instead of intercourse)

References

Bergmark, K., Avall-Lundqvist, E., Dickman, P.W., Henningsohn, L., & Steineck, G. (1999). Vaginal changes and sexuality in women with a history of cervical cancer. *New England Journal of Medicine, 340,* 1383–1389.

Cartwright-Alcarese, F. (1995). Addressing sexual dysfunction following radiation therapy for gynecological malignancy. *Oncology Nursing Forum, 22,* 1227–1232.

Chyle, V., Zagars, G.K., Wheeler, J.A., Wharton, J.T., & Delclos, L. (1996). Definitive radiotherapy for carcinoma of the vagina: Outcome and prognostic factors. *International Journal of Radiation Oncology, Biology, Physics, 35,* 891–905.

Greendale, G.A., Lee, N.P., & Arriola, E.R. (1999). The menopause. *Lancet, 353,* 571–580.

Heller, D.S., Kambham, N., Smith, D., & Cracchiolo, B. (1999). Recurrence of gynecologic malignancy at the vaginal vault after hysterectomy. *International Journal of Gynaecology and Obstetrics, 64,* 159–162.

Kirkbride, P., Fyles, A., Rawlings, G.A., Manchul, L., Levin, W., Murphy, K.J., & Simm, J. (1995). Carcinoma of the vagina—Experience at the Princess Margaret Hospital (1974–1989). *Gynecology Oncologic, 56,* 435–443.

Kusiak, J.F., & Rosenblum, N.G. (1996). Neovaginal reconstruction after exenteration using an omental flap and split-thickness skin graft. *Plastic and Reconstructive Surgery, 97,* 775–783.

Perez, C.A., Grigsby, P.W., Garipagaoglu, M., Mutch, D.G., & Lockett, M.A. (1999). Factors affecting long-term outcome of irradiation in carcinoma of the vagina. *International Journal of Radiation, Oncology, Biology, Physics, 44,* 37–45.

Chapter

83. Acute Renal Failure
Julie D. Painter, RNC, MSN, OCN®

I. Definition: Acute renal failure (ARF) is characterized by a rapid decrease in the glomerular filtration rate and the retention of nitrogenous waste products.

II. Physiology/Pathophysiology
   A. Normal
      1. Kidneys receive 20%–25% of the cardiac output and, therefore, are sensitive to blood supply changes.
      2. Function of the kidneys
         a) Maintain fluid and electrolyte balance when loss of functioning nephrons occurs.
         b) Excrete waste products: Normal healthy adults need a urine output of approximately 400 ml/24 hours to excrete waste products.
         c) Activate the renin-angiotensin-aldosterone system as an adaptive response.
            (1) When stimulated, peripheral and efferent arteriole vasoconstriction occurs, increasing perfusion pressure.
            (2) Activation of this system also causes aldosterone secretion, causing reabsorption of sodium and water with potassium excreted.
               (a) Sodium reabsorption leads to an increased plasma osmolality, which stimulates the hypothalamic osmoreceptor to release antidiuretic hormone (ADH).
               (b) ADH enhances water reabsorption from the distal tubules, thereby increasing intravascular volume and renal perfusion.
      3. The glomerular capillary bed lies between the afferent arteriole and the efferent arteriole. When resistance to blood occurs, an increase or decrease at either end alters the glomerular hydrostatic pressure.
      4. Autoregulation maintains glomerular hydrostatic pressure by dilation of the afferent arteriole and constriction of the efferent arteriole.
   B. Pathophysiology: Acute renal failure is categorized as prerenal, intrinsic (intrarenal), or postrenal.
      1. Prerenal failure: Results from inadequate perfusion of the kidneys, causing tubular damage, and is rapidly reversible with restoration of the renal blood flow and glomerular filtration pressure.

          a) If not restored in a timely fashion, ischemic renal parenchymal injury and intrinsic renal azotemia may result.

          b) Diminished glomerular filtration results in the accumulation of waste products as reflected by rising blood urea nitrogen (BUN) and creatinine levels within the blood (i.e., azotemia).

          c) In hypoperfusion, the kidneys activate two major adaptive responses—autoregulation and renin release.

  2. Intrinsic renal azotemia (intrarenal ARF)

          a) Most cases are caused by ischemia, secondary to renal hypoperfusion (ischemic ARF) or toxins (nephrotoxic ARF).

          b) Ischemic and nephrotoxic ARF often are associated with necrosis of the tubule epithelial cells and damage to the renal parenchyma. The mechanism of failure is not completely understood; therefore, only hypotheses are proposed.

              (1) Back leak theory proposes that glomerular filtrate backs up through damaged tubules into the peritubular circulation, leading to morphologic changes in the basement membrane of the glomerular capillary.

              (2) Another theory is the tubules become obstructed with cellular and protein debris.

              (3) Vascular theory relates to renal hypoperfusion, which results in cell death and tubular necrosis.

          c) This type of ARF does not resolve easily or quickly with restoration of renal perfusion but requires the removal of the causative factor, condition, or toxin.

  3. Postrenal failure (obstruction/postrenal azotemia): Obstruction of the urinary tract accounts for about 5% of acute renal failure, with obstruction of the bladder neck being the most common cause.

III. Clinical features: ARF usually is asymptomatic and is diagnosed on screening of patient's serum BUN and creatinine, showing increased values. ARF is usually reversible but remains a major cause of morbidity and mortality, most likely from the seriousness and acuity of the underlying disease process.

  A. Phases of acute renal failure

    1. During initial phase of injury, immediate intervention can reverse or prevent further damage.

    2. Oliguric phase has a duration of 8–14 days, during which the urine output is greatly reduced.

    3. Degree of azotemia development depends on the urine output and the degree of protein breakdown.

    4. Diuretic phase marks the recovery of the nephrons and ability to secrete urine over 10 days. Diuresis occurs before complete recovery so the patient remains azotemic.

    5. Recovery phase may last up to six months of renal improvement with the ability to concentrate urine being the last to recover.

  B. Risk factors

    1. Nephrotoxic agents administered

2. Age (i.e., elderly more susceptible)
3. Comorbidity (e.g., diabetes mellitus, chronic hypertension)
C. Etiology: Occurs in about 5% of acute care admissions and 30% of admissions to intensive care
   1. Prerenal causes
      a) Hypovolemia caused by
         (1) Hemorrhage, burns, dehydration
         (2) Gastrointestinal fluid loss
         (3) Renal fluid loss (i.e., from diuretics, diabetes mellitus)
         (4) Sequestration of fluid in extravascular space (i.e., from pancreatitis, burns, trauma, peritonitis, hypoalbuminemia)
      b) Low cardiac output caused by
         (1) Diseases of the myocardium, valves, and pericardium
         (2) Dysrhythmia
         (3) Cardiac tamponade
         (4) Pulmonary hypertension
         (5) Pulmonary emboli
         (6) Positive pressure mechanical ventilation
      c) Increased renal to systemic vascular resistance ratio from
         (1) Systemic vasodilatation caused by sepsis, antihypertensives, afterload reducers, anesthesia, and anaphylaxis
         (2) Renal vasoconstriction caused by hypercalcemia, norepinephrine, epinephrine, cyclosporine, amphotericin B
         (3) Cirrhosis with ascites
      d) Renal hypoperfusion with impairment of renal auto-regulatory responses caused by cyclooxygenase inhibitors (e.g., NSAIDs) or angiotensin-converting enzyme inhibitors
      e) Hyperviscosity syndrome: Rare, but causes include multiple myeloma, macroglobulinemia, and polycythemia
      f) Renovascular obstruction (bilateral or unilateral with one functioning kidney) caused by
         (1) Renal artery or vein obstruction
         (2) Atherosclerotic disease
         (3) Thrombosis
         (4) Embolism
         (5) Aneurysm
   2. Intrinsic renal
      a) Diseases of glomeruli or renal microvasculature caused by
         (1) Glomerulonephritis
         (2) Hemolytic uremic syndrome
         (3) Thrombotic thrombocytopenic purpura
         (4) Disseminated intravascular coagulopathy
         (5) Pregnancy—toxemia
         (6) Accelerated hypertension
         (7) Radiation nephritis

        (8) Scleroderma

        (9) Systemic lupus erythematosus

    b) Acute tubular necrosis caused by

        (1) Ischemia: Related to low cardiac output, abruptio placenta, renal vasoconstriction, systemic vasodilatation, postpartum hemorrhage

        (2) Exogenous toxins: Contrast media, cyclosporine, antibiotics (e.g., amphotericin B, aminoglycosides), chemotherapeutic agents (e.g., cisplatin), organic solvents (e.g., ethylene glycol), acetaminophen or illegal abortifacient

        (3) Endogenous causes: Rhabdomyolysis, hemolysis, uric acid, plasma cell dyscrasia (e.g., multiple myeloma)

    c) Interstitial nephritis

        (1) Allergic reaction caused by antibiotics (e.g., beta-lactam, sulfonamides, trimethoprim, rifampin), cyclooxygenase inhibitors, diuretics

        (2) Infections: Bacterial or viral

        (3) Infiltration of lymphoma, leukemia, sarcoidosis disease

        (4) Cholesterol emboli

    d) Intratubular deposition and obstruction: Myeloma proteins, uric acid, oxalate, acyclovir, methotrexate, sulfonamides

    e) Renal allograft rejection

  3. Postrenal failure

    a) Ureteric

        (1) Renal calculi

        (2) Blood clot, sloughed papillae, cancer, external compression, which may be caused by retroperitoneal fibrosis

    b) Bladder neck

        (1) Neurogenic bladder

        (2) Anticholinergic medications

        (3) Benign prostatic hypertrophy

        (4) Prostate cancer

        (5) Prostatitis

        (6) Calculi

        (7) Blood clots

    c) Urethra

        (1) Stricture

        (2) Congenital valve

        (3) Phimosis

D. History

  1. History of cancer and cancer treatment

  2. Current medications: Prescribed and over-the-counter

  3. History of presenting symptom(s): Precipitating factors, onset, and duration

  4. Changes in activities of daily living

  5. Past medical history: Diabetes mellitus, hypertension, benign prostate hypertrophy, blood transfusions, blood loss

E. Signs and symptoms

  1. Nausea and vomiting

2. Drowsiness, confusion, stupor, coma
3. Excessive thirst
4. Palpitations
5. Breathing difficulty (i.e., Kussmaul's repiration)
6. Minimal axillary perspiration
7. Decrease or increase in body weight of 5%–10%
8. Decreased urine output
9. Lower back pain (flank pain)
10. Swelling
11. Fever
12. Muscle aches, fever, and joint pain
13. Blood in urine, bladder pressure, and inability to urinate
14. Rash or skin changes

F. Physical exam
   1. Integument exam indicative of
     a) Prerenal
       (1) Palmar erythema, jaundice indicating chronic liver disease or portal hypertension
       (2) Poor skin turgor
     b) Intrinsic: Skin eruptions may be noted.
     c) Postrenal: Nonspecific
   2. Neurologic exam may reveal drowsiness, confusion, and coma caused by electrolyte imbalance or deterioration of renal function, resulting in the accumulation of metabolites.
   3. Vital signs and weight
     a) Increase or decrease in weight
     b) Hypertension: May be evident with fluid overload in postrenal or intrinsic renal failure
     c) Prerenal: Hypotension caused by volume depletion
   4. Cardiovascular exam
     a) Prerenal
       (1) Gallop indicative of cardiac failure
       (2) Hypotension and tachycardia indicative of loss of vascular volume
       (3) Flat jugular veins indicative of hypovolemia
     b) Intrinsic: Nonspecific
     c) Postrenal: Nonspecific
     d) Pericardial rub: May occur in each phase
   5. Pulmonary: Kussmaul's respiration may be evident in all phases from metabolic acidosis.
     a) Prerenal: Basilar lung crackles indicative of cardiac failure
     b) Intrinsic: Nonspecific
     c) Postrenal: Nonspecific
   6. Abdomen exam
     a) Prerenal: Ascites or splenomegaly indicative of portal hypertension or chronic liver disease

        b) Intrinsic: Nonspecific

        c) Postrenal

           (1) Flank pain radiating to groin may indicate acute ureteric obstruction.

           (2) Distended bladder may be present, indicating neurogenic bladder.

           (3) Pelvic mass may be palpated.

   7. Thorax exam: Costovertebral angle (CVA) tenderness

   8. Extremities exam

        a) Prerenal

           (1) Peripheral edema or coolness of extremities indicative of cardiac failure

           (2) Asterixis (i.e., involuntary muscle tremor)

        b) Intrinsic: Evidence of distal cholesterol emboli in extremities with atheroemboli renal failure

        c) Postrenal: Nonspecific

   8. Rectal

        a) Prerenal: Nonspecific

        b) Intrinsic: Nonspecific

        c) Postrenal: Enlarged prostate may indicate obstruction.

IV. Diagnostic tests: The healthcare provider should first determine if the patient is experiencing acute or chronic renal failure. Indicators for chronic failure are anemia, neuropathy, and radiologic evidence of renal osteodystrophy or small, scarred kidneys, yet anemia can occur in acute renal failure.

   A. Laboratory

     1. Urinalysis

        a) Prerenal

           (1) Sodium < 20, osmolarity > 500 (unless patient is on diuretics), otherwise normal

           (2) Specific gravity 1.020 or greater

           (3) Urine volume: Oliguria

        b) Intrinsic

           (1) RBC casts and proteinuria suggest glomerulonephritis or vascular inflammatory disease.

           (2) Pyuria with eosinophils on Wright stain or urinary sediment indicate interstitial nephritis.

           (3) Brown cellular casts and renal tubular epithelial cells in urine sediment suggest acute tubular necrosis.

           (4) Urine volume: Nonoliguria or oliguria

        c) Postrenal

           (1) Crystals may be present in urinary sediment if obstruction is a stone.

           (2) Early obstruction causes urinary indices identical to prerenal failure, yet progression will resemble acute tubular necrosis.

           (3) Specific gravity value variable

           (4) Urine volume: Oliguria, polyuria, or anuria

           (5) Osmolality increased or similar to plasma osmolality

2. Serum BUN and creatinine
   a) Prerenal: BUN/creatinine ratio—20:1 or greater
   b) Intrinsic: BUN/creatinine ratio—10:1 or less
   c) Postrenal: BUN/creatinine ratio usually elevated however can be normal
3. Electrolytes may reveal imbalances (see Chapters 144–148).
   a) Hyperkalemia
   b) Metabolic acidosis
   c) Increased phosphorus, decreased calcium
   d) Increased uric acid
4. CBC may reveal anemia.
B. Radiology: Ultrasonography of kidneys is recommended in most patients with acute renal failure to exclude obstructive uropathy.
C. Other: Renal biopsy may be needed to determine etiology in intrinsic renal disease.

V. Differential diagnosis
A. Chronic renal failure
B. Congestive heart failure (see Chapter 40)
C. Chronic hypertension (see Chapter 45)

VI. Treatment
A. Prevent the occurrence in situations of known risk factors (e.g., nephrotoxic agent use, contrast dye for radiologic exams).
   1. Maintain cardiovascular and intravascular volume.
   2. Monitor renal function before (baseline value), during, and after administration of pharmacologic agents considered to be nephrotoxic.
B. Evaluate for etiology (i.e., prerenal, intrinsic, postrenal) and correct.
   1. Prerenal: Reestablish perfusion of kidneys.
   2. Intrinsic: Remove causative factor (e.g., toxin).
   3. Postrenal: Remove the obstruction.
C. Attempt to establish urine output with volume challenge (e.g., 500–1,000 cc normal saline bolus).
D. Initiate conservative therapy.
   1. Measure intake and output, including daily weight.
   2. Titrate total amount of fluids according to clinical status.
   3. Correct electrolyte imbalances (see Chapter 144–148) and monitor daily.
   4. Transfuse blood products for support.
   5. Eliminate all causative factors (e.g., nephrotoxic agents).
E. Dialysis may be indicated for volume overload, pericarditis, bleeding, symptomatic uremia, severe hyperkalemia, or acidosis.

VII. Follow-up
A. Patient's follow-up should depend on the severity and resolution of symptoms.
B. Frequent assessment of renal function (i.e., BUN and creatinine values) will be necessary.

VIII. Referrals
    A. Urologist: For resolution of obstruction
    B. Nephrologist: If failure is not resolved

References

Andreoli, S.P. (1998). Renal manifestations of systemic diseases. *Seminars in Nephrology, 18,* 270–279.

Casperson, D.S., Zumsteg, M., & Mahon, S.M. (1995). Focus on oncology: Nephrotoxicity of chemotherapeutic agents for genitourinary cancers. *Journal of Urological Nursing, 14,* 1110–1119.

Liano, R., & Pascual, J. (1998). Outcomes in acute renal failure. *Seminars in Nephrology, 18,* 541–550.

Perazella, M.A. (1999). Crystal-induced acute renal failure. *American Journal of Medicine, 106,* 459–465.

Ritz, E. (1999). Nephropathy in type 2 diabetes. *Journal of International Medicine, 245*(2), 111–126.

Uribarri, J. (1999). Past, present and future of end-stage renal disease therapy in the United States. *Mt. Sinai Journal of Medicine, 66*(1), 14–29.

Vijayan, A., & Miller, S.B. (1998). Acute renal failure: Prevention and nondialytic therapy. *Seminars in Nephrology, 18,* 523–532.

84. Adrenal Metastasis

Laura M. Stempkowski, RN, MS, CUNP, AOCN®

I. Definition: Metastasis to the adrenal glands from solid tumors

II. Physiology/Pathophysiology
  A. Normal adrenal gland
    1. Paired organs lying atop each kidney, each structurally and functionally differentiated into two sections—the outer adrenal cortex and the inner adrenal medulla
    2. Function of the adrenal gland is to maintain metabolic homeostasis in the face of internal and external stressors.
    3. The adrenal cortex
      a) Makes up about 90% of the adrenal gland
      b) Synthesizes several corticosteroids (i.e., hormones) essential for life
        (1) Glucocorticoids (e.g., hydrocortisone)
          (a) Provide increased glucose in response to stress
          (b) Enhance skeletal and cardiac muscle contraction
          (c) Inhibit bone formation
          (d) Inhibit collagen synthesis
          (e) Increase vascular contractility
          (f) Produce anti-inflammatory effect
          (g) Regulate anti-immune system activity
          (h) Maintain normal glomerular filtration
        (2) Mineralocorticoids: Aldosterone is responsible for 95% of mineralocorticoid activity.
          (a) Maintain electrolyte homeostasis
          (b) In response to fluid loss, aldosterone induces the kidney to reabsorb sodium and water and decrease the reabsorption of potassium.
        (3) Gonadocorticoids (i.e, testosterone, estradiol)
          (a) Unlike glucocorticoid and mineralocorticoid, the production of these sex steroids is not essential for life.
          (b) In the normal individual, androgens and estrogens produced by the adrenal cortex are not as important in sexual development and function as those produced by the testes and ovaries.

        (4) Secretion into the circulation is regulated by negative feedback mechanisms responding to extreme stress or low levels of these hormones.

        (5) The release of hormones from the adrenal cortex is slow and the hormonal response long-lasting.

    4. The adrenal medulla synthesizes catecholamines (i.e., epinephrine, norepinephrine) responsible for the fight-or-flight reaction to stress.

       a) The secretion of catecholamines from the medulla is directly controlled by the sympathetic nervous system and occurs within seconds of a stressful event.

       b) Catecholamines have both a stimulatory and inhibitory effect on all body tissues.

       c) When stress is withdrawn, the catecholamines are taken up by the sympathetic nerve endings, returning homeostasis.

       d) A normal adrenal gland can compensate for the hypofunction of an abnormal adrenal gland and maintain homeostasis.

B. Pathophysiology

    1. Metastasis occurs by lymphohematogenous spread to the adrenals from the primary site of malignancy.

    2. Metabolic homeostasis is altered when abnormalities occur in the life-sustaining glucocorticoid and mineralocorticoid pathways.

III. Clinical features: Most adrenal metastases are asymptomatic and found incidentally. However, assessment for adrenal insufficiency is critical when there is bilateral involvement.

A. Etiology: The adrenals are potential sites of metastasis from solid tumors with the following incidence.

    1. Lung cancer: 58%

    2. Breast cancer: 42%

    3. Renal cell carcinoma: 19%

    4. Stomach cancer: 16%

    5. Colorectal cancer: 14%

    6. Adrenal metastasis involving both glands 50%: resulting in adrenal hormone insufficiency: 19%–33%

B. History

    1. History of cancer and cancer treatment

    2. Current medications: Prescribed and over-the-counter.

    3. History of presenting symptom(s): Precipitating factors, onset, and duration. Associated symptoms are nausea, loss of appetite, dizziness, pain, weakness, and anorexia

    4. Changes in activities of daily living

    5. Past medical history: Kidney disease, heart disease

C. Signs and symptoms

    1. Postural hypotension

    2. Nausea

    3. Anorexia/weight loss

    4. Asthenia

    5. Adrenal pain syndrome: Unilateral flank pain, back pain, and, less commonly, abdominal pain

  D. Physical exam
   1. Assess for weight loss of > 5% from baseline.
   2. Integument exam: Dry skin and mucous membranes
   3. Neurologic exam
       a) Assess orientation to persons, place, and time; may be disoriented with electrolyte imbalance
       b) Loss of deep tendon reflexes, indicating hyperkalemia
   4. Cardiovascular exam: Monitor blood pressure for orthostatic hypotension (i.e., > 15 mm Hg drop in systolic blood pressure from the supine to the upright position with a concomitant > 15 beats per minute increase in heart rate, both sustained for at least three minutes)
       a) Decreased heart rate may indicate electrolyte imbalance.
       b) Irregular heart rate may indicate dysrhythmia.
   5. Abdominal exam
       a) Abdominal tenderness or pain
       b) May have palpable abdominal mass
   6. Musculoskeletal exam: Decreased muscle strength, indicating hyperkalemia
   7. Lymph node assessment to rule out palpable adenopathy
   8. Overall decrease in performance status

IV. Diagnostic tests
  A. Laboratory
   1. Electrolytes: To evaluate for hyponatremia, hyperkalemia
   2. Endocrinologic testing: Recommended in all patients with bilateral adrenal metastasis who are symptomatic to evaluate adrenal reserve and determine the need for replacement therapy
       a) Adrenocorticotropic hormone (ACTH) stimulation is the test of choice to evaluate adrenal insufficiency.
       b) A baseline serum cortisol level is drawn followed by the IV administration of cosyntropin 0.25 mg. Cortisol levels are checked at 30 and 60 minutes.
       c) Failure to increase serum cortisol at least 5 ug/100 ml above the baseline level and at least to a level of 15 ug/100 ml at either 30 or 60 minutes is diagnostic of adrenal insufficiency.
  B. Radiology
   1. CT of abdomen with contrast: To evaluate disease status, extent of adrenal involvement
   2. MRI of the abdomen: May be more useful in differentiating between adrenal adenoma and adrenal metastasis
  C. Other: EKG to rule out arrhythmias; if hyperkalemia is present, may reveal increased T wave or a heart block

V. Differential diagnosis
  A. Adrenal adenoma
  B. Adrenal carcinoma (primary)
  C. Electrolyte imbalance (see Chapters 144–148)

D. Paraneoplastic syndrome from ACTH-producing tumors (e.g., bronchogenic carcinoma, small cell lung cancer, pancreatic cancer, colon cancer, medullary thyroid cancer see Appendix 12)

E. Medication-induced adrenal insufficiency
   1. Ketoconazole for the treatment of prostate cancer
   2. Aminoglutethimide for the treatment of prostate or breast cancer

F. Cardiac disease (e.g., dysrhythmia [see Chapter 43])

G. Renal disease (e.g., renal insufficiency/failure [see Chapter 83])

H. Medication-related hyperkalemia/hyponatremia (see Chapter 145–147)
   1. Potassium supplements
   2. Potassium-sparing drugs (e.g., spironolactone)
   3. Recent chemotherapy affecting fluid/electrolyte balance or kidney function (e.g., cisplatin, ifosfamide)

VI. Treatment
   A. Treat underlying malignancy.
   B. Implement supportive care for symptom management.
      1. Nausea (see Chapter 59)
      2. Anorexia (see Chapter 62)
      3. Pain (see Appendices 8a/b and 11)
      4. Ensure safety if patient is disoriented/has postural hypotension.
   C. Replacement therapy for coexisting adrenal insufficiency
      1. Glucocorticoid: Hydrocortisone 20 mg po every am and 10 mg po every pm
      2. Mineralocorticoid: Fludrocortisone 0.1–0.2 mg every day (an oral aldosterone analogue)
         a) Orthostatic hypotension and electrolyte imbalance often resolves with glucocorticoid replacement.
         b) Patients with concomitant aldosterone deficiency resulting in persistent hyperkalemia will require the addition of fludrocortisone.
         c) Symptoms related to adrenal insufficiency should resolve within a few days of initiating replacement therapy.
   D. Adrenalectomy (possibly laparoscopic) if adrenal metastasis is a solitary lesion and no other evidence of metastatic disease is present

VII. Follow-up: Depends on treatment plan and may vary considerably among patients
   A. If patients are on replacement therapy, follow up initially in one month and every three to six months thereafter if no concurrent problems.
   B. If widespread metastasis, follow-up depends on symptoms.

VIII. Referrals
   A. Endocrinologist: For endocrine testing/replacement therapy
   B. Medical oncologist: For consideration of chemotherapy/appropriate clinical trials
   C. Surgical oncologist: For consideration of adrenalectomy
   D. Home health or hospice: If widespread metastasis and multiple symptomatology

References

Aupetit-Faisant, B., Blanchouin-Emeric, N., Tenenbaum, F., Battaglia, C., Tabarin, A., Amar, J., Kutten, E., Warnet, A., Assayag, M., & Chamontin, B. (1995). Plasma levels of aldosterone versus aldosterone precursors: A way to estimate the malignancy of asymptomatic and nonsecretory adrenal tumors: A French retrospective multicentric study. *Journal of Clinical Endocrinology and Metabolism, 80,* 2715–2721.

Ayab, H., Tsuji, H., Hara, S., Tagawa, Y., Kawahara, K., & Tomita, M. (1995). Surgical management of adrenal metastasis from bronchogenic carcinoma. *Journal of Surgical Oncology, 58*(3), 149–154.

Barnes, R.D., Abratt, R.P., Cant, P.J., & Dent, D.M. (1995). Synchronous contralateral adrenal metastasis from renal cell carcinoma: A 7 year survival following resection. *Australian & New Zealand Journal of Surgery, 65,* 540–541.

Bernini, G., Miccoli, P., Moretti, A., Vivaldi, P., Iacconi, P., & Salvetti, A. (1998). Sixty adrenal masses of large dimensions: Hormonal and morphologic evaluation. *Urology, 51,* 920–925.

Elashry, O.M., Clayman, R.V., Soble J.J., & McDougall, E.M. (1997). Laparoscopic adrenalectomy for solitary metachronous contralateral adrenal metastasis from renal cell carcinoma. *Journal of Urology 157,* 1217–1222.

Ichikawa, T., Ohtomo, K., Uchigyama, G., Koizumi, K., Monzawa, S., Oba, J., Nogata, Y., Kachi, K., Toyama, K., & Yamaguchi, M. (1994). Adrenal adenomas: Characteristic hyperintense rim sign on fat-saturated spin-echo MR images. *Radiology, 193,* 247–250.

Novick, A.C., & Howards, S.S. (1996). The adrenals. In J.Y. Gillenwater, J.T. Grayhock, S.S. Howards, & J.W. Duckett (Eds.), *Adult and pediatric urology.* (3rd ed.) (pp. 587–615). St. Louis: Mosby.

Redman, B.G., Pazdur, M.D., Zingas, A.P., & Loredo, R. (1987). Prospective evaluation of adrenal insufficiency in patients with adrenal metastasis. *Cancer, 60,* 103–107.

Chapter

85. Benign Prostatic Hyperplasia

Julie D. Painter, RNC, MSN, OCN®

I. Definition: Noncancerous adenomatous hyperplasia of the prostate gland

II. Pathophysiology
   A. Benign prostatic hyperplasia (BPH) arises from nodular hyperplasia of the prostatic stromal and glandular tissue. Growth begins in periurethral glandular tissue.
   B. As the prostate gland enlarges, urethral resistance to urine flow increases, resulting in muscular hypertrophy of the bladder.
      1. As the urethra is impinged further, the bladder is unable to fully empty.
      2. Residual urine can result in an infection.
   C. Bladder herniation or saccule can form between the overlapping muscular bands that compose the detrusor muscle.
      1. Herniation allows for incomplete emptying of the bladder, predisposing one to infection.
      2. Because of inability of the detrusor muscle to exert enough pressure to overcome the urethral obstruction, bladder failure and urinary retention occur.
   D. Ureteral dilatation may occur in cases that are more advanced and where there is chronic urine retention because of increased pressure on the bladder.
      1. Hydronephrosis and renal deterioration may occur after ureteral dilatation.
      2. The hyperplastic prostate becomes vascular and predisposed to bleeding.

III. Clinical features: Symptomatology of BPH may occur long before patient seeks medical attention, usually because of an infection or frequent urination that becomes bothersome. Symptoms related to BPH rarely occur before age 50.
   A. Risk factor: Age (i.e., > 50)
   B. Etiology: Actual cause is unknown.
      1. Increased 5-alpha dihydrotestosterone, which is the active form of testosterone
      2. Increased levels of estrogen
      3. Stimulation of alpha-adrenergic nerve endings interfering with the opening of the bladder neck internal sphincter
      4. Further impairment of contractile function of the bladder may occur because of anticholinergic agents; increased outflow resistance may occur from sympathomimetic drugs.
      5. Androgenic changes at the cellular level may have a major influence.

C. History
1. History of cancer and cancer treatment
2. Current medications: Prescribed and over-the-counter
3. History of precipitating symptom(s): Precipitating factors, onset, location, and duration. Associated symptoms are pain, discomfort, hematuria, bone pain, anorexia, and weight loss.
4. Changes in activities of daily living
5. Past medical history: Genitourinary problems, diabetes mellitus, neurologic disease

D. Signs and symptoms
1. Urinary hesitancy
2. Loss of urinary stream force
3. Frequent urination
4. Nocturia
5. Sense of incomplete voiding
6. Stream interruption
7. Urinary dribbling, leaking, incontinence
8. Hematuria: May be an early sign of BPH, but malignancy must be ruled out

E. Physical exam
1. Abdominal exam: May reveal bladder distention and enlargement, tenderness, mass, renal tenderness, or flank pain
2. Digital rectal examination (DRE): To determine approximate size of the prostate gland, assess for nodules, induration, and other signs that may indicate cancer
    a) Normal prostate is 2.5–3.0 cm in vertical and transverse diameters.
    b) BPH causes the gland to be enlarged, firm, smooth, and symmetrical and results in the inability to palpate the median sulcus.
    c) Cancer is more likely to be asymmetric and nodular with a hard, fixed mass.
    d) Inability to palpate distal margins may indicate massive enlargement.

IV. Diagnostic tests
A. Laboratory
1. Urinalysis: To test for infection and hematuria
    a) Pyuria suggests infection.
    b) Hematuria
2. Serum creatinine: To assess renal function
3. Serum PSA: To rule out prostate cancer

B. Radiology: Renal ultrasound to rule out obstruction of the kidneys and urinary tract

C. Other
1. Postvoid residual and pressure flow urodynamic studies: Depend on symptomatology (residual volumes can be assessed fairly well with a bladder scanner; provide a cost-effective noninvasive ultrasonic mechanism of testing)
2. Urethrocystoscopy: To consider invasive treatment, include in evaluation

V. Differential diagnosis
A. Prostate cancer
B. Bladder outlet obstruction

      1. Urethral obstruction

      2. Vesical neck obstruction

  C. Neurogenic, myogenic, or psychogenic causes of impaired detrusor contractility

  D. Cystitis (see Chapter 91)

  E. Prostatitis (see Chapter 92)

VI. Treatment: Treatment decisions must be based on how the obstructive symptoms affect the patient's quality of life and renal function.

  A. Mild to moderate symptoms

      1. Assess and evaluate patient's symptoms at least annually.

      2. Discuss the use of behavior change to reduce symptoms.

         a) Limit fluid intake after dinner and before bedtime.

         b) Avoid the use of decongestants.

         c) Avoid the use of caffeine and alcohol-containing beverages.

         d) Avoid medications (e.g., anticholinergics, tranquilizers, antidepressants).

         e) Massage the prostate.

  B. Moderate to severe symptoms: Always check PSA and prostate exam before beginning any medication regimen.

      1. Medication

         a) Terazosin (Hytrin®, Abbott Laboratories, Inc., North Chicago, IL): 2–10 mg po every day; start with 0.5 mg at bedtime, and titrate to desired effect (alpha-blocker therapy)

         b) Prazocin (Minipress®, Pfizer Inc., New York, NY): 2–5 mg po every day (selective alpha-blocker)

         c) Doxazosin mesylate (Cardura®, Pfizer Inc.): Begin with 1 mg po every day; maximum of 16 mg po every day (selective long-acting alpha-blocker)

         d) Finasteride (Proscar®, Merck & Co., West Point, PA): Can decrease prostatic size, increase peak urine flow rate, and reduce symptoms; 5 mg po every day

         e) Other medications: GnRH agonist, progestational antiandrogen, flutamide, testolactone

      2. Balloon dilatation

      3. Surgery: Transurethral resection of the prostate (TURP), transurethral incision of the prostate (TUIP), or open prostatectomy

         a) Consider surgery for men with refractory urinary retention who have failed at least one attempt at catheter removal and medical therapy.

         b) Consider surgery for men who have recurrent urinary infections, recurrent gross hematuria, bladder or renal insufficiency clearly related to BPH.

      4. Newer treatments

         a) Laser

         b) Microwave thermal therapy

         c) Prostatic stents

VII. Follow-up

  A. Instruct patient to watch for signs and symptoms of obstruction, infection, and retention and report any of these to the medical provider as soon as noted.

B. Patients who desire observation rather than treatment must be seen on an annual basis or as symptoms necessitate.

C. Patients who have balloon dilatation or surgery should be followed up based on recommendations of the urologist or surgeon.

VIII. Referrals: Urologist for input on treatment plans

References

Anderson, R.J. (1998). Primary care management of benign prostatic hyperplasia. *Hospital Practice, 33*(3), 11–12, 15–16, 21.

Beduschi, R., Beduschi, M.C., &, Oesterling, J.E. (1998). Benign prostatic hyperplasia: Use of drug therapy in primary care. *Geriatrics, 53*(3), 24–28, 33–34, 37–40.

Heil, B.J. (1999). Treatment of benign prostatic hyperplasia. *Journal of American Academy of Nurse Practitioners, 11*(7), 303–310.

Holtgrewe, H.L. (1997). Benign prostatic hyperplasia. *Journal of Urology, 157,* 184.

Medina, J.J., Parra, R.O., & Moore, R.G. (1999). Benign prostatic hyperplasia (the aging prostate). *Medical Clinics of North America, 83,* 1213–1229.

Ziada, A., Rosenblum, M., & Crawford, E.D. (1999). Benign prostatic hyperplasia: An overview. *Urology, 53* (Suppl. 3a), 1–6.

86. Chlamydia

Julie D. Painter, RNC, MSN, OCN®

I. Definition: A sexually transmitted disease (STD) that is caused by the organism *Chlamydia trachomatis*

II. Pathophysiology
   A. An intracellular organism that has the properties of a virus and bacteria
      1. Occurs in the genital tract of women at the transition zone of the endocervix
      2. Can occur in other areas of the body (e.g., oral cavity, anal canal), depending on sexual practices
   B. Reproduces itself by parasitizing the adenosine triphosphate (ATP) of the infected cell
   C. Untreated infection can lead to tubal scarring, infertility, or the cause of an ectopic pregnancy.

III. Clinical features: One of the two most common causes of cervicitis; the other is *Neisseria gonorrhoeae*. In women, the cervix is infected in 75% of cases and the urethra in 50%; in men, infection occurs prominently in the urethra.
   A. Risk factor: Women are at greater risk for contracting chlamydia by receiving infected ejaculate or secretions from their partner's genital tract; men are exposed through the vaginal secretions and secretions of the genital tract.
   B. History
      1. History of cancer and cancer treatment
      2. Current medications: Prescribed and over-the-counter
      3. History of presenting symptom(s): Precipitating factors, onset, location, and duration. Associated symtpoms are dysuria, discharge, abnormal bleeding, pelvic pain, and dyspareunia.
      4. Changes in activities of daily living
      5. History of menstrual cycle and sexual history
      6. Past medical history of STDs and treatment
   C. Signs and symptoms: May be absent, mild, or nonspecific
      1. Men
         a) Acute scrotal pain and discomfort, indicating spread to epididymis
         b) Penile discharge or pyuria
      2. Women

          a) Mucopurulent discharge
          b) Bleeding
          c) Abdominal pain
      3. Dysuria
      4. Pelvic pain
   D. Physical exam
      1. Pelvic exam
          a) Inspect outer vulvovaginal areas.
          b) Assess cervix for mucopurulent discharge from the endocervix and for inflammation.
          c) Swab cervix for friability; easily bleeds upon mild scraping of surface.
          d) Cervix may be extremely erythematous.
          e) Conduct bimanual exam to assess for adnexal tenderness, uterine tenderness, and cervical motion.
      2. Lymph node exam: Inguinal nodes enlarged for women and men
      3. Genitalia exam: Reveals inflammation of urethra and epididymis

IV. Diagnostic studies
   A. Laboratory: Cell culture: Urogenital swabs for direct antigen test or fluorescent microscopy to confirm diagnosis
   B. Radiology: Not indicated

IV. Differential diagnosis
   A. Pelvic inflammatory disease
   B. Gonorrhea (see Chapter 87)
   C. Syphilis (see Chapter 95)
   D. Bacterial vaginitis (see Chapter 97)

V. Treatment
   A. Doxycycline: 100 mg bid orally for seven days (treatment of choice)
   B. Azithromycin: 1 g orally in single dose
   C. Alternative
      1. Erythromycin base: 500 mg orally qid for seven days
      2. Ethylsuccinate: 800 mg orally qid for seven days
      3. Ofloxacin: 300 mg orally bid for seven days
   D. Treat scxual partner(s).
   E. Advise patients to avoid sexual practice until they and their partner(s) are cured.

VII. Follow-up
   A. No follow-up necessary if treated with doxycycline, azithromycin, or ofloxacin; retesting is necessary within three weeks of completing other therapies.
   B. Annual pelvic examination and Pap smear is recommended

VIII. Referrals: No specific referrals unless patient is pregnant or immunocompromised

References

Ghinsberg, R.C., & Nitzan, Y. (1994). Chlamydia trachomatis direct isolation, antibody prevalence and clinical symptoms in women attending outpatient clinics. *New Microbiology, 17*(3), 231–242.

Mardh, P.A., Tchoudomirova, K., Elshibly, S., & Hellberg, D. (1998). Symptoms and signs in single and mixed genital infections. *International Journal of Gynaecology and Obstetrics, 63*(2), 145–152.

Nilsson, U., Hellberg, D., Shoubnikova, M., Nilsson, S., & Mardh, P.A. (1997). Sexual behavior risk factors associated with bacterial vaginosis and chlamydia trachomatis infection. *Sexually Transmitted Diseases, 34*(5), 241–246.

Roe, V.A., & Gudi, A. (1997). Pharmacologic management of sexually transmitted disease. *Journal of Nurse Midwifery, 43,* 275–289.

Chapter

87. Gonorrhea
Julie D. Painter, RNC, MSN, OCN®

I. Definition: An STD caused by *Neisseria gonorrhoeae*

II. Pathophysiology
   A. Gram-negative diplococcus that prefers to infect columnar and pseudo-stratified epithelium
   B. *Neisseria gonorrhoeae* are organisms that are present in exudate and secretions of infected mucous membranes. Organisms can gain access to the blood stream, causing systemic infections.

III. Clinical features: Transmission occurs with sexual practices. Incubation period is two to seven days. Common sites of infection in women are endocervix, urethra, upper genital tract, rectum, and pharynx. Disseminated disease most often occurs in women if contracted during menses or pregnancy; it infrequently occurs in men.
   A. History
      1. History of cancer and cancer treatment
      2. Current medications: Prescribed and over-the-counter
      3. History of presenting symptom(s): Precipitating factors, onset, location, and duration. Associated symptoms are women: pelvic/abdominal pain, vaginal discharge, dysuria, and abnormal bleeding; men: dysuria, urethral discharge, and rectal pain.
      4. Changes in activities of daily living
      5. History of menstrual cycle (women)
      6. History of sexual practices and STDs
   B. Signs and symptoms: Many women with infection are asymptomatic until other complications occur; most infections in men cause symptoms that prompt them to seek medical care.
      1. Women: Vaginal discharge, abnormal uterine bleeding, dysuria
      2. Men: Purulent urethral discharge, urinary frequency, dysuria
      3. Disseminated disease: Tenosynovitis, skin lesions, fever, polyarthritis
   C. Physical exam
      1. Vital signs: Assess for febrile state.
      2. Oral cavity: Assess pharynx for exudate.
      3. Lymph exam: Assess for adenopathy, especially femoral and cervical.

4. Abdominal exam: Assess for pain and tenderness, indicating peritonitis.
5. Pelvic examination
    a) Assess and inspect the Bartholin and Skene's glands for tenderness and enlargement.
    b) Assess the urethra for discharge.
    c) Assess and inspect the cervix for mucopurulent discharge; scrape the cervix to test for friability.
    d) Assess for labial edema and pain.
    e) Perform a bimanual examination to assess for adnexal tenderness, masses, uterine tenderness, and cervical motion tenderness.
        (1) Adnexal mass, fever, and chills indicate salpingitis.
        (2) Pelvic pain and vaginal bleeding indicate possible endometritis.
6. Perform genital exam (men).
    a) Assess for urethral discharge.
    b) Assess for scrotal edema and tenderness.
7. Rectal examination: Check for discharge, lesions, bleeding, and tenderness.
8. Assess joints for tenderness, edema, and warmth suggestive of polyarthritis or tenosynovitis.

IV. Diagnostic tests
    A. Laboratory
        1. Using modified Thayer-Martin or Transgrow media, culture cervix or other areas suspected for *Neisseria gonorrhoeae*.
            a) Organism is fragile and requires special handling.
            b) Organism is readily killed by drying; all cultures must be plated promptly.
            c) Streak the swab across in a Z-shaped pattern.
            d) In women, obtain an endocervix culture by inserting a swab into the cervical opening through a speculum lubricated with only water.
        2. Collect culture of cervix or from suspicious areas or perform an antigen detection test to rule out *Chlamydia trachomatis*.
        3. Test all patients for syphilis and offer HIV testing to rule out other diseases.
        4. Perform gram stain of urethral discharge in men; obtain cervical swab in women
            a) Considered positive when biscuit-shaped gram-negative polymorphonuclear leukocytes are present.
            b) Considered negative if no diplococci are seen.
            c) Test is less reliable in cervical, rectal, and pharyngeal infections.
        5. Culture anal canal and pharynx if oral and rectal sex are suspected.
    B. Radiology: Not indicated
    C. Other: With acute arthritis, culture joint fluid.

V. Differential diagnosis
    A. Pelvic inflammatory disease (PID)
    B. Chlamydia trachomatis (see Chapter 86)
    C. Candida
    D. Trichomoniasis (see Chapter 96)
    E. Ectopic pregnancy
    F. Appendicitis

    G. Endometriosis

    H. Proctitis

    G. Ovarian cyst

VI. Treatment

    A. Adults with uncomplicated gonococcal infections

        1. Ceftriaxone (Rocephin®, Roche Pharmaceutical Laboratories, Nutley, NJ): 125 mg IM in a single dose

        2. Cefixime: 400 mg orally in a single dose

        3. Ciprofloxacin: 500 mg orally in a single dose

        4. Ofloxacin: 400 mg orally in a single dose plus doxycycline 100 mg orally bid for seven days (or use another regimen effective against possible *Chlamydia trachomatis* coinfection)

    B. Alternative treatment

        1. Spectinomycin: 2 g IM in a single dose

        2. Ceftizoxime: 500 mg IM in a single dose

    C. If disseminated infection is present, the patient should be hospitalized for initial therapy of ceftriaxone 1 g IM or IV every 24 hours.

    D. Treatment of sexual partners

        1. Sex partners of symptomatic patients: Partners who have had sexual contact with the patient within 30 days of symptom onset should be evaluated and treated for *Neisseria gonorrhoeae* and *Chlamydia trachomatis* infections.

        2. Sex partners of asymptomatic patients: Partners who have had sexual contact with the patient within 60 days of diagnosis should be evaluated and treated.

        3. The patient's most recent sex partner should be treated if the last sexual contact was before any of these time periods.

VII. Follow-up

    A. If treatment failure: Rare if treated with combination of ceftriaxone and doxycycline therapy

    B. Post-treatment cultures are not necessary.

    C. Annual pelvic examination and Pap smear is recommended.

VIII. Referrals: All sexual partners should be referred for evaluation and treatment.

References

Goodfellow, A., Standley, T., & Ross, J.D. (1999). Predicting penicillin resistance in patients with gonorrhea. *Sexually Transmitted Diseases, 75*(3), 190.

Mahadani, J.W., Dekate, R.R., & Shrikhande, A.V. (1998). Cytodiagnosis of discharge per vaginum. *Indian Journal of Pathology and Microbiology, 41,* 403–411.

Roe, V.A., & Gudi, A. (1997). Pharmacologic management of sexually transmitted diseases. *Journal of Nurse Midwifery, 42,* 275–289.

Woodward, C., & Fisher, M.A. (1999). Drug treatment of common STDs: Part 1. Herpes, syphilis, urethritis, chlamydia, and gonorrhea. *American Family Physician, 60,* 1387–1394.

88. Hemorrhagic Cystitis

Roberta A. Strohl, RN, BSN, MN, AOCN®

I. Definition: An irritation of the bladder that ranges from microscopic hematuria to acute exsanguinating hematuria

II. Pathophysiology
   A. Urothelium of the bladder is injured by metabolites of alkylating agents (e.g., cyclophosphamide, ifosfamide, busulfan).
      1. Excreted acrolein (i.e., byproduct metabolite) binds to the bladder mucosa and results in ulceration, necrosis, hemorrhage, inflammation, erythema, and reduced bladder capacity.
      2. Lesions disrupt integrity of bladder mucosa, resulting in cystitis with microscopic or frank hemorrhage.
   B. Herpes simplex virus can alter the bladder mucosa, resulting in hemorrhagic cystitis.
   C. Acute urethral syndrome can cause submucosal hemorrhages or interstitial cystitis that may be caused by chlamydia infection.

III. Clinical features: Hemorrhagic cystitis may occur as an emergent event or may be preceded by a history of microscopic hematuria.
   A. Etiology
      1. Carcinoma of bladder
      2. Infection
      3. Chemotherapy
      4. Chronic interstitial cystitis
      5. Pelvic radiation
      6. Bone marrow transplantation
   B. History
      1. History of cancer and cancer treatment
      2. Current medications: Prescribed and over-the-counter
      3. History of presenting symptom(s): Precipitating factors, onset, and duration
      4. Changes in activities of daily living
   C. Signs and symptoms
      1. Hematuria
      2. Dysuria

        a) Burning
        b) Frequency
        c) Urgency
        d) Nocturia
        e) Incontinence
    3. Suprapubic pain
  D. Physical exam: Nonspecific
    1. Usually normal
    2. Abdominal exam may elicit suprapubic pain and distended bladder.

IV. Diagnostic tests
  A. Laboratory
    1. Urinalysis: RBCs in urine range from microscopic to gross blood with clots.
    2. Hemoglobin and hematocrit: Decrease with blood loss
  B. Radiology: Renal ultrasonography and/or IV urogram to rule out obstruction if source/
    etiology of bleeding cannot be determined

V. Differential diagnosis
  A. Cystitis (see Chapter 91)
  B. Benign prostate hypertrophy, chronic prostatitis (see Chapters 85 and 92)
  C. Carcinoma of bladder
  D. Renal cell carcinoma: Late sign indicating invasion of vascular or collecting system
  E. Calculous disease: Renal colic and hematuria are presenting signs
  F. Trauma
  G. Glomerular disease
  H. Sickle cell anemia (see Chapter 118)

VI. Treatment: Treat underlying etiology or disease.
  A. Discontinue chemotherapeutic agent or radiation.
  B. Administer mesna (a uroprotective agent) with chemotherapy to protect the bladder
    against cytotoxic effects of drugs
    1. Dose depends on chemotherapy dose—usually 60%–80% of total chemotherapy
      dose prior to chemo and repeated four and eight hours after chemo or as a continuous
      infusion
    2. Amifostine 200–500 mg/m^2 is being evaluated to lessen hemorrhagic cystitis as a
      urinary protectant.
  C. Implement continuous bladder irrigation with saline by a three-way indwelling catheter
    to decrease the bleeding episode.
  D. Administer hyperbaric oxygen to treat radiation-induced cystitis.
  E. Encourage fluid intake and frequent bladder emptying when patients are on cyclophospha-
    mide, especially during infusion; instruct patients to empty bladder before going to bed.
  F. Perform cystoscopy to cauterize bleeding vessels.
  G. Administer bladder instillation of carboprost 1 mg/dl q 6 hours or formalin 1%–4% for
    life-threatening hemorrhage; results in severe fibrosis and contraction.
  H. Cystectomy is last resort.

VII. Follow-up
A. Monitor urine frequently during treatment with chemotherapeutic agents known to cause bladder toxicity.
B. Long-term follow-up is recommended for patients who have received chemotherapy and/or pelvic radiation therapy for late bladder toxicity.

VIII. Referrals
A. Urologist: To assist patients with decreased bladder capacity related to radiation fibrosis and effects of chemotherapy
B. Specialist: For hyperbaric oxygen

References

Baronciani, D., Angelucci, E., Erer, B., Fabrizi, G., Galimberti, M., Giardini, C., Milella, D., Montesi, M., Polchi, P., Severini, A., et al. (1995). Suprapubic cystotomy as treatment for severe hemorrhagic cystitis after bone marrow transplantation. *Bone Marrow Transplantation, 27,* 267–270.

Cappelli-Schellpfeffa, M., & Gerber, G.S. (1999). The use of hyperbaric oxygen in urology. *Journal of Urology, 162,* 647–654.

Haselberger, M.B. & Schwinghammer, T.L. (1995). Efficacy of mesna for prevention of hemorrhagic cystitis after high-dose cyclophosphamide therapy. *Annals of Pharmacotherapeutics, 29,* 918–921.

Loughlin, K., & Richie, J. (1997). Invasive bladder cancer. In D. Raghavan, H. Scher, S. Leibel, & P. Lang (Eds.), *Principles and practice of genitourinary oncology* (pp. 955–965). Philadelphia: Lippincott-Raven.

Sommerkamp, H. (1998). Hemorrhagic cystitis after high dose chemotherapy: An interdisciplinary problem. *Urology, 37,* 516–521.

Srivastava, A., Nair, S.C., Srivastava, V.M., Balamurugan, A.N., Jeyaseelan, L., Chandy, M., & Gunasekaran, S. (1999). Evaluation of uroprotective efficacy of amifostine against cyclophosphamide-induced hemorrhagic cystitis. *Bone Marrow Transplantation, 23,* 463–467.

Yazawa, H., Nakada, T., Sasagawa, I., Miura, M., & Kubota, Y. (1995). Hyperbaric oxygen therapy for cyclophosphamide-induced hemorrhagic cystitis. *International Journal of Urology and Nephrology, 27,* 381–385.

Chapter

89. Herpes Simplex
Julie D. Painter, RNC, MSN, OCN®

I. Definition: Sexually transmitted disease caused by herpes simplex virus 2 (HSV-2); oral infection and disseminated disease is most likely associated with herpes simplex virus 1 (HSV-1)

II. Pathophysiology
   A. HSV contains an inner core of double-stranded DNA surrounded by a glycoprotein envelope.
   B. Epidermotropic viruses cause infection within keratinocytes.
   C. Transmission is only by direct contact with active lesions or by bodily secretions that contain the virus (e.g., saliva, vaginal/cervical secretions).
      1. Incubation period is approximately 2–12 days after the initial exposure of the mucous membranes or skin.
      2. After exposure, the virus takes about 48 hours to travel along afferent nerves and find a host ganglion.
         a) HSV-1 (oral virus) usually affects the trigeminal ganglia.
         b) HSV-2 (genital virus) affects the sacral ganglia.
   D. The virus can reactivate, causing a recurrence of the viral lesions.
      1. The lesion may occur at a different location than the original site, even though the original nerve root is still affected.
      2. The virus lies dormant in associated dorsal root ganglion.

III. Clinical features: About 30 million people in the United States may be infected with genital HSV infection. Viral shedding for the primary episode of infection is about 12 days; for recurrent infections, approximately 7 days. Healing of lesions with the primary infection is notably longer than recurrent episodes (i.e., 21 days as compared to 5 days for recurrent).
   A. Etiology
      1. HSV-1 generally causes infection of lips, mucous membranes of mouth, buccal mucosa, and throat.
      2. HSV-2 usually causes infection of the genitalia.
   B. History
      1. History of cancer and cancer treatment
      2. Current medications: Prescribed and over-the-counter

3. History of presenting symptom(s): Precipitating factors, onset, location, and duration. Associated symptoms are burning, itching, pain, paresthesia, fever, myalgia, malaise, headaches, and nausea.
4. Changes in activities of daily living
5. Social history of sexual practices

C. Signs and symptoms: Can be mild or asymptomatic
   1. Primary infection
      a) Hyperparesthesia, burning, itching, dysuria, pain, tenderness
      b) Fever
      c) Myalgia
      d) Malaise
      e) Headaches
   2. Recurrent infection
      a) Prodromal symptoms (e.g., paresthesia, itching, pain) can last approximately two days.
      b) Local mild symptoms may occur, but they are less severe than the first viral infection and may not last as long.

D. Physical exam
   1. Vital signs: Note fever.
   2. Oral cavity: Assess for pharyngitis.
   3. Integument, oral cavity, genital area exams: Examine lesions for characteristics, location, appearance, and distribution pattern.
   4. Lymph nodes: Assess for lymphadenopathy.
   5. Genital exam: Examine for lesion characteristics.

IV. Diagnostic tests
   A. Laboratory
      1. Viral culture: Most accurate
         a) Gather specimen by scraping lesion, then swab the vesicular fluid.
         b) Swab in appropriate viral transport media.
         c) Results may take seven days; test can be costly.
      2. Enzyme-linked immunoabsorbent assay (ELISA) testing is available but has lower sensitivity.
      3. Culture results vary with the activity of the lesion.
         a) Often, lesions that are vesicles and pustules give a positive reading.
         b) For lesions that are crusted and dry, the percentage of positive readings declines.
   B. Radiology: Not indicated

V. Differential diagnosis
   A. Syphilis (see Chapter 95)
   B. Chancroid
   C. Bacterial infection
   D. Inflammatory bowel disease
   E. Mononucleosis

VI. Treatment: No treatment available for cure; available treatment is self-limited.
 A. Acyclovir treatment
  1. Acyclovir ointment 5% is available and can be used on primary herpes lesions in the labial areas.
   a) Do not apply to vaginal areas, as the polyethylene glycol base can be irritating.
   b) Instruct patients to wear gloves when applying ointment to lesions to decrease spread of the virus.
   c) Ointment is not likely to be effective in people with recurrent infections.
  2. Oral acyclovir
   a) For first clinical infection with genital herpes: Acyclovir (Zovirax®, Glaxo Wellcome Inc., Research Triangle Park, NC) 200 mg po five times/day for 7–10 days or until resolution occurs
   b) For first clinical infection of herpes proctitis: Zovirax 400 mg po five times/day or until clinical resolution of the lesions
   c) Valtrex® (Glaxo Wellcome Inc.) may be used when convenience is needed with a bid dosing.
   d) Famciclovir 125 mg po bid x 5 days
  3. Recurrent infections: Initiate treatment during the prodromal period or within two days of lesion appearance.
   a) Acyclovir 200 mg po five times/day for five days
   b) Acyclovir 400 mg po three times/day for five days
   c) Acyclovir 800 mg po two times/day for five days
   d) Daily suppressive therapy is recommended for people with frequent recurrences (i.e., six or more/year).
    (1) Acyclovir 400 mg po two times/day
    (2) After one year of suppressive therapy, acyclovir should be stopped and then patient reassessed for recurrent episodes.
    (3) Suppressive therapy does not guarantee the elimination of symptomatic or asymptomatic viral shedding and the potential for transmission to others.
   e) Famciclovir 125 mg po bid x 5 days
 B. Management
  1. Advise people to abstain from sexual activity when lesions are present; discuss the use of barrier methods to reduce transmission.
  2. Advise that genital herpes can have recurrent episodes and viral shedding can occur when asymptomatic.
  3. Discuss the use of sitz baths, cool compresses, and other nonpharmacologic interventions for comfort.

VII. Follow-up
 A. None indicated unless further complications. If person has a history of HIV or other disease or is receiving treatment that may result in immunosuppression, follow-up may be indicated to verify response without further complications.
 B. For women: Annual pelvic examination and Pap smear is recommended.

VIII. Referrals: Gynecologist or infectious disease specialist if patient is receiving cancer treatment or has HIV.

References

Ashley, R.L. (1998). Genital herpes. Type-specific antibodies for diagnosis and management. *Dermatologic Clinics, 16,* 789–793.

Barton, S.E. (1998). Herpes management and prophylaxis. *Dermatologic Clinics, 16,* 799–803.

Sacks, S.L. (1999). Improving the management of genital herpes. *Hospital Practice, 34*(2), 41–49.

Stanberry, L., Cunningham, A., Mertz, G., Mindel, A., Peters, B., Reitano, M., Sacks, S., Wald, A., Wassilew, S., & Woodley, P. (1999). New developments in the epidemiology, natural history and management of genital herpes. *Antiviral Research, 42*(1), 1–14.

Wald, A. (1999). New therapies and prevention strategies for genital herpes. *Clinics of Infectious Diseases, 28*(Suppl. 1), S4–S13.

Chapter

90. Human Papilloma Infection (Genital Warts)

Julie D. Painter, RNC, MSN, OCN®

I. Definition: An STD caused by the human papillomavirus (HPV)

II. Pathophysiology
   A. More than 50 subtypes of HPV have been identified in humans.
      1. Ten of the HPV types infect the lower genital tract.
      2. HPV 6, HPV 11, HPV 16, and HPV 18 are more common; HPV 6 and 11 are most common and usually are associated with benign genital warts.
      3. HPV 16 and 18 are more likely to be associated with higher grades of cervical and intraepithelial neoplasia or invasive carcinoma.
   B. The DNA virus enters the body through an epithelial break and infects the stratified squamous epithelium of the lower genital tract.

III. Clinical features: The incubation period is relatively long and variable, ranging from three weeks to eight months. HPV may occur along with other STDs (e.g., gonorrhea); most commonly occurs during ages 16–25.
   A. History
      1. History of cancer and cancer treatment
      2. Current medications: Prescribed and over-the-counter
      3. History of presenting symptom(s): Precipitating factors, onset, location, and duration
      4. Changes in activities of daily living
      5. Social history of sexual practices
      6. Past medical history of STDs, HIV, HPV
   B. Signs and symptoms
      1. Lump in vulvar area and following presence of wart
         a) In women, spread of warts to urethra, vagina, and cervix is common and spread of warts to the labial areas is rare; in males, warts commonly develop on the penis.
         b) HPV presents as small, flesh-colored warts that begin as tiny pink areas and become pedunculated, spreading to the perineum and perianal area.
      2. Bleeding may occur from lesions that become irritated or inflamed.
   C. Physical exam
      1. External genitalia exam to assess for lesions
         a) Women: Assess the preclitoral, vestibular, perineal, and perianal areas.

b) Men: Assess the scrotum, penis, and perianal area.

2. Use of 3%–5% acetic acid to the vulvar and perianal areas: May assist in the visualization of warts; acetic acid creates acetowhitening of the wart areas.
3. Pelvic examination: Check vaginal walls and cervix for motion tenderness and perform a Pap smear.
4. Rectal examination: Assess for wart-like lesions.

IV. Diagnostic tests
   A. No specific diagnostics are needed if the lesion appearance is characteristic of HPV.
   B. If lesions are not characteristic of HPV, consider rapid plasma reagin test (RPR) to rule out syphilis.

V. Differential diagnosis
   A. Herpes simplex (see Chapter 89)
   B. Syphilis (see Chapter 95)
   C. Cervical dysplasia

VI. Treatment
   A. Patient's decisions should guide treatment.
      1. Cost
      2. Toxic effects
      3. Cosmetic effects (e.g., scarring)
   B. Recommended methods: Refer to the appropriate references and resources before implementing any treatment.
      1. Surgical excision of the wart
      2. Cryotherapy
         a) Treatment of choice for external and genital warts
         b) Liquid nitrogen or cryoprobe
            (1) Cryotherapy with liquid nitrogen can be used for vaginal warts, but use of the cryoprobe in the vagina is not recommended.
            (2) Cryotherapy may be used with liquid nitrogen or podophyllum 10%–25% in compound tincture of benzoin for urethral meatus warts.
            (3) Oral warts may be removed by cryotherapy with liquid nitrogen, electrode-siccation, or surgery.
      3. Chemical burning
         a) Podofilox 0.5%: For genital warts only
         b) Podophyllin 10%–25% in compound tincture of benzoin
         c) Trichloroacetic acid (TCA) 80%–90%: Alternative for treatment of external genitalia and perianal warts
      4. Laser vaporization
      5. Interferon (local or parenteral): For chronic lesions
      6. Sexual partners do not require treatment for genital warts; reinfection probability is low.

II. Follow-up
   A. No follow-up is necessary if the warts have responded to therapy.

B. Annual pelvic examination and Pap smear is recommended.

VIII. Referrals: To gynecologist for evaluation and treatment of cervical dysplasia if patient has cervical warts; referral to a practitioner with knowledge of appropriate treatment is critical, as some lesions may be located in areas such as rectum or clitoris. Referral must be made before beginning any treatment. If patient has extensive or refractory disease, refer to a gynecologist.

References

Hudson, C.P. (1999). Syndrome management for sexually transmitted diseases: Back to the drawing board. *International Journal of STD and AIDS, 10,* 423–434.

Mardh, P.A., Tchoudomirova, K., Elshibly, S., & Hellberg, D. (1998). Symptoms and signs in single and mixed genital infections. *International Journal of Gynaecology and Obstetrics, 63*(2), 145–152.

Roe, V.A., & Gudi, A. (1997). Pharmacologic management of sexually transmitted diseases. *Journal of Nurse Midwifery, 42,* 275–289.

Chapter

91. Lower Urinary Tract Infection— Cystitis

Diane G. Cope, PhD, ARNP-CS, AOCN®

I. Definition: Infection limited to the bladder and urethra

II. Pathophysiology
   A. Bacteria can enter the urinary tract through three pathways.
      1. Blood stream to the kidneys
      2. Lymphatic channels to the kidneys from possible bowel or pelvic sources
      3. Ascension from the urethra into the bladder, then up the ureters to the kidneys
   B. The majority of infections are caused by ascending microorganisms that originate from the gastrointestinal tract.
      1. Significant bacteriuria occurs when more than 10^5 pathogenic bacteria are present per milliliter of urine with or without symptoms.
      2. The most common infecting organism is *Escherichia coli*.

III. Clinical features
   A. Risk factors: The short female urethra and bladder catheterization promote entry of bacteria into urethra.
   B. History
      1. History of cancer and cancer treatment
      2. Current medications: Prescribed and over-the-counter
      3. History of presenting symptom(s): Precipitating factors, onset, and duration
      4. Changes in activities of daily living
      5. Past medical history: STDs, UTIs
      6. Social history: Sexual practices, birth control method
   C. Signs and symptoms
      1. Dysuria
      2. Frequency
      3. Urgency
      4. Suprapubic tenderness
      5. Malodorous urine
      6. Incontinence
      7. Nocturia
      8. Cloudy urine

         9. No fever, chills, or flank pain (if present, represents upper UTI).

      10. No vaginal or urethral discharge, unless concurrent vaginitis

  D. Physical exam

     1. Vital signs noting any elevation in temperature

     2. Abdomen

       a) Suprapubic tenderness

       b) Distended bladder

     3. Posterior thorax exam: No flank or costovertebral angle tenderness

     4. Pelvic exam (women) to rule out vaginitis

IV. Diagnostic tests

  A. Laboratory

     1. Urinalysis (abnormalities with cystitis)

       a) Color (usually dark yellow [concentrated] or amber [hematuria])

       b) Pyuria: > 2–5 WBCs per high power field indicative of cystitis

       c) Presence of one organism on high-power field represents clinically significant bacteriuria (> 10^5 organisms/ml)

       d) RBCs—tissue destruction

       e) Leukocytes: Finding not specific for cystitis, but majority of patients with infections have leukocytes.

       f) Nitrite: Formed when bacteria reduce the nitrate present in normal urine

     2. Urine culture: To delineate bacterial source

       a) If no response to treatment

       b) Recurrent infections

       c) Urethral symptoms (e.g., frequency, dysuria, urgency)

  B. Radiology

     1. Rarely performed in uncomplicated cystitis

     2. Indicated for

       a) Women with recurrent infections to evaluate for renal abnormalities

       b) Upper UTIs

       c) Unusual infecting organisms

       d) Coexistent hypertension

       e) Persistent microscopic hematuria

         (1) IV pyelogram: To identify renal function and structural defects

         (2) Cystometry: To evaluate filling and emptying pressures in the bladder

  C. Other: Cystoscopy to evaluate the bladder for source of cystitis

V. Differential diagnosis

  A. Vaginitis (see Chapter 97)

  B. Bladder obstruction

  C. Renal calculi

  D. Prostatitis (see Chapter 92)

  E. Acute pyelonephritis (see Chapter 93)

  F. Cervicitis

  G. Salpingitis

    H. Acute abdominal disorder (see Chapter 50)

    I. Urethritis (e.g., chlamydia, gonococcal infection, herpes simplex virus) (see Chapters 86, 87, and 89)

    J. Diabetes mellitus/insipidus (see Chapter 143)

    K. Chemotherapy-induced cystitis (see Chapter 88)

    L. Radiation-induced cystitis (see Chapter 88)

    M. Cancer

VI. Treatment

    A. Nonpharmacologic therapy

       1. Drink six to eight eight-ounce glasses of water every day.

       2. Cleanse the genital area before and after sexual intercourse.

       3. Cleanse the genital area from front to back to prevent contamination from the rectal area.

       4. Take showers instead of tub baths.

    B. Pharmacologic therapy: Depends on source (see Appendix 1)

       1. Trimethoprim (Trimpex®, Hoffman La-Roche Inc., Nutley, NJ): 100 mg po every 12 hours for three to five days

       2. Trimethoprim 160 mg/sulfamethoxazole 800 mg (Bactrim® DS, Roche Pharmaceutical Laboratories, Nutley, NJ; Septra® DS, Monarch Pharmaceuticals, Bristol, TN): One tablet po every 12 hours for three to five days

       3. Amoxicillin (Amoxil®, SmithKline Beecham Pharmaceuticals, Philadelphia, PA): 500 mg po every eight hours for three to five days

       4. Nitrofurantoin (Macrodantin®, Procter & Gamble Pharmaceuticals, Inc., Mason, OH; Furadantin®, Dura Pharmaceuticals, San Diego, CA): 100 mg po four times/day for three to five days

       5. Quinolones

         a) Ciprofloxacin: 500–750 mg po every 12 hours for three to five days

         b) Orofloxacin: 300 mg po every 12 hours for three to five days

         c) Levaquin® (Ortho-McNeil Pharmaceuticals, Raritan, NJ): 250 mg every day for three to five days

         d) Maxaquin® (Unimed Pharmaceuticals, Inc., Buffalo Grove, IL): 400 mg po every day for three to five days

       6. Analgesic: Phenazopyridine HCl (Pyridium®, Warner Chilcott Laboratories, Rockaway, NJ): 200 mg po three times/day for two days with antibiotic therapy

    C. Relapsed cystitis: Treat with 14-day course of therapy if relapse occurs within 7–14 days after initial therapy.

    D. Long-term treatment (maintenance therapy for six months if three or more recurrences per year)

       1. Trimethoprim (Trimpex): 100 mg po postcoital or nightly

       2. Nitrofurantoin (Macrodantin): 100 mg po postcoital or nightly

VII. Follow-up

    A. Short-term: Symptomatic relief in one to three days; a follow-up urine culture may be obtained in one to two weeks after discontinuation of therapy to detect relapses.

    B. Long-term: Urine cultures every one to two months while on maintenance therapy

VIII. Referrals
    A. Urologist: Recurrent infections, suspected obstructions or renal calculi, cystitis in young males
    B. Gynecologist: Vaginitis, STD

References

Bacheller, C.D., & Bernstein, J.M. (1997). Urinary tract infections. *Medical Clinics of North America, 81,* 719–730.

Hooten, T.M., Scholes, D., Hughes, J.P., Winter, C., Roberts, P.L., Stapleton, A.E., Stergachis, A., & Stamm, W.E. (1996). A prospective study of risk factors for symptomatic urinary tract infection in young women. *New England Journal of Medicine, 335,* 468–474.

Hooten, T.M., & Stamm, W.E. (1997). Diagnosis and treatment of uncomplicated urinary tract infections. *Infectious Disease Clinics of North America, 11,* 551–581.

Karlowicz, K.A. (1997). Pharmocologic therapy for acute cystitis in adults: A review of treatment options. *Urology Nurse, 17*(3), 106–114.

Rieber, J.M., & Goodman, R.L. (1995). Treatment of acute cystitis. *JAMA, 274,* 25–26.

Wisinger, D.B. (1996). Urinary tract infection. Current management strategies. *Postgraduate Medicine, 100,* 229–236.

Chapter

92. Prostatitis: Lower Urinary Tract Symptoms

Roberta A. Strohl, RN, BSN, MN, AOCN®

I. Definition: Infection and inflammation of the prostate gland

II. Pathophysiology
   A. Acute prostatitis: Result of obstructing urethral abnormalities with ascent of bacteria up the urethra
   B. Chronic prostatitis: May follow acute bacterial prostatitis or may be nonbacterial in origin

III. Clinical features: Acute prostatitis usually has a febrile illness with urinary tract infection and bacteremia. In the elderly, chronic inflammation leads to scarring and bladder neck contracture.
   A. Etiology
      1. Nonbacterial: May be related to *Chlamydia trachomatis* in young patients
      2. Bacterial: Related to gram-negative bacilli (*Escherichia coli*), enterococcus, and ureaplasma
      3. Obstruction may result from edema of prostate already enlarged by benign prostatic hypertrophy.
   B. History
      1. History of cancer and cancer treatment
      2. Current medications: Prescribed and over-the-counter
      3. History of presenting symptom(s): Precipitating factors, onset, location, and duration
      4. Changes in activities of daily living
      5. Past medical history: UTI, prostate disease, STD
   C. Signs and symptoms
      1. Pelvic tenderness
      2. Fever (low-grade)
      3. Difficulty voiding
         a) Slow stream
         b) Sense of incomplete voiding
         c) Nocturia
         d) Urgency
         e) Dribbling

    D. Physical exam
- 1. Vital signs: Fever
- 2. Prostate exam
  - *a)* Enlarged prostate: Vigorous exam is contraindicated if abscess is suspected, as massage may result in sepsis.
  - *b)* Prostate: Smooth, firm, tender
  - *c)* Rectal vault: Smooth without lesions or nodules
- 3. Abdominal exam: May reveal suprapubic pain

IV. Diagnostic tests
- A. Laboratory
  - 1. Urinalysis: Bacteria greater than five leukocytes per high-power field in the sediment of a centrifuged midstream urine specimen; *Escherichia coli* is usual organism
  - 2. Expressed prostatic secretions (obtained by digital massage): Reveal lipid-laden leukocytes
  - 3. CBC: WBCs may be increased.
- B. Radiology: Ultrasound of prostate to evaluate size and masses

V. Differential diagnosis
- A. Cystitis (see Chapter 91)
- B. Benign prostatic hypertrophy (see Chapter 85)
- C. Prostate cancer
- D. Urethral stricture
- E. Bladder carcinoma
- F. Neurogenic bladder

VI. Treatment
- A. Acute bacterial prostatitis
  - 1. Hydration: Oral fluids should be increased to three liters/day.
  - 2. Analgesics: Begin with NSAIDs unless contraindicated; opioids usually are not necessary (see Appendix 11).
  - 3. Stool softeners
  - 4. Antibiotics (e.g., ampicillin 500 mg po qid x two weeks or more in acute prostatitis) treatment are successful (see Appendix 1).
- B. Chronic prostatitis
  - 1. Bacterial: Fluoroquinolones (Cipro®, Bayer Corp. Pharmaceutical Division, West Haven, CT) 500 mg po bid; classification is lipid soluble-based, allowing diffusion across prostate epithelium
  - 2. Nonbacterial: Two weeks of tetracycline or doxycycline, which should be effective against *Chlamydia trachomatis*
  - 3. Oral antibiotics: Three to four weeks
    - *a)* Bactrim® DS (Roche Pharmaceutical Laboratories, Nutley, NJ): 160 mg/800 mg po bid (preferred)
    - *b)* Ampicillin: 500 mg po qid
    - *c)* Tetracycline: 500 mg po qid

      d) Doxycycline: 100 mg po bid

      e) Carbenicillin: 1 g po qid

      f) Ciprofoxcin: 500 mg po bid (may be better for chronic)

VII. Follow-up
   A. Patients are followed to assess response to therapy.
   B. Acute prostatitis responds rapidly to therapy; fever and symptoms resolve within three days of antibiotic therapy. Re-evaluate 48–72 hours after initial evaluation.
   C. Chronic prostatitis requires follow-up to distinguish these symptoms from the development of benign prostatic hypertrophy (BPH) and prostate cancer.
   D. Intractable pain, dehydration, or fever over 102°F (38.8°C) may require a brief hospital stay.

VIII. Referrals for refractory to treatment
   A. Urologist
   B. Internist
   C. Oncologist

References

Berry, D. (1996). Bladder disturbances. In S.L. Groenwald, M.H. Frogge, M. Goodman, & C.H. Yarbro (Eds.), *Cancer symptom management* (pp. 467–484). Boston: Jones & Barlett.

Criste, G. (1994). Prostatitis: A review of diagnosis and management. *Nurse Practitioner, 19*(7), 32–33, 37–38.

Fowler, J. (1996). Prostatitis. In J. Gillenwater, J. Grayhack, S. Howards, & J. Duckett (Eds.), *Adult and pediatric urology* (3rd ed.) (pp. 1715–1745). St. Louis: Mosby.

Mitsumorik, K., Tera, A., Yamamoto, S., Ishtoya, S., & Yoshida, O. (1999). Virulence characteristics of *Escherichia coli* in acute bacterial prostatitis. *Journal of Infectious Disease, 180*, 1378–1381.

Nickel, J.C., Nyberg, L.M., & Hennenfent, M. (1999). Research guidelines for chronic prostatitis: Consensus report from the First National Institutes of Health International Prostatitis Collaborative Network. *Urology, 54*, 229–233.

93. Pyelonephritis

Diane G. Cope, PhD, ARNP-CS, AOCN®

I. Definition: Infection and inflammation of the upper urinary tract, which includes the kidneys and renal pelvis

II. Pathophysiology
   A. Acute
      1. Tubule-interstitial inflammation with accumulation of leukocytes occurs.
      2. Abscesses and edema form in the renal parenchyma.
   B. Chronic
      1. Leukocytes, plasma cells, and macrophages infiltrate the interstitium of the kidney.
      2. Chronic inflammation causes fibrosis with atrophy of renal tissue and scarring.
      3. Normal renal tissue may become hypertrophic and appear to be a mass lesion on radiographic study.

III. Clinical features: Acute and chronic
   A. Etiology
      1. Acute: Generally the result of ascending bacterial infection with the most common organisms being *Escherichia coli*, proteus, and klebsiella
      2. Chronic: Caused by renal tract abnormalities or chronic infection
   B. History
      1. History of cancer and cancer treatment
      2. Current medications: Prescribed and over-the-counter
      3. History of presenting symptom(s): Precipitating factors, onset, location, and duration
      4. Changes in activities of daily living
      5. Past medical history: UTIs, sexual history
   C. Signs and symptoms
      1. Acute
         a) Dysuria
         b) Frequency
         c) Urgency
         d) Acute flank or back pain
         e) Severe abdominal or groin pain
         f) Fever higher than 102°F (38.8°C) with shaking chills

            g) Flushed skin; diaphoresis

            h) Nausea/vomiting

            i) Fatigue

            j) General ill feeling

            k) Cloudy, malodorous urine

            l) No vaginal or urethral discharge

    2. Chronic

        a) Dysuria

        b) Frequency

        c) Vague flank or abdominal discomfort

        d) Intermittent low-grade fevers

        e) Hypertension

D. Physical exam (acute and chronic)

    1. Vital signs: Note elevation in temperature or blood pressure.

    2. Abdominal exam

        a) Suprapubic tenderness

        b) Distended bladder

    3. Posterior thorax exam: Flank or costovertebral angle tenderness

    4. Pelvic exam: To rule out vaginitis (women)

IV. Diagnostic tests

A. Acute: Laboratory

    1. Urinalysis

        a) Color: Usually dark yellow or amber from bacteria acting on urea

        b) RBCs: Indicating tissue destruction

        c) Leukocytes: Increased WBCs and/or clumps suggesting infection

        d) Nitrite: Formed when bacteria reduce the nitrates present in normal urine

        e) Protein: May or may not be increased

        f) Presence of casts: Indicates proteinuria, increased urine concentration, and renal stasis

        g) Increased pH: Results from some bacteria acting on the urine

    2. Urine culture and sensitivity: Usually greater than 100,000 bacteria/ml; lower colony counts are sufficient for symptoms to occur.

B. Chronic: Laboratory

    1. Urinalysis

        a) Pyuria: May or may not be present

        b) White cell casts: Less commonly seen in urinalysis

    2. Chemistry panel

        a) Hyperkalemia

        b) Creatinine: 2–3 mg/dl

    3. Blood cultures: Indicated for patients appearing acutely ill to rule out bacteremia

C. Radiology

    1. Rarely performed in acute pyelonephritis

    2. IV pyelogram: Most definitive diagnostic procedure for chronic pyelonephritis to reveal

        a) Involved kidney as irregular

        b) Hydronephrosis
        c) Calyces clubbing
        d) Scarring of upper pole or entire kidney
    3. CT scan: To further evaluate chronic pyelonephritis to reveal
        a) Renal atrophy
        b) Wedge-shaped areas of decreased attenuation
        c) Fascial/tubular thickening
    4. Cystometry: To evaluate filling and emptying pressures in bladder
    5. Renal ultrasound: To evaluate for renal abnormalities; may be performed before CT scan

V. Differential diagnosis
    A. Vaginitis (see Chapter 97)
    B. Bladder obstruction
    C. Renal calculi
    D. Acute appendicitis
    E. Acute cholecystitis
    F. Nephrolithiasis
    G. Prostatitis (see Chapter 92)
    H. Cervicitis
    I. Salpingitis
    J. Acute abdominal disorder (see Chapter 50)
    K. Chlamydial urethritis (see Chapter 86)
    L. Gonococcal urethritis (see Chapter 87)
    M. Diabetes mellitus/insipidus (see Chapter 143)
    N. Chemotherapy-induced nephrotoxicity
    O. Radiation-induced nephrotoxicity

VI. Treatment: Less ill patients, treat for 10 days; 14 days for critically ill patients
    A. Outpatient pharmacologic therapy for acute pyelonephritis (mild symptoms): Based on organisms isolated (see Appendix 1)
        1. Trimethoprim (Trimpex®, Hoffman La-Roche Inc., Nutley, NJ): 100 mg po every 12 hours for 10–14 days
        2. Trimethoprim 160 mg/sulfamethoxazole 800 mg (Bactrim® DS, Roche Pharmaceutical Laboratories, Nutley, NJ; Septra® DS, Monarch Pharmaceuticals, Bristol, TN): One tablet po every 12 hours for 10–14 days
        3. Amoxicillin (Amoxil®, SmithKline Beecham Pharmaceuticals, Philadelphia, PA): 500 mg po every eight hours for 10–14 days
        4. Nitrofurantoin (Macrodantin®, Procter & Gamble Pharmaceuticals, Inc., Mason, OH; Furadantin®, Dura Pharmaceuticals, San Diego, CA): 100 mg po four times/day for 10–14 days
        5. Quinolones
           a) Ciprofloxacin: 500 mg po every 12 hours for 10–14 days
           b) Orofloxacin: 300 mg po every 12 hours for 10–14 days
           c) Levaquin® (Ortho-McNeil Pharmaceuticals, Raritan, NJ): 250 mg/day po for 10–14 days

       d) Maxaquin® (Unimed Pharmaceuticals, Inc., Buffalo Grove, IL): 400 mg/day po for 10–14 days

  B. Inpatient therapy for acute pyelonephritis (moderate to severe symptoms): IV fluids and parenteral therapy until patient clinically improves, then oral treatment for 10 days

    1. Ceftriaxone (Rocephin®, Roche Pharmaceutical Laboratories): 1–2 g every 24 hours; ampicillin: 1 g every four hours IV

    2. If aminoglycosides must be used, exercise caution.

  C. Chronic pyelonephritis

    1. Intrarenal abscesses may require drainage or prolonged antimicrobial therapy.

    2. Emphysematous pyelonephritis requires immediate nephrectomy.

    3. Treatment for renal calculi depends on stone size and location.

    4. Treatment for relapse or chronic pyelonephritis is four to six weeks of antibiotic therapy.

VII. Follow-up

  A. Short-term: Symptomatic relief in 48–72 hours; a follow-up urine culture may be obtained two and six weeks after discontinuation of therapy to detect relapses.

  B. Long-term: Relapse or chronic pyelonephritis; treat individuals with four to six weeks of antibiotic therapy.

VIII. Referrals: Urologist for recurrent infections, suspected obstructions or renal calculi, and cystitis in young males

References

Cruz, D.N., Perazella, M.A., & Mahnensmith, R.L. (1996). A middle-aged woman with back and flank pain. *Hospital Practice, 31*(9), 193–194.

Kawashima, A., Sandler, C.M., Goldman, S.M., Raval, B.K., & Fishman, E.K. (1997). CT of renal inflammatory disease. *Radiographics, 17,* 851–866.

Kim, E.D., & Schaeffer, A.J. (1994). Antimicrobial therapy for urinary tract infections. *Seminars in Nephrology, 14,* 551–569.

M\u1d9cMurray, B.R., Wrenn, K.D., & Wright, S.W. (1997). Usefulness of blood cultures in pyelonephritis. *American Journal of Emergency Medicine, 15*(2), 137–140.

Orenstein, R., & Wong, E.S. (1999). Urinary tract infections in adults. *American Family Physician, 59,* 1225–1234.

Pinson, A.G., Philbrick, J.T., Lindbeck, G.H., & Schorling, J.B. (1997). Fever in the clinical diagnosis of acute pyelonephritis. *American Journal of Emergency Medicine, 15*(2), 148–151.

Samm, B.J., & Dmochowski, R.R. (1996). Urologic emergencies. Conditions affecting kidney, ureter, bladder, prostate, and urethra. *Postgraduate Medicine, 100*(4), 177–180.

Smith, W.R., M\u1d9cClish, D.K., Poses, R.M., Pinson, A.G., Miller, S.T., Bobo-Mosley, L., Morrison, R.E., & Lancaster, D.J. (1997). Bacteremia in young urban women admitted with pyelonephritis. *American Journal of Medical Science, 313*(1), 50–57.

Chapter

94. Syndrome of Inappropriate Antidiuretic Hormone

Susan A. Ezzone, MS, RN, CNP

I. Definition: Abnormal production and secretion of antidiuretic hormone (ADH [i.e., vasopressin]) causing the kidneys to retain water and reduce serum osmolality

II. Physiology/Pathophysiology
   A. Normal
      1. Under normal conditions, ADH is released from the posterior pituitary gland in response to increased osmolality or decreased plasma volume and acts on the collecting ducts of the kidneys.
      2. ADH normally causes the kidneys to reabsorb water, thereby concentrating urine and normalizing serum osmolality.
   B. Pathophysiology
      1. Excess production of ADH results in increased water retention by the kidneys, increasing body water and causing moderate expansion of plasma volume.
      2. In syndrome of inappropriate antidiuretic hormone (SIADH), either primary excess of ADH (vasopressin) is present, increasing water retention and causing hyponatremia, or secondary stimulation of ADH (vasopressin) occurs by three mechanisms.
         a) ADH may be synthesized and autonomously released from tumors (see Appendix 12).
         b) Nontumorous tissue may synthesize and release ADH autonomously or stimulate ADH release by the pituitary gland.
         c) ADH may be released from the pituitary gland inappropriately because of inflammation, neoplasm, vascular lesions, or drugs (e.g., morphine).

III. Clinical features: SIADH is considered an isovolumic, hypotonic, hyponatremic condition.
   A. History
      1. History of cancer and cancer treatment
      2. Current medications: Prescribed and over-the-counter
      3. History of presenting symptom(s): Precipitating factors, onset, location, and duration
      4. Changes in activities of daily living
      5. History of fluid intake and output in the last 24 hours
   B. Signs and symptoms of SIADH depend on how quickly the syndrome develops and the degree of hyponatremia.

1. Symptoms of mild, moderate, and severe SIADH have been described (see Figure 94-1).
2. Other symptoms may include
    a) Weight gain without edema
    b) Thirst
    c) Headache
    d) Impaired memory
    e) Decreased urine output
    f) Coma if severe SIADH occurs.
C. Physical exam: Neurologic examination
    1. Change in level of consciousness: Confusion, irritability
    2. Deep tendon reflexes: Hyporeflexia

IV. Diagnostic tests
   A. Laboratory
       1. Serum osmolality: < 280 mOsm/kg
       2. Serum sodium concentration: < 130 mEq/l
       3. Urine sodium: > 25 mEq/l
       4. Urine osmolality: > 100 mOsm/kg
       5. Urine-specific gravity: Increased > 1.032
       6. Renal, thyroid, and adrenal function: Normal
       7. Plasma creatinine, BUN, uric acid, and phosphate: Low normal
   B. Radiology: CT scan of the head to evaluate for anatomical lesions

V. Differential diagnosis: Focuses on identifying the cause of SIADH (see Figure 94-2).
   A. Malignant tumors (see Appendix 12)
   B. CNS disorders
   C. Pulmonary conditions (e.g., pulmonary tuberculosis, pneumonia)
   D. Postoperative secondary to anesthetic agents.
   E. Drugs (e.g., diuretics, amitriptyline, vincristine, cyclophosphamide) may potentiate the release or action of ADH.

Figure 94-1. Signs and Symptoms of Syndrome of Inappropriate Antidiuretic Hormone

Mild	Moderate	Severe
• Sodium level 120 mmol/l or below	• Sodium level 110 mmol/l or below	• Sodium level 100 mmol/l or below
• Muscle cramps	• Irritability	• Seizure activity
• Anorexia/nausea/vomiting	• Disorientation	• Coma
• Fatigue	• Confusion	
	• Lethargy	
	• Extrapyramidal signs	
	• Abdominal cramps/diarrhea	

Note. Based on information from Rohaly-Davis & Johnston, 1996.

Figure 94-2. Ectopic Antidiuretic Hormone Secretion

Malignancies	Endogenous causes	Drugs
• Lung (oat cell)	• Central nervous system disorders	• Nicotine
• Lymphoma	- Brain tumors	• Carbamazepine (Tegretol®,
• Pancreas and	- Hemorrhagic states (subdural hematoma,	Novartis Pharmaceutical Corp.,
duodenum	cerebral vascular accident)	East Hanover, NJ)
	- Head trauma	• Chlorpropamide
	- Infections: Meningitis, encephalitis, brain	• Barbiturates
	abscesses	• Analgesics (e.g., morphine)
	- Guillain-Barré syndrome	• Antineoplastic drugs
	- Lupus erythematosus	• Anesthetics
	• Pulmonary conditions	• Tricyclic antidepressants
	- Positive-pressure mechanical ventilation	
	- Acute respiratory failure ($^-$ Po_2 - Pco_2)[a]	
	- Infection	
	- Viral pneumonia	
	- Tuberculosis	
	- Chronic obstructive pulmonary disease	
	- Lung abscesses	
	• Postoperative period	

[a]Po_2, partial pressure of oxygen; Pco_2, partial pressure of carbon dioxide

Note. From "Syndrome of Inappropriate Antidiuretic Hormone Secretion," by J. Batcheller, 1994, *Critical Care Nursing Clinics of North America, 6,* p. 688. Copyright 1994 by W.B. Saunders Co. Reprinted with permission.

VI. Treatment (see Chapters 147)

    A. Treatment of SIADH is aimed at disrupting the effects of ADH on the kidneys. Therapy is based on the severity of hyponatremia, symptomatology, and cause of SIADH.

    B. Treat the underlying cause. Chronic treatment may be necessary for SIADH caused by cancer.

    C. Fluid restriction of less than 500–1,000 ml/day may be used to treat acute (occurring in less than 48 hours) and is indicated for chronic (persisting for more than 48 hours) hyponatremia.

    D. IV fluid administration

        1. Administration of isotonic (0.9%) saline is adequate in most cases.

            a) Mild hyponatremia: Serum sodium is 126–134 mEq/l; infuse minimal hydration.

            b) Moderate hyponatremia: Serum sodium <125 mEq/l; may require administration of IV fluids, electrolytes, and diuretics.

        2. Administration of hypertonic (3%) saline solution may be used for severe symptomatic hyponatremia (serum sodium < 120 mEq/l). Correct sodium by 1–2 mEq/l per hour until normalization of sodium levels occurs and symptoms resolve.

        3. In symptomatic chronic SIADH, the rate of sodium replaced might be one mEq/l per hour for about five hours, followed by slowing therapy to allow raising the sodium level to 12–15 mEq/l in 24 hours.

        4. Too rapid correction of hyponatremia in patients with chronic hyponatremia (longer than 2 to 5 days) may lead to central pontine myelinolysis or demyelination, which

is caused by rapid loss of brain electrolytes and organic osmolytes. Stop hypertonic solution when level reaches 120 mEq/l.

E. Drug therapy may be initiated if hyponatremia continues despite fluid restriction or IV administration of saline solution.

   1. Loop diuretics (e.g., furosemide) may be administered if the patient is volume overloaded and may assist in reducing the renal response to ADH, causing electrolyte-free water excretion.

      a) Sodium loss through urinary excretion also occurs and needs to be replaced by IV infusion.

      b) Dosages may begin at 20–40 mg and be titrated according to fluid balance.

   2. Agent commonly used in SIADH is demeclocycline 300–600 mg/day orally; reduces the kidneys' response to ADH; used most often in chronic SIADH

F. Initiate seizure precautions if severe hyponatremia is present.

G. Initiate safety measures if altered mental status is present.

H. Implement frequent mouth care to minimize dryness and promote integrity of mucus membranes.

I. Avoid administration of hypotonic fluids (e.g., IV 5% dextrose), as it could potentiate water retention and hyponatremia.

J. Use normal saline to irrigate nasogastric or enteral tubes.

K. Avoid tap water or saline enemas.

L. Increase salt and protein intake.

VII. Follow-up

A. Frequently monitor serum sodium.

B. Schedule outpatient visits for history and physical examination for symptom monitoring.

VIII. Referrals

A. Nephrologist or endocrinologist: For diagnostic workup of hyponatremia and recommendations for management if etiology is unknown

B. Pharmacist: For drug and fluid management recommendations

References

Batcheller, J. (1994). Syndrome of inappropriate antidiuretic hormone secretion. *Critical Care Nursing Clinics of North America, 6,* 687–692.

Haapoja, S.I. (1997). Paraneoplastic syndromes. In S.L. Groenwald, M.H. Frogge, M. Goodman, & C.H. Yarbo (Eds.), *Cancer nursing: Principles and practice* (4th ed.) (pp. 702–708). Boston: Jones & Bartlett.

Faber, M.D., Kupin, W.L., Heilig, C.W., & Narins, R.G. (1994). Common fluid-electrolyte and acid-base problems in the intensive care unit: Selected issues. *Seminars in Nephrology, 14*(10), 8–22.

Keenan, A.M. (1999). Syndrome of inappropriate secretion of antidiuretic hormone in malignancy. *Seminars in Oncology Nursing, 15,* 160–167.

Rohaly-Davis, J., & Johnston K. (1996). Hematologic emergencies in the intensive care unit. *Critical Care Nursing Quarterly, 18*(4), 35–43.

Soupart, A., & Decaux, G. (1996) Therapeutic recommendations for management of severe hyponatremia: Current concepts on pathogenesis and prevention of neurologic complications. *Clinical Nephrology, 46*(3), 149–169.

Sterns, R.H., Ocdol, H., Schrier, R.W., & Narins, R.G. (1994). Hyponatremia: Pathophysiology, diagnosis, and therapy. In R.G. Narins (Ed.), *Maxwell and Kleeman's clinical disorders of fluid and electrolyte metabolism* (5th ed.) (pp. 583–615). New York: McGraw-Hill.

95. Syphilis

Julie D. Painter, RNC, MSN, OCN®

I. Definition: An STD that can potentially involve multiple organ systems caused by *Treponema pallidum*

II. Pathophysiology
   A. *Treponema pallidum* is an anaerobic spirochete, which is a thin, delicate organism.
   B. *Treponema pallidum* enters the bloodstream through apparent and inapparent breaks in abraded skin or mucous membrane during sexual contact, then multiplies and spreads rapidly to regional lymph nodes. The spirochetes enter the systemic blood stream within hours of transmission and are carried to other body tissues.

III. Clinical features: Congenital syphilis can occur from transplacental transmission of the organism. Incubation period for developing primary syphilis lesion is about three weeks but can range between 10–90 days after initial exposure.
   A. History
      1. History of cancer and cancer treatment
      2. Current medications: Prescribed and over-the-counter
      3. History of presenting symptom(s): Precipitating factors, onset, location, and duration. Associated symptoms are rash, mucous patches, and condylomata lata.
      4. Changes in activities of daily living
      5. Past medical history: STDs, HIV
      6. Social history: Illicit drug, tobacco, alcohol use, sexual practices
   B. Signs and symptoms: Varies according to clinical stages of primary, secondary, latent, and tertiary
      1. Primary syphilis: Characterized by appearance of chancre at site of entry of the organism; usually on the genitals approximately three weeks after exposure
         a) Genital lesions: Usually indurated and without pain
         b) Extragenital lesions: Painful
            (1) Can occur anywhere, depending upon sexual practices
            (2) Common sites: Anal canal, oral cavity, hands, nipples
         c) Chancre persists for one to five weeks and then heals spontaneously.
      2. Secondary syphilis: Occurs about six to eight weeks later

          a) Characterized by flu-like symptoms (e.g., headache, myalgia, arthralgia, fever, lymphadenopathy, rash)

          b) Most contagious stage

          c) Rash usually involves palms and soles.

              (1) Can be macular, papular, annular, or follicular

              (2) Remains about two to six weeks then resolves

          d) Mouth, throat, and cervix may have mucous patches.

          e) Pruritus

          f) Without treatment, healing occurs spontaneously in the first two stages and moves into the latent stage.

      3. Latent syphilis: Early latent is less than one year and is the infectious stage; late latent is greater than one year and is the noninfectious stage.

          a) Approximately one-third of infected people are asymptomatic.

          b) Symptoms include ataxic gait, general paresis, paresthesias

  C. Physical exam

    1. Pelvic or penile exam

          a) Primary: Lesion begins as small papule that enlarges and undergoes necrosis, forming an ulcer.

          b) Secondary: Lesions tend to be symmetric and uniform in size.

    2. Lymph node exam: Inguinal nodes are usually enlarged.

    3. Systemic disease

          a) Secondary

              (1) Oral cavity exam: May have mucous patches and split papules.

              (2) Neck exam: Nuchal rigidity may indicate aseptic meningitis.

              (3) Abdominal exam: Hepatomegaly may indicate hepatitis.

          b) Tertiary

              (1) Cardiovascular exam: Rub or murmur indicating aortic insufficiency

              (2) Neurologic exam: Dull affect, decreased intellectual function, ataxic gait, impaired pain and temperature sensation, hypoactive reflexes, and autonomic dysfunction

              (3) Integument exam: Gumma may be present; isolated slow, progressive lesions of skin that can be single or multiple with center necrotic surrounded by inflammation

IV. Diagnostic tests

  A. Laboratory

    1. Serologic tests used for initial screening and titers

          a) Nontreponemal-specific tests: Rapid plasma reagin (RPR) test yields high false-positive results.

          b) Venereal disease research laboratory (VDRL) test

              (1) A decline in the titer indicates response to therapy.

              (2) RPR is the most common test used today.

              (3) If desiring to correlate titer to response, the same test (i.e., VDRL or RPR) must be used each time.

    2. Treponemal-specific tests

         a) Fluorescent treponemal antibody absorption (FTA-ABS): Standard adult test

         b) Microhemagglutination assay for treponema pallidum antibodies (MHA-TP): Often used in testing neonates; treponemal tests are used to confirm diagnosis of syphilis in people with positive VDRL or RPR.

     3. Darkfield microscopy is useful with lesions that have active mobile spirochetes, such as in primary and secondary lesions.

  B. Radiology: Not indicated

  C. Other: Lumbar puncture to evaluate cerebral spinal fluid if neurologic exam indicates abnormalities or in patients with syphillis greater than one year

V. Differential diagnosis

  A. Sexually transmitted diseases (i.e., herpes, chancroid, lymphogranuloma venereum, scabies, balanitis)

  B. Secondary syphilis can mimic skin disruptions.

VI. Treatment: Based on the clinical and serological staging

  A. Primary, secondary, and early latent syphilis (of less than one year)

     1. Recommended regimen: Benzathine penicillin G 2.4 million units IM as single dose

     2. Alternative regimen: Penicillin-allergic and nonpregnant patients

         a) Doxycycline: 100 mg po twice a day for two weeks

         b) Tetracycline: 500 mg po four times a day for two weeks

  B. Late latent syphilis (of more than one year duration; gummas and cardiovascular syphilis)

     1. Recommended regimen: Benzathine penicillin G 7.2 million units total, adminis-tered as three doses of 2.4 million units IM given every week for three consecutive weeks

     2. Alternative regimen: Penicillin-allergic, nonpregnant patients

         a) Doxycycline: 100 mg po twice a day for four weeks

         b) Tetracycline: 500 mg po four times a day for four weeks

     3. If patient is penicillin-allergic, alternate drugs should be used only after lumbar puncture exam excludes neurosyphilis.

  C. Neurosyphilis

     1. Recommended regimen: Aqueous crystalline penicillin G 12–24 million units every four hours IV for 10–14 days

     2. Alternative regimen (if outpatient compliance unsure)

         a) Procaine penicillin 2–4 million units IM daily plus probenecid 500 mg po four times a day, both for 10–14 days

  D. Treat people exposed to those with infectious syphilis as for early-stage disease.

VII. Follow-up

  A. Monitor therapy with serial quantitative VDRL titers at 3, 6, 9, and 12 months after therapy for early syphilis.

  B. Patients with syphilis for greater than one year duration should also have VDRL titers done at 18 and 24 months post-therapy.

C. HIV-positive people should have more frequent follow-up, including serologic testing at 1, 2, 3, 6, 9, and 12 months.

D. Women should have an annual pelvic examination and Pap smear.

VIII. Referrals: Refer patient back to specialist if being treated for cancer, autoimmune disease, or HIV/AIDS for appropriate follow-up.

References

Mardh, P.A., Tchoudomirova, K., Elshibly, S., & Hellberg, D. (1998). Symptoms and signs in single and mixed genital infections. *International Journal of Gynaecology and Obstetrics, 63*(2), 145–152.

Roe, V.A., & Gudi, A. (1997). Pharmacologic management of sexually transmitted diseases. *Journal of Nurse Midwifery, 42,* 275–259.

Schmid, G.P. (1999). Treatment of chancroid, 1997. *Clinics of Infectious Diseases, 28*(Suppl. 1), S14–S20.

Woodward, C., & Fisher, M.A. (1999). Drug treatment of common STDs: Part I. Herpes, syphilis, urethritis, chlamydia and gonorrhea. *American Family Physician, 60,* 1387–1394.

Chapter

96. Trichomoniasis
Julie D. Painter, RNC, MSN, OCN®

I. Definition: Infection of the vagina by *Trichomonas vaginalis*

II. Pathophysiology: *Trichomonas vaginalis*, a unicellular flagellated protozoan, is the cause of this disease, which is primarily classified as sexually transmitted.

III. Clinical features: Incubation period is 4–20 days after exposure. Can be asymptomatic involving the Skene's ducts and lower urinary tract in women and the lower genitourinary tract in men. Symptoms may worsen immediately following menstruation and during pregnancy. Frequently occurs in presence of other STDs.
   A. History
      1. History of cancer and cancer treatment
      2. Current medications: Prescribed and over-the-counter
      3. History of presenting symptom(s): Precipitating factors, onset, location, and duration. Associated symptoms are dysuria, and dyspareunia.
      4. Changes in activities of daily living
      5. History of menstrual cycle
      6. Social history of sexual practices and STDs
   B. Signs and symptoms
      1. Major symptom: A pale-yellow to gray-green vaginal or penile discharge
      2. Amount of discharge: May vary; could be frothy or have a fishy odor
      3. Dysuria, increased frequency
      4. Abdominal pain
   C. Physical exam
      1. External genitalia exam: Assess for discharge pooling at introitus or posterior fourchette.
         a) Petechiae or hemorrhages of external genitalia
         b) Lesions, ulcerations, erythema
      2. Pelvic exam
         a) Edema and redness may be present in the vaginal tissue.
         b) Cervix may appear inflamed and friable.
         c) Rarely, punctate lesions on the cervix will have a "strawberry" appearance.
         d) Observe rectal area for edema and redness.

      3. In men, perform digital rectal exam to determine tenderness and enlargement of prostate; urethritis may be present.

IV. Diagnostic tests
    A. Laboratory
       1. Sample vaginal secretions; gather sample from anterior or lateral wall on a dry swab and apply to pH paper.
         a) Normal pH is 3.5-4.5; trichomoniasis has pH > 4.5.
         b) Under microscope, examine vaginal secretions mixed with a saline solution; observe for a motile organism with a whip-like flagella.
       2. In men, collect the first morning urine (about 5–30 ml), and examine for trichomonad under microscope.
    B. Radiology: Not indicated

V. Differential diagnosis
    A. Vaginitis: Bacterial vaginitis or vulvovaginal candidiasis (see Chapters 97 and 98)
    B. Cervicitis: Chlamydia or gonorrhea (see Chapters 86 and 87)
    C. Candida (see Chapter 98)
    D. Prostatitis (see Chapter 92)

VI. Treatment
    A. Metronidazole (Flagyl®, G.D. Searle & Co., Chicago, IL): 2 g po for one dose is treatment of choice.
       1. Single dose improves compliance, whereas other dosing regimens may result in less compliance. A single dose often is effective; however, in relapse, the single dose can be repeated.
       2. Alternative: Metronidazole (Flagyl) 500 mg po given twice daily for seven days
       3. If condition fails to resolve with the above regimens, retreat with metronidazole (Flagyl) 500 mg po twice daily for another seven days.
    B. Sexual partners should be treated with the single-dose regimen or the seven-day regimen.

VII. Follow-up
    A. No formal follow-up is necessary unless the treatment regimen is not effective in resolving the infection.
    B. Annual pelvic examination and Pap smear is recommended.

VIII. Referrals: Refer to gynecologist for refractory disease.

References

Mahadani, J.W., Dekate, R.R., & Shrikhande, A.V. (1998). Cytodiagnosis of discharge per vaginum. *Indian Journal of Pathology and Microbiology, 41,* 403–411.

Ries, A.J. (1997). Treatment of vaginal infections: Candidiasis, bacterial vaginosis, and trichomonia-sis. *Journal of the American Pharmacy Association, 37,* 563–569.

Roes, V.A., & Gudi, A. (1997). Pharmacologic management of sexually transmitted diseases. *Journal of Nurse Midwifery, 42,* 275–289.

Chapter

97. Vaginitis
Julie D. Painter, RNC, MSN, OCN®

I. Definition: A noninflammatory infection of the vagina

II. Pathophysiology
   A. Bacterial vaginosis (BV) is a condition that results from an overgrowth of both anaerobic bacteria and *Gardnerella vaginalis*.
   B. *Mobiluncus* is a curved bacterial rod that is highly motile and present in approximately 50% of BV cases.

III. Clinical features: About 40% of vaginal infections are the result of BV, and the majority are asymptomatic; incubation period is 5–10 days after exposure.
   A. Risk factors
      1. Although BV is associated with sexual activity, it is not exclusively considered a STD.
      2. BV in the nonsexually active woman is rare.
      3. BV is more likely in women with STDs, and their male partners will remain asymptomatic.
   B. Etiology
      1. Associated with *Gardnerella vaginalis*, *Mobiluncus*, and other newly discovered anaerobes
      2. Exact etiology is not known
   C. History
      1. History of cancer and cancer treatment
      2. Current medications: Prescribed and over-the-counter
      3. History of presenting symptom(s): Precipitating factors, onset, and duration
      4. Changes in activities of daily living
      5. Social history of sexual activity
   D. Signs and symptoms
      1. Vaginal discharge may be grayish-white.
      2. Discharge may be frothy.
      3. Discharge may have a fishy odor.
      4. Mild vaginal discomfort, burning, and itching typically are present.

E. Physical exam: Focuses on pelvic exam
    1. Examine introitus for discharge (85% of women have a grayish-white discharge).
    2. Observe for discharge coating vaginal walls; note odor.
    3. Assess for cervical motion tenderness (often indicative of pelvic inflammatory disease or other STD).

IV. Diagnostic tests
    A. Laboratory
        1. Clinical criteria must include three or more of the following to be diagnostic of bacterial vaginitis.
            a) Grayish-white, homogeneous, malodorous discharge that may be minimal or profuse
            b) Presence of clue cells on microscopic exam (i.e., vaginal cells with a stippled appearance because of bacilli adhered to their surfaces)
            c) Vaginal fluid with pH > 4.5
            d) Vaginal discharge with fishy odor before or after the addition of 10% potassium hydroxide with approximately 23 drops (i.e., whiff test)
            e) If these characteristics are present, there is minimal value in obtaining other laboratory tests.
        2. Gram stain: To determine the relative concentration of the bacterial morphotype characteristic of the altered flora of BV
        3. Wet mount: Reveals short, motile rods and characteristic clue cells
    B. Radiology: Not indicated

V. Differential diagnosis
    A. Other forms of vaginitis: Trichomoniasis, vulvovaginal candidiasis (see Chapters 96 and 98)
    B. Cervicitis: Chlamydia, gonorrhea (see Chapters 86 and 87)

VI. Treatment: Goal of therapy is to relieve symptoms; therefore, only symptomatic women require treatment.
    A. Treatment of choice is metronidazole (Flagyl®, G.D. Searle & Co., Chicago, IL) 500 mg po bid for seven days or 2 g metronidazole po (one dose).
    B. Alternative: Clindamycin 300 mg orally bid for seven days; metronidazole gel 0.75%, one full applicator (5 g) intravaginally bid for five days; or clindamycin cream 2%, one full applicator (5 g) intravaginally at bedtime for seven days.
    C. Treatment of sex partners not recommended.

VII. Follow-up
    A. Not indicated: Recurrence of BV is common; use alternative treatment regimens for recurrent disease.
    B. Annual pelvic examination and Pap smear is recommended.

VIII. Referrals: No specific referrals needed unless complications with pregnancy

References

Carr, P.L., Felsenstein, D., & Friedman, R.H. (1998). Evaluation and management of vaginitis. *Journal of Geriatric Internal Medicine, 13,* 335–336.

Centers for Disease Control. (1998). Sexually transmitted infections. *MMWR, 47*(RR-1).

Nagesha, C.N., & Rama, N.K. (1998). Clinical and microbiological aspects of vaginitis. *Indian Journal of Medicine Science, 52,* 526–532.

Ries, A.J. (1997). Treatment of vaginal infections: Candidiasis, bacterial vaginitis, and trichomoniasis. *Journal of American Pharmacy Association, NS37,* 563–569.

Sobel, J.D. (1997). Vaginitis. *New England Journal of Medicine, 337,* 1896–1903.

Sobel, J.D. (1999). Vulvovaginitis in healthy women. *Comprehensive Therapy, 25,* 335–346.

Williams, P.A. (1999). Nonscientifically validated herbal treatments for vaginitis. *Nurse Practitioner, 24*(8), 101, 102, 104.

Winefield, A.D., & Murphy, S.A. (1998). Bacterial vaginosis: A review. *Clinical Excellence in Nurse Practitioner, 2*(4), 212–217.

98. Vulvovaginal Candidiasis

Julie D. Painter, RNC, MSN, OCN®

I. Definition: An infection of the vulvovaginal area(s) caused by *Candida albicans*

II. Pathophysiology: An imbalance in the organisms that compose the normal vaginal flora results in an overabundance of *Candida albicans* (i.e., yeast).

III. Clinical features: Not considered an STD. *Candida albicans* is the most common yeast organism in vaginal flora; present in about 10% of vulvovaginal infections diagnosed.
   A. Risk factors
      1. Pregnancy
      2. Antibiotic therapy
      3. Chemotherapy
      4. Estrogen therapy
      5. Lower pelvic radiation
      6. Steroid therapy
      7. Immunosuppression
      8. Diabetes mellitus
   B. History
      1. History of cancer and cancer treatment
      2. Current medications: Prescribed and over-the-counter
      3. History of presenting symptom(s): Precipitating factors, onset, and duration. Associated symptoms are itching, dyspareunia, and dysuria.
      4. Changes in activities of daily living
      5. Social history of sexual practices, STDs, HIV
   C. Signs and symptoms: Rapid onset occurring prior to menstruation when vaginal pH falls
      1. Key symptom: Vulvar pruritus (i.e., extreme itching and burning)
      2. Vulvar erythema
      3. Edema and excoriated areas on the vulva
      4. Discharge: Usually odorless and has cheesy appearance
      5. Burning: May occur with discharge
   D. Physical exam
      1. Genital exam: Assess the external features of the vulva for edema, erythema, excoriation, and any form of discharge.

2. Pelvic exam
   a) Assess vagina for erythema, plaques, white patches.
   b) Note the odor of the secretions; *Candida albicans* should be odorless.
   c) Observe discharge; may be thick, white, and adherent (i.e., like cottage cheese)
   d) Assess for cervical motion, tenderness, pain, or lesions.

IV. Diagnostic tests
   A. Laboratory: During pelvic exam, obtain a specimen of vaginal secretions from the anterior and lateral walls of the vagina.
      1. Gather specimen on a dry swab, and apply the secretions to pH paper.
      2. If candidiasis, the pH of the secretions will be < 4.5 (normal pH of the vagina is 3.5–4.5).
      3. Examination of the secretions mixed with 10%–20% potassium hydroxide on a microscopic slide should reveal typical yeast and pseudohyphal forms.
      4. Women with recurrent infections (i.e., three or more symptomatic episodes per year of vulvovaginal candidiasis) should have cultures done, and findings should be documented.
      5. Diagnostic testing may be needed to determine HIV status.
   B. Radiology: Not indicated

V. Differential diagnosis
   A. Other forms of vaginitis: Bacterial vaginitis or trichomoniasis (see Chapters 96 and 97)
   B. Cervicitis: Chlamydia or gonorrhea (see Chapters 86 and 87)
   C. Pediculosis
   D. Chemical irritants
   E. Vulvar carcinoma

VI. Treatment: Immunocompetent women can be treated with over-the-counter antifungal vaginal creams.
   A. Butoconazole: 2% cream, 5 g intravaginally for three nights
   B. Clotrimazole: 1% cream, 5 g intravaginally for 7–14 nights
   C. Clotrimazole: 100 mg vaginal, two tablets for three nights
   D. Miconazole: 2% cream, 5 g intravaginally for seven nights
   E. Miconazole: 200 mg vaginal suppository, one suppository for three nights or 100 mg vaginal suppository for seven nights
   F. Tioconazole: 6.5% ointment, 5 g intravaginally in a single application
   G. Terconazole: 0.4% cream 5 g intravaginal for three or seven nights
   H. Terconazole: 80 mg suppository, intravaginal one suppository for three days
   I. Fluconazole: For immunocompetent patients; may be given in a one-time oral dose of 150 mg (available in doses of 50 mg, 100 mg, 150 mg, and 200 mg).
   J. Oral regimens are reserved for recurrent infections and women who are HIV positive or immunocompromised.
      1. Dosing of oral antifungal agent (i.e., fluconazole) 150 mg po qd for 14–21 days
      2. Many HIV patients may need to stay on prophylactic doses of Diflucan® (Pfizer Inc., New York, NY).

K. Treatment of sexual partners is not recommended unless the male partner is experiencing candidal balanitis.

L. If patient has normal immune function, discuss daily intake of yogurt to reduce the risk of candidasis developing when taking medications such as antibiotics and/or estrogen.

VII. Follow-up

A. None indicated unless the infection is recurrent

B. Annual pelvic examination and Pap smear is recommended.

VIII. Referrals: Refer to physician if patient has recurrent infections and candidiasis has unknown etiology or if referral will be needed if patient is HIV-positive.

References

Eckert, L.O., Hawes, S.E., Stevens, C.E., Koutsky, L.A., Eschenbach, D.A., & Holmes, K.K. (1998). Vulvovaginal candidiasis: Clinical manifestations, risk factors, management algorithm. *Obstetrics and Gynecology, 92,* 757–765.

Edelman, D.A., & Grant, S. (1999). One-day therapy for vaginal candidiasis. A review. *Journal of Reproductive Medicine, 44,* 543–547.

Elliott, K.A. (1998). Managing patients with vulvovaginal candidiasis. *Nurse Practitioner, 23*(3), 49–53.

Faro, S. (1999). Easy access to antifungal agents. *Infectious Diseases of Obstetrics and Gynecology, 7*(3), 125.

Haefner, H.K. (1999). Current evaluation and management of vulvovaginitis. *Clinics in Obstetrics and Gynecology, 42,*(2), 184–195.

Sobel, J.D. (1998). Vulvovaginitis due to *Candida glabrata.* An emerging problem. *Mycoses, 41*(Suppl. 2), 18–22.

Sobel, J.D. (1999). Vulvovaginitis in healthy women. *Comprehensive Therapy, 25,* 335–346.

Spinillo, A., Capuzzo, E., Acciano, S., DeSantolo, A., & Zara, R. (1999). Effect of antibiotic use on the prevalence of symptomatic vulvovaginal candidiasis. *American Journal of Obstetrics and Gynecology, 180*(1), 14–27.

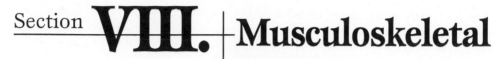

Section VIII. Musculoskeletal

Symptoms

Medical Diagnosis

99. Bone Pain

Karen E. Maher, ANP, MS, AOCN®

I. Definition: Somatic type pain of the bone

II. Pathophysiology
   A. Nociceptors and mechanoreceptors are activated and sensitized in the periphery (e.g., tumor compression or infiltration) or by chemical (e.g., epinephrine, serotonin, bradykinin, prostaglandin, histamine) stimuli.
   B. Nociceptors appear to be localized to connective tissue between muscle fibers and in blood vessel walls, tendons, the joint capsule, and periosteum.
   C. Neuropathic and bone pain frequently coexist, especially when vertebrae are involved with metastasis that expands the bone, causing compression of nerve roots or the spinal cord.

III. Clinical features: Bone is the most common type of cancer pain and is the site most frequently affected by metastatic cancer. Bone pain may or may not be accompanied by a neuropathic component, depending on the extent of disturbance of the highly innervated periosteum.
   A. History
      1. History of cancer and cancer treatment
      2. Current medications: Prescribed and over-the-counter
      3. History of presenting symptom(s): Precipitating factors, onset, location, and duration
      4. Elicit description of pain (e.g., sharp, dull, aching, burning, intermittent, continuous)
      5. Changes in activities of daily living
      6. History of recent trauma or falls
   B. Signs and symptoms
      1. Often localized, but can be diffuse in nature
      2. Characterized with multiple descriptions, including constant aching to a deep, boring sensation accompanied by episodes of stabbing pain
      3. May be worse at night; sleep or lying down may provide little relief.
      4. May occur around joints because of mechanical, chemical, or bony change
      5. Symptoms may depend on location and activity (i.e., increasing pain with ambulation in weight-bearing areas, such as hip and femur).
   C. Physical exam

    1. Musculoskeletal exam: Include pain assessment with percussion in painful areas, as identified by the patient.

    2. Neurologic exam: Assess for muscle strength and sensory deficits, especially in patients with vertebral pain and suspected nerve root compression and/or spinal cord compression.

IV. Diagnostic tests

  A. Laboratory

    1. Alkaline phosphatase may be increased.

    2. Calcium may be increased, phosphorus decreased.

    3. Test thyroid-stimulating hormone (TSH) to rule out hyperthyroidism or hypothyroidism.

  B. Radiology

    1. Plain radiograph in area of interest

      a) Blastic/lytic metastases often are identified with plain film; important in weight-bearing area (e.g., neck and proximal femur) to evaluate integrity of bone cortex.

      b) Assess for pathological fractures.

    2. Bone scan

      a) To identify bone metastasis, most sensitive to blastic lesions

      b) Lytic bone metastases (e.g., multiple myeloma) rarely absorb tracer and bone scan will not visualize well; if lytic metastasis is suspected, order plain films first.

      c) Other types of bone lesions or defects (e.g., past trauma, osteoporotic lesions) will be visualized on bone scan.

    3. CT and MRI: To further evaluate extent of bone involvement if metastasis is suspected; will visualize associated soft-tissue mass. MRI is preferred for evaluation of suspected or impending spinal cord compression.

V. Differential diagnosis

  A. Bone metastasis: Axial skeleton is the most common site (see Chapter 103).

  B. Bone marrow infiltration by tumor

  C. Sequelae from growth factors (e.g., granulocyte-colony-stimulating factor, granulocyte macrophage-colony-stimulating factor)

  D. Hypercalcemia (see Chapter 144)

  E. Hyperthyroidism (see Chapter 149)

  F. Osteopenia secondary to drug therapy

    1. Glucocorticoids: Dexamethasone, prednisone

    2. Post-transplant immunosuppression: Cyclosporine

  G. Hypertropic osteoarthropathy: Paraneoplastic syndrome (see Appendix 12)

  H. Acromegaly: Causes bony enlargement and soft-tissue thickening of fingers, toes, and scalp

  I. Pathological fractures (see Chapter 104)

  J. Arthritis (see Chapters 106 and 108)

  K. Hypothyroidism (see Chapter 150)

VI. Treatment: Refer to appropriate medical diagnosis section.

    A. Assist in maintaining adequate pain management (i.e., NSAIDs with appropriate opioid as indicated by etiology) (see Appendices 8a/b and 11).

    B. Pamidronate (Aredia®, Novartis Pharmaceutical Corp., East Hanover, NJ): 90 mg IV q four weeks; for diagnosis of bone metastasis; to prevent fracture, reduce pain, and strengthen bone

VII. Follow-up

    A. Refer to appropriate medical diagnosis section.

    B. Monitor pain regimen for adequate control.

    C. Monitor for potential neurologic compromise in patients with vertebral metastasis.

VIII. Referrals: Refer to appropriate medical diagnosis section. May include orthopedic surgeon, physical therapy, and rehabilitation services for evaluation of safety issues and mobility.

References

Coleman, R. (1997). Skeletal complications of malignancy. *Cancer, 80*(Suppl. 8), 1588–1594.

Coleman, R.E., Rubens, R.D., Hoskin, P.J., Atkinson, R.E., Owen, J., & Ahmedzai, S. (1995). Supportive care in oncology: Pain and bone problems. *Journal of Cancer Care, 4*(3), 121–126.

Fisher, G., Mayer, D.K., & Struthers, C. (1997). Bone metastases. Part I: Pathophysiology. *Clinical Journal of Oncology Nursing, 1,* 29–35.

Mayer, D.K., Struthers, C., & Fisher, G. (1997). Bone metastases. Part II: Nursing management. *Clinical Journal of Oncology Nursing, 1,* 37–44.

Mercandante, S. (1997). Malignant bone pain: Pathophysiology and treatment. *Pain, 69,* 1–18.

Payne, R. (1997). Mechanisms and management of bone pain. *Cancer, 80*(Suppl. 8), 1608–1613.

100. Joint Pain

Kimberly A. Rumsey, RN, MSN, CS

I. Definition: Monoarthralgia (one joint) and polyarthralgia (several joints)

II. Pathophysiology: Painful stimuli arising from degenerative, inflammatory, or noninflammatory factors of the joint

III. Clinical features
   A. History
      1. History of cancer and cancer treatment
      2. Current medications: Prescribed and over-the-counter
      3. History of joint pain: Precipitating factors, onset, location, and duration. Associated symptoms are fever, rash, diarrhea, and fatigue.
      4. Changes in activities of daily living
      5. Social history of alcohol use, IV drug abuse
      6. Past medical history: Tick bites, STDs, urethritis, uveitis
   B. Signs and symptoms
      1. Depend on the cause of the joint pain
      2. Pain may involve one joint (monoarthalgia) or several joints (polyarthalgia)
      3. Erythema
      4. Edema
      5. Decreased range of motion
   C. Physical exam
      1. Musculoskeletal exam: Assess joint for edema, erythema, warmth, tenderness, and limited range of motion.
      2. Complete physical exam is needed to detect extra-articular symptoms based on the review of systems.
         a) Rheumatoid arthritis
            (1) Auscultate heart (murmur) and lungs (pleural rubs)
            (2) Low-grade fever
         b) Systemic lupus erythematosus
            (1) Rash
               (a) Malar rash: Fixed, erythematous, flat, or raised rash over cheeks (e.g., "butterfly" rash).
               (b) Discoid rash: Erythematous raised areas with scaling
            (2) Oral ulcers

        c) Gout: Tophi (i.e., white lesions beneath the skin) typically found in the ears, hands, and feet

        d) Behcet's syndrome: Mouth ulcers

        e) Reiter's syndrome

           (1) Mouth ulcers

           (2) Conjunctivitis

        f) Psoriatic arthritis: Pitting of nails, psoriatic skin lesions

IV. Diagnostic tests

  A. Laboratory

    1. Specific lab tests based on the review of systems and physical exam findings

    2. The following lab tests may be appropriate.

      a) CBC: May help to differentiate between infectious and noninfectious or systemic and nonsystemic causes

      b) Erythrocyte sedimentation rate (ESR): May be used to screen for inflammatory disease

      c) Rheumatoid factor: Elevated in 80% of rheumatoid arthritis

      d) Antinuclear antibody (ANA): Elevated in systemic lupus erythematosus

      e) Uric acid level: Elevated in gout

      f) HIV testing: To rule out onset of HIV infection

      g) Lyme titer

      h) Synovial fluid evaluation

         (1) Gram stain and culture

         (2) Crystaline diseases (polarized microscopy)

         (3) Inflammation (synovial fluid WBC > 2,000)

  B. Radiology

    1. X-rays: Typically used to obtain baseline information

    2. MRI: To localize an infection or inflammatory process

    3. Bone scan: To rule out bone metastasis, osteomyelitis, osteonecrosis

V. Differential diagnosis

  A. Polyarthritis

    1. Rheumatoid arthritis (see Chapter 108)

    2. Systemic lupus erythematosus

    3. Polymyalgia rheumatica

    4. Fibromyalgia

    5. Gonococcal arthritis (scc Chapter 87)

    6. Lyme arthritis

    7. Rheumatic heart disease

    8. Ankylosing spondylitis

    9. Adrenal insufficiency

    10. Medication-induced

      a) Procainamide

      b) Antihypertensives

      c) Anticonvulsants

   d) Adrenergic blockers

   e) Estrogen

   f) Sulfonamides

   g) Taxanes

   h) Growth factors/colony-stimulating factors

  11. Malignancy

  12. Infections

   a) Childhood illness: Mumps, rubella, chickenpox

   b) Mononucleosis

   c) Hepatitis (see Chapter 69)

   d) Rocky Mountain spotted fever

   e) Enterovirus

   f) Lyme disease

 B. Monoarthritis

  1. Infection: Consider monoarthritis infection until proven otherwise.

   a) Septic arthritis: Usually related to disseminated gonorrhea or gram-positive bacteria

   b) Gram-negative infections: Immunosuppressed patients and patients who are IV drug users

   c) Tuberculous arthritis

  2. Trauma

  3. Osteonecrosis (secondary to trauma, sickle cell disease, or radiation therapy)

 C. Monoarthritis or polyarthritis

  1. Gout (see Chapter 105)

  2. Inflammatory bowel disease (e.g., ulcerative colitis, Crohn's disease)

  3. Psoriatic arthritis

  4. Behcet's disease

  5. Reiter's syndrome

  6. Hemarthrosis: Usually caused by a bleeding abnormality

  7. Osteoarthropathy: Paraneoplastic syndrome in non-small cell lung cancer (see Appendix 12)

  8. Osteoarthritis (see Chapter 106)

  9. HIV (see Chapter 156)

VI. Treatment

 A. Treatment is based on the known cause of the joint pain.

 B. Symptomatic treatment

  1. Rest the involved joint.

  2. Apply warm or cold therapy for 15 minutes, four times a day.

  3. Analgesia

   a) NSAIDs (see Appendix 11)

   b) Aspirin, except in suspected cases of gout

VII. Follow-up: Based on known cause of the joint pain

VIII.   Referrals: Based on known cause of the joint pain

References

Hench, P.K., & Willkens, R.F.   (1994).   Choosing the right NSAID for joint pain. *Patient Care, 28*(20), 76–90.

Jain, R., & Lipsky, P.E. (1997). Treatment of rheumatoid arthritis. *Medical Clinics of North America, 81*(1), 57–84.

Pisetsky, D.S. (1996). Beating joint pain: New strategies are very effective. *Health Confidentional, 10*(3), 11–13.

Schnitzer, T.J. (1998). Non-NSAID pharmacologic treatment options for the management of chronic pain. *American Journal of Medicine, 105*(1B), 45S–52S.

Willkens, R.F. (1993). Arthralgias: A quick guide to causes other than arthritis. *Consultant, 33*(2), 59–61.

101. Muscle Cramps
Kimberly A. Rumsey, RN, MSN, CS

I. Definition: Prolonged involuntary muscle contractions
  A. Contractures: Involuntary muscle contractions that occur during exertion
  B. Tetany: State of motor and sensory hyperactivity with muscle spasm and paresthesia

II. Pathophysiology
  A. Originates in the distal portion of the motor nerves
  B. Unknown whether nerves become hyperexcitable or are prone to repetitive activity

III. Clinical features: Painful and difficult to manage, but rarely reflect a serious underlying disease
  A. Etiology
    1. Neurologic disease
    2. Metabolic cause
    3. Other: Dehydration, familial disposition, idiopathic
  B. History
    1. History of cancer and cancer treatment
    2. Current medications: Prescribed and over-the-counter
    3. History of presenting symptom(s): Precipitating factors, onset, location, and duration (e.g., nocturnal pain). Associated symptoms are cold or heat intolerance, profuse sweating, and diarrhea.
    4. Changes in activities of daily living
    5. Past medical history: Leptomeningeal disease, renal disease, thyroid disease
  C. Signs and symptoms
    1. Acute onset of severe muscle pain: Most commonly occurs in the gastrocnemius muscle
    2. Pain with residual tenderness
    3. Twitching at the start and end of the cramp
    4. Occurs after trivial movement or at rest
    5. Alleviated by passive stretching of the muscle
  D. Physical exam
    1. Vital signs: Assess for decreased blood pressure or increased pulse.
    2. Musculoskeletal exam

a) Assess muscle for spasm, tightness, erythema, warmth, or tenderness.

b) Muscle may be easily palpable or visibly hardened.

  3. Neurologic exam

a) Complete neurologic exam to rule out neurologic causes.

b) Deep tendon reflexes may be absent or abnormal.

c) Trousseau's sign may indicate tetany (see Appendix 13).

IV. Diagnostic tests

  A. Laboratory

    1. Glucose to rule out hypoglycemia

    2. Sodium to rule out hyponatremia

    3. BUN and creatinine increased, indicating dehydration

    4. Magnesium to rule out hypomagnesemia

    5. Calcium to rule out hypocalcemia

    6. TSH level to rule out hypothyroidism

  B. Radiology: Typically not helpful in diagnosing

  C. Other: Nerve conduction study recording may show a high-frequency, high-amplitude discharge of potentials that resemble motor unit potentials; frequently preceded or accompanied by fasciculations in the same muscle.

V. Differential diagnosis

  A. Neurologic

    1. Peripheral neuropathy (see Chapter 131)

a) Chemotherapy-induced

b) Vitamin deficiency (B_{12}, B_1) (see Chapter 114)

c) Diabetes mellitus (see Chapter 143)

d) Hypothyroidism (see Chapter 150)

e) Paraneoplastic syndromes (see Appendix 12)

f) Uremia

    2. Nerve root or plexus pathology

a) Leptomeningeal disease

b) Compression or infiltration by tumor (see Chapter 138)

c) Radiation-induced

d) Surgically induced

e) Guillain Barre syndrome

    3. Anterior horn disorders

a) Radiation-induced

b) Amyotrophic lateral sclerosis

  B. Metabolic

    1. Electrolyte imbalance (e.g., sodium, potassium, magnesium, calcium) (see Chapters 144–148)

    2. Dehydration (see Chapter 147)

    3. Hemodialysis-induced

  C. Drug-induced

    1. Hormone therapy

    2. Chemotherapy
    3. Diuretics
    4. Amphotericin B
    5. Cimetidine
    6. Lithium
    7. Clofibrate
  D. Common nocturnal cramps

VI. Treatment
  A. Treat the underlying cause.
  B. Cancer treatment protocol may require alteration.
  C. Teach the patient to stretch the cramped muscle.
  D. Massage the involved muscle.
  E. Apply ice locally.
  F. Pharmacologic relief of cramps
    1. Quinine sulfate: 200–300 mg orally every night
    2. Phenytoin: 300–400 mg po every day and carbamazepine, 200 mg bid or qid, also have been used to alleviate muscle cramps.

VII. Follow-up
  A. Depends on the cause of the muscle cramp
  B. Frequent (every one to two months) monitoring of pharmacologic therapy and side effects (e.g., liver function tests)

VIII. Referrals: Depend on cause of muscle cramps

References

Haskell, S.G., & Fiebach, N.H. (1997). Clinical epidemiology of nocturnal leg cramps in male veterans. *American Journal of Medical Science, 313*(4), 210–214.

Levin, S. (1993). Investigating the cause of muscle cramps. *The Physician and Sportsmedicine, 21*(7), 111–113.

Man-Son-Hing, M., Wells, G., & Lau, A. (1998). Quinine for nocturnal leg cramps: A meta-analysis including unpublished data. *Journal of General Internal Medicine, 13,* 600–606.

McGee, S.R. (1990). Muscle cramps. *Archives of Internal Medicine, 150,* 511–518.

Siegal, T. (1991). Muscle cramps in the cancer patient: Causes and treatment. *Journal of Pain and Symptom Management, 6*(2), 84–91.

Schwade, S. (1996). Training. 20 crick fixes . . . muscle cramps. *Men's Health, 11*(2), 128–130.

102. Myalgia

Kimberly A. Rumsey, RN, MSN, CS

I. Definition: Generalized muscle aches

II. Pathophysiology: Damaged tissue releases bradykinin in response to trauma, which stimulates the muscle nociceptors.

III. Clinical features: Frequently associated with fever
   A. Etiology
      1. Fibromyalgia
      2. Chemotherapy-induced
         a) Taxanes
         b) Bleomycin
         c) Dacarbazine
      3. Biotherapy-induced (flu-like syndrome)
         a) Interferons
         b) Growth factors
         c) Interleukins
         d) Tumor necrosis factor
      4. Steroid withdrawal
      5. Fatty acid deficiency
   B. History
      1. History of cancer and cancer treatment
      2. Current medications: Prescribed and over-the-counter
      3. History of presenting symptom(s): Precipitating factors, onset, location, and duration. Associated symptoms are fever, shaking chills, fatigue, nonrestorative sleep, and headache.
      4. Changes in activities of daily living
      5. Past medical history: Irritable bowel syndrome, paresthesias, restless leg syndrome, cold sensitivity
   C. Signs and symptoms
      1. Generalized or localized muscle aches
      2. Edema
      3. Induration

    4. Fever

    5. Warm and flushed skin

    6. Tachycardia

    7. Shortness of breath

    8. Headache

    9. Thirst

D. Physical exam

    1. Vital signs: Assess for increased temperature, tacycardia, or tachypnea

    2. Musculoskeletal exam

      a) Assess muscle for edema, spasm, erythema, warmth, tenderness, and strength.

      b) Determine if myalgia is localized or generalized.

IV. Diagnostic tests

A. Laboratory

    1. CBC with differential: To evaluate for neutropenia and infectious causes

    2. Biochemical profile: Include

      a) Potassium to rule out hypo/hyperkalemia

      b) Magnesium to rule out hypomagnesemia

      c) Calcium to rule out hypocalcemia

      d) Sodium to rule out hypo/hypernatremia

      e) Phosphorus to rule out hypophosphatemia

      f) Creatine kinase (CK) level to evaluate for muscle inflammation or damage

    3. Urinalysis showing dipstick blood but no RBCs on microscopic examination—indicates rhabdomyolysis

    4. TSH level to rule out hypothyroidism

    5. Blood cultures if neutropenia suspected

B. Radiology: Not indicated

C. Other

    1. Electromyography: To differentiate myopathy from neuropathy

    2. Muscle biopsy: To differentiate specific myopathies

V. Differential diagnosis

A. Localized myalgia

    1. Neoplasm or metastasis

    2. Hematoma

    3. Ruptured tendon

    4. Thrombophlebitis (see Chapters 41 and 157)

    5. Pyomyositis

    6. Fasciitis

    7. Sarcoidosis

    8. Ischemia or infarct (i.e., diabetic muscular infarct)

    9. Acute alcoholic myopathy

   10. Exertional muscle damage

B. Generalized myalgia

    1. Primary fibromyalgia

    2. Inflammation (e.g., polymyositis, dermatomyositis)

    3. Neutropenic fever (see Chapters 121 and 140)

    4. Infection: Toxoplasmosis, trichinosis, influenza, herpes (see Chapter 20), gram-negative infection, toxic shock, Kawasaki's syndrome

    5. Electrolyte imbalance: Hypophosphatemia, hypo/hyperkalemia, hypomagnesemia, hypo/hypernatraemia, hypocalcemia (see Chapters 144-148)

    6. Hypothyroid (see Chapter 150)

    7. Drug-induced (e.g., steriod withdrawal)

    8. Amyloidosis

    9. Osteomalacia

    10. Guillain-Barré syndrome

    11. Polymyalgia rheumatica

    12. Fabry's disease

    13. Parkinson's disease

VI. Treatment

  A. Treat the underlying cause.

  B. Symptomatic treatment may include

    1. Massage of the involved muscle

    2. Local application of ice or heat

    3. Pharmacologic relief: NSAIDs (see Appendix 11).

VII. Follow-up: Depends on the cause of the myalgia

VIII. Referrals: Depend on the etiology of myalgia

References

Barsky, A.J., & Borus, J.F. (1999). Functional somatic syndromes. *Annals of Internal Medicine, 130,* 910–921.

Haeuber, D. (1995). The flu-like syndrome. In P.T. Rieger (Ed.), *Biotherapy: A comprehensive overview* (pp. 243–258). Boston: Jones & Bartlett.

Lamberg, L. (1999). Patients in pain need round-the-clock care. *JAMA, 281,* 689–690.

Simon, H.B. (1995). Evaluation of fever. In A.H. Goroll, L.A. May, & A.G. Mulley (Eds.), *Primary care medicine: Office evaluation and management of the adult patient* (3rd ed.) (pp. 48–53). Philadelphia: Lippincott.

Smith, A.J. (1998). The analgesic effects of selective serotonin reuptake inhibitors. *Journal of Psychopharmacology, 12,* 407–413.

Thompson, J.M. (1996). The diagnosis and treatment of muscle pain syndromes. In R.L. Braddom (Ed.), *Physical medicine and rehabilitation* (pp. 893–914). Philadelphia: Saunders.

103. Bone Metastasis

Roberta A. Strohl, RN, BSN, MN, AOCN®

I. Definition: Spread of primary cancer to the bone

II. Pathophysiology
   A. Hematogenous spread is primary route.
      1. Intravascular dissemination through normal venous system
      2. Batson's plexus
         a) Low-pressure valveless system throughout thoracolumbar spine and pelvis.
         b) Transmits multiple venous communications from the pelvis to the brain.
         c) Increased pressure allows metastatic disease to travel to specific skeletal sites without entering the vena cava.
   B. Tumor cells enter the red marrow.
      1. Malignant cells attach to the endothelial surface where the cells invade bony structures. Osteoclasts normally mediate bone resorption, which also is key to the growth of bone metastasis.
      2. Malignant cells grow to include cortical bone.
         a) Malignant cells secrete many factors that can stimulate the proliferation and activity of osteoclasts and produce osteolysis.
         b) Cancer cells can activate osteoclasts directly by the tumor cells or indirectly by tumor-stimulated immune cells.
            (1) Transforming growth factors
            (2) Prostaglandins
            (3) Tumor necrosis factor
            (4) Parathyroid hormone-related protein
            (5) Cytokines (e.g., interleukins)
   C. Certain cancers are known to stimulate osteoclast activity.
      1. Breast cancer secretes a parathyroid hormone-related peptide (PTHrP).
      2. Lymphomas produce interleukin-6 and PTHrP.
      3. Prostate cancer stimulates osteoblasts by secreting transforming growth factors beta- and protease-urokinase.

III. Clinical features
   A. Etiology: Metastatic tumors are the most common neoplasm in bone.

1. Three most common cancers to develop bone metastases are breast, prostate, and lung.
   a) Skeletal metastases develop in 50% of these patients
   b) Bone metastases also occur in thyroid and renal cell cancers.
2. Rib cage, spine, pelvis, limbs, and skull are common sites of bone metastases.
3. Bone metastases usually are confined in the bone and do not cross joint spaces. Complications include
   a) Pathological fractures: Greatest risk in weight-bearing bones
   b) Progressive immobility and crippling
   c) Pain.
4. Upper cervical spine metastases (C1 to C4) can damage the spinal cord.
5. Neurologic function can be compromised from extraosseous extension.
6. Refractory pancytopenia results from invasion into the bone marrow.

B. History
1. History of cancer and cancer treatment
2. Current medications: Prescribed and over-the-counter
3. History of presenting symptom(s): Precipitating factors, onset, location, and duration
4. Changes in activities of daily living

C. Signs and symptoms
1. Pain is the presenting sign of bone metastases and is described as
   a) Dull, boring
   b) Intermittent, then continuous.
2. Pain progresses during the day which distinguishes pain from arthritis or degenerative diseases.
3. Sudden increase in pain may indicate pathologic fracture.
4. Nausea, vomiting, constipation, fatigue, and change in mentation may indicate hypercalcemia.
5. Paresthesia indicates spinal cord compression with progression to sensory and motor loss of function, such as interruption of urinary/bowel function.

D. Physical exam
1. Musculoskeletal exam to identify all sites of disease
   a) Patient may report only the site of most severe pain.
   b) Assess for percussion tenderness over areas of disease.
2. Neurologic exam: Assess for sensory and motor changes indicating spinal cord compression (see Chapter 138).
   a) Decreased or absent deep tendon reflexes
   b) Decreased muscle strength
   c) Diminished pain and temperature sensation

IV. Diagnostic tests
A. Laboratory
1. Calcium to assess for hypercalcemia
2. Alkaline phosphatase may be elevated in bone metastases. Elevations reflect an osteoblastic (i.e., healing) response to tumor destruction.
B. Radiology

    1. Plain films: To rule out fracture

    2. Bone scan

       a) Small lesions may not be detected.

       b) Early metastatic disease without bone destruction may not elicit positive scan.

       c) Arthritis, trauma, and infection also can produce positive scan.

    3. CT/MRI

       a) To evaluate cortex and cortical integrity

       b) To identify bone lesions and soft-tissue masses, if present

       c) To detect spinal cord compression

V. Differential diagnosis

    A. Osteoarthritis (see Chapter 106)

    B. Compression fracture (see Chapter 104)

    C. Trauma

    D. Osteomalacia

    E. Paget's disease

    F. Spinal cord compression (see Chapter 138)

VI. Treatment

    A. Surgery: Performed based on prognosis and ability to tolerate procedure

       1. Surgical stabilization of impending pathologic fracture

         a) Goal is to pin the bone before fracture occurs.

         b) Follow with radiation.

       2. Surgical stabilization postfracture: In weight-bearing bone, fracture may be pinned.

       3. Surgical decompression laminectomy for spinal cord compression

    B. Radiation therapy

       1. External beam therapy

         a) Palliation of pain

         b) Usual protocol is 300 cGy fractions for 10 treatments.

         c) Single, larger fractions may be used depending on site of lesion.

         d) Larger volume may be treated (e.g., half-body therapy for extensive metastatic disease).

       2. Strontium 89/Samarium SM 153

         a) Analog of calcium that concentrates in osteoblastic bone lesions

         b) Used primarily to treat metastatic prostate cancer; has been used in metastatic disease from a variety of primary tumors

         c) Dose is 40 mCi/kg; mean dose 3 mCi; radiation dose is 20–40 Gy to metastatic sites.

         d) Major toxicity is hematologic (WBC and platelet nadir 2–12 weeks); mean percentage reduction 32% for WBC; 14% for Hgb; 40% for platelets

         e) External beam therapy can be given to residual sites of pain.

    C. Analgesics for pain management

       1. Narcotics (see Appendix 8)

       2. NSAIDs (see Appendix 11)

    D. Treatment of primary disease and sequelae

1. Therapy of primary tumor
   a) Radiation
   b) Chemotherapy
   c) Surgery
2. Management of hypercalcemia (see Chapter 144)

E. Pamedronate (Aredia®, Novartis Pharmaceutical Corp., East Hanover, NJ) 90 mg IV every four weeks for osteolytic bone lesions.

VII. Follow-up
   A. Evaluate response to therapy and development of further bone metastases (e.g., tumor markers).
   B. Follow pain as a measure of response and ensure adequate pain control.

VIII. Referrals
   A. Physical therapist: To assist in weight-bearing post fixation
   B. Surgeon (e.g., orthopedic or neurosurgery): For consideration for surgical procedure
   C. Radiation oncologist: For treatment of metastasis

References

Buckwalter, J., & Brandser, E. (1997). Metastatic disease of the skeleton. *American Family Physician, 55,* 1761–1768.

Fisher, G., Mayer, D., & Struthers, C. (1997). Bone metastases. Part 1: Pathophysiology. *Clinical Journal of Oncology Nursing, 1,* 29–35.

Krasnow, A., Hellman, R., Timins, M., Collier, D., Anderson, T., & Isitman, A. (1997). Diagnostic bone scanning in oncology. *Seminars in Nuclear Medicine, XXVII*(2, April), 107–141.

Lee, C., Aeppli, D., Unger, J., Boudreau, R., & Levitt, S. (1996). Strontium-89 chloride for palliative treatment of bony metastases: The University of Minnesota experience. *American Journal of Clinical Oncology, 19*(2), 102–107.

Mayer, D., Struthers, C., & Fisher, G. (1997). Bone metastases: Part II: Nursing management. *Clinical Journal of Oncology Nursing, 1,* 37–44.

McEwan, A. (1997). Unsealed source therapy of painful bone metastases: An update. *Seminars in Nuclear Medicine, 27*(2), 165–182.

104. Fractures

Kimberly A. Rumsey, RN, MSN, CS

I. Definition: A break in the continuity of a bone, classified as
   A. Closed or simple fracture: Bone is not exposed.
   B. Open or compound fracture: Bone is exposed.

II. Pathophysiology: Occurs when the bone is subjected to increased stress or decreased bone density

III. Clinical features
   A. Etiologies
      1. Trauma (e.g., direct blow, crushing force, sudden twisting motion)
      2. Severe muscle contraction
      3. Osteoporosis
      4. Bone metastasis (e.g., breast, prostate, thyroid, lung, renal cell cancers, Hodgkin's lymphoma)
      5. Multiple myeloma
   B. Types of fractures
      1. Greenstick: Break occurs on one side of the bone, and the other side is bent.
      2. Transverse: Break occurs straight through the bone.
      3. Oblique: Break occurs at an angle through the bone.
      4. Spiral: Break twists around the shaft of the bone.
      5. Comminuted: Break causes the bone to splinter into several fragments.
      6. Depressed: Break drives the bone fragments inward; frequently seen in skull and facial fractures.
      7. Compression: Break causes the bone to become compressed (e.g., vertebral fracture).
      8. Pathologic: Break is caused by an area of diseased bone (e.g., osteoporosis, bone metastasis, tumor).
      9. Avulsion: Ligament or tendon pulls away a fragment of bone.
      10. Epiphyseal: Break occurs through the epiphysis of the bone.
      11. Stress fracture
   C. History
      1. History of cancer and cancer treatment

    2. Current medications: Prescribed and over-the-counter

    3. History of presenting symptom(s): Precipitating factors, onset, location, and duration

    4. Changes of activities of daily living

  D. Signs and symptoms

    1. Acute onset of severe, continuous pain; may be associated with muscle spasm

    2. Localized edema

    3. Local discoloration

    4. Inability to bear weight on affected area, decreased mobility

  E. Physical exam

    1. Vital signs: Assess for signs of shock caused by blood loss (especially if caused by trauma) (i.e., hypotension)

    2. Cardiac exam: Palpate distal pulses, and assess for adequate tissue perfusion.

    3. Musculoskeletal exam

      a) Palpate area for deformity, crepitus (i.e., caused by bone fragments), and edema.

      b) Assess range of motion of extremity.

IV. Diagnostic tests

  A. Laboratory

    1. Usually not necessary

    2. CBC, including platelets if blood loss occurred

    3. If surgery indicated, CBC, clotting times, electrolytes as protocol indicates

  B. Radiology

    1. X-ray of affected area: To assess type of fracture

    2. Bone scan: If metastasis is suspected

V. Differential diagnosis

  A. Osteoporosis (see Chapter 107)

  B. Paget's disease

  C. Malignancy-related

    1. Bone metastasis (see Chapter 103)

    2. Multiple myeloma

    3. Osteosarcoma

  D. Trauma

  E. Osteomalacia

VI. Treatment

  A. Based on the underlying cause and type of fracture

  B. Some fractures do not require treatment (e.g., vertebral fractures without cord impingement or loss of function).

  C. Conservative measures

    1. Bed rest

    2. Analgesics

    3. Ambulation and daily exercise: Necessary when acute pain subsides

  D. Fracture reduction and immobilization: Approximately six to eight weeks for bone to heal

1. Open reduction (i.e., surgical fixation): Fracture parts are openly reduced and held in place by internally placed rods, plates, screws, and/or wires.
2. Closed reduction: Manipulation and manual traction are used to bring the bone fragments into apposition (i.e., ends in contact). Cast, splint, or other device is used to maintain the position.
3. Traction: A pulling force is applied to achieve fracture reduction and immobilization.

   E. Patient education: Avoid lifting and vigorous physical activity.

VII. Follow-up: Depends on the cause and type of fracture and treatment used

VIII. Referrals
   A. Orthopedist: Consult to assist in diagnosing and treating the fracture.
   B. Orthopedic surgeon: Referral may be indicated.
   C. Medical and radiation oncologist: Refer for cancer-related causes and treatment.

References

Carlson, D.C. (1988). Common fractures of the extremities: How to recognize and treat them. *Postgraduate Medicine, 83,* 311–317.

Fisher, G., Mayer, D.K., & Struthers, C. (1997). Bone metastases: Part I—Pathophysiology. *Clinical Journal of Oncology Nursing, 1,* 29–35.

Herron, D.G., & Nance, J. (1990). Emergency department nursing management of patients with orthopedic fractures resulting from motor vehicle accidents. *Nursing Clinics of North America, 25*(1), 71–83.

Kushwaha, V.P., & Garland, D.G. (1998). Extremity fractures in the patient with a traumatic brain injury. *Journal of the American Academy of Orthopedic Surgery, 6*(5), 298–307.

Lips, P. (1997). Epidemiology and predictors of fractures associated with osteoporosis. *American Journal of Medicine, 103*(2A), 3S–11S.

Mayer, D.K., Struthers, C., & Fisher, G. (1997). Bone metastases: Part II—Nursing management. *Clinical Journal of Oncology Nursing, 1,* 37–44.

McClung, B.L. (1999). Using osteoporosis management to reduce fractures in elderly women. *Nurse Practitioner, 24*(3), 26–27, 32, 35–38.

Wolinsky, P.R. (1997). Assessment and management of pelvic fracture in the hemodynamically unstable patient. *Orthopedic Clinics of North America, 28,* 321–329.

Chapter

105.

Gout

Kimberly A. Rumsey, RN, MSN, CS

I. Definition: A metabolic disorder caused by accumulation of uric acid deposits within the joint, resulting in acute inflammation of the joint

II. Pathophysiology
   A. Gout is the result of hyperuricemia, an increased level of uric acid in the blood and tissues. Uric acid is the end product of purine (adenine and guanine) catabolism and may not be excreted adequately by the kidneys.
   B. May be primary or secondary
      1. Primary hyperuricemia is caused by a congenital error in the production or excretion of uric acid.
      2. Secondary hyperuricemia may be caused by an increased rate of purine biosynthesis or reduced uric acid excretion related to an acquired disease
      3. Deposits of monosodium urate crystals develop in synovial lining cells and possibly cartilage.
      4. Polymorphonuclear cells (PMNs) initiate the inflammatory response when they ingest the urate crystals.
      5. Chronic gout leads to erosion of the cartilage, resulting in arthritis or deformed joints.

III. Clinical features: The joint develops inflammatory symptoms.
   A. Risk factors
      1. Male gender
      2. Middle-aged (i.e., > 40 years), postmenopausal women
      3. Alcohol abuse
      4. Obesity
      5. Family history (i.e., inherited predisposition)
      6. Drugs: Diuretics, salicylates, cyclosporine, chemotherapy agents
      7. Excessive consumption of purine-rich foods (e.g., liver, shellfish, beer)
      8. Other: Renal insufficiency, hypertension, hematologic malignancy, hemolytic anemia, cirrhosis
   B. History
      1. History of cancer and cancer treatment

2. Current medications: Prescribed and over-the-counter
3. History of presenting symptom(s): Precipitating factors, onset, location, and duration
4. Changes in activities of daily living
5. Social history of alcohol abuse, diet recall

C. Signs and symptoms
1. Acute onset of pain, usually in one joint (frequently affects the first metatarsophalangeal joint called podagra).
    a) More than 80% involve lower-extremity joints.
    b) Can occur in any joint
2. Typically, pain develops rapidly over 24–48 hours.
3. Involved joint is edematous, erythematous, warm, and tender.
4. Temperature may be elevated.
5. Chronic gout presents with tophi (i.e., white lesions beneath the skin), typically found in ears, hands, and feet.
6. Movements are restricted because of severe pain, but the joints are normal between attacks.

D. Physical exam
1. Vital signs: Assess for temperature elevation to 39°C.
2. Integument exam: Assess for tophi.
3. Musculoskeletal exam: Assess joint for edema, erythema, warmth, tenderness, and limited range of motion.

IV. Diagnostic tests
A. Laboratory
1. WBC count and erythrocyte sedimentation rate may be elevated.
2. Serum uric acid levels usually are elevated.
    a) Levels > 7.0 support the diagnosis of gout but alone are insufficient to make the diagnosis; levels are normal in 20% of patients during acute attack.
    b) May also be used to assess the risk for uric acid renal stones and the need for aggressive therapy to prevent nephrolithiasis.
3. Consider a 24-hour urine collection to measure uric acid excretion.

B. Radiology
1. X-rays of the affected area may be used to rule out other diagnoses.
2. X-rays are diagnostic only in advanced cases when the affected joint begins to punch-out areas in the bone.

C. Other: Synovial fluid aspirate for smear and culture to exclude infection

V. Differential diagnosis
A. Pseudogout: Presents with similar symptoms, but serum uric acid is normal.
B. Cellulitis (see Chapter 16)
C. Septic arthritis
D. Rheumatoid arthritis (see Chapter 108)
E. Bursitis related to a bunion
F. Chronic lead intoxication

G. Tumor lysis syndrome

VI. Treatment
  A. Acute phase
    1. Joint immobilization and decreased weight bearing
    2. Analgesics
      a) NSAIDs (see Appendix 11)
        (1) Drug of choice, but consider side effects before prescribing; risk of side effects is greatest in patients with renal or hepatic dysfunction.
        (2) Effective in reducing pain and inflammation
        (3) Most effective if initiated soon after the onset of the acute attack
        (4) Any NSAID will work, but the most commonly prescribed for gout are
          (a) Indomethacin: 50–75 mg po every eight hours for six to eight doses, then 25 mg po every eight hours until attack resolves.
          (b) Naproxen: 750 mg po initially, then 250 mg po every eight hours.
        (5) Taper medications over 24–48 hours after symptoms resolve.
      b) Colchicine
        (1) Optional choice in patients unable to take NSAIDs; most effective if given within 48 hours of onset
        (2) Inhibits crystal phagocytosis but has no effect on uric acid metabolism
        (3) Increased toxicity in patients with renal or hepatic dysfunction
        (4) Side effects include diarrhea, abdominal cramping, nausea, and vomiting.
        (5) Several dosing regimens available
          (a) Most commonly, 0.5–0.6 mg po every hour until the pain is relieved, side effects occur, or maximum dosage of 6 mg is reached. Diarrhea commonly occurs with this regimen.
          (b) IV dose 1–2 mg in 20 ml of NS, infused slowly over 20 minutes (rarely used). Should only be given by a physician with experience in this delivery route.
      c) Corticosteroids
        (1) Intra-articular injection of a corticosteroid is very effective in treating patients with monoarticular gout.
        (2) Systemic corticosteroid therapy can be used for patients with polyarticular gout or for whom NSAIDs or colchicine are contraindicated (i.e., increased creatinine).
          (a) Prednisone: 30 mg po bid; taper quickly over five to seven days.
          (b) Triamcinolone acetonide: 60 mg IM
          (c) Adrenocorticotropic hormone (ACTH): 20–80 units IM or IV; may repeat in 48–72 hours
        (3) The potential for rebound inflammation exists.
  B. Chronic phase
    1. Patients with three or more attacks per year or who are difficult to treat with the aforementioned therapies because of allergies or side effects are considered to be chronic.

2. Low doses of NSAIDs (e.g., naproxen 250 mg po bid or colchicine 0.5–1.0 mg po qd) may be continued.
3. The goal is to decrease serum uric acid concentration.
4. Do not initiate urate-lowering agents until four weeks after the onset of the acute attack and the patient has been on colchicine for four to six weeks. Continue colchicine until six to nine months after uric acid level is reduced.
5. Allopurinol
   a) Decreases synthesis of uric acid by inhibiting xanthine oxidase (i.e., enzyme required for uric acid synthesis)
   b) Initial dose is 100 mg po qd for one month, then increase based on uric acid level assessments.
   c) Typical dose is 300 mg po qd for patients with mild gout. May need 400–600 mg qd for moderate to severe gout but also may take less than 300 mg. Titrate dose to renal function and serum uric acid goal.
   d) Side effects: GI upset, headache, rash, marrow suppression, fever, liver and/or kidney failure, alopecia, lymphadenopathy
   e) Monitor treatment with urate-lowering drugs. May be discontinued when serum urate concentrations are < 6.0 mg/dl. However, intermittent therapy or withdrawal of drugs that decrease serum urate concentration leads to a recurrence of acute gout and tophi. Some clinicians believe that urate-lowering therapy should be lifelong.
6. Probenecid
   a) Increases uric acid excretion if creatinine clearance > 60 ml/minute
   b) 0.5 g/day po initially with gradual increases to 1–2 g/day
   c) Avoid use with salicylates (reverses action of probenicid).
   d) Side effects: GI upset, skin rash, nephrolithiasis
C. Asymptomatic hyperuricemia
   1. Identify risk factors, and make appropriate lifestyle changes.
   2. Consider pharmacologic therapy when
      a) Lifestyle changes do not change serum urate concentration to < 7.0 mg/dl.
      b) Patient has had two or four definite attacks of gout or has tophi.
   3. Medications as above
D. Patient education
   1. Dietary changes: Weight loss, reduction of alcohol intake
   2. Proper fluid intake: Increase to 2–3 l/day
   3. Symptoms of gout

VII. Follow-up
A. Patients with acute gout should return to clinic in 24 hours for assessment of pain relief, then again in four weeks to discuss prophylactic therapy.
B. Patients with chronic gout should have annual check of uric acid levels.

VIII. Referrals: Rheumatologist for aspiration of synovial fluid and/or intra-articular injection of a corticosteroid

References

Buckley, T.J. (1996). Radiologic features of gout. *American Family Physician, 54,* 1232–1238.

Emerson, B.T. (1996). The management of gout. *New England Journal of Medicine, 334,* 445–451.

George, T.M., & Mandell, B.F. (1996). Individualizing the treatment of gout. *Cleveland Clinic Journal of Medicine, 63*(3), 150–155.

Hasselbacher, P. (1996). Gout: The best understood form of arthritis? *Arthritis Care and Research, 9*(1), 74–77.

Jones, R.E., Ball, E.V., & Davis, J.S. (1999). Gout: Beyond the stereotype. *Hospital Practice, 34*(6), 95–102.

Pittman, J.R., & Bross, M.H. (1999). Diagnosis and management of gout. *American Family Physician, 59,* 1799–1806, 1810.

Simkin, P.A. (1999). Gout and hyperuricemia. *Current Opinions in Rheumatology, 9,* 268–273.

Chapter

106.

Osteoarthritis

Amy Crawford Minchin, RN, MNS, ANCC

I. Definition: A degenerative disease of the joints

II. Pathophysiology
   A. Hyaline articular cartilage, lining the bony ends of all synovial joints, is made of collagen II fibers, proteoglycans, chondrocytes, and water. Degeneration of the articular cartilage is the primary lesion in osteoarthritis (OA).
      1. OA leads to the depletion of the content of proteoglycans, which results in a decrease in water content and a loss of "shock absorption."
      2. The subchondral bone breaks down, resulting in hypertrophic repair. This results in sclerotic changes and the formation of osteophytes.
      3. Following tissue damage, cytokines (e.g., interleukin-1, enzymes) are released, which contribute to further destruction.
   B. The familial tendency to develop primary OA possibly is linked to a defect in a procollagen gene.

III. Clinical features: OA can be found in 80% of adults over age 65. It is not a systemic, inflammatory disease. A history of exercise without significant injury is not linked to the development of OA.
   A. Etiology
      1. Primary OA has no known cause.
      2. Secondary OA is a result of other disease mechanisms, including infection, injury, and metabolic disorders.
   B. History: The patient's history is helpful in diagnosing and differentiating between OA and other diseases affecting joints.
      1. History of cancer and cancer treatment
      2. Current medications: Prescribed and over-the-counter
      3. History of presenting symptom(s): Precipitating factors, onset, location, and duration. Associated symptoms are morning stiffness and warm, painful joints.
      4. Changes in activities of daily living
   C. Signs and symptoms
      1. Morning stiffness: May be present but is brief and limited to the affected joint
      2. No constitutional symptoms

    3. Pain: Generally present with movement and relieved by rest

    4. Rest not interrupted by pain unless cartilage degeneration is severe

    5. Joint involvement: Asymmetrical or symmetrical (e.g., hands in distal interphalangeal [DIP] and proximal interphalangeal [PIP] finger joints)

    6. Insidious onset of joint dysfunction

    7. In advanced disease: Pain on weight-bearing and joint instability

    8. Crepitus or discomfort on movement

    9. Decreased joint mobility

D. Physical exam: Musculoskeletal exam with attention to strength and range of motion

    1. No significant soft-tissue swelling or increased warmth should be present.

    2. Various joints may be involved.

        a) DIP and PIP joints (assess for Heberden's and Bouchard's nodes)

        b) First carpometacarpal joints (may have decreased grip)

        c) Hips (for internal rotation), knees, cervical and lumbar spine (for pain, paresthesia, and limited range of motion of spine)

        d) First metatarsophalangeal (for enlargement, decreased range of motion)

    3. Crepitus may be present.

    4. Bony enlargement and overgrowth from osteophyte formation

    5. Deformity of joints with malalignment

IV. Diagnostic tests

  A. Laboratory tests

    1. Erythrocyte sedimentation rate (ESR): Normal and helpful in excluding other diagnoses. ESR may be falsely elevated in the elderly.

    2. Baseline CBC, chemistry profile: Normal values are expected; must draw blood prior to starting medications, as some may cause changes in CBC and chemistry values because of toxicity.

  B. Radiology: Plain films of anterior-posterior and lateral views of joints reveal

    1. Joint-space narrowing

    2. Osteophytes (usually later in disease)

    3. Subchondral increase in bone density

    4. Subchondral cysts (in later stages of disease).

  C. Other: Joint aspiration is warranted if a joint is warm and erythematous and infection or gout is suspected. In OA, synovial fluid is noninflammatory. Check for crystals, infectious pathogens, and synovial fluid WBCs (200–2,000/mm^3).

V. Differential diagnosis

  A. Bursitis or tendonitis

  B. Gout (see Chapter 105)

  C. Trauma

  D. Sickle cell disease crisis (see Chapter 118)

  E. Psoriatic arthritis

  F. HIV-associated arthritis (see Chapter 156)

  G. Avascular necrosis

  H. Foreign body synovitis

  I. Osteoarthropathy (paraneoplastic syndrome) (see Appendix 12)

VI. Treatment
    A. Goals are pain control and maintenance of joint function.
    B. Weight reduction has been shown to reduce symptoms of OA; stress the importance of long-term weight loss to patients.
    C. Exercise program
    D. Medications
       1. Acetaminophen: Initial drug of choice; maximum dose (4 g daily) should be given for at least two weeks before changing medications.
       2. NSAIDs: Can be given in low doses in combination with acetaminophen; inhibition of prostaglandin synthesis is the primary mechanism of NSAIDs (see Appendix 11).
          a) Possible side effects: Gastric ulcers, GI bleeding, inhibited platelet aggregation, nephrotoxicity, confusion (in the elderly), hepatotoxicity
          b) With NSAIDs, consider misoprostol (Cytotec®, G.D. Searle & Co., Chicago, IL) 200 mcg po bid or qid or omeprazole 20–40 mg po qd to help to prevent peptic ulcers. Initial side effects from misoprostal include diarrhea, abdominal pain, and bloating (often resolve after using for a few weeks). Side effects can be lessened by starting at a lower dose of 100 mcg bid.
          c) When prescribing NSAIDs to the elderly, lower doses may be indicated because of reduced renal function or concomitant medications.
          d) Do not combine NSAIDs, as this raises toxicity without therapeutic benefit.
          e) Analgesics are most beneficial if taken before activities known to exacerbate pain.
       3. Systemic corticosteroids have no role in the treatment of OA.
       4. Use of narcotics, other than in limited doses for severe pain, is discouraged because of the chronicity of OA, as well as the potential for abuse and dependency.
       5. Intra-articular injections of corticosteroids are beneficial; recommended frequency is no more than once every three to four months.
       6. Intra-articular knee injections of hyaluronic acid may be beneficial; a series of three to five weekly injections (product-dependent) every six months is recommended.
    E. Topical therapies: Capsaicin, a derivative of chili peppers, is available as an over-the-counter ointment; trial of four weeks is needed to determine efficacy.
    F. Hot and cold therapy
       1. Cold packs: Help to reduce inflammation and swelling; instruct patient not to apply directly to skin.
       2. Heat therapy: Ideally as a hot bath or shower. Advise use of safety measures with heating pads or hot packs.
    G. Physical/occupational therapy
       1. Initial consultation upon diagnosis for counseling on body mechanics, devices to assist with activities of daily living, and range-of-motion exercises.
       2. Exercise to strengthen muscles supporting joints is an important element of joint protection.
    H. Surgery
       1. Arthroscopic debridement: Slows disease progression and reduces pain
       2. Joint arthroplasty (i.e., artificial joint replacement): Most artificial joints last 10–15 years. Joints most commonly replaced are hip and knee.

      3. Arthroscopic lavage using saline: Performed using local anesthesia in the office; currently used to alleviate pain and reduced function in knees
- I. Patient education: Provide material in writing whenever possible.
  1. Medication instructions, side effects, precautions
  2. Body mechanics
  3. Laboratory test and follow-up schedule

VII. Follow-up
- A. Obtain follow-up chemistry profile with liver function values one to two weeks after initiating treatment then every three to six months to detect any renal or hepatic toxicity.
- B. See patients as needed for joint dysfunction or worsening of pain.

VIII. Referrals
- A. Rheumatologist: Consultation is warranted at the time of diagnosis prior to beginning therapy and if the patient does not respond to treatment with NSAIDs or acetaminophen and exercise.
- B. Surgeon: Refer patients with persistent pain or disability for consideration of arthroscopy, joint replacement, or arthroscopic lavage.
- C. Physical/occupational therapist: Refer upon diagnosis to assess function, recommend assistive devices and exercises, and teach joint-preserving body mechanics.

References

Barth, W. (1997). Office evaluation of the patient with musculoskeletal complaints. *American Journal of Medicine, 102*(Suppl. 1A), 1A3S–1A9S.

Block, J., & Schnitzer, T. (1997). Therapeutic approaches to osteoarthritis. *Hospital Practice, 32*(2), 159–165.

Hochberg, M., Altman, R., Brandt, K., Clark, B., Dieppe, P., & Griffin, M. (1995). Guidelines for the medical management of osteoarthritis: Part I. Osteoarthritis of the hip. *Arthritis & Rheumatism, 38,* 1535–1539.

Hochberg, M., Attman, R., Brandt, K., Clark, B., Dieppe, P., & Griffin, M. (1995). Guidelines for the medical management of osteoarthritis: Part II. Osteoarthritis of the knee. *Arthritis & Rheumatism, 38,* 1541–1545.

Litman, K. (1996). A rational approach to the diagnosis of arthritis. *American Family Physician, 53,* 1295–1310.

Ross, C. (1997). A comparison of osteoarthritis and rheumatoid arthritis: Diagnosis and treatment. *Nurse Practitioner, 22*(9), 20–38.

Schumacher, R. (1995). Arthritis of recent onset. *Arthritis, 97*(4), 52–63.

Totemchokchyakarn, K., & Ball, G. (1996). Arthritis of systemic disease. *American Journal of Medicine, 101,* 642–647.

107. Osteoporosis

Kimberly A. Rumsey, RN, MSN, CS

I. Definition: A metabolic disorder characterized by decreased bone mass and mechanical support of the skeleton

II. Pathophysiology
   A. Osteoporosis results from an accelerated imbalance in the normal cycle of bone resorption and formation.
   B. Several different biochemical factors cause this imbalance, which results in decreased bone mass.
      1. Decreased plasma concentration of calcium causes an increase in parathyroid hormone secretion.
         a) Osteoclastic activity is increased, resulting in increased resorption of bone.
         b) Calcium and phosphate move from the bone to extracellular fluid.
      2. Vitamin D deficiency causes a decrease in the intestinal absorption of calcium and decreased plasma calcium concentration.
      3. An increase in calcitonin inhibits the osteoclastic activity, decreasing the rate of bone resorption, which results in decreased serum calcium and phosphate.

III. Clinical features: Decreased bone mass leads to an increased incidence of fractures, which most commonly occur in the sacral and lumbar vertebrae, hip, humerus, and wrist.
   A. Risk factors
      1. Inadequate calcium and/or vitamin D intake
      2. Excessive intake of coffee, alcohol, salt, and protein
      3. Age
      4. Menopause
      5. Small bone frame
      6. Inactivity (i.e., prolonged bed rest, lack of weight-bearing exercise)
      7. Family history
      8. Female gender
      9. Hyperthyroid state
      10. Medications: Steroids, anticonvulsants, thyroid replacement, barbiturates, heparin
   B. History
      1. History of cancer and cancer treatment

2. Current medications: Prescribed and over-the-counter (corticosteroids, anti-convulsants, thyroid medications, barbiturates, and heparin can increase risk of osteoporosis).
3. History of presenting symptom(s): Precipitating factors, onset, location, and duration. Associated symptoms are chronic back pain, loss of height, and exercise intolerance.
4. Changes in activities of daily living
5. Family history of osteoporosis
6. Social history: Tobacco, alcohol, caffeine, and calcium
7. Menstrual history (women)

C. Signs and symptoms
1. Loss of height (generally indicates vertebrae compression)
2. Backache
3. Spontaneous fracture

D. Physical exam: May be no physical findings, unless a fracture is present.
1. Vital signs: Measure height and compare to previous measurements.
2. Musculoskeletal exam
   a) Assess back for kyphosis or "dowager's hump."
   b) Assess for paravertebral muscle spasm, point tenderness, and tenderness upon deep palpation or percussion.
   c) Assess all muscle groups for strength.
3. Neurologic exam:
   a) Assess for gait disturbance and mobility.
   b) Assess for spinal cord compression.

IV. Diagnostic tests
A. Laboratory
1. Alkaline phosphatase may be elevated in the presence of a healing fracture.
2. Calcium, phosphate, vitamin D, and parathyroid hormone are within normal limits.

B. Radiology
1. Usually not necessary unless fracture is suspected. Obtain plain films.
   a) Able to detect bone loss in excess of 25%–40% (i.e., osteopenia)
   b) May show anterior wedging of thoracic vertebral bodies or widening of intervertebral bodies.
   c) Characteristic finding is the loss of horizontal vertebral trabeculae, which accentuates the end plates and results in biconcave "codfish" vertebrae.
2. If bone metastasis is suspected, a bone scan may be necessary.
3. Quantitative CT
   a) Can be used to differentiate between cortical and trabecular bone.
   b) Exposes the patient to higher levels of radiation than the dual-photon absorptiometry.

C. Other: Dual-energy absorptiometry (i.e., bone density test)
1. Provides a measure of bone mineral content in the lumbar spine and intertrochanteric regions of the hip and wrist

2. Expensive; only should be used as a screening tool in the general population if risk factors are present and/or therapy decisions depend on the results
3. Should be performed on symptomatic patients as a baseline prior to initiating pharmacologic therapy
4. Also may be used to evaluate the effects of pharmacologic therapy

V. Differential diagnosis
  A. Metastatic bone disease (see Chapter 103)
  B. Glucocorticoid excess
  C. Multiple myeloma
  D. Leukemia
  E. Hypercalcemia (see Chapter 147)
  F. Hyperthyroidism (see Chapter 149)
  G. Hyperparathyroidism
  H. Diabetes mellitus (see Chapter 143)
  I. Chronic renal failure
  J. Liver disease
  K. Rheumatoid arthritis (see Chapter 108)
  L. Cushing's syndrome
  M. Chronic heparin use
  N. Anorexia nervosa (see Chapter 62)
  O. Paget's disease

VI. Treatment
  A. Goals
    1. Increase bone mineral density.
    2. Decrease risk of osteoporotic fractures.
  B. Pharmacologic
    1. Hormone replacement therapy (HRT) (see Chapter 151)
      a) Currently, HRT is the most common treatment.
      b) Use is controversial in patients with gynecologic or breast cancer.
      c) Estrogen and progestin are used in women with an intact uterus to decrease the risk of endometrial cancer (several regimens are available).
      d) Estrogen alone is used in women without a uterus.
      e) Therapy must be initiated at the onset of menopause.
      f) Therapy should be continued indefinitely, as bone loss resumes upon discontinuation.
    2. Alendronate (Fosamax®, Merck & Co., Inc., West Point, PA): Dose is 10 mg po every morning; patient should take with eight ounces of water while sitting up for at least 30 minutes prior to consumption of another food or beverage.
    3. Salmon calcitonin
      a) 50–100 IU/day: Subcutaneous injection daily or every other day
      b) 200 IU intranasal daily: One puff in one nostril, alternating nostrils each day
    4. Pamidronate (Aredia® Novartis Pharmaceuticals, East Hanover, NJ): 90 mg IV every four weeks; although not indicated for treatment of osteoporosis, has been indicated to decrease bone-mass loss and fracture occurrence

    5. Etidronate (Didronel®, Procter & Gamble Pharmaceuticals, Inc., Mason, OH): 400 mg po qd for 14 days; repeat every three months with calcium and vitamin D held during the 14-day treatment.

    6. Tamoxifen (Nolvadex®, Astra Zeneca Pharmaceuticals, Inc., Wilmington, DE): 10 mg po bid or 20 mg po qd; although not indicated in treatment of osteoporosis, has been indicated to decrease bone-mass loss and fracture occurrence

    7. Raloxifene (Evista®, Eli Lilly and Co., Indianapolis, IN): 60 mg po daily; although not indicated in the treatment of osteoporosis, has been indicated to decrease bone-mass loss and fracture occurrence

C. Increase physical activity to include at least 30 minutes or more of moderate-intensity physical activity five days a week.

D. Supplements
    1. Calcium: 1,000–1,500 mg daily
    2. Vitamin D: 400–800 IU daily to achieve a 25-hydroxy vitamin D level of 35–55

E. Avoid lifting and other weight-bearing stresses.

VII. Follow-up
  A. Women who are prescribed HRT and salmon calcitonin should return in one to two months and have regular follow-up visits annually. Annual mammogram and pelvic exam with Pap smear is recommended.
  B. All patients should be followed at least every six months.

VIII. Referrals
  A. Endocrinologist or rheumatologist: Patient may require referral for initial diagnosis and initiation of therapy.
  B. Orthopedist or neurologist: Refer patients with vertebral fracture and signs of spinal cord compression.

References

Beauchesne, M.F., & Miller, P.F. (1999). Etidronate and alendronate in the treatment of postmenopausal osteoporosis. *Annuals of Phamacotherapy, 33,* 587–599.

Burki, R.E. (1999). Trends in osteoporosis management. *The Clinical Advisor,* 22–29.

Daly, P.A. (1995). Office management of osteoporosis: A guide for the primary care provider. *Comprehensive Therapy, 21,* 565–574.

Kanis, J. (1999). Strategies for osteoporosis treatment. *Bulletin of the World Health Organization, 77,* 431–432.

Kessenich, C.R. (1996). Update on pharmacologic therapies for osteoporosis. *Nurse Practitioner, 21*(8), 19–24.

Kessenich, C.R. (1996). The pathophysiology of osteoporotic vertebral fractures. *Rehabilitation Nursing, 22*(4), 192–195.

Lin, E.M., Aikin, J.L., & Good, B.C. (1999). Premature menopause after cancer treatment. *Cancer Practice, 7*(3), 114–121.

Mahon, S.M. (1998). Osteoporosis: A concern for cancer survivors. *Oncology Nursing Forum, 25,* 843–851.

Matkovic, V., Ilich, J.Z., Skugor, M.M., & Saracoglu, M. (1995). Primary prevention of osteoporosis. *Physical Medicine and Rehabilitation Clinics of North America, 6,* 595–627.

Recker, R.R., Davies, K.M., Dowd, R.M., & Heaney, R.P. (1999). The effect of low-dose continuous estrogen and progesterone therapy with calcium and vitamin D on bone in elderly women. A randomized controlled trial. *Annals of Internal Medicine, 130,* 897–904.

108. Rheumatoid Arthritis

Amy Crawford Minchin, RN, MSN, ANCC

I. Definition: A systemic autoimmune disease involving joints

II. Pathophysiology
   A. Rheumatoid arthritis (RA) is considered to be a T cell-mediated disease.
   B. The interaction of T cells with antigen-presenting cells initiates destructive changes. This leads to tissue destruction through the release of cytokines, particularly interleukin-1 (Il-1) and tumor necrosis factor (TNF).
   C. Il-1 and TNF act to stimulate the production of degradative enzymes by cells in the joints and promote further inflammatory cells into the joint.

III. Clinical features: RA frequently progresses and is characterized by constitutional symptoms as well as joint inflammation; a minority of cases develop abruptly. RA can cause pulmonary and cardiovascular destruction, reducing the life expectancy of women and men by three and seven years, respectively (see Figure 108-1).

Figure 108-1. 1987 American Rheumatology Association Criteria for Rheumatoid Arthritis Diagnosis

---

Symptoms
- Morning stiffness lasting longer than one hour for six weeks
- Swelling involving wrist, metacarpophalangeal joints, proximal intraphalangeal joints, ankle, or metatarsophalanages for six weeks or more
- Swelling of three or more joints for six weeks or more

Physical examination
- Rheumatoid nodules

Laboratory
- Elevated rheumatoid factor
- Increased erythrocyte sedimentation (sed) rate

Radiography
- Bony demineralization or erosions in joints of hands and wrists

---

Note. Based on information from Barth, 1997; Guidelines for the Management of Rheumatoid Arthritis, 1996.

A. Risk factors
   1. Age: Young or middle-aged
   2. Gender: Female
   3. History of autoimmune (e.g., type II collagen) disease
   4. Infection
B. Etiology: Although etiology remains undetermined, environmental factors and genetic predisposition are considered to be important factors.
C. History: Some diagnoses of RA are largely based on history alone.
   1. History of cancer and cancer treatment
   2. Current medications: Prescribed and over-the-counter
   3. History of presenting symptom(s): Precipitating factors, onset, location, and duration. Associated symptoms are painful joints, morning stiffness, fever, weight loss, and sleep disturbances.
   4. Changes in activities of daily living
D. Signs and symptoms: Begins insidiously but may be abrupt in some cases
   1. Musculoskeletal symptoms
      a) Symmetrical joint pain
      b) Morning stiffness lasting one hour or longer for six weeks
      c) Pain occurring with movement and rest
      d) Swelling involving wrist, metacarpophalangeal, proximal interphalangeal, ankle, or metatarsophalangeal joints
      e) Swelling of three or more joints for six or more weeks
      f) Muscle weakness
   2. Constitutional symptoms
      a) Rest is interrupted by pain.
      b) Acute onset RA may be preceded by a period of emotional distress.
      c) Depression
      d) Anorexia, weight loss
      e) Malaise
      f) Fatigue
      g) Low-grade fever
   3. Extra-articular manifestations
      a) Subcutaneous nodules
      b) Shortness of breath
E. Physical exam
   1. Vital signs and weight: Assess for low-grade fever and weight loss.
   2. Cardiac exam: Assess for extra or distant heart sounds or rub, indicating pericarditis or pericardial effusion.
   3. Pulmonary exam: Assess for decreased breath sounds and dullness, indicating pleural effusion or fibrosis.
   4. Musculoskeletal exam
      a) Rheumatoid nodules: Generally appear on extensor surfaces (e.g., fingers, elbows)
      b) Warm, boggy, swollen, tender joints
      c) Crepitus

      d) Decreased range of joint motion

      e) Observe for symmetric joint involvement, especially in peripheral joints.

   5. Extremities: Assess for cutaneous infarcts, indicating vasculitis. Numbness and tingling indicate neuropathy.

IV. Diagnostic tests

  A. Laboratory

    1. Rheumatoid factor: Elevated finding alone is not diagnostic of RA, as this value often is elevated in other inflammatory conditions.

      a) Approximately 20% of patients with RA have a negative rheumatoid factor.

      b) Presence of an elevated rheumatoid factor in a symptomatic patient predicts a more aggressive disease course.

    2. Antinuclear antibody titer: Positive with high titers in 30% of RA patients; draw if systemic lupus erythematosus is suspected.

    3. Baseline CBC: To assess for anemia and to confirm adequate bone marrow function

    4. Baseline chemistry and urinalysis: To assess hepatic and renal function

    5. Erythrocyte sedimentation rate (ESR): Typically elevated but not diagnostic of RA, nor does a normal ESR exclude RA

  B. Radiology: With RA on plain films, changes showing bony demineralization around or erosion in joints of the hands and feet generally are bony erosion, joint-space narrowing, soft-tissue swelling, and periarticular demineralization (i.e., osteopenia).

  C. Other: Joint aspiration, if a joint is warm and erythematous and infection or gout is suspected, aspiration is imperative to exclude infection.

    1. Check for crystals, infectious pathogens, and WBCs.

    2. If RA, synovial fluid WBC values will be elevated (2,000–50,000/mm^3).

V. Differential diagnosis

  A. Systemic lupus erythematosus

  B. Gout (see Chapter 105)

  C. Trauma (if monoarticular presentation)

  D. Sickle cell disease crisis (see Chapter 118)

  E. Psoriatic arthritis

  F. HIV-associated arthritis (see Chapter 156)

  G. Scleroderma

  H. Osteoarthropathy (see Appendix 12)

  I. Ankylosing spondylitis

  J. Reiter's syndrome (i.e., syndrome of unknown cause; consists of urethritis, conjunctivitis, subcutaneous lesions, and arthritis)

VI. Treatment: A significant portion of the erosive damage caused by RA often occurs during the first two years after onset; therefore, early treatment upon diagnosis is desirable. However, treatment of symptoms, with the exception of septic arthritis, should be avoided until other systemic conditions have been ruled out, which will prevent masking symptoms (e.g., fever) of other diseases.

A. Pharmacologic management of RA is categorized as first- and second-line agents.
   1. It is universally agreed upon that second-line agents should be instituted if relief is not achieved after a two- or three-month trial of NSAIDs (see Appendix 11).
   2. The most recent research supports early initiation of second-line agents to minimize joint damage.
   3. Second-line agents usually are administered with, rather than to replace, NSAIDs; full therapeutic effect can take weeks to months.
   4. With NSAIDs, consider misoprostol (Cytotec®, G.D. Searle & Co., Chicago, IL) 200 mcg po bid up to qid or omeprazole 20–40 mg po qd to help to prevent peptic ulcers. Initial side effects of misoprostol may include diarrhea, abdominal pain, and bloating (often resolve after using for a few weeks). Side effects can be lessened by starting at a lower dose of 100 mg bid.
B. Disease-modifying antirheumatic drugs (DMARDs) second-line agents: Consultation with a rheumatologist is recommended.
   1. Hydroxychloroquine (Plaquenil®, Sanofi Pharmaceuticals, Inc., New York, NY): 200 mg po bid; patients must have baseline ophthalmologic exam and serial eye exams every 6–12 months because of possible retinal toxicity.
   2. Sulfasalazine (Azulfidine®, Pharmacia & Upjohn, Peapack, NJ): 500 mg po bid up to 1.5 g bid; obtain CBC and liver function tests (LFTs) every three weeks for the first three months to monitor for bone marrow and hepatotoxicity, then extend to every six weeks.
   3. Oral gold (auranofin): 3 mg po bid up to tid; obtain CBC and urinalysis every month.
   4. Gold sodium injections (Solganal®, Schering Corp., Kenilworth, NJ): IM to a maximum dose of 1,000 mg; obtain a CBC and urinalysis before each injection.
   5. D-penicillamine: 125–150 mg po qd; escalated at monthly intervals by 250 mg qd to a target dose of 500–750 mg po qd.
   6. Methotrexate (Rheumatrex®, Lederle Laboratories, Pearl River, NY): 7.5–15 mg po weekly; obtain CBC, creatinine, and LFTs monthly to monitor for bone marrow suppression, hepatotoxicity, and nephrotoxicity. Instruct patients to avoid ethanol while on methotrexate.
   7. Prednisone: 5–10 mg po qd; temporary therapy until DMARDs become effective.
   8. Popular combinations of the above include methotrexate/hydrocholoroquine, gold/hydrochloroquine, and methotrexate/sulfasalazine.
   9. Narcotics are approved only if severe pain occurs while waiting for other medications' effectiveness to build; long-acting narcotics such as oxycodone are recommended (see Appendix 8).
C. Tumor necrosis factor (TNF) inhibitors: Indicated for patients with poor response to DMARD therapy. Synovial levels of TNF are five times the normal value (1–2 ng/ml) in patients with RA; TNF inhibitors provide a synthetic receptor for TNF, thus inhibiting excess production. Etanercept (Enbrel®, Wyeth-Ayerst Pharmaceuticals, Philadelphia, PA): 25 mg SC biweekly; instruct patient to rotate injection sites, immediately report any infections, and avoid pregnancy during therapy. Monitor CBC every other month. Medication must be refrigerated at all times.
D. Leflunomide (Arava®, Hoechst Marion Roussel, Kansas City, MO): Immunologic agent that inhibits enzymes involved in the synthesis of pyrimidine; loading dose is 100

mg po for three days, then maintenance dose of 20 mg po. Check liver enzymes at baseline and monitor monthly. Advise women to avoid pregnancy during therapy and for three months following. Side effects include gastritis, diarrhea, and anorexia. Drug is contraindicated in patients with known alcoholism or liver function abnormalities.

E. Hot and cold therapy
 1. Cold packs: Help to reduce inflammation and swelling; instruct patient to avoid applying directly to skin.
 2. Heat therapy: Ideal as a hot bath or shower. Advise patient on safety measures with heating pads or hot packs.

F. Occupational therapy
 1. Appropriate for patients with joint deformity and/or functional difficulties
 2. Can recommend assistive devices for fine-motor activities

G. Surgery
 1. Synovectomy (open or arthroscopic): Slows disease progression and reduces pain
 2. Joint arthroplasty (i.e., artificial joint replacement): Most artificial joints last 10–15 years.

H. Patient education: Provide material in writing whenever possible.
 1. Medication instructions, side effects, and precautions
 2. Body mechanics
 3. Laboratory test and follow-up schedule
 4. Activity: Balance between rest and activity

VII. Follow-up
 A. When starting medications or during an exacerbation, see patient every two or three weeks.
 B. Obtain labs based on patient's drug therapy (see Treatment).
 C. Follow-up intervals are based on patient's condition and therapy.

VIII. Referrals
 A. Rheumatologist: Consultation is warranted at the time of diagnosis prior to beginning therapy or if patient appears to need second-line therapy.
 B. Clients on DMARD therapy can be managed in collaboration with a rheumatologist.
 C. Physical therapist: Initial consultation upon diagnosis to counsel on body mechanics, devices to assist with activities of daily living, range-of-motion exercises, and thermal modalities (e.g., paraffin baths).

References

Barth, W. (1997). Office evaluation of the patient with musculoskeletal complaints. *American Journal of Medicine, 102*(Suppl. 1A), 1A3S–1A9S.

Cox, L. (1997). Update on rheumatoid arthritis. *Radiologic Technology, 69*(1), 11.

Grahame, R., & West, J. (1996). The role of the rheumatology nurse practitioner in primary care: An experiment in the further education of the practice nurse. *British Journal of Rheumatology, 35,* 581–588.

Guidelines for the management of rheumatoid arthritis. American College of Rheumatology Ad Hoc Committee on Clinical Guidelines. (1996). *Arthritis & Rheumatism, 39,* 713–722.

Guidelines for monitoring drug therapy in rheumatoid arthritis. American College of Rheumatology Ad Hoc Committee on Clinical Guidelines. (1996). *Arthritis & Rheumatism, 39,* 723–731.

Litman, K. (1996). A rational approach to the diagnosis of arthritis. *American Family Physician, 53,* 1295–1310.

Ross, C. (1997). A comparison of osteoarthritis and rheumatoid arthritis: Diagnosis and treatment. *Nurse Practitioner, 22*(9), 20–38.

Schiff, M. (1997). Emerging treatments for rheumatoid arthritis. *American Journal of Medicine, 102*(Suppl. 1A), 1A11S–1A15S.

Schumacher, R. (1995). Arthritis of recent onset. *Arthritis, 97*(4), 52–63.

Totemchokchyakarn, K., & Ball, G. (1996). Arthritis of systemic disease. *American Journal of Medicine, 101,* 642–647.

Section **IX.** Lymph

Symptoms

Medical Diagnosis

Chapter

109. Lymphadenopathy

Joanne Lester, MSN, RNC, OCN®, CNP

I. Definition: Lymph node enlargement

II. Physiology/Pathophysiology
   A. Normal physiology
      1. The lymphatic system is comprised of collecting ducts, lymph fluid, and tissues located in
         a) Lymph nodes throughout the body
         b) Organs, including the spleen, tonsils, Peyer's patches of the mesentery, and thymus gland
         c) Aggregates in the bone marrow, lung, and gastric and appendiceal mucosa.
      2. Functions
         a) Transport of lymph fluids and proteins for return to cardiovascular system
         b) Maturation of lymphocytes (B and T cells)
         c) Production of antibodies in response to microorganisms
         d) Phagocytosis
         e) Absorption of fat from the intestine; filtration of debris or dead cells from general circulation
   B. Pathophysiology
      1. Lymphadenopathy occurs as a result of filtration of aggregates, causing swelling of the affected lymph nodes.
      2. When interstitial fluid pressure increases, the flow from lymphatic capillaries into the lymphatics increases, causing edema or enlarged lymph nodes.

III. Clinical features
   A. Etiology
      1. Small lymph nodes palpable in neck, axilla, or groin or present on radiographic studies (e.g., mammogram, chest x-ray, scans) measuring < 1 cm are usually benign.
      2. Lymph nodes palpable or present on radiographic studies measuring > 1 cm often indicate bacterial, viral, or neoplastic etiology; a tissue biopsy must pathologically confirm diagnosis.

3. Lymph nodes palpable or present on radiographic studies measuring > 3 cm usually indicate neoplastic disease. Unless a diagnosis of a neoplastic disease has already been made, biopsy is necessary.

4. Lymphangitis presenting as erythema, pain, warmth, and red streaks along a lymphatic chain originating from a wound or area of cellulitis suggests acute inflammation or infection.

   a) Frequent etiology is staphylococci or hemolytic streptococci.

   b) Typically presents in a limb distal to a lymph node(s) dissection or body part drained by specific lymph chain (e.g., breast).

5. Lymphedema presenting as swelling, discomfort, and mild erythema in a limb distal to a lymph node(s) dissection or body part drained by specific lymph chain (e.g., breast) can be transient or permanent (see Chapter 110).

B. History

   1. History of cancer and cancer treatment

   2. Current medications: Prescribed and over-the-counter

   3. History of presenting symptom(s): Precipitating factors, location, and duration. Associated symptoms are fever, rash, sore throat, weight loss, and night sweats.

   4. Changes in activities of daily living

   5. Associated factors: Pet or animal exposure, recent foreign travel, infectious process, exposure to tuberculosis, recent body piercing or tattoo

C. Signs and symptoms

   1. Weight loss or gain

   2. Fever, chills, malaise

   3. Presence of inflammation or infection: Neutropenic patient may progress rapidly to septicemia

   4. Unusual sweating (particularly night sweats)

   5. Skin changes (e.g., rash, erythema, inflammation, abrasions)

   6. Sternal tenderness: May signify mediastinal pressure from node enlargement

   7. Abdominal swelling: Secondary to hepatosplenomegaly

   8. Edema or swelling of extremity

   9. Arthralgia, myalgia

D. Physical exam

   1. Skin: Include all areas adjacent to the lymphadenopathy; edema distal to the involved nodes often indicates obstruction.

   2. Lymph nodes exam:

      a) Location and symmetry

      b) Size (e.g., dimensions in centimeters, shape): Matted nodes usually indicate malignancy or metastasis.

      c) Surface characteristics (e.g., smooth, nodular, irregular)

      d) Consistency (e.g., hard, firm, soft, resilient, spongy, cystic)

         (1) Soft, rubbery nodes often indicate non-Hodgkin's lymphoma.

         (2) Firm, hard nodes may indicate Hodgkin's or disease metastasis.

      e) Fixation or mobility of underlying or overlying tissue: Fixed usually indicates malignancy.

  f) Tenderness or pain (e.g., direct, referred, rebound): Tenderness indicates acute inflammation or excessive manipulation.

  g) Erythema or warmth: May indicate infection

  h) Increased vascularity and transillumination (i.e., of scrotum): May be useful in distinguishing tumor, lymphadenopathy, or infection

IV. Diagnostic tests

 A. Laboratory

  1. CBC with differential: To evaluate for leukocytosis, leukopenia, anemia, elevated hemoglobin, thrombocytosis, and thrombocytopenia and changes in differential

   a) Increased granulocytes may indicate pyogenic infection or myeloproliferative condition.

   b) Increased eosinophils may indicate hypersensitivity/allergic reaction, parasitism, or underlying neoplastic condition.

   c) Left shift is indicative of infection.

   d) Increase in lymphocytes may indicate viral process or lymphoproliferative condition.

  2. Throat culture: If symptoms of pharyngitis, or cervical or submandibular adenopathy are present

  3. Urethral or cervical culture and sensitivity: If symptoms of genital disease or inguinal adenopathy (e.g., lymphogranuloma venereum, granuloma inguinale) are present

  4. Serologic tests: For syphilis, HIV, antibody titers (depending on suspected causative agent), antinuclear antibodies, rheumatoid arthritis factor

  5. Blood chemistries: Specifically liver and renal panels if malignancy is suspected; in the presence of unexplained lymphadenopathy, an elevated uric acid may indicate lymphoma or other hematologic cancer.

  6. Peripheral smear review: May be extremely useful and may indicate other tests to order

 B. Radiology

  1. Chest x-ray, PA and lateral: To evaluate evidence of infection or hilar lymphadenopathy

  2. Cardiac axial tomography scan: If generalized lymphadenopathy or organomegaly is present

 C. Other

  1. Bone marrow aspiration and biopsy: If leukemia or lymphoma is suspected

  2. Lymph node biopsy via needle aspiration or excisional biopsy: For tissue confirmation

  3. Purified protein derivative/Mantoux test with mumps control: To evaluate for tuberculosis

V. Differential diagnoses

 A. Generalized lymphadenopathy

  1. Infections: Acute (e.g., infectious mononucleosis, toxoplasmosis, cytomegalovirus, generalized dermatitis [see Chapters 18 and 19], common communicable diseases); chronic (e.g., syphilis [see Chapter 93], tuberculosis [see Chapter 34], sarcoidosis); AIDS (see Chapter 156).

   2. Hypersensitivity reactions and connective tissue diseases: Serum sickness, drug reactions (i.e., with phenytoin), vasculitis, rheumatoid arthritis (see Chapter 108), systemic lupus erythematosus
   3. Endocrine disorders: Hyperthyroidism (see Chapter 149), hypoadrenalism, hypopituitarism, lipidosis
   4. Primary lymphoproliferative diseases: Leukemia (e.g., chronic lymphatic leukemia, acute lymphocytic leukemia, blast crisis of chronic myelogenic leukemia), Waldenstrom's macroglobulinemia, Hodgkin's disease, non-Hodgkin's lymphoma
   5. Dermatopathic lymphadenitis
   6. Metastatic cancers: Most commonly breast, lung, gastrointestinal
   7. Superficial thrombophlebitis (see Chapter 157)
   8. Venous thrombosis (see Chapter 41)
 B. Localized lymphadenopathy
   1. Anterior or posterior auricular: Viral conjunctivitis (see Chapter 7), rubella, scalp infection
   2. Submandibular or unilateral cervical: Buccal cavity infection, pharyngitis (see Chapter 4), nasopharyngeal, thyroid, or head/neck malignancy
   3. Bilateral cervical: Mononucleosis, sarcoidosis, toxoplasmosis, pharyngitis (see Chapter 4), cytomegalovirus, Epstein-Barr virus, malignancy
   4. Supraclavicular: Pulmonary, mediastinal, esophageal, gastrointestinal, lymphoma, breast, intra-abdominal, renal, testicular, ovarian, or breast malignancy; Virchow's node in the left supraclavicular area may be the result of either abdominal or thoracic malignancy.
   5. Axillary: Upper extremity infection, lymphoma, melanoma, or breast malignancy or infection
   6. Epitrochlear: Syphilis (bilateral [see Chapter 95]), hand infection (unilateral), rheumatoid arthritis (see Chapter 108), sarcoidosis, malignancy (particularly breast)
   7. Inguinal: Syphilis (see Chapter 93), genital herpes (see Chapter 89), lymphogranuloma venereum, chancroid, lower extremity or local infection, lymphoma, pelvic, or metastatic cancer
   8. Any region: Cat-scratch fever, Hodgkin's disease, non-Hodgkin's lymphoma, leukemia, metastatic cancer, sarcoidosis, Epstein-Barr virus, granulomatous infections
   9. Hilar: Fungal infection, sarcoidosis, lymphoma, bronchogenic malignancy, tuberculosis (see Chapter 34)

VI. Treatment: Depends on etiology, extent of lymphadenopathy
 A. Observation: Resolution with time
 B. Antibiotic therapy: For streptococcus coverage or hemolytic streptococci (e.g., broad spectrum penicillin, cephalosporin [see Appendix 1]), depending on organism isolated
 C. Antiviral agents (e.g., acyclovir): For known viral infection
 D. Tissue biopsy: Warranted if initial treatment does not resolve the lymphadenopathy
 E. Appropriate cancer treatment: Surgery, chemotherapy, or radiation, depending on histology

VII. Follow-up
    A. Short-term: Based on the etiology and treatment of lymphadenopathy. For viral or infectious condition, marked resolution should occur within 48–72 hours of treatment initiation; progression of symptoms warrants further investigation.
    B. Long-term: Depends on the etiology

VIII. Referrals
    A. Patients who improve significantly within 48–72 hours (without evidence of underlying disease) generally do not require a physician referral. It is important to re-examine the patient two to four weeks after cessation of antibiotic treatment to ensure complete resolution of lymphadenopathy. All patients exhibiting symptoms of a malignancy should be referred to a physician or oncologist for evaluation and treatment.
    B. Patients who do not improve within 48–72 hours, or who progress, require a physician referral.
    C. All patients with persistent lymphadenopathy should be referred for a tissue biopsy.

References

Connolly, A.A., & MacKenzie, K. (1997). Pediatric neck masses—A diagnostic dilemma. *Journal of Laryngology & Otology, 111,* 541–545.

Dean, S.S. (1994). Otolaryngology head and neck surgery: A review of malignancies. *Australian Family Physician, 23,* 2130–2136.

Golledge, C. (1997). A lump in the neck. *Australian Family Physician, 26,* 483.

Miller, L.T. (1994). Lymphedema: Unlocking the doors to successful treatment. *Innovations in Oncology Nursing, 10,* 53–62.

110.

Lymphedema

Diane G. Cope, PhD, ARNP-CS, AOCN®

I. Definition: Obstruction of the lymphatic system that causes overload of lymph fluid in interstitial spaces

II. Pathophysiology: Blockage or destruction of the lymphatic vessels causes an increase in the interstitial fluid hydrostatic and colloid oncotic pressures.
  A. Increased pressure causes leaking of fluid and proteins into the interstitial spaces.
  B. Collagen accumulation and fibrosclerosis cause brawny skin changes with edema.

III. Clinical features
  A. Etiology
    1. Primary lymphedema occurs without any obvious etiology.
      a) More common in women
      b) More common in lower extremities
      c) May be familial or congenital: Lymphedema congenita occurs at birth; lymphedema praecox occurs late in life; lymphedema tarda occurs after age 35.
    2. Secondary lymphedema is caused by injury, scarring, or excision of the lymph nodes.
      a) Injury (e.g., caused by central venous catheter placement)
      b) Lymph node dissection for malignancy
      c) Scarring from a vesicant extravasation
      d) Burns
  B. History: Patient's pain, onset of swelling, extent of edema, skin changes, muscle strength, range of motion, sensory deficits, precipitating factors, and exercise/activity levels
    1. History of cancer and cancer treatment
    2. Current medications: Prescribed and over-the-counter
    3. History of presenting symptom(s): Precipitating factors, location, and duration
    4. Changes in activities of daily living
    5. Past medical history: Burns, extravasation, chronic inflammation, cellulitis, diabetes mellitus
  C. Signs and symptoms
    1. Sudden onset: May occur for the first time after traumatic injury, infection, excessive physical exertion, or airplane travel (especially with suboptimal pressurization of cabin)

2. Gradual onset: Usually begins in the distal portion of the extremity and later involves the proximal area, occurring over a three-month period
   a) Edema
   b) Tightness of clothing, watch, or jewelry
   c) Weakness of the involved extremity
   d) Decreased range of motion
   e) Stiffness
   f) Pain
   g) Numbness or paresthesia of the extremity
   h) Erythema
   i) Weight gain
   j) Heavy extremity (subjective finding)
D. Physical exam
   1. Vital signs: Fever may be present, indicating infection.
   2. Integument exam: Inspect tissue for
      a) Thickening, pitting, and erythema (usually unilateral, but can be bilateral)
      b) Chronic lymphedema becomes indurated with nonpitting edema
      c) Hyperpigmentation
      d) Stasis dermatitis
      e) Superficial veins
   3. Extremity measurements (compared to contralateral unaffected extremity)
      a) Mild lymphedema: 1–3 cm discrepancy
      b) Moderate lymphedema: 3–5 cm discrepancy
      c) Severe lymphedema: For > 5 cm discrepancy, measure upper extremities 10 cm above or below olecranon process; for lower extremities, measure instep, ankle, calf, knee, lower thigh, and upper thigh.
   4. Lymph node exam: Evaluate for enlargement.

IV. Diagnostic tests
   A. Laboratory: Not indicated.
   B. Radiology
      1. Doppler ultrasound: Evaluate venous patency.
      2. CT scan or MRI: Evaluate bulky tumor involvement or obstruction.

V. Differential diagnosis
   A. Disease recurrence (e.g., lymphoma)
   B. Tumor involvement
   C. Lymphangitis
   D. Cellulitis (see Chapter 16)
   E. Deep vein thrombosis (see Chapter 41)
   F. Superficial thrombosis
   G. Phlebitis (see Chapter 157)

VII. Treatment
   A. Prevention: Patient should avoid

 1. Blood drawing, injections, intravenous administration, vaccinations, and blood pressure monitoring in affected or at-risk extremity
 2. Weight gain
 3. Laceration, abrasion, and injury to extremity
 4. Constricting clothing and jewelry
 5. Heat (e.g., saunas, hot baths, overexposure to sunlight)
 6. Lifting or moving objects heavier than 15 pounds
 7. Strenuous exercise
 8. Prolonged dependency of extremity.
B. Maintenance nonpharmacological therapy
 1. Elevation of extremity
 2. Elastic garment (requires measuring by physical or occupational therapist)
 3. Weight management counseling
 4. Massage therapy
 5. Pneumatic compression devices (e.g., Jobst™ pump, Jobst Institute, Toledo, OH)
 6. Complete decongestive physiotherapy (e.g., manual lymph massage drainage, compression bandages)
C. Pharmacological therapy
 1. Dexamethasone (e.g., 4 mg po bid short-term)
 2. Low-dose Dilantin® (Parke-Davis, Morris Plains, NJ) (e.g., 100 mg po daily)
 3. Trials with benzopyrones to enhance lymphatic flow: Studies have shown coumarin to be beneficial, but it is not approved in the United States for this indication).
 4. Antibiotic therapy for staphylococcus and hemolytic streptococcus
   a) Cephalexin (Keflex®, Dista Products Company, Indianapolis, IN) 500 mg po q 12 hours for 7–14 days
   b) Any agent directed against gram-positive organisms (see Appendix 1)
   c) Antibiotics early in course to decrease scarring of lymphatic channels, which increase the risk for lymphedema

VII. Follow-up: Every one to two weeks during acute phase undergoing massage therapy or if cellulitis occurs; referral to a skilled lymph drainage therapist may be necessary

VIII. Resources
A. The National Lymphedema Network (800-541-3259, phone; www.lymphnet.org, Web site)
B. Susan G. Komen Breast Cancer Foundation (800-462-9273, phone; www.komen.org, Web site)
C. American Cancer Society (800-227-2345, phone; www.cancer.org, Web site)
D. National Cancer Institute (800-4-CANCER, phone; www.cancernet.nci.nih.gov, Web site)

References

Boris, M., Weindorf, S., Lasinski, B., & Boris, G. (1994). Lymphedema reduction by noninvasive complex lymphedema therapy. *Oncology, 8*(9), 95–106.

Carter, B.J. (1997). Women's experiences of lymphedema. *Oncology Nursing Forum, 24,* 875–882.

Hornsby, R. (1995). The use of compression to treat lymphoedema. *Professional Nurse, 11*(2), 127–128.

Humble, C.A. (1995). Lymphedema: Incidence, pathophysiology, management, and nursing care. *Oncology Nursing Forum, 22,* 1503–1511.

Loprinzi, C.L., Kugler, J.W., Sloan, J.A., Rooke, T.W., Quella, S.K., Novotny, P., Mowat, R.B., Michalak, J.C., Stella, P.J., Levitt, R., Tschettr, L.K., & Windschitl, H. (1999). Lack of effect of coumarin in women with lymphedema after treatment for breast cancer. *New England Journal of Medicine, 340,* 346–350.

Marcks, P. (1997). Lymphedema: Pathogenesis, prevention and treatment. *Cancer Practice, 5*(1), 32–38.

Petrek, J.A., & Lerner, R. (1996). Lymphedema. In J. Harris, M. Lippman, M. Morrow, & S. Hellman (Eds.), *Diseases of the breast* (pp. 896–903). Philadelphia: Lippincott-Raven.

Section **X.**

Hematologic

Symptoms

Medical Diagnosis

Chapter

111.

Overview of Anemia

Mary Pat Lynch, CRNP, MSN, AOCN®

I. Definition: A reduction in either the red blood cell (RBC) volume or concentration of hemoglobin or the number of erythrocytes in the blood

II. Physiology/Pathophysiology
   A. Normal
      1. RBCs originate in the bone marrow, which resides in the sternum, ribs, vertebrae, pelvis, and proximal ends of the femur and humerus in adults.
      2. A feedback mechanism initiated by decreased oxygen tension at the level of the kidney causes an increased release of erythropoietin from the kidney, which stimulates the production of RBCs.
   B. Pathophysiology (see each type of anemia)
      1. Blood loss
      2. Inadequate production: Occurs when there are defects in stem cell proliferation or differentiation, deoxyribonucleic acid (DNA) synthesis, hemoglobin synthesis, or a combination of these deficiencies
      3. Excessive destruction: Occurs from membrane disorders, abnormal hemoglobin, enzyme deficiencies, and a host of extrinsic problems (e.g., mechanical disruption, antibody-mediated injury)

III. Classifications/Etiologies
   A. Anemia can be divided into three categories according to the size of the RBC, as determined by the mean corpuscular volume (MCV). Examples of the most common anemias are
      1. Microcytic: Small size
         a) Iron deficiency
         b) Anemia of chronic disease (ACD)
         c) Thalassemia minor
         d) Sideroblastic anemia
      2. Normocytic: Normal size
         a) Hemolytic anemia
            (1) Drug-induced
            (2) Autoimmune (e.g., idiopathic, collagen disease, lymphoma)

           (3) Cold agglutinin-induced (e.g., viral infection, lymphoma)
           (4) Hemoglobinopathy (e.g., sickle cell disease, glucose-6-phosphate dehydrogenase deficiency [G6PD])
           (5) Hereditary spherocytosis
           (6) Microangiopathy (e.g., vasculitis, disseminated intravascular coagulation, heart valve)
        b) Aplastic anemia
        c) Renal failure
        d) Hypothyroidism
        e) ACD
    3. Macrocytic: Large size
        a) Vitamin B_{12} deficiency
        b) Folate deficiency
        c) Liver disease
        d) Myelodysplastic syndromes: Heterogenous group of clonal neoplastic hematologic disorders characterized by varying degrees of bone marrow failure, abnormal hematopoiesis, and proliferation of myeloid blast cells. Five subtypes are
           (1) Refractory anemia
           (2) Refractory anemia with ringed sideroblast
           (3) Refractory anemia with excess blasts
           (4) Refractory anemia with excess blasts in transformation
           (5) Chronic myelomonocytic leukemia.
  B. Anemia can also be classified by the reticulocyte count.
    1. Low reticulocyte count: State of decreased RBC production (e.g., aplastic, ACD, iron deficiency, B_{12} deficiency, and folate deficiency)
    2. High reticulocyte count: State of increased RBC destruction (e.g., hemolysis, recovery phase of iron)

IV. Clinical presentation: Depends on abruptness of onset, severity, age, and ability of the cardiopulmonary system to compensate for the decrease in blood volume and oxygen-carrying capacity.

References

See page 681.

112. Anemia of Chronic Disease

Mary Pat Lynch, CRNP, MSN, AOCN®

I. Definition: A normocytic, normochromic anemia with low reticulocyte count

II. Pathophysiology: Etiology and mechanisms of anemia of chronic disease (ACD) are not clearly understood. Theories include
   A. Iron is not released from storage but remains in the reticuloendothelial system (often seen in inflammatory conditions and myelodysplasia).
   B. Erythropoietin is inadequately released from the kidneys in response to the degree of anemia (usually seen in patients with chronic renal insufficiency or AIDS).
   C. Erythropoietin fails to stimulate red blood cell (RBC) production with mild hemolysis.

III. Clinical features: Despite the term "chronic disease," the characteristics of ACD may occur very quickly (e.g., following an acute infection); most common type of anemia in hospitalized patients.
   A. Etiology
      1. Chronic infection
      2. Inflammatory disease
      3. Neoplastic disease
      4. Cancer treatments
   B. History
      1. History of cancer and cancer treatment
      2. Current medications: Prescribed and over-the-counter
      3. History of presenting symptom(s): Precipitating factors, onset, and duration
      4. Changes in activities of daily living
      5. Past medical history: Infection, inflammation (including collagen vascular disorders), trauma
   C. Signs and symptoms: Fewer and milder symptoms than most anemias
      1. Fatigue
      2. Weakness
      3. Dyspnea on exertion
      4. Other signs and symptoms related to underlying disease (e.g., infection, trauma)
   D. Physical exam: Nonspecific (e.g., skin pallor)

IV. Diagnostic tests
   A. Laboratory (see Tables 112-1 and 112-2)
      1. Mildly decreased hemoglobin: If < 9 g/dl, consider other causes.
      2. RBC indices: If normochromic and normocytic but hypochromic, microcytic features develop as ACD progresses and are associated with defective utilization of iron.
      3. Decreased reticulocyte count
      4. Decreased serum iron
      5. Decreased or normal total iron binding capacity
      6. Normal or increased serum ferritin
   B. Radiology: Not indicated

V. Differential diagnosis
   A. Aplastic anemia (see Chapter 113): May be distinguished from ACD by the usual association of thrombocytopenia and neutropenia.
   B. Pure red cell aplasia: May be associated with signs and symptoms of parvovirus infection (e.g., rash, arthralgia).
   C. Malignant invasion of the bone marrow caused by myelodysplasia: Distinguished by the presence of teardrop for myelodysplasia and leukoerythroblastic changes.
   D. Drug-induced marrow suppression or hemolysis: History of associated medication ingestion.
   E. Anemia of chronic renal failure: Distinguished by low erythropoietin level and increased creatinine.

VI. Treatment
   A. No treatment may be necessary for this mild anemia.
   B. Once treatment with erythropoietin growth factor has begun, ferritin usually drops quickly, and the patient becomes iron deficient. Therefore, ferrous sulfate (e.g., 325 mg po tid) is usually started along with the erythropoietin.
   C. Blood transfusions: Performed only if patient is symptomatic (usually not necessary unless the patient has poor cardiac reserve).
   D. A trial of erythropoietin (20,000–40,000 units SC weekly) may be helpful.
      1. May take two to four weeks to increase red blood cells. If no increase in four weeks, increase the dose by 10,000 units.
      2. Reticulocyte count should increase in two to four weeks. Hemoglobin should increase in four to six weeks.
      3. If no increase in hematocrit in seven to eight weeks after increasing the dose, erythropoietin usually will not be helpful.
   E. Patient education: Instruct patient on the importance of adequate nutritional intake and rest; provide instruction on self-injection for erythropoietin if necessary.

VII. Follow-up
   A. Short-term: Repeat hemoglobin when underlying process has resolved (hemoglobin should correct itself within a few months).
   B. Long-term
      1. When underlying process cannot be resolved, monitor hemoglobin (monthly transfusion is rarely needed).

2. For patients receiving erythropoietin, monitor reticulocyte count and hemoglobin monthly (reticulocyte count should increase within two to four weeks, hemoglobin should increase within six weeks).

   a) Continue erythropoietin if observed to be effective in a seven-week therapeutic trial.

   b) Ensure patient has adequate iron (iron stores must be normal, or increased, for erythropoietin to be effective); vitamin C (approximately 60 mg) is necessary for iron absorption.

VII. Referrals: Refer to appropriate specialist for treatment when workup reveals underlying inflammatory, infectious, or neoplastic disease for treatment.

References

See page 681.

Table 112-1. Laboratory Assessment of Anemia: Normal Values (Adults)

Laboratory Test	Normal Value
Red blood cell count	Male: 4.7–6 mi/ccmm; Female: 4.2–5.4 mi/ccmm
Hemoglobin	Male: 13.5–18 g/dl; Female: 12–16 g/dl
Hematocrit	Male: 42%–52%; Female: 37%–47%
Mean corpuscular volume (MCV)	78–100 fl
Mean corpuscular hemoglobin (MCH)	27–31 pg/cell
Red cell distribution width (RDW)	11.5%–14%
Reticulocyte count	0.5%–1.85% of erythrocytes
Ferritin	Male 20–300 ng/ml; Female 15–120 ng/ml
Serum iron	Male 75–175 ug/dl; Female 65–165 ug/dl
Total iron binding capacity (TIBC)	250–450 ug/dl
Serum erythropoietin level	Male 17.2 mU/ml; Female 18.8 mU/ml
Coomb's test (direct and indirect)	Negative
Serum B$_{12}$	190–900 ng/ml
Serum folate	> 3.5 ug/

Note. Based on information from Wallach, 1996.

Table 112-2. Laboratory Assessment of Anemia: Results of Tests

Type of Anemia	MCV[a]	Retic	Ferritin	Iron	TIBC[b]	Bili	B12	Folate
Iron deficiency*	D	D	D	D/N	I	N	N	N
Thalassemia	D	I/N	I/N	I/N	N	I	N	N\D
Sideroblastic	D	I/N	I	I	NA	NA	NA	NA
Aplastic anemia*	N	D	NA	NA	NA	NA	NA	NA
Anemia of chronic disease*	D/N	D/N	I/N	D	D	N	N	N\D
B12 deficiency*	I	D/N	I	I	N	N	D	N
Folate deficiency*	I	D/N	I	I	N	N	N	D
Acute blood loss	N	I	NA	NA	NA	NA	NA	NA
Sickle cell*	N	I	NA	NA	NA	NA	NA	NA
G6PD deficiency	N	I	NA	NA	NA	NA	NA	NA
Hemolytic: Warm	N	I	NA	NA	NA	NA	NA	NA
Hemolytic: Cold	N	I	NA	NA	NA	NA	NA	NA

I, increased; D, decreased; N, normal; NA, not applicable
[a] Mean corpuscular volume; [b] total iron binding capacity
*Located in this section.
Note. Based on information from Wallach, 1996.

Chapter

113. Aplastic Anemia

Mary Pat Lynch, CRNP, MSN, AOCN®

I. Definition: A marrow failure syndrome characterized by peripheral pancytopenia and marrow hypoplasia

II. Pathophysiology: The reduction in functional marrow mass is initiated by multiple forms of injury to the marrow stem cells or their microenvironment because of fatty replacement.

III. Clinical features
   A. Etiology
      1. Hereditary causes (e.g., Fanconi's anemia, dyskeratosis congenita)
      2. Idiopathic (occurs in about 65% of patients)
      3. Acquired
         a) Chemicals (e.g., benzene and related compounds)
         b) Drugs (e.g., gold salts, penicillamine, phenylbutazone, carbamazepine, hydantoin, chloramphenicol, quinacrine, acetazolamide)
         c) Radiation
         d) Viruses (e.g., Epstein-Barr virus, hepatitis)
         e) Miscellaneous (e.g., connective tissue disorders, pregnancy)
   B. History
      1. History of cancer and cancer treatment
      2. Current medications: Prescribed and over-the-counter
      3. History of presenting symptom(s): Precipitating factors, onset, and duration
      4. Changes in activities of daily living
   C. Signs and symptoms
      1. Fatigue
      2. Bleeding
      3. Infections
   D. Physical exam
      1. Vital signs: Fever
      2. Skin exam
         a) Pallor
         b) Petechiae
         c) Purpura

      3. HEENT exam: Retinal hemorrhages
      4. Lymphadenopathy
      5. Abdominal exam: Splenomegaly

IV. Diagnostic tests
    A. Laboratory (see Tables 112-1 and 112-2)
      1. Complete blood count
        a) Pancytopenia
        b) Elevated mean corpuscular volume (MCV)
        c) Low absolute neutrophil count (ANC)
      2. Iron studies
        a) Increased serum iron
        b) Increased ferritin
      3. Bone marrow aspirate and biopsy (may be hypocellular)
      4. Low reticulocyte count
      5. Sucrose hemolysis test to rule out paroxysmal nocturnal hemaglobinurea (PNH)
      6. Increased erythropoietin level
    B. Radiology: Not indicated

V. Differential diagnosis
    A. Hypoplastic myelodysplastic syndrome
    B. PNH
    C. Hypoplastic acute lymphocytic leukemia
    D. Hairy-cell leukemia
    E. Myelofibrosis
    F. Metastatic cancer

VI. Treatment
    A. Untreated patients with severe aplastic anemia have a median survival of three to six months.
    B. Allogeneic bone marrow transplantation is only curative treatment.
      1. Human lymphocyte antigen (HLA) matched sibling donor is preferred.
      2. Approximately 80% of previously untransfused patients achieve cure; approximately 60% who received multiple transfusions will be cured.
    C. Immunosuppressive therapy is not curative.
      1. Antithymocyte globulin (ATG) IV: Given for 4–10 days (serum sickness common; 50% response rate)
      2. Cyclosporine: given daily by mouth for four to six months (25% response rate)
      3. Combination therapy with ATG + cyclosporine
    D. Supportive care
      1. Instruct patient in measures to reduce risk of infection and bleeding.
      2. Minimal or no transfusions are given to potential transplant recipients.
        a) If needed, do not use family members as donors.
        b) Potential antibodies can develop, increasing the risk for patient to be refractory to blood products.

3. Use single-donor platelets to decrease development of antibodies.
   a) Use Amicar® (Immunex Corporation, Seattle, WA) to control bleeding.
   b) Administer loading dose of 5 g, followed by 1 g/hour IV or 2 g every two hours orally (usually discontinued after 8–24 hours; contraindicated in renal failure).
4. Promptly institute broad-spectrum antibiotics for fever (see Chapter 140)
5. Use hematopoietic growth factors to stimulate white blood cell and red blood cell counts if necessary (e.g., granulocyte colony-stimulating factor, granulocyte-macrophage-colony-stimulating factor, erythropoietin).

VII. Follow-up
   A. Short-term: Aplastic anemia requires frequent visits to check blood counts and evaluate for signs and symptoms of infection or bleeding.
   B. Long-term: Required with transplant team following bone marrow or stem cell transplant

VII. Referrals
   A. Aplastic anemia should always be managed in collaboration with an oncologist or hematologist.
   B. Refer patient and potential sibling donors to transplant center for evaluation immediately following diagnosis and once patient is stabilized.

References

See page 681.

Chapter

114. Cobalamin (Vitamin B$_{12}$) Deficiency

Mary Pat Lynch, CRNP, MSN, AOCN®

I. Definition: A megaloblastic, macrocytic, normochromic anemia caused by a deficiency of vitamin B$_{12}$

II. Physiology/Pathophysiology
   A. Normal
      1. Intrinsic factor (IF) is a glycoprotein secreted by parietal cells of the stomach.
      2. IF is necessary for cellular transport of cobalamin (vitamin B$_{12}$).
      3. Cobalamin is required for the production of myelin-based proteins.
   B. Pathophysiology
      1. Interference with DNA synthesis is caused by the lack of vitamin B$_{12}$, which is required for metabolism of folate.
      2. Deficiency usually results from impaired absorption of B$_{12}$ or deficiency of IF.
      3. Deficiency of B$_{12}$ results in a demyelinating condition causing mixed motor and sensory peripheral neuropathy.

III. Clinical features: Common in Caucasians of northern European descent; usually occurs in sixth decade of life, yet can occur in younger patients.
   A. Etiology
      1. Pernicious anemia: Atrophy causes gastric mucosa to fail to secrete IF.
      2. Gastrectomy syndrome: After a partial or total gastrectomy, IF ceases to secrete within five to six years.
      3. Insufficient diet: Although it occurs rarely, it usually is experienced by vegetarians who avoid dairy products and eggs.
   B. History
      1. History of cancer and cancer treatment
      2. Current medications: Prescribed and over-the-counter
      3. History of presenting symptom(s): Precipitating factors, onset, and duration
      4. Changes in activities of daily living
      5. Past surgical history: Partial or total gastrectomy
      6. Review dietary intake: Diet recall
   C. Signs and symptoms
      1. Weakness

        2. Sore throat

        3. Paresthesia of extremities (e.g., numbness, tingling, burning)

        4. Swelling of legs

        5. Dizziness

        6. Dementia in advanced stages of B_{12} deficiency

    D. Physical exam

        1. HEENT exam

            a) Slightly icteric skin and sclera

            b) Smooth, beefy, red tongue

        2. Cardiovascular: Systolic murmur

        3. Neurological exam

            a) Decreased position sense

            b) Poor or absent vibratory sense in lower extremities

            c) Ataxia

            d) Increased or decreased deep tendon reflexes

            e) Mental status changes (e.g., confusion and lethargy)

IV. Diagnostic tests

    A. Laboratory (see Tables 112-1 and 112-2)

        1. CBC (i.e., increased mean corpuscular volume [MCV > 100])

        2. Decreased or normal reticulocyte count

        3. Decreased B_{12} level

        4. Normal or increased serum folate

        5. Schilling test: Measures urinary radioactivity after ingestion of oral dose of radioactive cobalamin; detects lack of IF to rule out pernicious anemia or malabsorption disorders

        6. Increased lactic dehydrogenase (LDH) and total bilirubin

        7. Increased homocysteine levels

        8. Other blood tests that may be ordered to further delineate diagnosis

            a) Increased holotranscobalamin II level (can detect early B_{12} deficiency)

            b) Increased serum or urine methylmalonic acid levels

            c) Anti-intrinsic factor antibodies

    B. Radiology: Not indicated

V. Differential diagnosis

    A. Folate deficiency (see Chapter 115)

    B. Anemia of chronic disease (see Chapter 112)

    C. Myelodysplastic syndrome

VI. Treatment

    A. Vitamin B_{12} (i.e., cobalamin): 100–1,000 mcg IM daily over two weeks, then weekly until hemoglobin normalizes

    B. Should receive a total of 2,000 mcg of vitamin B_{12} during the first six weeks

    C. Transfusion if prompt alleviation of anemia symptoms is necessary; to alleviate hemodynamic instability

    D. Patient education regarding the nature of the disease, need for lifelong replacement, injection technique, and diet

VII. Follow-up
   A. Short-term
      1. Reticulocyte count: Should increase in three to five days, indicating marrow response to B$_{12}$ replacement; recovery phase may be associated with a temperature spike.
      2. Hemoglobin: Should normalize in one to two months.
      3. Serum potassium levels: Severe hypokalemia may develop after B$_{12}$ deficiency because of rapid incorporation into cells that have previously had an arrest of maturation.
   B. Long-term
      1. Once replete, patient takes vitamin B$_{12}$ 100–1,000 mcg monthly for life.
      2. Conduct appropriate follow-up for increased risk for gastric cancer in patients with pernicious anemia.

VIII. Referrals: Consult physician if pernicious anemia is suspected and further testing (e.g., gastric analysis, bone marrow biopsy, GI radiographic studies) is indicated.

References

See page 681.

Chapter

115. Folate Deficiency

Mary Pat Lynch, CRNP, MSN, AOCN®

I. Definition: A macrocytic, normochromic, megaloblastic anemia caused by folic acid deficiency

II. Physiology/Pathophysiology
   A. Normal: Folic acid is needed for DNA synthesis, red blood cell maturation, and maintenance of gastric mucosa.
      1. Serum folate levels reflect the recent oral intake of folate.
      2. Within five weeks of inadequate oral folate intake, serum folate levels will decline to the subnormal range.
   B. Pathophysiology: Unable to absorb folic acid or a decreased intake of folic acid

III. Clinical features: Folic acid reserves are small; deficiency can develop rapidly. Signs and symptoms closely resemble B_{12} deficiency without the presence of neurologic symptoms.
   A. Etiology
      1. Inadequate diet is the principle cause of folic acid deficiency because folate is absorbed from food throughout the small intestine.
      2. Impaired absorption (i.e., spruc)
      3. Increased requirements (i.e., during pregnancy, infancy, chronic hemolytic anemia)
      4. Alcohol can depress folic acid levels and impair folic acid utilization.
      5. Drugs that may cause decreased folic acid levels
         a) Phenytoin (Dilantin®, Parke-Davis, Morris Plains, NJ)
         b) Antimalarial agents
         c) Oral contraceptives
         d) Chloramphenicol
         e) Phenobarbital
         f) Methotrexate
         g) Trimethoprim-sulfamethoxazole
   B. History
      1. History of cancer and cancer treatment
      2. Current medications: Prescribed and over-the-counter
      3. History of presenting symptom(s): Precipitating factors, onset, and duration

       4. Changes in activities of daily living

       5. Diet: Types of food and food processing

       6. Social history: Alcohol intake

   C. Signs and symptoms

       1. Fatigue

       2. Dyspnea on exertion

       3. Dizziness

       4. Pallor

       5. Weakness

       6. Headache

       7. Angina

   D. Physical exam

       1. No overt signs if anemia is mild

       2. Integument exam

          a) Pallor

          b) Brittle nails

          c) Fine hair

       3. Oral exam

          a) Angular cheilitis

          b) Stomatitis

       4. Cardiovascular exam

          a) Tachycardia

          b) Systolic murmur

IV. Diagnostic tests

   A. Laboratory (see Tables 112-1 and 112-2)

       1. CBC

          a) Increased mean corpuscular volume (MCV)

          b) Leukopenia and thrombocytopenia

       2. Normal or decreased reticulocyte count

       3. Decreased serum folic acid level

       4. Normal serum B_{12}

       5. Peripheral smear: Presence of megaloblastic cells and oval macrocytes

       6. Increased homocysteine

   B. Radiology: Not indicated

V. Differential diagnosis

   A. Pernicious anemia (see Chapter 114)

   B. Myelodysplastic syndrome

   C. Megaloblastic anemia caused by drugs such as

       1. Methotrexate

       2. Pyrimethamine

       3. Trimethoprim

       4. Sulfasalazine

       5. Triamterene

      6. Acyclovir
      7. 5-fluorouracil
      8. Zidovudine
      9. Hydroxyurea
    10. Cytarabine
    11. Phenytoin
    12. Phenobarbital

VI. Treatment
  A. Folate: 1 mg po daily, up to 5 mg po daily; duration depends upon etiology of deficiency. May be used if deficiency is related to sprue.
  B. When possible, eliminate underlying cause.
  C. Teach patient dietary sources of folic acid (e.g., asparagus, bananas, fish, green leafy vegetables, peanut butter, oatmeal, red beans, beef liver, wheat bran).
     1. Encourage daily intake of these foods.
     2. Instruct patient in food preparation (i.e., overcooking can destroy folic acid).

VII. Follow-up
  A. Short-term
     1. Check hemoglobin and reticulocyte count for response (increase) in one to two weeks.
     2. Evaluate for vitamin B_{12} deficiency; failure to assess B_{12} status can result in nontreatment of this deficiency associated with cognitive impairment and neuropathy.
  B. Long-term
     1. Check hemoglobin and reticulocyte count every 6–12 months while on treatment.
     2. Check folate level in four months to evaluate repletion.

VIII. Referrals: Consult physician if a coexisting iron deficiency, thalassemia trait, or inflammation is suspected.

References

See page 681.

116.

Iron-Deficiency Anemia

Mary Pat Lynch, CRNP, MSN, AOCN®

I. Definition: A microcytic, hypochromic anemia caused by insufficient iron for hemoglobin synthesis

II. Pathophysiology
   A. The result of inadequate intake of iron
   B. The result of excessive loss of iron
   C. Inadequate absorption of dietary iron (i.e., from interference of gastric contents, abnormal mucosa, alteration in intestinal transit time)
      1. Delayed intestinal transit time increases iron absorption.
      2. Ascorbic acid promotes the absorption of nonheme iron.
   D. When iron supply is decreased, stores of iron are first depleted, followed by a reduction in hemoglobin formation.

III. Clinical features: Frequently occurs in young children, women during the childbearing years, and the elderly. Iron deficiency is the most frequent cause of anemia.
   A. Etiology
      1. Inadequate intake (< 1–2 mg/day)
      2. Inadequate absorption (after partial gastrectomy)
      3. Excessive loss of iron
         a) Uterine bleeding
         b) Gastrointestinal bleeding
         c) Urinary tract bleeding
   B. History
      1. History of cancer and cancer treatment
      2. Current medications: Prescribed and over-the-counter
      3. History of presenting symptom(s): Precipitating factors, onset, and duration. Associated symptoms are black tarry stools and pica (i.e., cravings for nonfood substances such as clay, ice, starch)
      4. Changes in activities of daily living
      5. Menstrual blood loss (if appropriate): Include type and number of pads used (i.e., super versus light pads).
      6. Past medical history: Gastric surgery, ulcers, gastritis

    C. Signs and symptoms: Depend on etiology, degree, and rapidity of onset of anemia
1. Fatigue
2. Shortness of breath, dyspnea on exertion
3. Pica
4. Burning of the tongue
5. Paresthesia
6. Brittle nails
7. Exercise intolerance
8. Angina pectoris
9. Palpitations
10. Intolerance to cold
    D. Physical exam
1. Integument exam
   a) Pallor
   b) Koilonychia (i.e., spoon nails)
2. HEENT
   a) Conjunctiva pale
   b) Oral exam
      (1) Papillary atrophy of the tongue
      (2) Glossitis
      (3) Angular cheilitis
3. Cardiovascular exam: May reveal tachycardia or symptoms of congestive heart failure

IV. Diagnostic tests
    A. Laboratory: See Tables 112-1 and 112-2 for common diagnostic tests and normal values.
1. CBC
   a) Decreased hemoglobin and hematocrit
   b) Low mean corpuscular volume (MCV) and mean corpuscular hemoglobin concentration (MCHC)
   c) Increased red (cell) distribution width (RDW)
   d) Decreased reticulocyte count
2. Iron studies
   a) Decreased ferritin
   b) Low or normal serum iron concentration
   c) Increased total iron binding capacity
3. Stool for occult blood
    B. Radiology: Upper and lower endoscopy in any male or postmenopausal female to rule out gastrointestinal malignancy or ulcer
    C. Other: Bone marrow biopsy to check iron stores if diagnosis is unclear; evaluate for any concurrent processes.

V. Differential diagnosis
    A. Thalassemia

B. Anemia of chronic disease (see Chapter 112)
C. Sideroblastic anemia
D. Lead toxicity

VI. Treatment
  A. Treat the underlying cause.
  B. Replete with ferrous sulfate ($FeSO_4$) 325 mg po tid for six months.
      1. Side effects of iron therapy include nausea, constipation, diarrhea, and black stools.
      2. If side effects are significant, consider starting iron daily for one week, twice daily for the next week, and three times daily the following week.
  C. Red blood cell transfusions not usually needed.
  D. Instruct patient to take iron between meals for better absorption; must take approximately 60 mg of vitamin C to absorb iron.
  E. Foods high in iron include organ and lean meats, egg yolk, shellfish, apricots, peaches, potatoes, prunes, grapes, raisins, green leafy vegetables, and iron-fortified breads and cereals.
  F. May need IV iron infusion if oral supplementation does not begin to correct deficiency within six weeks.

VII. Follow-up
  A. Short-term
      1. Repeat CBC and reticulocyte count in two weeks and monthly until corrected.
      2. Response indicated by increase in reticulocyte count in one to two weeks, correction of anemia in two to four months, and reaccumulation of iron stores in four to six months.
  B. Long-term
      1. Iron supplementation may be stopped when hemoglobin and ferritin have normalized, provided the underlying source of iron deficiency has been treated.
      2. May need long-term or lifetime iron replacement if unable to resolve the cause of the iron deficiency.

VIII. Referrals
  A. Consult physician if positive fecal occult blood or unexplained bleeding occurs.
  B. Refer to hematologist if patient fails to respond to iron supplementation.
  C. Consider IV iron infusion if no response to oral iron supplementation.

References

See page 681.

Chapter

117. Microangiopathic Hemolytic Anemia

Mary Pat Lynch, CRNP, MSN, AOCN®

I. Definition: Intravascular hemolysis caused by fragmentation of normal erythrocytes passing through abnormal arterioles

II. Pathophysiology
   A. Usually initiated with intravascular coagulation with deposition of platelets and fibrin in small arterioles
   B. Erythrocytes stick to fibrin and are fragmented by force of blood flow.
   C. Results in both intravascular and extravascular hemolysis

III. Clinical features
   A. Etiology
      1. Antineoplastic drugs (e.g., mitomycin, bleomycin, daunorubicin with cytosine arabinoside, cisplatin)
      2. Post-transplantation of kidney or liver, post allogeneic or autologous bone marrow transplant
      3. Generalized vasculitis
      4. Localized vascular disorders
      5. Invasive carcinomas
   B. History
      1. History of cancer and cancer treatment
      2. Current medications: Prescribed and over-the-counter
      3. History of presenting symptom(s): Precipitating factors, onset, and duration
      4. Changes in activities of daily living
   C. Signs and symptoms: Related to the underlying process
      1. Dyspnea on exertion
      2. Chest pain
      3. Fatigue and weakness
      4. Oliguria
      5. Anuria
   D. Physical exam: Related to the underlying process
      1. Integument exam
         a) Petechiae

   b) Pallor
   c) Edema
   2. Bleeding

IV. Diagnostic tests (see Tables 112-1 and 112-2)
   A. Laboratory
      1. Reticulocyte count increased
      2. Serum lactase dehydrogenase (LDH) increased
      3. Serum haptoglobin level decreased
      4. Peripheral smear reveals schistocytes, helmet cells, and burr cells
      5. Ferritin decreased secondary to iron deficiency because of urinary loss
      6. Direct Coombs test usually negative
   B. Radiology: Not indicated

V. Differential diagnosis
   A. Paroxysmal nocturnal hemoglobinuria (PNH)
   B. Paroxysmal cold hemoglobinuria
   C. Autoimmune hemolytic anemia
   D. Disseminated intravascular coagulation (see Chapter 119)
   E. Malignant hypertension (see Chapter 45)
   F. Thrombotic thrombocytopenic purpura (normal coagulation studies)
   G. Hemolytic uremic syndrome (normal coagulation studies)

VI. Treatment
   A. Directed toward management of underlying process
      1. If idiopathic thrombocytopenic purpura is confirmed, plasmapheresis or prednisone 60–80 mg/day po can be beneficial.
      2. Splenectomy is necessary in patients who fail other measures.
   B. Red blood cell transfusions
   C. Platelet transfusions if bleeding is caused by thrombocytopenia
   D. Heparin use is controversial because it can cause further bleeding.

VII. Referrals
   A. Hematologist: Management of hemolysis
   B. Appropriate specialist: Treatment of underlying process

References

See page 681.

118. Sickle Cell Anemia

Mary Pat Lynch, CRNP, MSN, AOCN®

I. Definition: Sickle cell anemia is a chronic, hereditary, hemolytic anemia characterized by sickle-shaped red blood cells (RBCs).

II. Pathophysiology
  A. Autosomal recessive genetic disorder, homozygous for hemoglobin S (Hb S)
  B. Abnormal Hb (Hb S) develops in place of normal Hb (Hb A).
  C. Patients with sickle cell trait are heterozygous and have approximately 25% Hb in abnormal form (Hb S); the remaining is normal (Hb A).
  D. Tissue injury secondary to obstruction of capillary flow from sickled erythrocytes

III. Clinical features: Marked by periods of wellness interspersed with episodes of deterioration; severity of symptoms varies widely among patients.
  A. Risk factors
    1. Prevalent in Africans and African Americans
    2. Lower frequency in people of Mediterranean ancestry
    3. Gene is present in all populations that have endured generations of exposure to malaria; patients with sickle cell trait have a selective advantage in surviving malarial infection.
    4. Excessive mortality has been reported among military recruits with sickle cell trait; extreme exertion is associated with higher risk of acidosis.
  B. History
    1. History of cancer and cancer treatment
    2. Current medications: Prescribed and over-the-counter
    3. History of presenting symptom(s): Precipitating factors (e.g., pain), onset, and duration
    4. Changes in activities of daily living
    5. Family history: Sickle cell anemia or trait, malaria exposure
    6. Past medical history: Vaso-occlusive crisis, anemia
  C. Signs and symptoms
    1. Patients with sickle cell trait are essentially asymptomatic except in cases of severe hypoxia.
    2. Vaso-occlusive crises are seen in patients with sickle cell.

      a) Precipitated by hypoxia, infection, high altitudes, stress, surgery, blood loss, dehydration; occasionally occur spontaneously

      b) Associated with sudden onset of acute pain in back, chest, and extremities that may last a few hours to a few days.

  D. Physical exam

    1. Acute: May be no physical findings

      a) Tachycardia

      b) Flow murmurs secondary to anemia

    2. Chronic

      a) Skin ulcers: Usually involve malleolus of ankles

      b) Splenomegaly: Unusual in homozygous sickle cell disease because of auto-infarction of spleen during childhood; seen in high sickle cell disease

      c) Hematuria

      d) Hepatomegaly

      e) Priapism (abnormal, painful, continued penile erection)

      f) Visual loss

IV. Diagnostic tests

  A. Laboratory (see Tables 112-1 and 112-2)

    1. CBC

      a) Normocytic, normochromic anemia

        (1) Common; typically no symptoms

        (2) Hematocrit usually 21%–31%

      b) Leukocytosis

      c) Thrombocytosis

    2. Peripheral smear

      a) Variation in RBC size and shape

      b) Sickle cells and target cells on smear

    3. Elevated reticulocyte count: If not elevated and hematocrit has dropped, suspect aplastic crisis.

    4. Hb electrophoresis: Presence of Hb S in sickle cell anemia; presence of Hb S and Hb A in sickle cell trait

  B. Radiology: Not indicated

V. Differential diagnosis

  A. Acute pulmonary infection (see Chapter 35)

  B. Acute hepatitis (see Chapter 69)

  C. Cholecystitis

VI. Treatment

  A. Therapy for vaso-occlusive crisis includes supportive care

    1. IV fluids, preferably with normal saline. Avoid lactated ringers because of risk of lactic acid.

    2. Analgesics (see Appendix 8a/b)

        a) Morphine sulfate is drug of choice: True allergy is rare, although itching is common.

        b) Diphenhydramine (Vistaril®, Pfizer Inc., New York, NY) may be used.

    3. Antibiotics: Give according to infectious source (see Appendix 1).

    4. Oxygen: Give only if oxygen saturation is less than 90%; routine oxygen supplementation should not be used because of risk of depressing erythropoiesis.

    5. RBC transfusion to replace prematurely destroyed red cells and to diminish percentage of Hb S in circulation in presence of severe anemic complications.

  B. Prevent vaso-occlusive crisis with hydroxyurea 10–30 mg/kg/day po. This works by enhancing fetal Hb (Hb F) production.

  C. Experimental treatment includes bone marrow transplant.

  D. Patient education includes pain control and genetic counseling for sickle cell trait.

VII. Follow-up

  A. Short-term: Determined by provider

  B. Long-term: Requires lifelong management of the disease, especially during exacerbation

VIII. Referrals: Sickle cell specialist or hematologist for evaluation and treatment

References

Baynes, R.D., & Cook, J.D. (1996). Current issues in iron deficiency. *Current Opinion in Hematology, 3*(2), 145–149.

Colon-Otero, G., Menke, D., & Hook, C.C. (1992). A practical approach to the differential diagnosis and evaluation of the adult patient with macrocytic anemia. *Medical Clinics of North America, 76,* 581–597.

Erickson, J.M. (1996). Anemia. *Seminars in Oncology Nursing, 12,* 2–14.

Fonseca, R., Tefferi, A. (1997). Practical aspects in the diagnosis and management of aplastic anemia. *American Journal of the Medical Sciences, 313,* 159–169.

Frenkel, E.P., Bick, R.L., & Rutherford, C.J. (1996). Anemia of malignancy. *Hematology-Oncology Clinics of North America, 10,* 861–873.

Kumpf, V.J. (1996). Parenteral iron supplementation. *Nutrition in Clinical Practice, 11*(4), 139–146.

Moliterno, A.R., & Spivak, J.L. (1996). Anemia of cancer. *Hematology-Oncology Clinics of North America, 10,* 345–363.

Moses, P.L., & Smith, R.E. (1995). Endoscopic evaluation of iron deficiency anemia. A guide to diagnostic strategy in older patients. *Postgraduate Medicine, 98,* 219–224.

Richer, S. (1997). A practical guide for differentiating between iron deficiency anemia and anemia of chronic disease in children and adults. *Nurse Practitioner, 22*(4), 82–103.

Rodgers, G.P. (1997). Overview of pathophysiology and rationale for treatment of sickle cell anemia. *Seminars in Hematology, 34*(Suppl. 3), 2–7.

Sears, D.A. (1992). Anemia of chronic disease. *Medical Clinics of North America, 76,* 567–577.

Steinberg, M.H. (1996). Sickle cell disease: Present and future treatment (Review). *American Journal of the Medical Sciences, 312,* 166–174.

Storb, R. (1997). Aplastic anemia. *Journal of Intravenous Nursing, 20,* 317–322.

119. Disseminated Intravascular Coagulation

Susan A. Ezzone, MS, RN, CNP

I. Definition: A disorder in which the coagulation pathways are excessively stimulated by various causes, resulting in thrombosis and hemorrhage

II. Physiology/Pathophysiology
   A. Normal
      1. Intrinsic (i.e., endothelial cell damage) and extrinsic (i.e., tissue injury) coagulation pathways are responsible for formation of fibrin clots and blood clotting, thereby maintaining hemostasis (see Figure 119-1).
      2. When the coagulation cascade is activated, plasmin and thrombin circulate, causing bleeding and clot formation, respectively.
   B. Pathophysiology
      1. Disseminated intravascular coagulation (DIC) results from abnormal procoagulant activation, fibrinolytic activation, inhibitor consumption, and biochemical evidence of end organ damage or failure.
      2. During rapid turnover of tumor or leukemic cells, a procoagulant is released from the cell and initiates the coagulation pathway, resulting in abnormal clotting and bleeding. Hemorrhage and/or microvascular or large-vessel thrombosis may occur, leading to ischemia and end organ damage.
      3. Platelet consumption with coagulation factor depletion occurs with stimulation of fibrinolysis.

III. Clinical features: DIC may be fulminant or low-grade, depending on the disease associated with triggering this syndrome.
   A. Etiology
      1. The intrinsic pathway can be activated by septicemia, urinary tract infection, hypotension, and acidosis.
      2. The extrinsic pathway can be activated by tissue injury caused by obstetrical complications, trauma, and hematologic or solid tumors.
      3. Solid tumor malignancies in which DIC occurs in 10% of patients include lung, pancreas, prostate, stomach, colon, ovary, gall bladder, breast, and kidney.
      4. The most common leukemia in which DIC occurs in about 85% of patients is acute promyelocytic leukemia.

Figure 119-1. Intrinsic and Extrinsic Pathways of the Blood Clotting Cascade

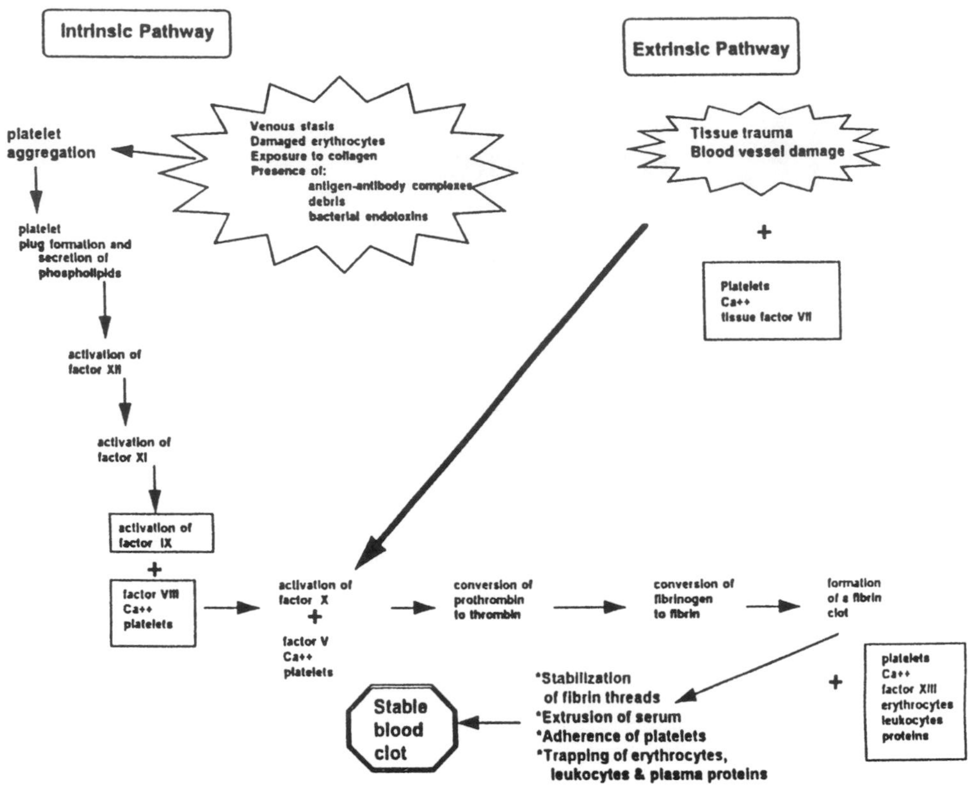

Intrinsic Pathway

Extrinsic Pathway

platelet aggregation

Venous stasis
Damaged erythrocytes
Exposure to collagen
Presence of:
    antigen-antibody complexes
    debris
    bacterial endotoxins

Tissue trauma
Blood vessel damage

platelet plug formation and secretion of phospholipids

+

Platelets
Ca++
tissue factor VII

activation of factor XII

activation of factor XI

activation of factor IX

+

factor VIII
Ca++
platelets

activation of factor X
+
factor V
Ca++
platelets

conversion of prothrombin to thrombin

conversion of fibrinogen to fibrin

formation of a fibrin clot

platelets
Ca++
factor XIII
erythrocytes
leukocytes
proteins

+

Stable blood clot

*Stabilization of fibrin threads
*Extrusion of serum
*Adherence of platelets
*Trapping of erythrocytes, leukocytes & plasma proteins

Note. From "Anticoagulants and Thrombolytics: What's the Difference?" by L.M. Workman, 1994, *AACN Clinical Issues, 5*(1), p. 30. Copyright 1994 by American Association of Critical-Care Nurses. Reprinted with permission.

    5. DIC can be manifested as acute or chronic.
        a) Acute: Bleeding occurs simultaneously from at least three sites associated with shock, respiratory failure, or renal failure.
        b) Chronic: Usually manifested with minimal bleeding and frequently seen in malignancy-induced condition.
  B. History
    1. History of cancer and cancer treatment
    2. Current medications: Prescribed and over-the-counter
    3. History of presenting symptom(s): Precipitating factors, onset, and duration
    4. Changes in activities of daily living
    5. Past medical history: Hepatitis, HIV, recent viral infection, recent burn, cardiovascular disease, autoimmune disease, renal disorder
  C. Signs and symptoms: From underlying disease
    1. Integument: Purpura, ecchymosis

    2. Gingival bleeding

    3. Epistaxis

    4. Hemoptysis

    5. Urine and stool with blood

    6. Heavily prolonged vaginal bleeding

    7. Peripheral edema secondary to fluid overload

D. Physical exam: Focus on hemodynamic stability and instability.

    1. Vital signs

        a) Tachycardia; weak, thready pulse

        b) Hypotension

        c) Narrow pulse pressure

        d) Tachypnea

    2. Integument exam

        a) Wounds, IV sites, and central lines for bleeding

        b) Ecchymosis, petechiae, purpura, and skin breakdown

        c) Sluggish capillary refill

        d) Cool, clammy skin

    3. HEENT exam

        a) Scleral hemorrhage

        b) Gingival or mucosal bleeding from oral cavity

        c) Epistaxis

    4. Abnormal sounds in lungs (e.g., rales), indicating signs of pulmonary edema from hemorrhage; respiratory compromise (e.g., accessory muscle use)

    5. Decreased peripheral pulses

    6. Neurologic exam every two to four hours

        a) Altered mental status, changes in level of consciousness

        b) Pupil reaction

    7. Abdominal exam: Tenderness and distention

IV. Diagnostic tests

A. Laboratory

    1. CBC

        a) Thrombocytopenia with platelet count < 50,000 mm^3

        b) Leukocytosis with a shift to the immature white blood cells

    2. Peripheral blood smear: Schistocytes (i.e., red blood cell fragments) may be present, indicating intravascular hemolysis.

    3. Increased reticulocyte count indicating presence of immature red blood cells: important because it suggests bone marrow synthetic ability and increased production in response to blood loss or destruction.

    4. Coagulation studies

        a) Prothrombin time/international normalized ratio (PT/INR): Shortened, normal, or prolonged

        b) Partial thromboplastin time (PTT): Shortened, normal, or prolonged

        c) Fibrinogen level < 150 mg/dl: usually decreased (normal = 195–365 mg/dl) *d)* Fibrinogen degradation products (FDPs)/fibrin split products (FSPs) > 40: usually elevated (normal = 10–40)

       e) Protamine sulfate test positive for fibrin

       f) Decreased antithrombin level: Thrombin and clotting factors complex with antithrombin

       g) Decreased plasminogen: Measure of fibrinolytic system activation by immunologic methods (normal = 10–20 mg/dl)

    5. Newer tests that may be used in the future for measuring DIC

       a) D-dimer assay: Elevated; specific for FDPs; measures a neoantigen, which is made when thrombin stimulates fibrinogen to form fibrin

       b) Fibrinopeptide A level: Elevated; procoagulant activation

       c) Plasmin: Elevated; measure of fibrinolytic system activation

       d) Prothrombin fragment (F I and II): Elevated; procoagulant activation

       e) Platelet factor IV: Elevated; measure of platelet reactivity and release

    6. Other: Guiac stool, emesis, and nasogastric tube secretions

  B. Radiology: Chest radiography (PA and lateral) to rule out acute respiratory distress syndrome

V. Differential diagnosis (see Figure 119-2)

Figure 119-2. Accepted Disease Entities Generally Associated with Disseminated Intravascular Coagulation

Fulminant DIC		Low-grade DIC

• Obstetric accidents
  - Amniotic fluid embolism
  - Placental abruption
  - Retained fetus syndrome
  - Eclampsia
  - Abortion
• Intravascular hemolysis
  - Hemolytic transfusion reactions
  - Minor hemolysis
  - Massive transfusions
• Septicemia
  - Gram-negative (endotoxin)
  - Gram-positive (mucopolysaccharides)
• Viremias
  - HIV
  - Hepatitis
  - Varicella
  - Cytomegalovirus
	• Metastatic malignancy
	• Leukemia
	  - Acute promyelocytic (M-3)
	  - Acute myelomonocytic (M-4)
	  - Many others
	• Burns
	• Crash injuries and tissue necrosis
	• Trauma
	• Acute liver disease
	  - Obstructive jaundice
	  - Acute hepatic failure
	• Prosthetic devices
	  - LeVeen or Denver shunts
	  - Aortic balloon assist devices
	• Vascular disorders
		• Cardiovascular diseases
		• Autoimmune diseases
		• Renal vascular disorders
		• Hematologic disorders
		• Inflammatory disorders
		• Cancer of the prostate

Note. From "Disseminated Intravascular Coagulation: Objective Clinical and Laboratory Diagnosis, Treatment, and Assessment of Therapeutic Response," by R.L. Bick, 1996, *Seminars in Thrombosis and Hemostasis,* 22(1), p. 70. Copyright 1996 by Thieme New York. Reprinted with permission.

VI. Treatment
   A. Treat underlying cause or disease process (e.g., infection, malignancy).
   B. Eliminate the triggering cause (e.g., septicemia, shock, obstetrical complications, chemotherapy, other therapies) such as antibiotic therapy for treatment of sepsis
   C. Outpatient treatment of chronic DIC
      1. Subcutaneous heparin may be used at doses of 80–100 units/kg every four to six hours.
      2. Administer 10 mg prophylactic medroxyprogesterone acetate (Provera®, Pharmacia & Upjohn, Peapack, NJ) po every day to prevent vaginal bleeding.
      3. Avoid medications that interfere with platelet function (e.g., aspirin-containing products, nonsteroidal anti-inflammatory drugs).
   D. Acute-care setting treatment of DIC
      1. Monitor hemodynamic status and vital signs frequently and maintain blood pressure ≥ 90 mm Hg systolic.
         a) Vital signs: Monitor every one to two hours; use IV vasopressor (e.g., dopamine) to maintain pressure (give doses of 5–20 mcg/kg/minute).
         b) Central venous pressure: Monitor and maintain at 5–12 mm Hg by administration of IV fluids or diuretics.
         c) Monitor daily weight, intake, and output to avoid dehydration or fluid overload.
      2. Heparin therapy
         a) Heparin therapy may be used to treat DIC to
            (1) Inhibit action of thrombin, which interrupts the clotting cycle and conversion of fibrinogen to fibrin.
            (2) Block intrinsic and extrinsic pathways by inhibiting Factor X, slowing clot formation.
         b) Heparin therapy is contraindicated in acute promyelocytic leukemia because of the increased risk of death related to hemorrhage. These patients should be treated with all-transretinoic acid and supported through their coagulopathy with platelets and plasma.
         c) IV heparin titrated to maintain the PTT at 1½–2 times normal.
            (1) Usually initiated at 100–200 units/kg/24 hours or 20,000–30,000 units/24 hours.
            (2) Various doses have been reported.
      3. Antithrombin concentrates may be used for moderate to severe DIC and administered every eight hours.
         a) Dose calculation total units needed = (desired level – initial level) x total body weight (kg).
         b) Clinical trials are necessary to determine efficacy for use in DIC.
      4. Epsilon-aminocaproic acid (EACA) IV infusions at 1 g/hour are controversial because EACA inhibits the fibrinolytic system and can lead to organ failure from large vessel thrombosis.
         a) The initial dose of EACA is 5–10 g IV push, then 2–4 g/hour.
         b) Therapy is continued for 24 hours or until bleeding stops.
      5. Newer agents used in DIC include recombinant hirudin, tranexamic acid, defibrotide, and gabexate, but clinical experience is limited.

6. Antifibrinolytic therapy may be used in acute promyelocytic leukemia or if bleeding continues despite other treatments.
7. Administer diuretics for treatment of fluid overload as necessary.
8. Replace fluid/volume (e.g., normal saline) as needed for hypovolemia.

E. Transfuse platelets as needed.
   1. Maintain platelet count > 50,000/mm³; usually platelet product will increase total platelets by at least 25,000 units.

F. Red blood cells may be administered to maintain a hemoglobin > 8 g if the patient is at risk for hemodynamic compromise.

G. Transfusion of blood components that contain fibrinogen (e.g., fresh frozen plasma, cryoprecipitate, whole blood) should be avoided, as they may be associated with increased hemorrhage and thrombosis during acute DIC.

H. Administer medications (e.g., antiemetics, cough suppressants) to control symptoms of nausea, vomiting, and cough, which may increase intracranial pressure causing scleral or intracranial hemorrhage.

VII. Follow-up
   A. Patients most often require hospitalization for close monitoring of signs and symptoms of acute bleeding or thrombosis.
   B. Patients with chronic DIC may be closely monitored in the outpatient setting through PT, PTT, fibrinogen, and antithrombin levels.

VIII. Referrals: Consult hematologist if
   A. Bleeding persists despite interventions.
   B. DIC is diagnosed during initial evaluation; referral is based on underlying condition.

References

Bick, R.L. (1996). Disseminated intravascular coagulation: Objective clinical and laboratory diagnosis, treatment, and assessment of therapeutic response. *Seminars in Thrombosis and Hemostasis, 22*(1), 69–88.

Kurtz, A. (1993). Disseminated intravascular coagulation with leukemia patients. *Cancer Nursing, 16,* 456–463.

Rohaly-Davis, J., & Johnson, K. (1996). Hematologic emergencies in the intensive care unit. *Critical Care Nursing Quarterly, 18*(4), 35–43.

Workman, L.M. (1994). Anticoagulants and thrombolytics: What's the difference? *AACN Clinical Issues, 5*(1), 26–35.

Chapter

120. Idiopathic Thrombocytopenic Purpura

Mary Pat Lynch, CRNP, MSN, AOCN®

I. Definition: An acquired disease characterized by a low platelet count, a normal marrow, and absence of evidence for other diseases

II. Pathophysiology
   A. Thrombocytopenia appears to be immune-mediated and caused by destruction of platelets and splenic sequestration (platelet dyscrasia).
      1. Most patients have either normal or decreased platelet production.
      2. Antiplatelet antibodies bind to megakaryocytes and cause ineffective thrombocytopoiesis.
   B. Platelet destruction may be due to binding immunoglobulin G (IgG) autoantibodies to circulating platelets resulting in platelet destruction by phagocytes in the spleen and liver.

III. Clinical features: In children, idiopathic thrombocytopenic purpura (ITP) is acute in onset and resolves spontaneously within six months; in adults, ITP is insidious in nature and rarely resolves spontaneously.
   A. Etiology: In 15%–20% of patients, thrombocytopenia is associated with an underlying disease and may be considered secondary ITP.
      1. Excess levels of paraproteins in patients with lymphoma, multiple myeloma, and Waldenstrom's macroglobulinemia can cause thrombocytopenia.
      2. Overt bleeding is rare.
   B. History
      1. History of cancer and cancer treatment
      2. Current medications: Prescribed and over-the-counter
      3. History of presenting symptom(s): Precipitating factors, onset, and duration
      4. Changes in activities of daily living
   C. Signs and symptoms
      1. Greater than two-month history of purpura
      2. Petechiae
      3. Menorrhagia (heavy menstrual bleeding)
      4. Epistaxis
      5. Oral cavity bleeding
   D. Physical exam

1. Integument exam
   a) Petechiae, often in dependent regions
   b) Purpura
   c) Ecchymosis
2. Gingival bleeding
3. Splenomegaly strongly suggests ITP, however, is <u>not</u> the cause of thrombocytopenia.

IV. Diagnostic tests (see Table 112-1)
   A. Laboratory
      1. CBC
         a) Decreased platelet count, less than 20,000 mm^3
         b) White blood cell and hemoglobin usually are normal.
      2. Peripheral blood smear: To rule out pseudothrombocytopenia (i.e., a laboratory phenomenon caused by clumping of platelets and EDTA, the preservative found in the blood tubes)
      3. Coagulation studies
         a) Normal: Evaluate bleeding time
         b) Abnormal: Consider disseminated intravascular coagulation (DIC) or Von Willebrand's disease
      4. Bone marrow studies: Increased megakarocytes in the bone marrow is the classic finding.
   B. Radiology: Not indicated

V. Differential diagnosis
   A. Acute infection
   B. Myelodysplasia
   C. Chronic DIC (see Chapter 119)
   D. Drug-induced thrombocytopenia (i.e., chemotherapy-induced) (see Chapter 123)
   E. Congenital thrombocytopenia

VI. Treatment
   A. Spontaneous remissions are rare in adults but occur frequently in children.
   B. Asymptomatic mild or moderate thrombocytopenia
      1. Follow with observation and without treatment.
      2. Evaluate for underlying cause (e.g., autoantibodies).
   C. Severe thrombocytopenia with acute bleeding
      1. Platelet transfusions for platelet counts less than 10,000 mm^3 and/or bleeding
         a) Recheck count six hours after transfusion.
         b) Single-donor platelets are preferable to reduce the risk of sensitization to platelet proteins.
      2. IV IgG single infusion 0.4–0.1 g/kg followed immediately by platelet transfusion
      3. High-dose glucocorticoid (e.g., methylprednisolone) 1 g IV daily for three days followed by prednisone 1–2 mg/kg po daily; alternatively, dexamethasone 40 mg IV daily for four days every month

    4. Aminocaproic acid (Amicar®, Immunex Corporation, Seattle, WA) to help control acute bleeding given IV and po
       a) 5 g loading dose IV then 1 g/hour IV or 2 g every two hours po
       b) Usually stopped after 8–24 hours
  D. Splenectomy: Offers complete, permanent responses in 60% of patients; short course of radiation therapy to spleen recommended for those who cannot tolerate surgery
  E. Chronic, refractory ITP
    1. IV IgG may be helpful, especially when a situation requires a transient increase in the platelet count.
       a) Given 2 g/kg over two to five days, platelet count will usually increase after several days and return to pretreatment level in several weeks.
       b) This may cause a transient drop in hematocrit.
       c) Implement maintenance therapy with single infusion of 60 g when count falls below 20,000 mm^3.
    2. Rhogam (WinRho SDF™, Nabi®, Boca Raton, FL) used for maintenance therapy with success seen in AIDS and ITP.

VII. Follow-up: Short-term
  A. Monitor platelet count closely if severe thrombocytopenia (see above).
  B. Monitor platelet count monthly for mild to moderate thrombocytopenia.

VIII. Referrals
  A. Hematologist: Consult for appropriate diagnostic work-up and treatment plan.
  B. Physician: May manage patient collaboratively long-term

References

Diagnosis and treatment of idiopathic thrombocytopenic purpura. American Society of Hematology ITP Practice Guideline Panel. (1996). *American Family Physician, 54,* 2451–2452.

Diehl, L.F., & Ketchum, L.H. (1998). Autoimmune disease and chronic lymphocytic leukemia: Autoimmune hemolytic anemia, pure red cell aplasia, and autoimmune thrombocytopenia. *Seminars in Oncology, 25,* 80–97.

George, J.N. (1996). Diagnosis, clinical course and management of idiopathic thrombocytopenic purpura. *Current Opinion in Hematology, 3,* 335–340.

Gillis, S. (1996). The thrombocytopenic purpuras. Recognition and management. *Drugs, 51,* 942–953.

Warkentin, T.E., & Smith, J.W. (1997). The alloimmune thrombocytopenic syndromes. *Transfusion Medicine Reviews, 11,* 296–307.

Chapter

121.

Neutropenia

Mary Pat Lynch, CRNP, MSN, AOCN®

I. Definition: An absolute neutrophil count (ANC) of < 1,000 cells/mm^3

II. Physiology/Pathophysiology
   A. Normal physiology
      1. Neutrophils are produced from the myeloid stem cell, as well as eosinophils, basophils, and monocytes (i.e., macrophages), and collectively are called granulocytes.
      2. Lymphoid stem cells produce T-lymphocytes and B-lymphocytes, which are responsible for the role of specific immunity cell-mediated and humoral immunity, respectively.
      3. The primary role of granulocytes is to ingest and destroy microorganisms and release chemical mediators that enhance and prolong the inflammatory response.
         a) Neutrophils make up 50%–60% of all circulating white blood cells (WBCs) and are vital components in the nonspecific immune response.
         b) Neutrophils act through phagocytosis and the stimulation of other WBCs.
   B. Pathophysiology: The decrease of neutrophils impairs nonspecific immunity resulting in infection.

III. Clinical features: The frequency of infection increases as the ANC falls below 500 and the longer the patient remains neutropenic.
   A. Risk factors
      1. Disease-related conditions
         a) Comorbid conditions (e.g., diabetes mellitus, chronic obstructive pulmonary disease)
         b) Poor performance status
      2. Poor nutritional status
      3. Treatment-related conditions
         a) Implanted devices
         b) High dose, combination, and dose-intensive chemotherapy
         c) Multimodality treatment
      4. Prolonged neutropenia (> 7 days) increases risk of fungal infections.
   B. Etiology: Neutropenia can be classified as
      1. Disorder of neutrophil production

    2. Disorder of neutrophil distribution

    3. Drug-induced neutropenia

    4. Neutropenia associated with infectious diseases.

        a) Febrile neutropenia is considered a potentially life-threatening emergency. Mortality rates during the first 48 hours range from 18%–40%.

        b) Gram-negative bacteria are the most common cause of infection in patients with cancer.

            (1) Other causes include gram-positive bacteria, viruses, fungi, and protozoa.

            (2) More than 80% of infections are from the patient's endogenous flora, usually acquired during hospitalization.

        c) Half of neutropenic patients have unexplained fever with negative evaluation.

        d) Most common sites of infection include

            (1) Respiratory tract

            (2) Gastrointestinal tract (i.e., *Escherichia coli*)

            (3) Genitourinary tract

            (4) Skin and mucous membranes

            (5) CNS

            (6) Systemic

            (7) Implanted devices

C. History

    1. History of cancer and cancer treatment

    2. Current medications: Prescribed and over-the-counter

    3. History of presenting symptom(s): Precipitating factors, onset, and duration

    4. Changes in activities of daily living

D. Signs and symptoms

    1. Fever: Temperature of 100.5°F (38.8°C) or greater is considered a fever in a neutropenic patient.

    2. Confusion or somnolence

    3. Productive cough

    4. Headache

    5. Dysuria

    6. Vaginal discharge

    7. Skin lesions with swelling and tenderness

    8. Diarrhea

    9. Sore throat

    10. Discomfort at site of indwelling catheters

    11. Neck stiffness

E. Physical exam

    1. Vital signs

        a) Fever

        b) Hypotension and tachycardia suggest sepsis

    2. Subtle change in mental status (e.g., restlessness, irritability, somnolence, confusion)

    3. Integument exam

        a) Open lesions (e.g., stomatitis)

        b) Edema, erythema, and/or tenderness of skin, especially at pressure areas, biopsy sites, and sites of venous access devices

        c) Perianal

    4. HEENT: Sinus tenderness

    5. Lungs: Decreased breath sounds, crackles, egophony, bronchial breath sounds

    6. Abdominal tenderness

    7. Costovertebral angle (CVA) tenderness

IV. Diagnostic tests

  A. Laboratory

    1. Decreased WBC count

        a) ANC < 1,000 cells per cubic millimeter

        b) ANC = total WBC x (% segmented neutrophils + % bands)

    2. Peripheral blood smear: Evaluate for atypical lymphocytes, abnormal cells that induced the depression in neutrophils

    3. Bone marrow exam: To rule out leukemia and myelodysplasia; may show fibrosis, hypoplasia, or atypical cells

    4. Blood chemistries: To evaluate electrolytes, renal and hepatic function; to rule out hemolysis, obstruction

    5. Arterial blood gases: If sepsis suspected to assess for associated metabolic acidosis

    6. Blood culture

        a) One set of aerobic and one set of anaerobic cultures obtained from at least two different peripheral sites

        b) Patients with vascular access devices should have one set taken from each lumen.

    7. Urinalysis and urine culture, even if asymptomatic

    8. Stool for WBC, ova and parasites, culture, *Clostridium difficile* antigen if patient has diarrhea

  B. Radiology

    1. Chest x-ray

        a) Pulmonary infiltrates are commonly seen in pneumonia; however, an infiltrate requires the presence of neutrophils to mount a response.

        b) Pulmonary infiltrates will often appear on follow-up x-rays when WBC has risen.

    2. Kidneys, ureter, and bladder (KUB) x-ray is performed to assess bowel gas pattern if patient is symptomatic. Typhlitis may occur in patients with prolonged neutropenia and is 80% fatal; this diagnosis is suggested by gaseous distention and/or the presence of gas in the bowel wall.

  C. Other

    1. Lumbar puncture: If CNS source is suspected

    2. Culture skin lesions

    3. Fungal and viral cultures: For patient with persistent febrile neutropenia without an identified source

    4. Gram stains of lesion or body fluid: To assess for bacterial infection

    5. Consider culture for acid-fast bacilli: If TB suspected

6. Patients with prolonged neutropenia and interstitial pulmonary infiltrates should be assessed for herpes zoster and cytomegalovirus.

V. Differential diagnosis
   A. Leukemia
   B. Aplastic anemia (see Chapter 113)
   C. Myelodysplastic syndrome
   D. Drug-induced conditions
     1. Phenothiazine
     2. Antithyroid drugs
     3. Chloramphenicol
     4. Chemotherapy
   E. Radiation treatment (especially to chest and large bones)
   F. Benign cyclic neutropenia
   G. Chronic idiopathic neutropenia
   H. Nutritional deficits, B_{12} (see Chapter 114), folate (see Chapter 115), copper (rare)
   I. Autoimmune neutropenia
   J. HIV disease (see Chapter 156)

VI. Treatment
   A. Initial treatment focuses on hemodynamic stabilization of the patient and eradication of organism.
   B. Once fever workup is complete; a course of empiric antibiotics is started within one hour of admission without waiting for culture results.
     1. When results are available, therapy can be modified to treat the identified organism (see Table 121-1).
     2. Usually consists of broad-spectrum antibiotics directed at both gram-positive and gram-negative organisms. Possible treatment plans: Antibiotic regimens vary widely with institutional and geographic location.
       a) Two beta-lactam antibiotics (e.g., aztreonam + ceftazidime)
       b) A beta-lactam and an aminoglycoside (e.g., piperacillin + tobramycin)
         (1) Avoid aminoglycosides if patient received nephrotoxic chemotherapy.
         (2) A quinolone can be substituted for an aminoglycoside, which provides adequate coverage.
       c) Monotherapy with an extended spectrum cephalosporin (e.g., ceftazidime) or carbapenem (e.g., imipenem)
       d) Commonly used beta-lactam antibiotics include extended spectrum penicillin, extended spectrum cephalosporins, and monobactam.
       e) Use of a third drug has not been shown to increase efficacy.
     3. Continue empiric therapy until resolution of the neutropenia or negative blood culture. If positive blood culture occurs, obtain follow-up blood cultures every 24–48 hours to ensure organism has been adequately treated.
   C. Persistent fevers that fail to respond to antibacterial drugs usually require empiric treatment with antifungal agents. Amphotericin B, at least 1 mg/kg/day IV; total dose determined upon clinical status, infection resolution, and marrow recovery.

Table 121-1. Commonly Used Antibiotics for Managing Infection in Patients With Cancer

Class of Antibiotic	Agent(s)	Spectrum	Usual Daily Dose
Third-generation cephalosporins	Ceftazidime	Gram −, some gram +, pseudomonas	100 mg/kg divided q8h IV
Third-generation cephalosporins	Ceftriaxone	Gram −, gram + except enterococci	1–2 g/d or 1–2 g/bid IV or IM
Carbapenums	Imipenum/cilastatin	Most gram +, gram −, including pseudomonas	50 mg/kg divided q6h IV
Monobactams	Azetreonam	Gram − aerobes only, including pseudomonas	100–150 mg/kg divided q6h IV
Extended spectrum penicillins	Piperacillin	Enteric aerobes, including pseudomonas, enterobacter; anaerobes	300 mg/kg divided q4h IV
Aminoglycosides	Gentamicin	Gram −, including pseudonomas, some gram + w/penicillin	1.0–1.7 mg/kg IV or IM q8h; adjust for renal function
Aminoglycosides	Tobramycin	Similar to gentamicin; more active versus pseudonomas	Same as gentamicin
Glycopeptides	Vancomycin	Gram + only, including MRSA[a], C. difficile[b]	25–40 mg/kg divided q6–12 h IV,
Quinolones	Trovafloxacin	Broad spectrum	100–200 mg IV over 60 minutes, then 100–200 mg po qd for 7–14 days

[a] MRSA – methicillin-resistant *Staphylococcus aureus*
[b] *C. difficile* – *Clostridium difficile*

   D. American Society of Clinical Oncology (ASCO) guidelines for use of filgrastim (Neupogen®, Amgen, Inc., Thousand Oaks, CA) growth factor to increase WBC count
     1. Recommended for use as prophylaxis with dose-intensive chemotherapy associated with a high incidence of febrile neutropenia
     2. Recommended for use as prophylaxis with subsequent cycles after one episode of febrile neutropenia if chemotherapy doses are not reduced
     3. Not recommended for neutropenic but afebrile patients
     4. Not recommended for use during febrile neutropenia except for those patients with poor prognostic factors
     5. Dose 5 mcg/kg/day SC or IVuntil ANC > 5,000 (available in 300 or 480 mcg vials)
   E. Outpatient management of febrile neutropenia is feasible alternative for selected low-risk patients with ANC > 1,000.
     1. Minimal or no documented site of infection
     2. No high-risk comorbidity (e.g., diabetes mellitus, COPD)
     3. Short duration of neutropenia anticipated

4. No symptoms of hard chills
5. Blood cultures and urine cultures should be obtained; patient should be started on the same antibiotic principles listed above, usually selecting the long-acting antibiotics.

VII. Follow-up: Short-term
A. For inpatients, evaluate daily and review vital signs, physical exam and lab values, fever curve, culture results.
B. For outpatients, call patient daily, recommend office visit at least two to three times per week for physical exam, lab values, culture results, and antibiotic levels, if appropriate.

VIII. Referrals
A. Physician: For evaluation, diagnostic work-up, treatment plan
B. May manage the patient collaboratively with the physician

References

Abramowicz, M. (Ed.). (1998). The choice of antibacterial drugs. *The Medical Letter, 40, 1023,* 33–42.

DeLalla, F. (1997). Antibiotic treatment of febrile episodes in neutropenic cancer patients. Clinical and economic considerations. *Drugs, 53,* 789–804.

Elting, L.S., Rubenstein, E.B., Rolston, K.V., & Bodey, G.P. (1997). Outcomes of bacteremia in patients with cancer and neutropenia: Observations from two decades of epidemiological and clinical trials. *Clinical Infectious Diseases, 25,* 247–259.

Engervall, P., & Bjorkholm, M. (1996). Infections in neutropenic patients. II: Management. *Medical Oncology, 13*(1), 63–69.

Malik, I.A., Khan, W.A., & Karim, M. (1995). Feasibility of outpatient management of fever in cancer patients with low-risk neutropenia: Results of a prospective randomized trial. *American Journal of Medicine, 98,* 224–231.

Meisenberg, B., Gollard, R., Brehm, T., McMillan, R., & Miller, W. (1997). Prophylactic antibiotics eliminate bacteremia and allow safe outpatient management following high-dose chemotherapy and autologous stem cell rescue. *Supportive Care in Cancer, 4,* 364–390.

Pizzo, P. (1993). Drug therapy: Management of fever in patients with cancer and treatment-induced neutropenia. *New England Journal of Medicine, 328,* 1323–1332.

Rubenstein, E.B, Rolston, K., Benjamin, R.S., Loewy, J., Escalante, C., Manzullo, E., Hughes, P., Moreland, B., Fender, A., Kennedy, K., et al. (1993). Outpatient treatment of febrile episodes in low risk neutropenic patients with cancer. *Cancer, 71,* 3640–3646.

Rubin, R.H., & Ferraro, M.J. (1993). Understanding and diagnosing infections in the immuno-compromised host. *Hematology Oncology Clinics of North America, 7,* 795–812.

122. Polycythemia Vera

Mary Pat Lynch, CRNP, MSN, AOCN®

I. Definition: A clonal disorder of the hematopoietic stem cells associated with proliferation of red cells, white cells, and platelets, with the erythroid series being the predominant cell line
  A. Polycythemia vera is one of the three myeloproliferative disorders.
  B. Other disorders include myelofibrosis with myeloid metaplasia and essential thrombocytopenia.

II. Pathophysiology
  A. Marrow-derived erythroid colonies develop without the stimulation of added erythropoietin.
  B. May evolve into idiopathic myelofibrosis, myelodysplasia, and/or acute leukemia.

III. Clinical features: Thrombotic events occur in 30% of patients prior to diagnosis and in 40%–60% over first 10 years. This is the cause of 40% of cases of unexplained hepatic vein thrombosis (i.e., Budd-Chiari syndrome).
  A. Risk factors
    1. More common in Eastern European Jewish people
    2. Insidious onset (average age 60) but may occur in children or young adults
  B. Phases of polycythemia
    1. Erythrocytic phase: Persistent erythrocytosis that necessitates regular phlebotomies; lasts 5–25 years; signs and symptoms depend on comorbid conditions.
    2. Burned out phase: Need for phlebotomies is greatly reduced, patient enters a long period of apparent remission, spleen increases in size but little marrow fibrosis is present.
    3. Myelofibrotic phase: Develops in 10% of patients; increases over the course of polycythemia vera; when cytopenia and progressive splenomegaly develop, the clinical manifestations and course become similar to myelofibrosis with myeloid metaplasia.
    4. Terminal phase: In 35%–50% of patients with polycythemia vera, death results from thrombotic or hemorrhagic complications.
  C. History
    1. History of cancer and cancer treatment
    2. Current medications: Prescribed and over-the-counter

3. History of presenting symptom(s): Precipitating factors, location, and duration. Associated symptom is pruritus after bathing, which occurs in 40% of patients and is a specific complaint suggesting the diagnosis.
4. Changes in activities of daily living
5. Family history: Familial incidence has been reported occasionally.
6. Past medical history: For peptic ulcer disease and gout, which are both associated disorders

D. Signs and symptoms: Vary depending on clinical course
   1. Predominant in early phase: Plethora—secondary to increased red cell mass, the over fullness of blood vessels, or the total quantity of any fluid in the body.
   2. Hyperviscosity will result in
      a) Headache
      b) Weakness
      c) Pruritus, especially after bathing
      d) Dizziness
      e) Sweating
      f) Vertigo
      g) Diplopia
   3. Hemorrhagic
      a) Epistaxis
      b) Easy bruising
   4. Erythromelalgia: Painful burning of finger tips

E. Physical exam
   1. Integument exam
      a) Petechiae
      b) Ecchymosis
      c) Dry skin, excoriation from itching
   2. Abdominal exam
      a) Splenomegaly
      b) Hepatomegaly
   3. Facial plethora

IV. Diagnostic tests
   A. Laboratory
      1. CBC
         a) Elevated erythrocyte count: May be out of proportion to the hemoglobin and hematocrit in patients who have had gastrointestinal blood loss or phlebotomy
         b) Red cell mass elevated in proportion to the hematocrit
         c) Absolute neutrophilia in approximately 60% of patients
         d) Platelet count increased in most patients
      2. Reticulocyte count slightly increased
      3. Prothrombin time/partial thromboplastin time/International Normalized Ratio (PT/PTT/INR) may appear prolonged if the amount of anticoagulant used in the test is not adjusted for the increased hematocrit.
      4. Elevated B_{12} level

     5. Increased serum uric acid level

     6. Normal or near-normal arterial oxygen saturation

     7. Check blood carboxyhemoglobin level (should be < 5%) in patients who smoke or have history of chronic lung disease.

  B. Radiology: Not indicated except to demonstrate the presence of splenic enlargement by abnormal ultrasound

V. Differential diagnosis

  A. Secondary polycythemia (secondary to high altitude acclimatization, pulmonary disease, cardiovascular disease, tissue hypoxia)

  B. Pure erythrocytosis

VI. Treatment

  A. Early-phase treatment focuses on controlling symptoms, decreasing risk of hemorrhage, and/or thrombotic events.

  B. Phlebotomy: 450–500 ml to target hematocrit < 42%–47%

     1. Induces iron deficiency but iron supplementation may result in rapid reappearance of polycythemia.

     2. Phlebotomy may be utilized for years.

  C. Myelosuppressive agents may be used for patients with advanced age, extreme thrombocytosis, thrombotic or bleeding complications, and severe systemic complaints not responding to phlebotomy with control observed in two to four months.

     1. Hydroxyurea 15–30 mg/kg/d po: Short duration, requires continuous monitoring of patient

     2. Other treatments

        a) Alpha interferon three to five million units SC three to five times per week

        b) Radioactive phosphorus

  D. Supportive care

     1. Treatment of pruritus (see Chapter 14)

        a) Cool water showers and baths

        b) Avoidance of vigorous skin rubbing

        c) H_1 or H_2 blockers such as ranitidine, diphenhydramine

        d) Ultraviolet light therapy

     2. Erythromelalgia: Treat with aspirin, indomethacin, and cytotoxic drugs to reduce platelet count.

     3. Anticoagulation therapy (see Chapter 41)

  E. Late phase is associated with anemia, progressive splenomegaly, signs of myelofibrosis and myeloid metaplasia, thrombosis, and hemorrhage.

     1. Extramedullary hematopoiesis may be a frequent finding as myelofibrosis progresses.

     2. Treatment is supportive/symptomatic only.

VII. Follow-up

  A. Short-term

     1. Monitor hematocrit every one to two weeks after each phlebotomy.

   2. Monitor hematocrit every month while on hydroxyurea until stable, then every two to three months.
  B. Long-term
   1. Follow hematocrit monthly.
   2. Prognosis is generally good with long-term survival.

VIII. Referrals: Hematologist: For complete evaluation and treatment plan; collaborate for long-term care.

References

Barbui, T., & Finazzi, G. (1997). Risk factors and prevention of vascular complications in polycythemia vera. *Seminars in Thrombosis and Hemostasis, 23,* 455–461.

Bilgrami, S., & Greenberg, B.R. (1995). Polycythemia rubra vera. *Seminars in Oncology, 22,* 307–326.

Elliott, M.A., & Tefferi, A. (1997). Interferon-alfa therapy in polycythemia vera and essential thrombocythemia. *Seminars in Thrombosis and Hemostasis, 23,* 463–472.

Knoop, T. (1996). Polycythemia vera. *Seminars in Oncology Nursing, 12,* 70–77.

Tefferi, A., Elliott, M.A., Solberg, L.A., & Silverstein, M.N. (1997). New drugs in essential thrombocythemia and polycythemia vera. *Blood Reviews, 11*(1), 1–7.

Chapter

123. Thrombocytopenia
Mary Pat Lynch, CRNP, MSN, AOCN®

I. Definition: A decreased number of platelets in the circulating blood

II. Physiology/Pathophysiology
   A. Normal physiology: Platelets are developed in the bone marrow from megakarocytes.
      1. Platelets prevent blood loss by adhesion with other platelets to block small breaks in blood vessels and capillaries.
      2. Platelets secrete chemicals (e.g., prostaglandins) that cause the broken vessel to constrict and partially close the broken area and initiate coagulation of the blood.
   B. Pathophysiology: Thrombocytopenia results from
      1. Deficient production of platelets
      2. Accelerated platelet destruction
      3. Abnormal distribution or pooling of the platelets within the body.

III. Clinical features
   A. Etiology
      1. Deficient production of platelets
         a) Marrow injury by myelosuppressive drugs
         b) Marrow injury from radiation
         c) Aplastic anemia
      2. Accelerated platelet destruction: Most common cause of thrombocytopenia
         a) Idiopathic thrombocytopenic purpura (ITP)
         b) Drug-induced antibodies
         c) Hemolytic anemia
         d) Systemic lupus erythematosus
         e) Isoantibody from transfusion
         f) Disseminated intravascular coagulation (DIC)
         g) Thrombotic thrombocytopenic purpura
      3. Abnormal distribution or pooling of the platelets within the body
         a) Various disorders associated with splenomegaly
            (1) Malignancy (e.g., non-Hodgkin's lymphoma, chronic lymphocytic leukemia)
            (2) Infection

   (3) Congestive or infiltrative processes

   (4) Chronic liver disease

  b) Platelet production is normal or increased, but most of the platelets are seques-tered in the enlarged spleen.

B. History

 1. History of cancer and cancer treatment

 2. Current medications: Prescribed and over-the-counter

 3. History of presenting symptom(s): Precipitating factors, onset, and duration

 4. Changes in activities of daily living

 5. Family history: Hereditary thrombocytopenia

 6. History of drug ingestion or exposure to toxic substances

C. Signs and symptoms: The following spontaneous hemorrhagic manifestations are usually seen only when the platelet count drops below $20,000/\text{mm}^3$.

 1. Petechiae: Often in dependent regions and over bony prominences

 2. Ecchymoses: Particularly on back and thighs

 3. Hemorrhagic vesicles or bullae inside mouth and on other mucous membranes

 4. Gingival bleeding

 5. Epistaxis

 6. Menorrhagia

 7. Hematuria

 8. Gastrointestinal bleeding (e.g., melena, hematemesis)

 9. Prolonged bleeding from injection sites

D. Physical exam

 1. Integument exam

  a) Petechiae

  b) Purpura

  c) Ecchymoses

  d) Changes in mucous membranes of mouth or palms: Ecchymosis usually presents as darkening of the skin in people of color.

 2. HEENT exam

  a) Gingival bleeding

  b) Icterus

 3. Abdominal exam

  a) Splenomegaly

  b) Hepatomegaly

 4. Lymph nodes: Lymphadenopathy

 5. Neurological exam: Assess for changes in mental status indicating intracranial hemorrhage.

IV. Diagnostic tests

A. Laboratory

 1. CBC

  a) Thrombocytopenia

  b) Low hematocrit and hemoglobin if large blood loss has occurred

  c) Normal white blood cell count and differential

    2. Peripheral blood smear
       a) Abnormalities of platelet size and morphologic characteristic (e.g., giant forms, bizarre shapes, deeply stained forms)
       b) Rule out pseudothrombocytopenia (i.e., platelet clumping from a reaction with the EDTA, a preservative found in the test tube used to collect the blood)
       c) Schistocytes in large volume blood loss
    3. Mean platelet volume increased with high numbers of large platelets
    4. Platelet distribution width increased with abnormal degree of platelet anisocytosis
    5. Normal coagulation studies in uncomplicated thrombocytopenia
    6. Increased lactic dehydrogenase (LDH) if large volume of red blood cell loss (i.e, in hemolytic anemia)
    7. Platelet antibody testing for isoimmune, drug-induced thrombocytopenia
    8. Confirmation of cause of thrombocytopenia with DIC screen exhibiting three of the following
       a) Increased fibrin split products or D-dimer
       b) Prolonged prothrombin time
       c) Prolonged partial thromboplastin time
       d) Prolonged thrombin time
       e) Decreased fibrinogen level.

V. Differential diagnosis
  A. Pseudothrombocytopenia
  B. Myelodysplasia
  C. Liver disease (see Chapters 64 and 69)
  D. Occult carcinoma
  E. Sarcoidosis
  F. Systemic lupus erythematosus
  G. Sepsis (see Chapters 121 and 140)
  H. Aplastic anemia (see Chapter 113)
  I. Primary disorder of the spleen (see Chapter 61)
  J. Severe iron-deficiency anemia (see Chapter 116)
  K. Vitamin B_{12} or folate deficiency (see Chapters 114 and 115)
  L. AIDS (see Chapter 156)

VI. Treatment: Depends on the underlying cause of the thrombocytopenia; selected causes will be briefly discussed.
  A. ITP with asymptomatic mild, or moderate thrombocytopenia (see Chapter 120)
    1. Follow without treatment.
    2. Evaluate for underlying cause (e.g., hypersplenism).
  B. ITP with severe thrombocytopenia with acute bleeding (see Chapter 120)
    1. Platelet transfusions for platelet count < 10,000 mm³ and bleeding
    2. IV IgG followed immediately by platelet transfusion
    3. High-dose glucocorticoid
    4. Aminocaproic acid to help control acute bleeding
    5. Splenectomy: Offers complete, permanent response in two-thirds of patients

      6. Short course of radiation to spleen for those who cannot tolerate surgery

C. Drug-induced thrombocytopenia
   1. No therapy may be needed if withdrawal of drug is followed by recovery; normal platelet count is usually achieved within one week.
   2. Platelet transfusions and steroids (e.g., prednisone 60–80 mg/day po) may be used for life-threatening thrombocytopenia while awaiting recovery of platelet counts.

D. Thrombotic thrombocytopenic purpura: Characterized by disseminated thrombotic occlusions of the microcirculation and a syndrome of hemolytic anemia, thrombocytopenia, neurologic symptoms, fever, and renal dysfunction
   1. Exchange plasmapheresis and plasma infusions.
   2. If seriously ill, concomitant antiplatelet drugs (e.g., aspirin, dipyridamole, sulfinpyrazone, dextran) and corticosteroids would be used in collaboration with the physician.
   3. If no response (approximately 20% of patients), splenectomy performed with dextran and corticosteroids.
   4. Diagnosis is made by clinical presentation and peripheral smear review.

E. DIC (see Chapter 119)
   1. Remove the precipitating factor or underlying cause, if possible.
   2. Take supportive measures.
      a) Control of active bleeding
      b) Platelet transfusions
      c) Fresh frozen plasma for hypofibrinogenemia
      d) Prevention of organ failure with vasopressor, dialysis, and ventilator
      e) Adequate hydration for renal perfusion
   3. Administer heparin (in some cases).
      a) Heparin inactivates thrombin, which will inhibit the clotting process and thereby inhibit fibrinolysis.
      b) In most cases of acute DIC, heparin has not been shown to decrease mortality rates.
      c) DIC caused by malignancy often responds to IV heparin followed by long-term SC heparin. The most important intervention is to treat the malignancy.

F. Splenic pooling of platelets
   1. Therapy seldom indicated for thrombocytopenia alone.
   2. Splenectomy or embolic occlusion of the splenic artery may alleviate pancytopenia or severe thrombocytopenia.

VII. Follow-up
A. Short-term
   1. Response to platelet infusions usually seen within six hours of transfusion; may last only a short time.
   2. Response to IV IgG usually occurs with rise in platelet count after several days and return to pretreatment level in several weeks.
   3. Maintenance treatment with IgG when count falls below 20,000
      a) IgG 2 g/kg over two to five days initially

        b) Maintenance dose of 60 g can be given monthly, every six weeks, or when platelets drop below 20,000.

  B. Long-term: Mild to moderate asymptomatic thrombocytopenia
     1. Check platelet count monthly
     2. Instruct patient to call for signs of bleeding.

VIII. Referrals
  A. Physician: Consult for diagnostic workup and treatment plan for most forms of thrombocytopenia; the advanced practice nurse may manage the patient in collaboration with the physician.
  B. Refer any hemorrhagic, life-threatening cases of thrombocytopenia to physician.

References

Alving, B.M., & Krishnamurti, C. (1997). Recognition and management of heparin-induced thrombocytopenia (HIT) and thrombosis. *Seminars in Thrombosis and Hemostasis, 23,* 569–574.

Chang, J.C. (1996). Postoperative thrombocytopenia: With etiologic, diagnostic and therapeutic consideration (Review). *American Journal of the Medical Sciences, 311,* 96–105.

Doyle, B., & Porter, D.L. (1997). Thrombocytopenia. *AACN Clinical Issues, 8,* 469–480.

Goldstein, K.H., & Abramson, N. (1996). Efficient diagnosis of thrombocytopenia. *American Family Physician, 53,* 915–920.

Rutherford, C.J., & Frenkel, E.P. (1994). Thrombocytopenia: Issues in diagnosis and therapy. *Medical Clinics of North America, 78,* 555–575.

Section **XI.** Neurologic

Symptoms

Medical Diagnosis

Chapter

124. Ataxia/Incoordination

Karen E. Maher, ANP, MS, AOCN®

I. Definitions
   A. Ataxia: Loss of muscular coordination causing disturbance of gait and inability to maintain proper posture
      1. Static ataxia: Incoordination when supine
      2. Kinetic ataxia: Incoordination only on standing or moving
   B. Incoordination: Inability to produce voluntary, harmonious, rhythmic muscular coordination

II. Physiology/Pathophysiology
   A. Normal physiology
      1. The corticospinal (i.e., cerebral cortex and spinal cord) and corticobulbar (i.e., cerebral cortex and upper portion brain stem) tracts are the most important pathways used in the initiation of voluntary motor movements. The corticospinal and corticobulbar tracts also are referred to as the pyramidal system because these tracts are present in the medullary pyramid.
      2. The extrapyramidal system applies to motor disorders associated with lesions involving the basal ganglia (i.e., four masses of gray matter containing cell bodies that regulate and integrate motor activity originating in the cerebral cortex), without reference to the particular motor pathways affected.
      3. Voluntary movements require contraction and relaxation of muscles in proper sequence.
         a) The mechanisms for programming these complex events include the posterior parietal lobe, supplementary motor cortex, and the premotor cortex (see Figure 124-1).
         b) The total integration of these movements is called coordination, partially mediated through efferent and afferent tracts of the cerebellum.
      4. The pattern generator for locomotion is contained within the neural circuitry of the spinal cord.
         a) Separate pattern generators exist for each limb.
         b) The activity of these generators allows for coordinated and precise movements of limbs.
      5. Sensory subsystems involved with coordinated movements include the vestibular apparatus and proprioceptive mechanisms.

Figure 124-1. Cortical Regions Involved in the Programming of Movements

The arrows show some of the interconnections of these regions. The numbers refer to Brodmann's areas.

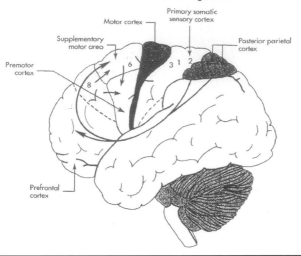

Note. From *Principles of Physiology* (p. 155) by R.M. Berne and M.N. Levy, 1996, St. Louis: Mosby, Inc. Copyright 1996 by Mosby, Inc. Reprinted with permission.

    B. Pathophysiology
        1. The hierarchic organization of the motor system can be demonstrated by the effects of lesions at different levels of the neuraxis (i.e., brain and spinal cord).
        2. A lesion can result in a particular effect by abolishing functions or allowing an action to occur by removing an inhibitory influence.

  III. Clinical features: Cerebellar lesions produce symptoms on the ipsilateral (i.e., same) side of the lesion, in contrast to cerebral lesions, which invariably produce contralateral effects.
    A. History
        1. History of cancer and cancer treatment
        2. Current medications: Prescribed and over-the-counter
        3. History of presenting symptom(s): Precipitating factors, onset, location, and duration. Associated symptoms are change in hearing or vision (e.g., diplopia), headaches, paresthesias, hemiparesis, or weakness of extremities.
        4. Changes in activities of daily living
    B. Signs and symptoms
        1. Disequilibrium (i.e., sensation of feeling drunk, unsteady on one's feet, imbalance)
        2. Vomiting that may not be preceded by nausea, especially with positional change
        3. Dysarthria (i.e., defective speech)
        4. Hemiparesis (i.e., one-sided paralysis)
        5. Diplopia (i.e., double vision)
        6. Splinting of affected extremity or body part
    C. Physical exam

1. Vital signs: Assess blood pressure for orthostatic hypotension (i.e., decreased blood pressure with increased heart rate with positional change from lying to sitting to standing).

    a) Observe temporal membrane for loss of landmarks, erythema, or bulging to rule out otitis or other findings of vestibular dysfunction.

    b) Assess for visual field defects, presence of nystagmus, extraocular muscle function, and ophthalmoscopic evaluation with attention to presence of papilledema that may indicate increased intracranial pressure.

2. Neurologic exam: Exam findings will determine location of lesion causing ataxia. Potential etiologies include abnormalities in the areas of sensory, strength, or proprioception; cerebellum; or basal ganglia.

    a) Mental status exam: Evaluate patient awareness, orientation, and cognitive abilities.

    b) Motor exam (see Appendicies 5 and 13)

        (1) Strength: Assess strength in all muscle groups for symmetry and tremor.

        (2) Coordination: Assess cadinance and tremor.

            (a) Rapid rhythmic, alternating hand movements

            (b) Finger-to-finger test

            (c) Finger-to-nose test

            (d) Heel-to-shin test

            (e) Observe gait for shuffling, widely placed feet, or toe walking and ability to execute tandem gait.

                i) Cerebellar ataxia: Feet wide-based, staggering, swaying of the trunk

                ii) Sensory ataxia: Wide-based gait, feet forward and outward, which brings heels down first, then toes; positive Romberg test

                iii) Ataxia: Uncontrolled falling

        (3) Balance

            (a) Romberg test

            (b) Heel-to-toe test

    c) Sensory exam: Assess for proprioception.

        (1) Pin-prick sensation or light touch

        (2) Two-point discrimination or vibration

    d) Evaluation of cortical sensory function (stereognosis): Place familiar object in patient's hand to assess ability to recognize objects by touch.

    e) Reflexes

        (1) Test each reflex, comparing response to corresponding side.

        (2) Absent reflex indicates neuropathy, lower motor neuron disorder.

        (3) Hyperactive reflex indicates upper motor neuron disorder.

IV. Diagnostic tests

    A. Laboratory: Comprehensive metabolic panel to include calcium and magnesium, BUN, creatinine to assess for dehydration or electrolyte imbalance that can result in neurologic/muscular dysfunction

B. Radiology: CT/MRI; site determined by clinical symptoms and physical exam findings
  1. If brain metastases are suspected, a head CT/MRI is appropriate.
  2. If weakness is caused by another condition (e.g., superior sulcus tumor), a CT of neck and chest will be helpful.
C. Other
  1. Audiologic evaluation: If vestibular cause is suspected
  2. Angiography: If vascular etiology is suspected

V. Differential diagnosis: In assessing the neurologic significance of ataxia/incoordination, exclude painful and restrictive conditions of joints, muscles, and other structures.
A. Malignancy-related
  1. Brain metastasis (see Chapter 134)
  2. Bone/soft tissue metastasis causing nerve root compression
  3. Paraneoplastic syndromes (see Appendix 12)
    a) Syndrome of inappropriate antidiuretic hormone (SIADH) (see Chapter 94)
    b) Hypercalcemia (see Chapter 144)
    c) Eaton-Lambert syndrome
    d) Hypercoagulable state, causing thrombosis of cerebral venous structures
  4. Primary malignancy of the nervous system
B. Vestibular disorders, including acoustic neuroma
C. Fluid and electrolyte imbalance
  1. Dehydration (see Chapter 147)
  2. Hypernatremia, hypophosphatemia, hypo/hyperkalemia, hypercalcemia (see Chapters 144–147)
D. Infectious disorders of the nervous system
  1. Meningitis (see Chapter 136)
  2. Encephalitis
  3. Reye's syndrome
E. Iatrogenic
  1. Drug-induced: Steroids (proximal muscle weakness), opioids, antibiotics (e.g. aminoglycosides), antiseizure (e.g., phenytoin, phenobarbital, carbamazepine)
  2. Chemotherapy (e.g., high-dose cytarabine, ifosfamide, 5-fluorouracil, vinca alkaloids, hexamethamelamine, busulfan)
F. Hypothyroidism (see Chapter 149)
G. Alcoholic cerebellar degeneration
H. Post-viral complications; status post herpes zoster
I. Drug abuse
J. Tabes dorsalis: Sclerosis of posterior columns of the spinal cord caused by *Treponema pallidum*
K. Connective tissue disease: Rheumatoid arthritis (see Chapter 108), systemic lupus, cerebral vasculitis
L. Vitamin deficiency: Vitamin B_{12} (see Chapter 114), vitamin E
M. Whipple's disease
  1. Multisystem infectious disorder of presumed etiology

2. Suspect in patients with AIDS.
N. Cerebral vascular accident (CVA)

VI. Treatment: Refer to appropriate medical diagnosis section; educate patients regarding safety to prevent falls.

VII. Follow-up: Refer to appropriate medical diagnosis section. Depends on cause.

VIII. Referrals: Physical/occupational therapists for evaluation of assistive devices and rehabilitation as indicated; refer difficult cases to neurologist.

References

Aminoff, M.J. (1994). Nervous system. In L.W. Tierney, Jr., S.J. McPhee, & M.A. Papadakis (Eds.), *Current medical diagnosis and treatment* (pp. 798–854). Norwalk, CT: Appleton & Lange.

Aminoff, M.J. (1995). *Neurology and general medicine* (2nd ed.). New York: Churchill Livingstone.

Bastian, A.J. (1997). Mechanisms of ataxia. *Physical Therapy, 77,* 672–675.

DeGowan, R.L. (1989). *Bedside diagnostic examination* (5th ed.). New York: Macmillan.

John, W.J., Patchell, R.A., & Foon, K.A. (1997). Paraneoplastic syndromes. In V.T. DeVita, S. Hellman, & S.A. Rosenberg (Eds.), *Cancer: Principles and practice of oncology* (5th ed.) (pp. 2397–2422). Philadelphia: Lippincott.

Trueblood, P.R., & Rubenstein, L.Z. (1991). Assessment of instability and gait in elderly persons. *Comprehensive Therapy, 17*(8), 20–29.

Chapter

125. Blurred Vision

Giselle J. Moore-Higgs, ARNP, MSN

I. Definition: Disorder of visual acuity in which difficulty seeing is described as blurring of the defined edges of items in the visual field

II. Pathophysiology: The result of a disorder that affects the ocular muscle, one or more cranial nerves (i.e., visual or ocular motor pathways in the brain), changes in the refracting surface of the eye, or opacification of the transparent ocular media

III. Clinical features: Most common visual complaint
   A. History
      1. History of cancer and cancer treatment
      2. Current medications: Prescribed and over-the-counter
      3. History of presenting symptom(s): Precipitating factors, onset, and duration. Associated symptoms are diplopia, unstable visual images (floaters), facial sensations, weakness, ataxia, and aphasia.
      4. Changes in activities of daily living
      5. Past medical history: Hereditary causes, demyelinating disease, ischemic disease, hematologic disorder, vascular disease, inflammatory disease, ocular trauma
      6. Social history: Exposure to toxic substances
   B. Signs and symptoms
      1. Blurred vision in central or peripheral vision in one or both eyes
      2. Headache
   C. Physical exam: To evaluate for visual deficits using a comprehensive neuro-ophthalmology exam
      1. Visual acuity testing: Snellen chart exam to identify approximate visual acuity deficit without visual apparatus (e.g., glasses, contacts)
      2. Visual field testing: To evaluate central and peripheral visual loss
      3. Fundoscopic exam: To evaluate for papilledema (swelling of the optic disk caused by active inflammation or passive congestion associated with increased intracranial pressure)
      4. Cranial nerve exam (see Appendix 5)
         a) Oculomotor (III): Lesions result in partial abduction (i.e., inability to adduct, elevate, and depress the eye); ptosis and nonreactive pupil may occur.

      b) Trochlear (IV): Lesions result in defective depression of the adducted eye.

      c) Abducens (VI): Lesions result in lateral rectus palsy with impaired abduction of the affected eye.

IV. Diagnostic tests
  A. Laboratory: The choice of hematologic studies depends on the suspected cause of the blurred vision.
  B. Radiology
    1. MRI of the head to evaluate for tumor or lesion of the brain
    2. MRI of the eye/orbit to evaluate for tumor or lesion of optical apparatus

V. Differential diagnosis
  A. Hereditary disease
    1. Optic atrophy
    2. Leber's disease
  B. Demyelinating disease
    1. Optic neuritis
    2. Multiple sclerosis
    3. Neuromyelitis
  C. Ischemic disease
    1. Hypotension (see Chapter 46)
    2. Transient ischemic attacks (adult and children)
    3. Temporal arteritis
    4. Systemic disease-related ischemia—diabetes mellitus (see Chapter 143)
    5. Fibromuscular dysplasia
    6. Dysautonomia
  D. Hematologic and vascular disease
    1. Chronic anemia (see Chapter 112)
    2. Vascular hypotension
    3. Blood dyscrasia
    4. Cortical blindness
      a) Arteriosclerosis
      b) Carbon monoxide poisoning
      c) Trauma
      d) Neoplasm
      e) Infection
    5. Intracranial aneurysm
  E. Inflammatory disease
    1. Intraocular or orbital inflammation
    2. AIDS (see Chapter 156)
    3. Lyme disease
    4. Radiation retinopathy
    5. Intracranial inflammation
  F. Tumor
    1. Ocular tumor

      a) Melanoma

      b) Lymphoma

  2. Leukemia and multiple myeloma: Increased blood viscosity results in vascular occlusive disease.

  3. Extraocular tumor: Results in increased intracranial pressure

  4. Paraneoplastic syndrome (see Appendix 12): May result in peripheral neuropathy, subacute cerebellar degeneration, and/or brain stem and limbic encephalitis

G. Toxic agents

  1. Tobacco

  2. Alcohol and methyl alcohol

  3. Cocaine

  4. Lead

  5. Ketogenic diets

H. Trauma

 I. Opacities of the media

  1. Cataracts

  2. Dislocation of the lens

  3. Vitreous degeneration

  4. Hemorrhage

  5. Corneal opacities

  6. Retinal disease

VI. Treatment: Depends on the accurate diagnosis and treatment of the underlying cause

VII. Follow-up: Depends on the underlying cause of the blurred vision and its treatment

VIII. Referrals: Complete retinal evaluation by an ophthalmologist

References

Adamczyk, D.T. (1996). Visual phenomena, disturbances, and hallucinations. *Optometry Clinics, 5,* 33–52.

Aminoff, M.J., Greenberg, D.A., & Simon, P. (1996). *Clinical neurology* (3rd ed.). Norwalk, CT: Appleton & Lange.

Freeman, W.R. (1989). Prevalence and significance of AIDS-related microvasculopathy. *American Journal of Opthalmology, 107,* 299.

Weibers, D.O., Dale, A.J.D., Kokmen, E., & Swanson, J.W. (1998). *Mayo Clinic examinations in neurology* (7th ed.). St. Louis: Mosby.

Chapter

126. Confusion/Delirium

Deborah McCaffrey Boyle, RN, MSN, AOCN®, FAAN

I. Definition: No clear and concise definition is used consistently.
   A. Terms "delirium" and "acute confusion" are used interchangeably.
   B. Delirium is a transient organic brain syndrome of acute onset that results in behavioral changes (e.g., disordered attention, changes in cognition and psychomotor activity, disruption of the sleep-wake cycle).
   C. End-of-life confusion refers to cognitive failure caused by widely metastatic cancer and, thus, systems failure.

II. Pathophysiology: Pathogenesis is poorly understood. Major theories include
   A. Reduction of cerebral oxidative metabolism
   B. Damaged neuronal enzyme synthesis
   C. Neurotransmitter imbalance
   D. Neuronal loss.

III. Clinical features: With age, the brain is more vulnerable to confusion. Most confusion is acute and reversible. Once the underlying etiology is determined and corrected, symptoms should resolve.
   A. Etiology
      1. Singular etiology is rare. The cause most often is multifocal in nature, particularly in elderly patients with cancer.
      2. Possible etiologies
         a) Electrolyte imbalance
         b) Infection
         c) Hypoxia
         d) Drugs with known central anticholinergic effects (e.g., atropine-containing drugs, opioids)
         e) Cancer
            (1) End-of-life, terminal phase
            (2) Metastatic disease
            (3) Brain tumors
         f) Nutritional deficiencies
         g) Sleep and sensory deprivation

    h) Fever
    i) Renal failure
    j) Hepatic failure
    k) Dehydration
  B. History (should be solicited from family member)
   1. History of cancer and cancer treatment
   2. Current medications: Prescribed and over-the-counter
   3. History of presenting symptom(s): Precipitating factors, onset, pattern, and duration
   4. Changes in activities of daily living
  C. Signs and symptoms (see Table 126-1)
   1. Hypoactive behavior (i.e., retardation, slowing, somnolence)
   2. Hyperactive behavior (i.e., restlessness, pacing, searching, picking)
   3. Presence of a delusional/paranoid component
   4. Forgetfulness, poor memory
   5. Lack of concentration

Table 126-1. Characteristics of Delirium

Classification	Primary Criteria	Clinical Manifestations
A	Disturbance in consciousness (reduced clarity of environment awareness) with impaired ability to focus or shift attention	Questions must be repeated because patient's attention may wander or patient may dwell on the answer to a previous question rather than appropriately shift attention. Patient is easily distracted by irrelevant stimuli. It is difficult to engage patient in conversation.
B	Change in cognition (memory impairment, disorientation, language disturbance) or the development of perceptual disturbance that is not better accounted for by a preexisting, established, or evolving dementia	Recent memory is impaired, as evidenced by inability to recall brief sentence or several unrelated objects after several minutes of distraction; disorientation to time (thinking morning is night) and to place (thinking is at home vs. hospital); language disturbance may be manifested as impaired ability to name objects or to write; speech may ramble or be irrelevant or incoherent; switches subject; perceptual disturbance includes misinterpretation of events, illusions, or hallucinations.
C	Disturbance evolves over a short period of time (hours to days) and fluctuates during the course of the day.	Periods of clarity, lucidness alter with periods of agitation, incoherence.
D	Evidence is derived from the history, physical exam, or lab findings that the disturbance is caused by physiologic consequences of a general medical condition.	Multicausal etiologies are evident, including systemic infections, metabolic disorders, fluid or electrolyte imbalances, hepatic or renal disease, thiamin deficiency, postop states, hypertensive encephalopathy, postictal states, sequela of head trauma, focal lesions of parietal lobe, and/or inferomedial surface of occipital lobe.

Note. Based on information from American Psychological Assocation, 1994.

6. Personality change
7. Alteration in daily routine (i.e., habits, self-care)

D. Physical exam: Essential to rule out focal neurologic findings that imply structural abnormalities

  1. Brief cognitive assessment (i.e., mini-mental status exam)

    a) Orientation

      (1) Time: Ask patient year, season, month, date, day.

      (2) Location: Ask patient state, county, town, hospital, floor/clinic.

    b) Memory: Name three unrelated objects and have patient repeat.

    c) Attention and calculation: Ask patient to recite serial numbers in sevens from 100.

    d) Recall: Ask patient to recall three items given by examiner.

    e) Language

      (1) Ask patient to identify two items (e.g., pencil, wristwatch).

      (2) Ask patient to repeat a short sentence (e.g., "No ifs, ands, or buts").

      (3) Ask patient to complete a three-stage command (e.g., take a paper in the right hand, fold it in half, and put on the table).

      (4) Ask the patient to write a sentence.

      (5) Ask the patient to copy a sentence.

  2. Wrong answers to the above questions only depict presence, not severity, of confusion and should be used only as a screening mechanism.

  3. Cardiovascular exam: To rule out abnormal heart sounds or rhythms

  4. Pulmonary exam: To rule out adventitious sounds

IV. Diagnostic tests

A. Laboratory

  1. Chemistry panel: To evaluate for metabolic abnormalities (e.g., hypercalcemia, hyponatremia, hypomagnesemia, hypo/hyperglycemia)

  2. Complete blood count: To assess for infection, anemia, and thrombocytopenia

  3. Therapeutic drug levels: To rule out toxic drug levels; consider digoxin, lithium, alcohol, toxin screen, antiepileptic medications

  4. Ammonia level: To rule out elevation

B. Radiology: CT/MRI of the head to evaluate for brain metastases, brain hemorrhage

C. Other

  1. Oxygen saturation level: To evaluate hypoxia

  2. Lumbar puncture (LP): To determine central nervous system cancer involvement or meningitis

  3. EEG: To rule out subclinical status

V. Differential diagnosis: To distinguish among delirium, dementia, and depression (see Table 126-2)

A. Electrolyte abnormalities (see Chapters 144–148)

B. Dehydration (see Chapter 147)

C. Renal failure (see Chapter 83)

D. Cirrhosis (see Chapter 64)

E. Sepsis (see Chapters 104 and 121)

Table 126-2. Differential Diagnosis of Delirium, Dementia, and Depression

Feature	Delirium	Dementia	Depression
Onset	Acute or subacute depends on cause; often occurs at twilight	Chronic, insidious	Coincides with life changes; often is abrupt
Course	Short; diurnal fluctuations in symptoms worse at night, in the dark, and on awakening	Long; no diurnal effects; symptoms progressive yet relatively stable over course of day	Diurnal effects typically worse in the morning; situational fluctuations occur but less than with delirium
Progression	Abrupt	Slow but even	Varies from rapid to slow but uneven
Duration	Hours to less than one month or several weeks	Months to years	At least two weeks but can be several months to years
Awareness	Reduced	Clear	Clear
Alertness	Fluctuates with lethargy or hypervigilance	Usually normal	Minimal impairment with distractibility
Attention	Impaired with lack of direction; selectivity, distractibility fluctuate	Relatively unaffected	Selective disorientation
Orientation	Generally impaired but fluctuates in severity; patient tends to mistake unfamiliar for familiar places and people	May be impaired	Selective or patchy impairment (i.e., "islands" of intact memory)
Memory	Immediate and recent often impaired	Recent and remote impaired	Intact but with themes of hopelessness, helplessness, or self-deprecation
Thinking	Disorganized, distorted, and fragmented with slow or accelerated incoherent speech	Patient exhibits persistence, difficulty with abstraction, impaired judgment, difficulty in finding words, and perseveration and confabulation.	Intact; delusions and hallucinations absent except in severe cases
Perception	Often distorted; illusions, delusions, and hallucinations present; patient has difficulty distinguishing between reality and misperceptions	No misperception	Intact; delusions and hallucinations absent except in severe cases
Speech	Incoherent, hesitant, slow, or rapid	Patient has difficulty in finding words; neologisms	Unaffected
Sleep-wake cycle	Always disrupted	Fragmented	Disturbed, early morning waking occurs often

(Continued on next page)

Table 126-2. Differential Diagnosis of Delirium, Dementia, and Depression *(Continued)*

Feature	Delirium	Dementia	Depression
Psychomotor behavior	Variable, hypokinetic, hyperkinetic, or mixed	Normal; patient may have apraxia	Variable; patient may exhibit psychomotor retardation or agitation
Mental status testing	Patient distracted from task	Failings highlighted by family; patient frequently "near misses" answers and struggles with finding appropriate reply	Failings highlighted by the patient; patient frequently does not know and will not attempt to find answers, acts indifferent and frequently gives up
Physical illness or drug toxicity	Either or both present	Often absent, especially with Alzheimer's disease	Variable

Note. From "Delirium (Acute Confusional States)," by Z.J. Lipowski, 1987, *JAMA, 285,* pp. 1789–1792. Copyright 1987 by American Medical Association. Reprinted with permission.

    F. Hypothermia or hyperthermia

    G. Drug-induced state (see Table 126-3)

    H. Meningitis (see Chapter 136)

VI. Treatment

    A. Correct/manage causative factors (e.g., electrolyte imbalance, medication regimen).

    B. Provide orientation cues (i.e., calendar, clock, nightlight, items from home, family pictures, reintroduction of staff and place).

    C. Enhance safety

       1. Lower bed; place call bell in patient's reach.

       2. Offer assistance with toileting, ambulation, and positioning.

       3. Inquire about thirst, dry mouth, indigestion, hunger, discomfort, and hypo/hyperthermia.

       4. Encourage family presence; plan alternating schedule of sitters.

       5. Ensure that patient uses hearing aids and glasses if necessary.

       6. Ensure that patient refrains from driving.

    D. Offer verbal reassurances (i.e., "We're going to try to find out what is making you feel mixed up. It must be frustrating not being able to remember things correctly.").

    E. Reduce symptom intensity via pharmacologic intervention.

       1. Haloperidol (Haldol®, Ortho-McNeil Pharmaceutical, Raritan, NJ) is preferred neuroleptic.

          a) Mild confusion: Give Haldol 0.5–1.0 mg bid po, IV, or IM.

          b) Agitated confusion: May give 1–2 mg Haldol q 30–60 minutes until agitation is controlled; assess amount required over 24 hours, then adjust to a twice daily dose. This should only be required until underlying cause is identified and corrected.

          c) Terminal confusion: If cause cannot be determined or corrected, treat around the clock with low-dose Haldol, as for mild confusion.

Table 126-3. Common Medications Causing Delirium in the Aged

Disorder	Medication Type	Common Examples
Cardiovascular	Antiarrhythmics	Procainamide, propranolol, quinidine, lidocaine
Gastrointestinal	Antihypertensives	Clonidine, methyldopa, reserpine
	Cardiac glycosides	Digitalis
	Antidiarrheals	Atropine, belladonna, homatropine, hyoscyamine, methantheline
	Antiematics	Phenothiazine
	Antispasmodics	Phenothiazine, scopolamine
	Antiulcer agents	Propantheline, cimetidine, ranitidine, metoclopramide
Musculoskeletal	Anti-inflammatory agents	Corticosteroids, indomethacin, phenylbutazone, salicylate
	Muscle relaxants	Carisoprodol, diazepam
Neurological-psychiatric	Anticonvulsants	Barbiturates, phenytoin
	Antiparkinsonian agents	Amantadine, benztropine, bromocriptine, levodopa, trihexyphenidyl, selegiline
	Hypnotics and sedatives	Barbiturates, bromides, chloral hydrate, glutethimide, hydroxyzine
	Psychotropics	Benzodiazepine, lithium salts, neuroleptic, antidepressants
Respiratory/allergic	Antihistamines	Brompheniramine, chlorpheniramine, cyproheptadine, diphenhydramine, tripelennamine
	Bronchodilators	Theophylline
Miscellaneous	Analgesics	Narcotics
	Antidiabetic agents	Insulin, oral hypoglycemics
	Antineoplastic agents	Methotrexate, mitomycin, procarbazine
	Anti-infectives	Acyclovir, amphotericin B, cotrimoxazole, isoniazid, ketoconazole, rifampin

Note. From *Pharmacological Considerations in Gerontological Nursing: Concepts and Practice* (2nd ed.) (p. 746), 1997, by E.S. McConnell, A.D. Linton, and J.T. Hanlon, Philadelphia: W.B. Saunders Co. Copyright 1997 by W.B. Saunders Co. Reprinted with permission.

2. Lorazepam (Ativan®, Wyeth-Ayerst Pharmaceuticals, Philadelphia, PA) is the benzodiazepine of choice in treating confusion associated with alcohol withdrawal and hepatic encephalopathy.
   a) Dose is 0.5–2.0 mg q 1–4 hours po, IV, or IM.
   b) May worsen confusion and induce paradoxical excitement in the elderly.

3. Other pharmacologic agents with limited use
   a) Phenothiazine (e.g., chlorpromazine (Thorazine®, SmithKline Beecham Pharmaceuticals, Philadelphia, PA): Recommended for severe symptoms when sedation is required; dose is 12.5–50 mg q 4–12 hours po, IV, or IM; puts patient at risk for hypotension.
   b) Diazepam (Valium®, Roche Pharmaceuticals, Roche Products, Inc., Manati, Puerto Rico): Long half-life and active metabolites can cause profound, prolonged sedation; must be used with caution; dose is 2–10 mg po or IV 2–4 times a day; not recommended for geriatric use.
   c) Midazolam (Versed®, Roche Pharmaceuticals, Roche Laboratories, Inc., Nutley, NJ): Used for extreme agitation only when other treatments fail to control symptoms; short half-life allows for easy titration; dose is 1–4 mg/hour as continuous IV/SC infusion; puts patient at risk for hypotension.

VII. Follow-up
  A. Short-term
     1. Evaluate effectiveness of drug regimen to treat confusion over first 24–48 hours.
     2. Evaluate the number of prn doses required to determine scheduled dose requirements.
     3. Expect clearing of acute confusion once underlying cause is corrected/managed; thus, drug therapy to manage confusion often is short-term.
     4. Consider safety measures to reduce risk for falls and self-injury (i.e., use of sitters, restraints).
     5. For end-of-life, terminal-stage confusion, balance sedation with wakefulness and clarity to facilitate patient/family communication.
  B. Long-term: Closely follow patients with metastatic disease who are more at risk for systems compromise that may cause metabolic and other physiologic etiologies of confusion.

VIII. Referrals
  A. Psychiatrist: Consultation is necessary if the nature of confusion is in question, there is concern about medication dose, or the patient has a premorbid history of psychiatric problems.
  B. Home care: Consultation necessary if cognitive impairment in the home setting is particularly difficult for the family to manage; team planning is necessary.
  C. Hospice: Appropriate for patients in the terminal stage of cancer.

References

American Psychological Association. (1994). *Diagnostic and statistical manual of mental disorders* (4th ed.). Washington, DC: Author.

Boyle, D.M., Abernathy, G., Baker, L., & Wall, A.C. (1998). Oncologic implications of end-of-life confusion. *Oncology Nursing Forum, 25,* 1335–1343.

Breitbart, W., Bruera, E., Chochinov, H., & Lynch, M. (1995). Neuropsychiatric syndromes and psychological symptoms in patients with advanced cancer. *Journal of Pain and Symptom Management, 10*(2), 131–141.

Inouye, S.K., Bogardus, S.T., Jr., Charpentier, P.A., Loe-Summers, L., Acampore, D., Holford, T.R., & Cooney, L.M., Jr. (1999). A multicomponent intervention to prevent delirium in hospitalized older patients. *New England Journal of Medicine, 340*, 669–676.

Ludwick, R. (1999). Clinical decision-making: Recognition of confusion and application of restraints. *Orthopaedic Nursing. 18*(1), 65-72.

Smith, M.J., Breitbart, W.S., & Platt, M.M. (1995). A critique of instruments and methods to detect, diagnose, and rate delirium. *Journal of Pain and Symptom Management, 10*(1), 35–77.

Trzepacz, P.T. (1994). The neuropathogenesis of delirium. *Psychosomatics, 35*, 374–391.

Weinrich, S., & Sarna, L. (1994). Delirium in the older person with cancer. *Cancer, 74*, 2079–2091.

Chapter

127. Dizziness/Vertigo

Karen E. Maher, ANP, MS, AOCN®

I. Definition: Faintness or a sensation of passing out
   A. Nonvertiginous dizziness differs from true vertigo in that the patient does not feel a rotary movement sensation (i.e., vertigo).
   B. Vertigo is a subjective sensation of movement (i.e., feeling as though one is revolving in space or as though objects in the environment are moving).

II. Pathophysiology: Dizziness/vertigo may result from lesions of the labyrinth, cranial nerve VIII, the brain stem, or the cerebral cortex. Thus, they can be divided into three main physiological categories: peripheral vestibular disorders, CNS diseases, and systemic diseases (see Table 127-1).
   A. Peripheral vestibular etiology: Abnormality occurs at some point along the course of the vestibular nerve other than at its origin in the brain stem; most often occurs at the nerve termination in the inner ear (labyrinth).
   B. CNS lesions/diseases: Any disease that disrupts the pathway between the vestibular apparatus and the brain; interruption can occur at two locations.
      1. Impulses from the vestibular apparatus are disrupted as they proceed through cranial nerve VIII to the vestibular nuclei of the brain stem.
      2. Impulses from the brain stem to the cerebellum and cerebral cortex are disrupted.
   C. Systemic diseases: Disorders in any organ system causing dizziness; spatial orientation depends on the complex interaction of adequate sensation, central integration, and the proper motor response.
   D. Cerebrovascular disease can cause interruption of blood supply, resulting in ischemia to the labyrinth.

III. Clinical features
   A. Etiology (see Table 127-1)
   B. History: The history should clearly elucidate what the patient means by specific terms used and specific symptoms reported to differentiate between nonvertiginous dizziness and vertigo.
      1. History of cancer and cancer treatment
      2. Current medications: Prescribed and over-the-counter

Table 127-1. Mechanism and Common Causes of Different Types of Dizziness

Type	Mechanism	Common Causes
Vertigo	Imbalance of tonic vestibular signals	Benign positional vertigo, Menière's disease, neurolabyrinthitis, vertebrobasilar insufficiency
Presyncopal lightheadedness	Diffuse cerebral ischemia	Orthostatic hypotension, vasovagal episode, cardiac arrhythmia, hyperventilation
Psychophysiologic dizziness	Impaired central integration of sensory signals	Anxiety, panic attacks, phobias
Disequilibrium	Loss of vestibulospinal, proprioceptive, or cerebellar function	Ototoxicity, peripheral neuropathy, stroke, cerebellar atrophy
Ocular dizziness	Visual-vestibular mismatch caused by impaired vision	Correction of astigmatism, change in magnification, oculomotor paresis
Multisensory dizziness	Partial loss of multiple sensory systems	Diabetes mellitus, aging
Physiologic dizziness	Sensory conflict caused by unusual combination of sensory signals	Motion sickness, height vertigo, mal de debarquement

Note. From "Approach to the Evaluation of the Dizzy Patient," by R.W. Baloh, 1995, *Otolarngology-Head and Neck Surgery, 112*(1), p. 4. Copyright 1995 by Lippincott-Raven. Reprinted with permission.

 3. History of presenting symptom(s): Precipitating factors, onset, and duration. Associated symptoms are positional change, cough, nausea, vomiting, diaphoresis, tinnitus, and hearing loss.
 4. Changes in activities of daily living
 5. Past medical history: Anemia
 6. Social history: Emotional and physical stress
C. Signs and symptoms: Certain words and phrases commonly are used to describe dizziness and vertigo.
  1. Nonvertiginous dizziness
   a) Described as sensation of spinning inside the head (i.e., light-headed, floating, giddy, swimming) while the environment remains still.
   b) Symptoms tend to be continuous.
   c) Episodes occur in specific situations (i.e., driving on a freeway, entering a crowded room, shopping in a busy supermarket).
   d) Nausea and vomiting are uncommon.
  2. Vertigo: Patients often will liken the sensation to that of being drunk or having motion sickness (i.e., feelings of imbalance like falling or tilting to one side).
   a) A sensation of spinning outside the head nearly always indicates a vestibular disorder; nausea and vomiting usually are present.
   b) Symptoms tend to be episodic and may include auditory (e.g., tinnitus, hearing loss) or neurologic (e.g., ataxia, imbalance) signs that are aggravated by head movements and positional change.

      c) Patients with CNS diseases almost always will have other CNS symptoms (e.g., facial numbness, hemiparesis, diplopia).

  3. Psychophysiologic dizziness

      a) The sensation that one has "left the body" is a characteristic symptom.

      b) Patients report feeling dizzy from morning to night without change for months to years at a time.

      c) Patient experiences multiple symptoms of acute and chronic anxiety.

      d) Hyperventilation occurs.

  4. Duration of common causes of vertigo

      a) Benign positional vertigo usually lasts a matter of seconds.

      b) Vertebrobasilar insufficiency or migraine can last minutes.

      c) Menière's disease can induce vertigo for hours.

      d) Vertigo lasting for days can be the result of viral neurolabyrinthitis; infarction of labyrinth, brain stem, or cerebellum; or labyrinthine trauma.

D. Physical exam

  1. Measure vital signs: Assess for orthostatic blood pressures.

  2. Ear examination: Observe tympanic membrane for loss of landmarks, erythema, or choleastoma (cystic process that can occlude the middle ear) and cerumen impaction.

      a) Perform whisper test to assess for hearing acuity.

      b) Perform Rinne test to assess bone and air conduction (see Appendix 13).

      c) Perform Weber test to assess lateralization of sound (see Appendix 13).

  3. Cardiovascular exam: Include auscultation for carotid bruits and effect of carotid sinus massage; irregularity of heartbeat suggests cerebrovascular disease or dysrhythmias.

  4. Neurologic exam: To evaluate for central lesion, primarily of cerebellum and brain stem

      a) Nystagmus is objective marker for new-onset vertigo.

        (1) Look for spontaneous nystagmus in five positions of gaze. Normally, minimal nystagmus movement of limiting lateral gaze will exist, and nystagmus should not occur on elevation and depression of the eyes, even at extremes.

        (2) Reproduce nystagmus with Nylen-Bárány maneuver (see Figure 127-1): Have patient sit, turning head to right and quickly lowering it to supine position over edge 30° below horizontal level; observe for nystagmus, and repeat on other side.

          (a) In benign positional vertigo, nystagmus usually is noted only on one side.

          (b) The response will resolve quickly; after patient repeats maneuver two to three times, response will not occur.

        (3) Brain stem lesions: Horizontal or vertical nystagmus or both

      b) Cranial nerve evaluation (see Appendix 5): Cranial nerve deficit/dysfunction may indicate a brain stem lesion; a large acoustic neuroma can affect nerves V, VII, and X.

      c) Romberg test: To test cerebellar function; test is positive in sensory ataxia (decreased conduction of sensory impulses, especially proprioception).

      d) Visual acuity evaluation: To assess for deficits, check extraocular movements for nystagmus (cranial nerves III, IV, VI).

Figure 127-1. Nylen-Bárány Maneuver

	Peripheral	Central
Intensity of vertigo	Severe	Mild or absent
Latency of onset	Yes; but nystagmus usually begins within 2–10 seconds	None; nystagmus begins immediately
Fatigue of nystagmus	Yes; nystagmus gradually abates	No; nystagmus persists
Habituation	Yes; cannot elicit nystagmus (or nystagmus lessens) after one or more maneuvers	No; nystagmus reproducible repetitively
Common causes	Labyrinthitis; otitis; benign positional vertigo	None common but multiple sclerosis, brain stem tumor occasional cause

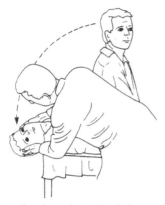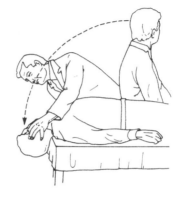

Patients are first observed, seated, with the eyes straight ahead. Any spontaneous nystagmus at rest, on horizontal gaze (no more than 30 degrees from the midline), or on vertical gaze is noted and analyzed. Extraocular movements are tested.

Patients turn their head 30–45 degrees to one side and are then lowered quickly backward to the supine position, such that the head is extended down over the end of the examining table to about a 30 degree subhorizontal angle (see Figure). The patient is now lying down, head turned to one side, and inclined backward, one ear facing the floor, with the examiner supporting the patient's head and neck. This position is maintained for 30 seconds. The patient's eyes are observed while in the midline and while looking down toward the floor. Induction of nystagmus is often accompanied by the onset of vertigo and a frantic urge to get up (especially when peripheral vestibular disease is the problem). The patient is then brought back to the upright position,

the eyes are observed for 30–60 seconds (nystagmus may then occur again), and the maneuver is repeated, turning the head now down to the opposite side.

During the Nylen-Bárány maneuver, remember that *positional nystagmus should be observed for:*
1. Direction of slow/fast components
2. The head position that elicits nystagmus
3. The latency of onset of nystagmus (the time between assumption of the head position and the onset of nystagmus)
4. The persistence of fatigue of nystagmus (Does nystagmus wane as the head position is maintained or does it continue unabated?)
5. The intensity of vertigo induced
6. The presence or absence of habituation (Does repeating the test in the vulnerable position cause a lesser or absent nystagmus response—habituation—or not?)

Note. From *Practical Strategies in Outpatient Medicine* (p. 204), by B.M. Reilly, 1991. Philadelphia: W.B. Saunders Co. Copyright 1991 by W.B. Saunders Co. Reprinted with permission.

    5. Neck exam: Assess relationship between symptoms and neck range of motion; may be vestibular etiology, visual etiology, or cervical spine integrity.

    6. Reproduce symptoms through hyperventilation: Ask patient to blow vigorously for three minutes on a paper towel held six inches from the mouth; may cause some circumoral and digital numbness as well as reproduce the patient's dizziness.

IV. Diagnostic tests
    A. Laboratory: To evaluate for unclear etiology (e.g., TSH test to assess for thyroid disorders, complete blood count to assess for anemia)
    B. Radiology

      1. Cervical spine x-rays: To assess vertebral integrity and rule out pathologic fracture, compression fracture, or abnormality (i.e., disc protrusion or tumor) that may cause nerve compression

      2. CT and/or MRI: Needed if more comprehensive imaging is indicated based on patient's history and physical examination

      3. Contrast angiography or contrast cisternography (i.e., injection of radionuclide by LP to assess altered flow and reabsorption of cerebral spinal fluid): May demonstrate specific intracranial lesions

C. Other

      1. Audiometry tests: To detect abnormalities with acoustic neuroma and Menière's disease.

      2. Vestibular function tests: Caloric stimulation to test vestibular portion of cranial nerve VIII (not done if possibility of acute middle ear infection or perforated eardrum)

        a) Ask patient to sit with head tilted 60° in extension position.

        b) Irrigate against eardrum with 10 cc ice water for 20 seconds (procedure may cause nausea and vomiting).

        c) Test one ear at a time.

        d) Abnormalities include bilateral unequal nystagmus with prolonged nausea and dizziness.

      3. Electronystagmography: To differentiate brain stem and cerebellar lesions

      4. LP: To assess for increase in abnormal proteins, as in demyelinating diseases

      5. Doppler examination of carotid and vertebral arteries: If clinical picture suggests transient ischemia attack

V. Differential diagnosis (see Table 127-1)

  A. Vestibular disorders

      1. Acute labyrinthitis

      2. Chronic labyrinthitis (Menière's disease)

      3. Toxic labyrinthitis

      4. Traumatic labyrinthitis

      5. Labyrinthine ischemia

      6. Benign positional vertigo

      7. Acoustic neuroma

  B. Cerebrovascular disease, especially vertebrobasilar insufficiency

  C. Cardiovascular disease, with special reference to rhythm disturbances; orthostatic hypotension (see Chapters 43 and 46)

  D. Cervical osteoarthritis and spondylosis

  E. Visual disturbances, especially cataracts

  F. Cerebral cortical lesions (rare causes of vertigo)

  G. Malignancies

      1. Brain metastasis with cerebral edema (see Chapter 134)

      2. Primary brain tumor

  H. Medications, especially opioids

    I. Sinusitis (see Chapter 10)

    J. Diabetes mellitus (see Chapter 143)

    K. Psychologic etiology: Anxiety, depression, psychosis (see Chapters 152 and 154)

    L. Otitis (see Chapters 8 and 9)

    M. Dehydration, hypovolemia, electrolyte imbalance (see Chapters 144–148)

VI. Treatment: Refer to appropriate medical diagnosis section.

    A. Benign paroxysmal positional vertigo

        1. Drug therapy

            a) Meclizine (Antivert®, Pfizer Inc., New York, NY): 12.5–25 mg po tid or qid with dosage tapered as symptoms improve

            b) Dimenhydrinate (Dramamine®, Richardson-Vicks Inc., Cincinnati, OH): 50 mg po tid or qid

            c) Antiemetics (see Appendix 3)

                (1) Prochlorperazine (Compazine®, SmithKline Beecham Pharmaceuticals, Philadelphia, PA): 5–10 mg po every four hours prn; spansule, 15–30 mg po in the am or 10–15 mg bid; suppositories, 25 mg rectally bid

                (2) Thiethylperazine maleate (Torecan®, Roxane Laboratories, Inc., Columbus, OH): 10 mg po tid prn

        2. Bed rest

        3. Exercise program to promote vestibular compensation

    B. Menière's disease: Difficult to treat with often short-term responses

        1. Drug therapy: Diuretic and the same medications prescribed for benign paroxysmal vertigo (i.e., hydrochlorothiazide 50–100 mg po qd)

        2. Vestibular desensitization exercises may be helpful.

    C. Peripheral vestibulopathy (i.e., acute viral labyrinthitis, vestibular neuronitis)

        1. May use medications as listed above.

        2. Symptoms usually resolve in three to six weeks with no residual deficits.

    D. Otitis media/serous otitis (see Chapters 8 and 9)

    E. Treat depression and anxiety as indicated (see Chapters 152 and 154) with antidepressants and anxiolytics (see Appendix 2).

    F. Stop nonessential medications as appropriate to diagnosis.

    G. Exercise safety concerns, especially in elderly patients.

VII. Follow-up

    A. Short-term: Recheck patient in three to six weeks.

    B. Long-term: May need appropriate medical referral for further evaluation and intervention

VIII. Referrals

    A. Physicians: May include neurologist, surgeon, otolaryngologist, or psychiatrist

    B. Physical/occupational therapists: Evaluate for exercise and activity programs that provide strengthening, gait training, and identification of specific activities that may trigger symptoms; possible referral for assistive devices and rehabilitation.

References

Baloh, R.W. (1995). Approach to the evaluation of the dizzy patient. *Otolaryngology-Head and Neck Surgery, 112,* 3–7.

Ruckstein, M.J. (1995). A practical approach to dizziness. *Postgraduate Medicine, 9*(3), 70–81.

Sloane, P.D. (1996). Evaluation and management of dizziness in the older patient. *Clinics in Geriatric Medicine, 12,* 785 801.

Weinstein, B.E., & Devons, C.A.J. (1995). The dizzy patient: Stepwise workup of a common complaint. *Geriatrics, 50*(6), 42–49.

128. Dystonia

Giselle J. Moore-Higgs, ARNP, MSN

I. Definition
   A. Dystonia is abnormal posture of one or more parts of the body involving co-contraction of agonist and antagonist muscles and, possibly, flexion-extension or lateral deviation.
   B. Torsion is the condition of being twisted; usually present with dystonic movement.

II. Pathophysiology
   A. Dystonia is a group of movement disorders that results from dysfunction of deep subcortical gray matter structures (i.e., basal ganglia).
   B. In some movement disorders, a discrete site of pathology within the circuitry of the basal ganglia can be identified. In other cases, the precise anatomic abnormality may be unknown.

III. Clinical features: Dystonia usually occurs without an identifiable precipitant and presents as focal (i.e., one limb involved), segmental (i.e., two contiguous body areas), or generalized. Dystonia may vary with change of posture, may disappear with sleep, and may be modified by tactile or proprioceptive input. Dystonia may worsen with stress and improve with relaxation or hypnosis.
   A. History
      1. History of cancer and cancer treatment
      2. Current medications: Prescribed and over-the-counter
      3. History of presenting symptom(s): Precipitating factors, onset, location, and duration. Associated symptoms are sensory or motor behaviors, such as tics, tremors, and paresthesia.
      4. Changes in activities of daily living
   B. Signs and symptoms
      1. Dystonia frequently is associated with other forms of adventitious movements and can seriously affect gait, which may be the first manifestation.
      2. Movement descriptors
         a) Movements usually are of a twisting nature (torsion spasms).
         b) Brisk movements occur from the beginning to the peak of the contraction.
         c) Movements can be phasic, rapid, and repetitive.
         d) Dystonic positions can be prolonged but usually only last a second or less.

      e) As dystonia worsens, involuntary contractions appear during rest and may lead to permanent deformity.

      f) Lateralized dystonia may relate to focal intracranial disease.

C. Physical exam: Complete neurologic exam: To evaluate for coexisting disorders

   1. Cognitive function exam to evaluate for orientation, concentration, memory, language, and speech.

   2. Cranial nerve exam with visual fields (see Appendix 5)

   3. Motor exam with gait and stance: Describe dystonic movements as focal, segmental, or general.

   4. Deep tendon reflexes: Increased or decreased movement depends on etiology.

   5. Sensory exam: Increased or decreased awareness depends on etiology.

IV. Diagnostic tests

A. Laboratory: The choice of the diagnostic tests depends on the suspected cause of the dystonia.

B. Radiology: Perform MRI of the brain to evaluate for mass, caudate atrophy, and basal ganglia abnormalities.

V. Differential diagnosis

A. Idiopathic dystonia: No known cause; not associated with a specific brain lesion

B. Hereditary dystonia

C. Symptomatic: Genetic

   1. Wilson's disease

   2. Huntington's chorea

   3. Parkinson's disease

D. Symptomatic: Nongenetic

   1. Perinatal injury: Cerebral palsy

   2. Trauma

   3. Reye's syndrome

   4. Encephalitis

   5. AIDS (see Chapter 156): Opportunistic infections

   6. Multiple sclerosis

   7. Focal vascular disease

   8. Hypoparathyroidism

   9. Neoplasm: Paraneoplastic syndrome (see Appendix 12) or intracranial mass

   10. Drugs

      a) H_2 receptor antagonists

      b) Levodopa

      c) Bromocriptine

      d) Ergot

      e) Anticonvulsant

      f) Antipsychotics (phenothiazine)

      g) Metoclopramide

      h) Tricyclic antidepressants

      i) Diazepam

11. Chemicals
    a) Methane
    b) Carbon monoxide

VI. Treatment: Depends on the accurate diagnosis and treatment of the underlying cause
   A. Eliminate causative agent.
   B. Treatment of dystonia is directly related to the underlying disorder; no specific treatment is recommended.
   C. Several drugs, including anticholinergic agents, dopamine agonists and antagonists, benzodiazepines, and catecholamine agonists and antagonists, have been used with varying success in decreasing symptoms. A local injection of Type A botulinum toxin or lidocaine has been used for focal dystonia.
      1. Benztropine mesylate: 0.5–2 mg/day po
      2. Levodopa: 250 mg po bid to qid with food, then increase total daily dose by 100–750 mg/three to seven days until optimum dosage reached (not to exceed 8 g/day).
      3. Carbidopa/levodopa: 10 mg/100 mg po tid to qid; increase by one tablet every one to two days until total dose is eight tablets per day.
      4. Baclofen 5 mg po tid: May titrate upwards as needed (not to exceed 20 mg qid).

VII. Follow-up: Related to the underlying cause and treatment

VIII. Referrals: Depends on the suspected underlying cause
   A. Neurology
   B. Physical therapy: To assist with ambulation
   C. Occupational therapy: To assist with learning alternative methods to conduct activities of daily living

References

Aminoff, M.J., Greenberg, D.A., & Simon, R.P. (1996). *Clinical neurology* (3rd ed.). Norwalk, CT: Appleton & Lange.

Crabb, L. (1994). What is dystonia? *Professional Nurse, 9,* 812–815.

Mastaglia, F.L. (1995). Iatrogenic (drug-induced) disorders of the nervous system. In M.J. Aminoff (Ed.), *Neurology and general medicine* (2nd ed.) (pp. 587–614). New York: Churchill Livingston.

Weibers, D.O., Dale, A.J.D., Kokmen, E., & Swanson, J.W. (1998). *Mayo Clinic examinations in neurology* (7th ed.). St Louis: Mosby.

Chapter

129.

Foot Drop

Karen E. Maher, ANP, MS, AOCN®

I. Definition: Loss of ankle dorsiflexion because of weakness or paralysis of the anterior muscles of the lower leg

II. Physiology/Pathophysiology
   A. Normal
      1. Fibers from the fourth and fifth lumbar nerves and the first to the fourth sacral nerves form the sacral plexus. It is located in the pelvis on the anterior surface of the sacrum on the piriformis muscle.
      2. Nerves that emerge from the sacral plexus include the common peroneal nerve that innervates the peroneus longus muscle that performs
         a) Motor function: Ankle dorsiflexion
         b) Sensory function: Lateral surface of leg and dorsal surface of foot
      3. The peroneus longus muscle originates at the upper fibula and lateral condyle of the tibia and inserts at the internal cuneiform and first metatarsal. This muscle controls ankle dorsiflexion, eversion, and abduction.
   B. Pathophysiology
      1. Alteration in motor, sensory, and autonomic function may be present with lesions at the level of the nerve roots, plexus, or peripheral nerves.
      2. Chronic pressure at the fibular head can lead to an entrapment neuropathy and secondary foot drop.

III. Clinical features
   A. History
      1. History of cancer and cancer treatment
      2. Current medications: Prescribed and over-the-counter
      3. History of presenting symptom(s): Precipitating factors, onset, location, and duration (e.g., recent trauma, leg crossing, low back pain)
      4. Changes in activities of daily living
   B. Signs and symptoms: Categorized as motor weakness or incoordination secondary to sensory dysfunction
      1. Dragging of toes and high lifting of knees (see Figure 129-1)
      2. Slapping of foot to the ground when walking

Figure 129-1. Steppage or Footdrop Gait

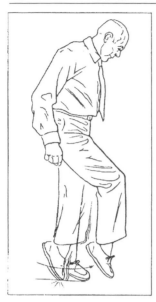

Steppage or footdrop gait. To avoid dragging his toes against the ground (since he cannot dorsiflex the foot), the patient lifts his knee high and slaps the foot to the ground on advancing.

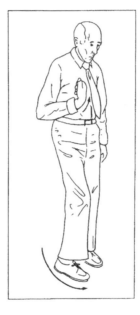

Hemiplegic (hemiparetic) gait. The arm is carried across the trunk, adducted at the shoulder. The forearm is rotated; the arm is flexed at elbow and wrist and the hand at the metacarpophalangeal joints. The leg is extended at the hip and knee. The patient swings his affected leg outward in a circle (circumduction).

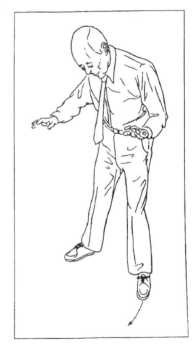

Ataxic gait. In cerebellar ataxia the patient has poor balance and a broad base; therefore, he lurches, staggers, and exaggerates all movements. In sensory ataxia the patient has a broadbased gait and, because he cannot feel his feet, slaps them against the ground and looks down at them as he walks. In both types of ataxias, the gait is irregular, jerky, and weaving.

To avoid dragging his toes against the ground (because he cannot dorsiflex the foot), the patient lifts his knee high and slaps the foot to the ground on advancing.

Note. From *Clinical Diagnosis: A Physiologic Approach* (p. 495), by R.D. Judge, G.D. Zuidema, and F.T. Fitzgerald, 1989, Boston: Little, Brown and Co. Copyright 1989 by Little, Brown and Co. Reprinted with permission.

      3. Decreased sensation of plantar surface of foot or extremity

      4. Lumbosacral back pain with radicular component in peroneal nerve distribution

      5. Atrophy of foot and/or distal extremity

  C. Physical exam

      1. Neurologic exam: Include sensory and motor evaluation of lumbosacral area, guided by specific symptoms/signs.

         a) Observe gait for dragging of toes, high lifting of knees or slapping of foot.

         b) Inability to heel-walk

         c) Test for sensory alteration of affected extremity.

            (1) Two-point discrimination unrecognizable

            (2) Unable to distinguish hot, cold, sharp, or dull

            (3) Unable to distinguish location of stimuli

            (4) Unable to distinguish position of toe joint

         d) Depressed or absent Achilles deep tendon reflex

      2. Musculoskeletal exam

         a) Muscle strength decreased in ankle dorsiflexion

         b) May have decreased strength of lower legs

IV. Diagnostic tests: Neurologic exam may be diagnostic.

  A. Laboratory: To confirm specific diseases or risks elicited in the history

      1. BUN and creatinine: To assess for renal failure

      2. Hemoglobin A_{1C}: Specific for diabetes mellitus

      3. Serum/urine protein electrophoresis: Specific for paraproteinemia

      4. Vitamin B_{12} and folate levels: To rule out deficiencies

  B. Radiology: CT, MRI, or myelography for suspected intracranial, vertebral, or spinal cord pathology; to evaluate for herniation or lateral neuroforaminal encroachment

  C. Other

      1. EMG and nerve conduction velocity (NCV) testing: To evaluate suspected lesion affecting the anterior horn cells, muscle, and peripheral nerves

      2. LP: To obtain cytology, cell count, glucose, and cultures

V. Differential diagnosis

  A. Chemotherapy-induced peripheral neuropathy (see Chapter 131): Drugs include vinca alkaloids, cisplatin, taxanes, cytarabine (primarily high-dose), hexamethylmelamine, procarbazine, and fludarabine.

  B. Peroneal nerve compression secondary to tumor

      1. Primary tumors: Schwannomas and neurofibromas

      2. Metastatic intrapelvic tumor

  C. Systemic disease-induced

      1. Diabetes mellitus (see Chapter 143)

      2. HIV/AIDS (see Chapter 156)

      3. Multiple sclerosis

      4. Chronic renal failure

      5. Stroke

      6. Cachexia (see Chapter 62)

      7. Collagen disease (principally the primary and secondary vasculitis syndrome)

      8. Amyotrophic lateral sclerosis (ALS)

      9. Post-polio syndrome

   D. Metabolic or toxic etiologies

      1. Alcoholism

      2. Uremia

      3. Vitamin deficiencies (e.g., thiamin [B_1]) (see Chapter 114)

      4. Heavy metal exposure (e.g., lead)

      5. Bacterial toxins (e.g., botulinum, tetanus)

   E. Fracture or trauma (see Chapter 104)

      1. Vertebrae

      2. Tibia/femur

      3. Knee (total knee replacement, patellectomy, tears of lateral collateral ligament)

      4. Femoral head dislocation

   F. Lumbar disc herniation

   G. Nerve compression secondary to

      1. Immobilization devices (e.g., knee-high elastic stockings or wraps, pneumatic compression boots, casts)

      2. Prolonged bedrest without foot support

      3. Heparinization, which predisposes a stretched nerve to intraneural bleeding

      4. Chronic pressure from crossing legs

   H. Idiopathic polyneuritis

      1. Guillain-Barré syndrome

      2. Paraproteinemias and macroglobulinemia

   I. Myelopathy secondary to radiation to sacral plexus (late effect seen one to two years after radiation)

VI. Treatment: Refer to appropriate medical diagnosis section.

   A. Pain management, including adjuvant drugs for neuropathic pain (see Appendix 10a/b)

   B. Patient education to maintain full function

   C. Foot drop splint

   D. Range-of-motion exercises to prevent contractures

   E. Orthotic/orthopedic brace

VII. Follow-up: Depends on etiology and treatment plan

VIII. Referrals

   A. Physical/occupational therapist: For assistive devices for ambulation

References

Delattre, J.Y., & Posner, J.B. (1995). Neurological complications of chemotherapy and radiation therapy. In M.J. Aminoff (Ed.), *Neurology and general medicine* (pp. 421–445). New York: Churchill Livingstone.

Duman, S., & Ginsburg, S.H. (1996). Weakness of neuromuscular origin. In H.H. Friedman (Ed.), *Problem-oriented medical diagnosis* (pp. 413–417). Boston: Little, Brown & Co.

Fisher, M.A. (1994). Peripheral neuropathy. In W.J. Weiner & C.G. Goetz (Eds.), *Neurology for the non-neurologist* (pp. 154–170). Philadelphia: Lippincott.

Haerer, A.F. (1992). *DeJong's the neurologic examination*. Philadelphia: Lippincott.

Ludwig, L.M. (1995). Preventing footdrop. *Nursing95, 25*(8), 32c–32j.

Chapter

130. Paresthesia

Giselle J. Moore-Higgs, ARNP, MSN

I. Definition: Abnormal spontaneous sensation of the skin, described as burning, tingling, or "pins and needles" sensation

II. Pathophysiology
   A. Disorders of somatic sensation result from a lesion in a nerve root in the spinal cord, brain stem, thalamus, or sensory cortex and may consist of diminished, increased, or distorted sensations.
   B. Hyperfunction of the sensory system is characterized by a lowered threshold to stimulation (i.e., hyperesthesia) or by spontaneous discharge leading to distortion of sensory input (i.e., paresthesia).

III. Clinical features
   A. History: Obtain a clear description of the paresthesia.
      1. History of cancer and cancer treatment
      2. Current medications: Prescribed and over-the-counter
      3. History of presenting symptom(s): Precipitating factors, onset, location, and duration
      4. Changes in activities of daily living
   B. Signs and symptoms: Location and characteristics of symptoms may provide information as to the origin.
      1. Focal site involvement: Peripheral cutaneous nerve or nerve root lesion or entrapment
      2. Single limb or hemibody involvement: Central brain, spinal cord, or brain stem lesion
      3. Involvement of all limbs: Peripheral neuropathy, cervical cord or brain stem lesion, or metabolic disorder
   C. Physical exam: Perform complete neurologic exam to evaluate for coexisting disorders.
      1. Cognitive function exam: Orientation, concentration, memory, language, and speech
      2. Cranial nerve exam: Visual fields (see Appendix 5)
      3. Motor exam: Gait and stance
      4. Deep tendon reflexes: Increased or decreased, depending on etiology
      5. Sensory exam: Nature and distribution of sensory change
         a) Mononeuropathy (disease of a single nerve) versus polyneuropathy (disease of multiple nerves)
         b) Lhermitte's sign: Paresthesia occurs in the extremities with neck flexion because of inflammation or lesion in posterior column of cervical spinal cord; also may

occur one to six months after radiotherapy to this region and usually resolves gradually.

    c) Glove-and-stocking sign: Systemic sensory loss is greater distally than proximally.

    d) Carpal tunnel syndrome: Median nerve compression occurs beneath the transverse carpal ligament at the wrist.

6. Evaluate for pain distribution using dermatome pattern (see Appendix 17).
7. Evaluate for autonomic disturbances.

    a) Postural hypotension

    b) Extremity coldness

    c) Impaired thermoregulation: Intolerance of cold or heat extremes, decreased ability to sweat

    d) Distended bladder or bowel: Indicates disturbances of bowel and bladder function.

IV. Diagnostic tests: The choice of diagnostic tests depends on the suspected cause of the paresthesia.

  A. Laboratory: If metabolic disorder is suspected

  B. Radiology

    1. MRI of the involved site: Evaluate for nerve compression.

    2. MRI of spinal cord and/or brain: Evaluate for mass or nerve compression.

  C. Other: Electromyography; evaluate for evidence of denervation in affected muscles.

V. Differential diagnosis

  A. Metabolic disorders

    1. Diabetes mellitus: Polyneuropathy (see Chapter 143)

    2. Hypothyroidism (see Chapter 150)

    3. Uremia

    4. Chronic liver disease

    5. Vitamin B deficiency (thiamin, B_{12}, folic acid [see Chapter 114], or pyroxidine deficiency [see Chapter 115] or overdose)

    6. Sarcoidosis

    7. Collagen vascular disease

    8. Vasculitis

    9. Myxedema

    10. Multiple sclerosis

    11. Guillain-Barré syndrome

    12. Chronic inflammation demyelinating polyradiculoneuropathy

    13. Chronic and recurrent immunologically mediated neuropathy

  B. Neoplastic disorders

    1. Metastasis

    2. Paraneoplastic syndromes (see Appendix 12)

    3. Chemotherapy-induced peripheral neuropathy (see Chapters 131 and 137)

      a) Platinum-based compounds

      b) Vinca alkaloids

     c) Paclitaxel
     d) Docetaxel
    4. Paraproteinemia: Distal symmetric sensorimotor polyneuropathy associated with multiple myeloma and Waldenstromm macroglobulinemia
    5. Surgery-induced neuropathy caused by severing of nerves
     a) Axillary node dissection
     b) Neck dissection
     c) Thoracotomy
     d) Mastectomy
    6. AIDS-related neuropathy (see Chapter 156)
    7. Herpes zoster radiculopathy (see Chapter 20)
  C. Drug-induced or toxic disorders
    1. Alcohol
    2. Heavy metals (e.g., lead, arsenic, thallium)
     a) Industrial solvents (e.g., hexacarbons, organophosphate)
     b) Insecticides/herbicides
    3. Isoniazid
    4. Hydralazine
    5. Phenytoin
    6. Gold
    7. Chloroquine
    8. Recreational drugs (e.g., glue, nitrous oxide, cocaine, heroin)

 VI. Treatment: Depends on the accurate diagnosis and treatment of the underlying cause.
  A. Eliminate causative agent.
  B. Treat underlying cause.
  C. Administer medications to relieve symptoms (see Appendix 10).
    1. Amitriptyline: 25–50 mg po qd
    2. Gabapentin: 300 mg po tid
    3. Nortriptyline: 50 to 150 mg po q hs

 VII. Follow-up: Depends on the underlying cause of the paresthesia and its treatment

VIII. Referrals
  A. Neurologist
  B. Neurosurgeon: To evaluate for surgical decompression
  C. Physical/occupational therapist: To assist with alternative methods of ambulation and activities of daily living if neuropathy persists

References

Aminoff, M.J., Greenberg, D.A., & Simon, R.P. (1996). *Clinical neurology* (3rd ed.). Norwalk, CT: Appleton & Lange.

Bowen, J., Gregory, R., Squirer, M., & Donaghy, M. (1996). The post irradiation lower motor neuron syndrome: Neuronopathy or radiculopathy? *Brain: Journal of Neurology, 119*(Part 5), 1429–1439.

Braverman, D.L., Ku, A., & Nagler, W. (1997). Herpes zoster polyradiculopathy. *Archives of Physical Medicine and Rehabilitation, 78,* 880–882.

Mastaglia, F.L. (1995). Iatrogenic (drug-induced) disorders of the nervous system. In M.J. Aminoff (Ed.), *Neurology and general medicine* (2nd ed.) (pp. 587–614). New York: Churchill Livingston.

Novak, C.B., & Mackinno, S.E. (1997). Repetitive use and static postures: A source of nerve compression and pain. *Journal of Hand Therapy, 19*(2), 151–159.

131. Peripheral Neuropathy

Deborah McCaffrey Boyle, RN, MSN, AOCN®, FAAN

I. Definition: Pathologic changes and functional disturbance in the peripheral nervous system and nerve root, which results in sensory, motor, autonomic, or cranial nerve dysfunction

II. Physiology/Pathophysiology
   A. Normal physiology
      1. Peripheral nervous system is located outside the CNS.
         a) Twelve pairs of cranial nerves with branches connect to the rest of the body (see Appendix 5)
            (1) Nerves arise from the brain rather than the spinal cord.
            (2) Each nerve has motor or sensory function; four have parasympathetic function to assist in conserving body resources and in maintaining day-to-day body functions (e.g., digestion, elimination).
         b) Thirty-one pairs of spinal nerves with branches connect to the rest of the body.
            (1) Sensory and motor fibers of each spinal nerve supply and receive information from a specific body distribution (i.e., dermatome) (see Appendix 17)
            (2) Multiple peripheral nerves originate from nerve plexi located on the anterior branches of several spinal nerves (e.g., brachial, cervical, lumbar, sacral plexi).
      2. Motor and sensory nerves and ganglia are located outside the CNS.
         a) Each nerve separates within the spinal cord into ventral and dorsal roots.
         b) Ventral root: Motor fibers of the ventral root carry impulses from the spinal cord to the muscles and glands of the body.
         c) Dorsal root: Sensory fibers of the dorsal root carry impulses from sensory receptors of the body to the spinal cord. Impulses then travel to the brain for interpretation by the cerebral sensory cortex, and reflex is initiated.
   B. Pathophysiology: Exact mechanism unknown
      1. May result from *direct* damage from neurotoxic drugs.
         a) Mitotic inhibition from vinca alkaloid therapy is thought to impede microtubule function in the axon transport system, resulting in axonal degeneration.
         b) Heavy metal compounds (e.g., cisplatin) produce segmental demyelination of large sensory nerves.
         c) Paclitaxel precipitates axonal degeneration and demyelination by increasing microtubular accumulation within the nerve.

2. Indirect damage occurs from compression of a nerve associated with metastasis, herniated disc, or compression fracture.

III. Clinical features: Dysfunction occurs from inflammation, injury, or degeneration to the peripheral nervous system. Direct damage to nerves and microvasculature results in varying levels of discomfort and pain.
  A. Risk factors
    1. High-dose chemotherapy or cumulative doses of neurotoxic drugs
    2. Age (> 60 years)
    3. Concurrent use of neurotoxic drugs (see Table 131-1)
    4. Radiotherapy to the spinal fields that results in 50% permanent neurological damage
    5. Underlying neuropathy (i.e., from diabetes mellitus or hereditary factor)
    6. Specific multiagent and multimodal regimens: May increase incidence of neuropathy because of their additive or synergistic effects (i.e., cisplatin + paclitaxel or radiation to the spine + methotrexate)
    7. Malnutrition with vitamin deficiency (especially B complex)
    8. Administration route of chemotherapy
  B. Etiology
    1. Symptoms occurring for years: Suggest hereditary cause
    2. Symptoms occurring for weeks to months: Suggest drug-related toxicity or metabolic cause
    3. Symptoms occurring for days: Suggest chemotherapy toxicity or Guillain-Barré syndrome
  C. History
    1. History of cancer and cancer treatment
    2. Current medications: Prescribed and over-the-counter
    3. History of presenting symptom(s): Precipitating factors, location, and duration
    4. Changes in activities of daily living: Difficulty handling keys, tying shoes, buttoning shirt; tripping or falling
    5. Past medical history: Diabetes mellitus, severe malnutrition, alcohol abuse
  D. Signs and symptoms: Insidious in onset and progression
    1. Motor/sensory
      a) Symptoms most often felt in hands and feet (i.e., glove-and-stocking presentation); usually bilateral and worse in lower extremities.
      b) Symptoms described as numbness, tingling (i.e., pins and needles sensation), burning.
      c) Radiation-induced spinal myelopathy may cause "electric shock" sensations in the spine and extremities.
      d) Pain can be sequential in nature (i.e., myalgia precedes painful paresthesias of the hands and feet).
    2. Autonomic
      a) Constipation
      b) Incontinence
      c) Urinary retention
      d) Acute abdominal distress (could represent adynamic ileus)

Table 131-1. Drugs Reported to Cause Peripheral Neuropathy

Drug Group	Predominantly Sensory Neuropathy	Mixed Sensorimotor Neuropathy	Predominately Motor Neuropathy
Antimicrobial agents	Chloramphenicol	Chloroquine	Amphotericin B
	Colistin	Ethambutol	Dapsone
	Ethionamide	Isoniazid	Sulfonamides
	Nalidixic acid	Metronidazole	
	Thiamphenicol	Nitrofurantoin	
		Streptomycin	
Anticonvulsants	Sulthiame	Phenytoin	
Antidepressants	Phenelzine	Amitriptyline	Amitriptyline
			Imipramine
Antimigraine drugs	Ergotamine		
	Methysergide		
Antirheumatic drugs		Chloroquine	Gold
		Colchicine	
		Penicillamine	
		Gold	
		Indomethacin	
		Phenylbutazone	
Cardiovascular drugs	Hydralazine	Amiodarone	
		Clofibrate	Cimetidine
		Disopyramide	
Gastrointestinal drugs		Chlorpropamide	
Oral hypoglycemics		Tolbutamide	

Note. From *Ellenhorn's Medical Toxicology: Diagnosis and Treatment of Human Poisoning* (2nd ed.) (p. 20), by M.J. Ellenhorn, 1997, Baltimore: Williams and Wilkins. Copyright 1997 by Williams and Wilkins. Reprinted with permission.

3. Cranial nerves
    a) Blurred vision (cranial nerve II)
    b) Hearing loss (cranial nerve VIII)
    c) Tinnitus (cranial nerve VIII)
    d) Jaw pain (cranial nerve V)
    e) Facial palsy (cranial nerve VII)
    f) Changes in taste sensation (cranial nerve VII)

        g) Hoarseness (cranial nerves IX, X)

        h) Dizziness (cranial nerve VIII)

E. Physical exam

  1. Sensory

      a) Decreased vibratory sensation

      b) Decreased superficial pain (i.e., patient unable to distinguish between sharp and dull)

      c) Lost position of joints: Test by holding and raising or lowering the great toe or finger and asking patient to state the position.

      d) Try superficial touch decreased with a cotton wisp or fingertip.

  2. Motor

      a) Deep tendon reflexes

          (1) Absence indicates neuropathy of the lower motor neuron or profound sensory loss.

          (2) Hyperactivity indicates upper neuron damage (CNS).

      b) Gait

          (1) Inability to perform heel-toe walking with broad base stance indicates sensory ataxia with profound neuropathy.

          (2) Steppage gait is common and can occur with foot drop. Occurs when the hip and knee are elevated excessively high to lift the foot; the foot is brought down to the floor with a "slap" (see Figure 129-1).

      c) Fine motor skills will be uncoordinated or unable to perform. Evaluation cannot be performed in the presence of weakness (see Appendix 13).

          (1) Rapid alternating movements

              (a) Pat knees with both hands, alternating palm and back hand.

              (b) Touch thumb to each finger of the same hand rapidly.

          (2) Finger-to-nose test: Ask patient to alternate touching nose with touching the examiner's finger.

          (3) Heel-to-shin test

  3. Autonomic

      a) Abdomen: Bowel sounds may be hypoactive and abdomen distended, indicating an ileus.

      b) Cranial nerves: Most neuropathies are bilateral (see Appendix 5).

          (1) Optic nerve: Check visual acuity using the Snellen chart for decrease in vision.

          (2) Optic fundi: Assess ophthalmoscopically to rule out papilledema or optic neuritis.

          (3) Cranial nerves III, IV, and VI: Assess together by evaluating pupillary reactions, extraocular movements, and ptosis.

              (a) Oculomotor (cranial nerve III): Shows ptosis, dilated pupil.

              (b) Trochlear (cranial nerve IV): Head often tilts slightly to the side opposite the eye with diplopia.

              (c) Trigeminal (cranial nerve V): Involvement is evident when patient complains of acute jaw pain.

(4) Facial (cranial nerve VII): Facial weakness, fasciculation, facial asymmetry, peripheral facial palsy

(5) Acoustic (cranial nerve VIII): Decreased hearing acuity

(6) Glossopharyngeal (cranial nerve IX) and vagus (cranial nerve X)

(a) May be affected when hoarseness is present because of vocal cord paralysis.

(b) Asymmetry of the palate and pharynx may occur.

(c) Patients will be unable to enunciate a difficult phrase that requires precise articulation (i.e., "The rain in Spain stays mainly on the plain.").

IV. Diagnostic tests
  A. Laboratory: Not indicated.
  B. Radiology: Not indicated.
  C. Other
    1. Baseline audiometric testing: Required for patients receiving high-dose ototoxic drugs (e.g., cisplatin), especially those with preexisting hearing loss; evaluates pure tone hearing and high- and low-frequency hearing
    2. Electromyography: To detect axonal neuropathy after four to six weeks (deinnervation changes) and muscle atrophy
    3. MRI of the spine: To evaluate intradural or extradural lesion resulting from cord edema from radiation necrosis, scarring, or tumor
    4. Nerve conduction studies: To identify location and severity of the neuropathy

V. Differential diagnosis
  A. Diabetes mellitus (see Chapter 143)
  B. Alcoholism
  C. Malignancy
    1. Primary brain cancer
    2. Spinal cord tumor
    3. Neoplastic meningitis (see Chapter 136)
    4. Paraneoplastic syndrome (see Appendix 12)
    5. Spinal cord compression (see Chapter 138)
  D. Vitamin deficiency (see Chapter 114)
  E. Idiopathic
  F. Guillain-Barré syndrome
  G. Amyloidosis
  H. Medication-induced damage: Nonchemotherapy drugs (see Table 131-1); chemotherapy drugs (see Table 131-2)
  I. Radiation therapy: Spinal myelopathy

VI. Treatment
  A. Medication discontinuation: Can reverse symptoms; however, the time of symptom resolution is variable and may be irreversible (see Appendix 9)

Table 131-2. Chemotherapy Agents Associated With Peripheral Neurotoxicity

Antineoplastic Agent	Sensory Neuropathy	Motor Neuropathy	Cranial Neuropathy	Autonomic Neuropathy
Carboplatin	X		X (rare)	X
Carmustine (BCNU)			X	X
Cisplatin	X	X	X	
Cytarabine (Ara-C)	X	X	X	
5-dFUrd (Doxifluridine)	X	X		
Etoposide (VP-16)	X	X		
5-fluorouracil (5-FU)		X (rare)		
Hexamethylmelamine	X	X		
Methotrexate	X	X	X	
Paclitaxel	X	X (mild)		X (mild)
Procarbazine	X	X		
Docetaxel	X	X (mild)		X (mild)
Teniposide (VM-26)	X	X		
Vinblastine	X	X	X	X
Vincristine	X	X	X	X
Vindesine	X	X	X	X
Vinorelbine	X	X	X	X (mild)

Note. Based on information from Armstrong, Rust, & Kohtz, 1997; Brogden & Nevidjon, 1995; McKeage, 1995; Wilkes, 1996.

1. Dose reduction or drug discontinuation is often required if the cause is medication-related and the neuropathy is significant.
2. Pyridoxine (vitamin B$_6$) may decrease the intensity of symptoms.
3. Additional measures depend on the type and nature of the symptom.
    a) Hearing loss: May require hearing aid; speak to patient in environment that minimizes extraneous noise, and look directly at patient when speaking.
    b) Vision impairment: Do not use color description in patient education (i.e., identifying pills by color); discourage abrupt head movements (e.g., quick turning).
B. Bowel management: Prophylactic bowel program is indicated at the initiation of chemotherapy with vinca alkaloids (see Chapter 52).
C. Incontinence: Encourage regularly scheduled fluid intake and bladder evacuation; discourage delaying of urination cues.
D. Pain: Use opioid and nonopioid analgesics (see Appendix 8a/b).
E. Tactile changes: Encourage patient to

    1. Avoid extreme temperatures.

    2. Protect hands and feet in cold weather.

    3. Wear gloves when washing dishes.

    4. Use a pot holder when cooking.

  F. Gait changes: Evaluate safety precautions for each patient.

VII. Follow-up

  A. Short-term: Ongoing neurologic examination

    1. Motor weakness resolution may take months; sensory loss resolution may take years.

    2. Reversibility of symptoms more problematic in the elderly.

  B. Long-term

    1. Consider neurotoxic potential of chemotherapy in monitoring for ongoing sensory, motor, cranial, and autonomic changes after cancer therapy is completed.

    2. Consider potential for spinal cord compression based on the primary tumor and history of bone metastases.

VIII. Referrals

  A. Rehabilitation specialist or occupational therapist: To assist with activities of daily living

  B. Occupational therapist/physical therapist: For muscle strengthening, range of motion skills, and provision of assistive devices

  C. Neurologist: For neurologic evaluation

References

Almadrones, L.A., & Arcot, R. (1999). Patient guide to peripheral neuropathy. *Oncology Nursing Forum, 26,* 1359–1362.

Armstrong, T., Rust, D., & Kohtz, J.R. (1997). Neurologic, pulmonary, and cutaneous toxicities of high-dose chemotherapy. *Oncology Nursing Forum, 24*(Suppl. 1), 23–33.

Brogden, J.M., & Nevidjon, B. (1995). Vinorelbine tartrate (Navelbine®): Drug profile and nursing implications of a new vinca alkaloid. *Oncology Nursing Forum, 22,* 635–645.

McCoy, A.M., & Borger, D.L. (1996). Selected critical care complications of cancer therapy. *AACN Clinical Issues, 7*(1), 26–36.

McKeage, M.J. (1995). Comparative adverse effect profiles of platinum drugs. *Drug Safety, 13*(4), 228–244.

Wilkes, G.M. (1996). Neurological disturbances. In S. Groenwald, M. Frogge, M. Goodman, & C. Yarbro (Eds.), *Cancer symptom management* (pp. 324–355). Boston: Jones & Bartlett.

Chapter

132. Syncope
Giselle J. Moore-Higgs, ARNP, MSN

I. Definition: Sudden, transient loss of consciousness and postural tone with spontaneous recovery

II. Pathophysiology
   A. Loss of consciousness occurs in response to an acute reduction in the cerebral blood flow, sufficient to deprive the cerebral reticular neurons of oxygen.
   B. CNS hypoperfusion may be the result of a vasovagal reflex, orthostatic hypotension, decreased cardiac output, or cerebrovascular occlusion.

III. Clinical features: The degree and duration of impaired consciousness depends on the severity and duration of the reduction of cerebral blood flow. The clinical features of syncope can be correlated with the underlying stimulus.
   A. Etiology
      1. Vasovagal syncope: A sudden decrease in arterial blood pressure and heart rate combine to produce CNS hypoperfusion.
         a) Most common type of syncope
         b) May occur in all age groups
         c) May be precipitated by emotional or visual stimulus, pain, fatigue, a medical procedure, blood loss, micturition, Valsalva maneuver, cough, or prolonged motionless standing
      2. Orthostatic hypotension-induced syncope: Hypotension that results in a syncopal episode when an individual rises rapidly to a standing position, stands after prolonged recumbency, or stands motionless for a prolonged period of time
         a) Occurs more often in men than women
         b) Common in the sixth and seventh decades of life
         c) May be precipitated by a systemic condition (e.g., dehydration, sepsis, hemorrhage) or use of drugs (e.g., diuretics, vasodilators) that decreases blood volume
         d) May result from an autonomic nervous system dysfunction caused by effects of anticholinergics (e.g., tricyclic antidepressants), sympathetic drugs, autonomic neuropathy (e.g., platinum compounds, vinca alkaloids), or a CNS disorder affecting sympathetic pathways in the hypothalamus, brain stem, or spinal cord

        e) May result from hypotension associated with some biological response modifiers (e.g., recombinant tumor necrosis factor [TNF], interleukin-2, bacillus Calmette-Guérin [BCG]).

        f) May result from anaphylaxis from chemotherapy (e.g., bleomycin, cisplatin, paclitaxel, 5-fluorouracil, etoposide)

        g) Common in terminal illness because of hypoglycemia and hypotension associated with malnutrition, dehydration, anemia, and/or sepsis

    3. Cardiovascular syncope: A loss of consciousness caused by an abrupt decrease in cardiac output with subsequent cerebral hypoperfusion; usually occurs when an individual is in a recumbent position or during or following physical exertion

        a) Dysrhythmia

        b) Cardiovascular flow obstruction

        c) Aneurysm

        d) Cardiomyopathy

        e) Viral myocarditis

        f) Graft-versus-host disease

        g) Acute pulmonary embolus

        h) Cardiac arrest

B. History

    1. History of cancer and cancer treatment

    2. Current medications: Prescribed and over-the-counter

    3. History of presenting symptom(s): Precipitating event, onset, and duration. Associated symptoms are tics, tremors, dystonia, numbness, seizures, and pain.

    4. Changes in activities of daily living

C. Signs and symptoms

    1. Vasovagal syncope

        a) Usually preceded by a prodromal episode that may last 10–90 seconds and includes lassitude, lightheadedness, nausea, pallor, diaphoresis, salivation, blurred vision, decreased visual fields, and tachycardia

        b) Followed by loss of consciousness during which the individual has bradycardia, pale skin, diaphoresis, and dilated pupils

        c) Abnormal movement, usually tonic or opisthotonic, and urinary incontinence may occur.

        d) Recovery is usually rapid, but residual nervousness, dizziness, headache, nausea, pallor, and diaphoresis may be present.

        e) Syncope may reoccur, especially if the individual attempts to stand within the following 30 minutes.

    2. Cardiovascular syncope

        a) Usually the loss of consciousness is quick.

        b) Seizure-like activity and urinary and fecal incontinence may be seen as the duration of cerebral hypoperfusion increases.

    3. Orthostatic hypotension syncope

        a) Loss of consciousness occurs when a drop in blood pressure of at least 20–30 mm Hg systolic or 10 mm Hg diastolic occurs when the patient moves from lying to standing.

        b) Usually an absence of a prodromal episode but may have pallor and sweating

    D. Physical exam
- 1. Vital signs: Orthostatic measurements of blood pressure in supine and standing positions and in both arms every 10 minutes
- 2. Skin: Pallor or ecchymoses from trauma
- 3. Cardiac examination
  - *a)* Presence of dysrhythmias (e.g., ventricular tachycardia, bradycardia) pulse irregularities
  - *b)* Cardiac valve abnormalities (e.g., murmurs)
  - *c)* Vascular obstruction in the neck (e.g., carotid bruits)
- 4. Complete neurologic exam: To evaluate for coexisting signs indicating structural brain or peripheral nerve abnormalities
  - *a)* Cognitive function exam: To evaluate for orientation, concentration, memory, language, and speech
  - *b)* Cranial nerve exam with visual fields (see Appendix 5)
  - *c)* Motor exam with gait and stance: Upright tilt-table test used to evaluate vasovagal syncope
  - *d)* Deep tendon reflexes: Could be increased or decreased depending on etiology
  - *e)* Sensory exam: Could be decreased depending upon etiology

IV. Diagnostic tests: The choice of diagnostic tests depends on the suspected cause of the syncope.
    A. Laboratory
- 1. CBC with differential: To rule out sepsis and anemia
- 2. Metabolic profile: To evaluate for dehydration, malnutrition, and hypoglycemia
- 3. Urine analysis and culture: To rule out sepsis
- 4. Blood cultures: To rule out sepsis
- 5. Serum drug screen: To screen for barbiturate or sedative use

    B. Radiology
- 1. MRI of brain: To evaluate for brain lesion or tumor
- 2. Chest x-ray: To evaluate for cardiomegaly or pleural effusion

    C. Other
- 1. Electrocardiogram: To evaluate for cardiac dysrhythmias; Holter monitor for extended testing
- 2. Electroencephalogram: To evaluate for seizure disorder
- 3. LP: To rule out meningitis or meningeal metastasis

V. Differential diagnosis
    A. Decreased cerebral blood flow
- 1. Vasodepressor (for vasovagal response)
- 2. Transient cardiac dysrhythmia (see Chapter 43)
- 3. Orthostatic hypotension (see Chapter 46)
- 4. Carotid sinus syndrome
- 5. Obstruction to flow
  - *a)* Aortic/pulmonic valve stenosis

    b) Hypertrophic cardiomyopathy (see Chapter 39)
    c) Prosthetic valve dysfunction
    d) Atrial myxoma
    e) Pulmonary embolus (see Chapter 33)
    f) Pulmonary hypertension
   6. Situational syncope
    a) Micturition
    b) Cough (see Chapter 22)
    c) Defecation (see Chapter 52)
  B. Altered composition of blood
   1. Hypoglycemia
   2. Anemia (see Chapters 111–116)
   3. Sepsis (see Chapter 121)
   4. Hypothyroidism (see Chapter 150)
  C. Cardiovascular disease
  D. Other
   1. Psychogenic
   2. Migraine headaches (see Chapter 135)
   3. Hyperventilation
   4. Glossopharyngeal neuralgia
   5. Vertebrobasilar insufficiency
   6. Carotid artery compression by tumor
   7. Subclavian or innominate artery stenosis (e.g., scarring from surgery, radiotherapy, embolic event)
   8. Takayasus or Menière's disease

VI. Treatment: Depends on the accurate diagnosis and treatment of the underlying cause
  A. Eliminate causative agent.
  B. Treat underlying cause.
  C. Instruct patient on safety from falls or injury related to loss of consciousness.
   1. Stand gradually.
   2. Avoid alcohol.
   3. Eliminate conditions that favor pooling of blood.

VII. Follow-up: Depends on the suspected underlying cause of the syncope and its treatment

VIII. Referrals: Depends on the suspected underlying cause of the syncope
  A. Cardiologist
  B. Neurologist

References

Aminoff, M.J., Greenberg, D.A., & Simon, R.P. (1996). *Clinical neurology* (3rd ed.). Norwalk, CT: Appleton & Lange.

Flowers, A. (1996). Seizures and syncope. In V.A. Levin (Ed.), *Cancer in the nervous system* (pp. 314–333). New York: Churchill Livingstone.

Mastaglia, F.L. (1995). Iatrogenic (drug-induced) disorders of the nervous system. In M.J. Aminoff (Ed.), *Neurology and general medicine* (2nd ed.) (pp. 587–614). New York: Churchill Livingstone.

Chapter

133. Tremor

Giselle J. Moore-Higgs, ARNP, MSN

I. Definition: Any involuntary, rhythmic movement across a joint

II. Pathophysiology
   A. Tremors result from alternating contractions of opposing muscle groups or from simultaneous contractions of agonist and antagonist muscles, with one group acting more forcefully than the other.
   B. Movement disorders, including tremors, impair the regulation of voluntary motor activity without directly affecting strength, sensation, or cerebellar function. This includes hypokinetic and hyperkinetic disorders, which result from dysfunction of deep subcortical gray matter structures (basal ganglia).
   C. In some movement disorders, a discrete site of pathology within the circuitry of the basal ganglia can be identified. In other cases, the precise anatomic abnormality may be unknown.

III. Clinical features: Tremors are the most common type of involuntary movement disorder. The fixed recurring interval between movements differentiates tremor from other repetitive movements and are classified depending on the pathophysiology. Tremors of the extremities are divided into four categories: rest, postural, action, and intention. With the exception of Parkinson's rest tremor, the significance of tremor cannot be determined out of context with other neurologic signs.
   A. History
      1. History of cancer and cancer treatment
      2. Current medications: Prescribed and over-the-counter
      3. History of presenting symptom(s): Precipitating factors, location, and duration
      4. Changes in activities of daily living
      5. Past medical history: Birth trauma, psychiatric disorders
      6. Family history: Tremors
   B. Signs and symptoms: Rhythmic oscillatory movement in one or more limbs
   C. Physical exam: Perform complete neurologic exam to assess the nature of the abnormal movements, extent of neurologic involvement, and presence of a coexisting disease
      1. Cognitive function exam: To evaluate for orientation, concentration, memory, language, and speech

2. Cranial nerve exam with visual fields (see Appendix 5)
3. Motor exam including gait and stance: To characterize tremors
    a) Rest tremor: Have patient place arms in lap when sitting or at side while lying down.
        (1) Tremor in a limb while at rest
        (2) Usually slow (3–7 Hz)
        (3) Diminished with purposeful movement of the extremity
        (4) Associated with increased muscle tone
    b) Postural tremor: Have patient stretch arms out in front of body or use hands to raise cup to mouth; evaluate handwriting and ability to copy spirals.
        (1) Tremor occurs in a limb during sustained posture or during movement (increases toward the end of the movement).
        (2) Usually rapid (7–11 Hz)
        (3) More severe in the distal part of the extremity than in the proximal part
        (4) May occur during subsequent movement but should not increase in severity
    c) Action tremor: Have patient do finger-to-nose maneuver. Tremor increases or is precipitated by purposeful activity.
4. Deep tendon reflexes: Increased or decreased depending on etiology
5. Sensory exam: Increased or decreased depending on etiology

IV. Diagnostic tests
    A. Laboratory: Toxicology studies may reveal excessive amounts of medications or alcohol.
    B. Radiology: MRI of the brain to evaluate for mass, basal ganglia abnormalities, and caudate atrophy.
    C. Other
        1. Electromyography: To evaluate for nerve conduction abnormalities
        2. Electroencephalograph: To evaluate for evidence of seizure activity

V. Differential diagnosis
    A. Essential tremors: Postural tremor accentuated by voluntary movement
    B. Cerebellar tremor: Tremor that usually includes side-to-side movement of arms and legs that interrupts an involuntary action, especially at the extremes of reach, and is absent at rest
    C. Parkinson tremor: Resting tremor that begins unilaterally in an upper or lower extremity
    D. Drug-induced tremor resulting from
        1. Sympathomimetic agents
        2. Bronchodilator (theophylline)
        3. Levodopa
        4. Corticosteroid
        5. Thyroxine
        6. Tricyclic antidepressants
        7. Hypoglycemic agents

      8. Benzodiazepine
      9. Lithium
    10. Cimetidine (may increase essential tremors)
    11. Terfenadine (may increase essential tremors)
    12. Caffeine
    13. Beta-adrenergic agonists
    14. Calcium channel blockers
    15. Epinephrine
    16. Amphetamines
    17. Carbon monoxide
    18. Heavy metals (e.g., mercury, lead, arsenic)
    19. Cyclosporin

  E. Rubral (midbrain) tremor
    1. An uncommon tremor that consists of a combination of rest and postural tremors caused by a lesion in the vicinity of the red nucleus (e.g., tumor, abscess, demyelination)
    2. Usually associated with other midbrain neurologic deficits, including third cranial nerve palsy and hemiparesis

  F. Peripheral neuropathy tremor: Irregular, rhythmic, proximal, or distal tremors

  G. Psychogenic tremors

VI. Treatment: Depends on the accurate diagnosis of the underlying causative factor. Treatment usually is not effective if the underlying cause cannot be treated; however, some treatments may effectively reduce the tremors and improve quality of life

  A. Essential tremor
    1. Beta-adrenergic blockers
      a) Propranolol: 120–240 mg/day po
      b) Metoprolol: 100–200 mg/day po
    2. Primidone: 50 mg/day po (may increase in 50 mg increments to a maximum of 250 mg/day po in divided doses)
    3. Ethanol (in small amounts)
    4. Behavioral therapy (e.g., psychotherapy, biofeedback, hypnosis)
    5. Surgical intervention (e.g., stereotaxic thalamotomy)

  B. Cerebellar tremor: Difficult to treat—surgical intervention (e.g., stereotaxic thalamotomy)

  C. Parkinson tremor
    1. Levodopa: 0.5–1 g/day po in divided doses
    2. Carbidopa/levodopa: 10/100 to 25/250 po tid
    3. Bromocriptine: 2.5–10 mg/day po
    4. Amantadine: 100 mg po bid
    5. Pergolide: titrate up to 1 mg po tid
    6. Selegiline: 5 mg po bid
    7. Trihexyphenidyl: 6–20 mg/day po
    8. Benztropine: 1–6 mg/day po
    9. Procyclidine: 7.5–30 mg/day po

10. Orphenadrine: 150–400 mg/day po
D. Drug-induced tremor: Eliminate the causative agent and consider alternative drugs.
E. Rubral tremor: Symptomatic treatment only
F. Peripheral neuropathic tremor: Treatment directed at underlying cause of neuropathy (see Chapter 131)
G. Psychogenic tremor: Treatment of underlying psychiatric disorder

VII. Follow-up: Depends on the cause of the tremor and its treatment

VIII. Referrals: Depend on the suspected underlying cause of the tremor
A. Neurologist
B. Pharmacotherapist
C. Psychiatrist
D. Occupational and physical therapists

References

Aminoff, M.J., Greenberg, D.A., & Simon, R.P. (1996). *Clinical neurology* (3rd ed.). Norwalk, CT: Appleton & Lange.

Eible, R.J., & Koller, W.C. (1990). *Tremor*. Baltimore: Johns Hopkins University Press.

Gillespie, M.M. (1991). Tremor. *Journal of Neuroscience Nursing, 23*(3), 170–174.

Pryse-Phillips, W., & Murray, T.J. (1992). *Essential neurology* (4th ed.). New York: Medical Examiner Publishers.

Taft, J.M. (1997). Tremor: When is it a sign of disease? *Journal of American Academy of Physician Assistants, 19*(8), 49–60.

Chapter

134.

Brain Metastasis

Terri S. Armstrong, RN, MS, NP, CS

I. Definition: Neoplasm that originates in tissues outside of the brain and spreads secondarily to the brain or brain coverings. Single or solitary brain metastasis refers to an apparently single cerebral lesion with no implication regarding the extent of cancer elsewhere in the body.

II. Pathophysiology: Cancer can invade or compress the brain tissue by hematogenous spread or by direct extension.
   A. Direct extension occurs when a lesion in the skull or other structure located close to the intracranial cavity (e.g., nasal sinus) invades the brain.
   B. Hematogenous spread usually occurs through the arterial circulation.
      1. Neoplastic cells detach from the primary tumor and migrate into the bloodstream.
      2. In the circulating bloodstream, clumps of tumor (i.e., tumor emboli) become lodged in cerebral capillaries, progressing through the basement membrane, and form a secondary tumor (or metastasis). These metastases are commonly found in the area directly beneath the gray-white junction because of the narrowing of blood vessels or at the watershed areas of arterial circulation (the zones on the border of or between the territories of the major cerebral vessels).

III. Clinical features: Metastases can be solid, cystic, or hemorrhagic. Slow-growing neoplasms can result in cerebral metastases from 1–15 years from the time of the initial diagnosis (i.e., the average length of time to development is three years for breast cancer and four months for non-small cell lung cancer; the diagnosis of leptomeningeal metastasis is usually made six months to three years after diagnosis of the primary tumor).
   A. Etiology
      1. Metastases occur more commonly in the larger areas of the brain with the larger volume of blood supply.
         a) Cerebral hemispheres (80%)
         b) Cerebellum (15%)
         c) Brain stem (5%)
      2. Most common primary tumors to metastasize to the brain
         a) Lung: Primary lung tumors account for 30%–60% of all brain metastases with small-cell being the most common histologic type.

        b) Breast

        c) Melanoma

        d) Gastrointestinal tract (colon)

        e) Renal carcinoma

    3. Other metastatic patterns

        a) Metastasis to the skull occurs most commonly with cancer of the breast or prostate, although prostate cancers rarely invade the brain.

        b) Spread to the spinal fluid is uncommon; sometimes occurs with leukemia and lymphomas

        c) Twenty to twenty-five percent of patients with brain metastases involving the posterior fossa will develop leptomeningeal spread.

        d) Metastasis can develop insidiously and progress to disability over a few weeks to months, depending on tumor location, extent of surrounding brain edema, and occurrence of rapid changes within the tumor (i.e., hemorrhage, stroke, necrosis).

B. History

    1. History of cancer and cancer treatment

    2. Current medications: Prescribed and over-the-counter

    3. History of presenting symptom(s): Precipitating factors, location, and duration

    4. Changes in activities of daily living

    5. Past medical history: Stroke, brain aneurysm, head trauma

C. Signs and symptoms: The onset of symptoms may occur suddenly as a result of seizure or hemorrhage or may be gradual, although onset usually does not exceed six months.

    1. Headache: Most common symptom (reported in 33%–50% of patients at diagnosis).

        a) Usually mild, not debilitating, and located ipsilateral to the tumor or bifrontal.

        b) Seventy-seven percent of headaches are reported to be "tension-type."

    2. Seizures: Occur in 15%–30% of patients at presentation. Most common in patients with melanoma, renal cell, and choriocarcinoma.

    3. Global loss of cognitive function: Varies in presentation; may include depression, loss of memory, worsening of intellect, or dementia.

    4. Aphasia: May present with difficulty naming objects, forming words, or understanding written or spoken words.

    5. Focal weakness: Patient may notice symptoms, or they may be appreciable only upon exam.

        a) Tumors of the cerebral hemispheres cause weakness contralateral to the lesion.

        b) Tumors of the cerebellum cause lack of coordination ipsilateral to the location of the lesion.

    6. Dizziness, ataxia, and tremor: Reported to occur in 62% of those with cerebellar metastases.

    7. Cranial nerve dysfunction: Common in tumors affecting the skull base, brain stem, or leptomeninges. Can present as ophthalmoplegia, causing double vision; facial droop, causing difficulty with speech; or inability to control the tongue or swallow, causing dysarthria or potentially aspiration (see Appendix 5).

    8. Vomiting, headache, and decreased level of consciousness: Caused by increased intracranial pressure.

D. Physical exam (see Table 134-1)

IV. Diagnostic tests
    A. Laboratory
        1. Lumbar puncture (LP): To determine, via spinal fluid, if tumor has spread; CT scan of brain should precede LP to rule out mass lesion and potential for herniation in patients with neurologic dysfunction.
        2. Spinal fluid should be tested for
            a) Glucose: Normal or reduced
            b) Protein: Normal or slightly elevated
            c) Cell count
            d) Cytology (identification of tumor histology): May require multiple LPs to obtain positive cytology.
    B. Radiology
        1. Contrast-enhanced MRI: Best diagnostic test for brain metastasis
        2. Contrast-enhanced CT scan: Useful in evaluating for bleeding if sudden neurologic worsening occurs; good for imaging bone, especially to evaluate metastases to the skull.

V. Differential diagnosis
    A. Vascular disorders
        1. Hypercoagulability (e.g., infarct, emboli)
        2. Hypocoagulability (e.g., hemorrhage)
    B. Cerebral abscess
    C. Infectious meningitis (see Chapter 136)
    D. Metabolic encephalopathy (e.g., hypoxemia, uremia, hepatic encephalopathy, hypothyroidism)
    E. Psychological reactions (see Chapters 152 and 154)

Table 134-1. Potential Physical Exam Findings From Brain Metastasis

Tumor Location	Potential Physical Exam Findings
Frontal lobe	Cognitive dysfunction (worsened intellect); behavioral changes (depression, mania, or indifference); weakness (contralateral to the tumor location); increased reflexes (contralateral to the tumor location)
Temporal lobe	Impairment of short-term memory; dominant hemisphere: receptive aphasia; association area in dominant hemisphere: dementia
Parietal lobe	Disruption of sensation on side of body contralateral to the lesion dominant hemisphere: loss of visual-spatial relations; inability to recognize fingers (finger agnosia) or discern left from right; difficulty with math calculations
Occipital lobe	Loss of part of visual field in both eyes (i.e., homonymous hemianopsia is loss of half of visual field); visual agnosia (loss of ability to recognize objects which are seen)
Cerebellum	Loss of balance (truncal or limb ataxia); dysarthria; nystagmus
Brain stem	Cranial nerve dysfunction; weakness; loss of sensation; hemodynamic instability; symptoms of increased intracranial pressure

F. Neurotoxicity (see Chapter 137)

G. Paraneoplastic disorders (see Appendix 12)

H. Cerebrovascular disease

I. Multiple sclerosis

VI. Treatment: The prognosis for patients with brain metastasis is poor. Untreated patients have a median survival of approximately one month. Factors to consider when determining the ideal treatment for each patient include extent of systemic disease, the patient's neurologic status, and the number and sites of metastasis.

A. Corticosteroids: Steroids are not tumoricidal for most types of tumors but act to reduce symptoms by reducing peritumoral edema.

1. More than 70% of patients will have improved symptoms after starting steroid therapy.

2. The clinical effects of steroids are noticeable within 6–24 hours after the first dose and reach a maximum effect in 3–7 days.

3. Various corticosteroid agents may be used (e.g., Medrol® [Pharmacia & Upjohn, Peapack, NJ], prednisone, dexamethasone).

a) Dosage will be determined by the size of the lesion, associated swelling, and symptoms.

b) Common dosages include dexamethasone IV bolus of 10–100 mg followed by 8–50 mg per day.

4. Corticosteroids usually are maintained through the initiation of therapy (i.e., surgery, radiation). Tapering is based on patient's symptomatic improvement, with most requiring maintenance of steroids through the completion of radiation and often for several weeks after.

B. Anticonvulsants: Seizures occur in 30% of patients with metastatic brain lesions.

1. Most authorities recommend using anticonvulsants prophylactically in patients whose tumors are known to spontaneously hemorrhage (i.e., melanoma, renal cell, choriocarcinoma).

2. Anticonvulsants generally are given to patients only if seizures occur.

3. Several anticonvulsants are available, although phenytoin (Dilantin®, Parke-Davis, Morris Plains, NJ) is the most commonly used (see Chapter 139).

a) Dilantin is started with a loading dose of 18 mg/kg po given over 24 hours and then dosed daily or twice daily at 300–400 mg/day.

b) Carbamazepine (Tegretol®, Novartis Pharmaceuticals Corporation, East Hanover, NJ) and valproic acid (Depakote®, Abbott Laboratories, Inc., North Chicago, IL) can be associated with thrombocytopenia when concurrent chemotherapy is administered.

C. Surgery: Craniotomy is generally reserved for special circumstances for metastatic brain lesions.

1. The best results are achieved in those patients with a single surgically accessible lesion and either no remaining systemic disease or controlled systemic cancer limited to the primary site.

2. Surgical treatment may be indicated for those patients without known systemic cancer (to obtain a tissue diagnosis) and for patients for whom death is imminent because of impending cerebral herniation.

        a) One clinical study showed the important finding that 11% of patients with known systemic malignancy and a solitary brain lesion were found not to have metastatic brain tumors when tissue was obtained via biopsy or resection.

        b) The lesions were found to be primary brain tumors, abscesses, or inflammatory processes.

  D. Radiotherapy: Whole brain radiotherapy (WBRT) is the treatment of choice for most patients with brain metastasis.

    1. Typical radiation treatment schedules for brain metastases consist of short courses (7–15 days) of whole-brain irradiation using high doses (150–400 cGy/day) with total doses in the range of 3,000–5,000 cGy.

    2. WBRT increases median survival to three to six months.

    3. Complications of radiotherapy include short-term symptoms (e.g., transient worsening of symptoms, alopecia, hearing loss, scalp drying/infection) and long-term symptoms (e.g., dementia, ataxia, urinary incontinence [develop in 10% of patients]).

  E. Stereotactic radiosurgery: Allows higher doses of radiation to be delivered to the tumor bed by sparing surrounding brain tissue.

    1. The dose is given at one time and may require a one-day hospital stay.

    2. Use is generally limited to patients with smaller, well-defined tumors and usually not more than three lesions within the brain.

  F. Chemotherapy: The efficacy of chemotherapy in the management of brain metastasis has not been demonstrated.

    1. Intrathecal chemotherapy: Used for patients with no leptomeningeal metastasis

    2. Intrathecal methotrexate, cytarabine, and thiotepa: Most commonly used; response rates reported as approximately 20%

VII. Follow-up

  A. About 50% of patients treated with surgery and WBRT for brain metastasis experience recurrence; 63% of metastases will be local and occur within six months of initial diagnosis.

  B. Anticonvulsants, if started, should be maintained and blood levels closely monitored based on seizure control and other concomitant therapies.

  C. Serial follow-up MRIs are recommended at least every three months based on symptom presentation.

    1. Worsening of neurologic symptoms may indicate changes within the tumor, necessitating intervention.

    2. Symptoms may include increased edema, requiring increased steroids; tissue necrosis, requiring surgical removal; or tumor recurrence, necessitating further treatment.

  D. Corticosteroids: Should be maintained as long as necessary to control neurologic symptoms. Tapering should occur slowly (two to four mg per week if neurologically stable); assessment of adrenal function, including a cortisol stimulation test, should occur before steroids are tapered in any patient taking them for three months or longer. If the patient fails the cortisol stimulation test, physiologic doses (e.g., hydrocortisone 20 mg q am and 10 mg q pm) must be maintained for life.

VIII. Referrals

  A. Neurosurgeon: If biopsy, resection, or stereotactic radiosurgery are indicated

B. Radiation oncologist: For standard treatment of brain metastases
C. Physical/occupational therapist: If neurologic deficits (e.g., weakness, gait abnormalities) exist
D. Speech therapist: If aphasia or cranial nerve deficits exist
E. Neurologist: If seizures are uncontrolled or difficult to manage
F. Oncologist: For assessment/management of systemic malignancies

References

Arbit, E., & Wronski, M. (1996). Clinical decision making in brain metastases. *Neurosurgery Clinics of North America, 7,* 447–457.

DeAngelis, L. (1994). Management of brain metastases. *Cancer Investigation, 12*(2), 156–165.

Fleming, D., Goldsmith, G., Stevens, D., & Herzig, R. (1999). Dose intensive chemotherapy for breast cancer with brain metastases: A case series. *American Journal of Clinical Oncology, 22,* 371–374.

Johnson, J., & Young, B. (1996). Demographics of brain metastases. *Neurosurgery Clinics of North America, 7,* 337–344.

Kemp, C. (1998). Metastatic spread and common symptoms. Part one: Introduction bladder cancer and brain cancer. *American Journal of Hospital Palliative Care, 15,* 355–366.

Patchell, R. (1996). The treatment of brain metastases. *Cancer Investigation, 14*(2), 169–177.

Posner, J. (1996). Brain metastases: 1995. A brief review. *Journal of Neuro-Oncology, 27,* 287–293.

Takahasji, J., Llena, J., & Hirano, A. (1996). Pathology of cerebral metastases. *Neurosurgery Clinics of North America, 7,* 345–366.

Chapter

135. Headache
Roberta A. Strohl, RN, BSN, MN, AOCN®

I. Definition: Pain referred to the surface of the head from deep structures

II. Pathophysiology: The brain itself is almost totally insensitive to pain; however, damage to the venous sinuses or to the membranes covering the brain can cause intense pain.

III. Clinical features: The clinical features of headache are related to the type of headache. History should elicit previous headache patterns to determine if headaches are directly related to a disease and/or its treatment. Table 135-1 describes the clinical characteristics of a variety of headaches.
   A. Etiology
      1. Depends upon the type of headache (see Figure 135-1)
      2. Cancer-related headache
         a) Headache related to brain tumor may be the result of increased intracranial pressure from mass effect or associated edema, which distorts nerve endings in the pain-sensitive dura.
         b) Headache related to brain edema has been reported as a side effect of high-dose cranial radiation.
         c) Headache has been reported as a side effect of intrathecal therapy.
         d) Headache presents in 35% of people with brain tumors or brain metastasis; 70% of patients with cancer develop headaches during the course of the disease.
   B. History
      1. History of cancer and cancer treatment
      2. Current medications: Prescribed and over-the-counter
      3. History of presenting symptom(s): Precipitating factors, location, and duration. Associated symptoms are nausea, syncope, and vision changes.
      4. Changes in activities of daily living
   C. Signs and symptoms: Table 135-1 describes signs and symptoms of a variety of headaches. Brain tumors or metastasis can present with the following.
      1. Headache is worse in the morning that initially eases during the day, then becomes persistent
      2. Awakens patient
      3. Moderately severe pain described as "dull"

Table 135-1. Differential Diagnosis of Headaches

Headache Variety	Localization	Age/Sex	Time of Day	Duration	Characteristics	Provoking Factors	Accompanying Symptoms
Migraine without aura	Hemicrania, temporal	Puberty Women > men	Morning	12–72 hours	Pulsating, stabbing	Alcohol, stress, weekends	Nausea, vomiting, photophobia, phonophobia
Migraine with aura	Hemicrania, temporal, frontal	See above	Morning	12–36 hours	See above	See above	Visual field defects, dysesthesia, nausea, vomiting
Cluster headache	Unilateral, retroorbital	>20 years 80% men	Mostly night	30–120 minutes	Unbearable, stabbing, gnawing	Alcohol, nitrates	Ptosis, miosis, lacrimination, rhinorrhea, motoric restlessness
Tension-type headache	Diffuse, frontal, parietal	Women > men	Daytime	12–16 hours	Dull, oppressive	Alcohol	Sleep disturbances, undirected vertigo
Drug-induced headache	Diffuse	Adults (10:1) Women > men	Morning	Daily	Dull, oppressive, stabbing	Withdrawal of analgesics	Gray tinge, anemia, ergotism, renal damage
Post-traumatic headache	Diffuse	All ages	All	Daily, weeks, months	Dull, oppressive	Bending, pressing	Frequent intake of analgesics
Postpunctional headache	Diffuse, occipital	No infants, > 65 years	All	3–7 days	Dull, knocking	Being in upright position	Tinnitus, vertigo, reduction of hearing, nausea
Temporal arteritis	Bitemporal, frontal	> 60 years	All	Weeks, months	Dull, stabbing	Chewing	ESR, fever, leucocytosis, arthopathis
Trigeminal neuralgia	Unilateral V2 > V3	Women > men elderly	Daytime	Seconds	Very intense, stabbing, burning	Eating, chewing, touching, swallowing	Weight loss, inability to talk
Atypical facial pain	Unilateral cheek	Women > men elderly	Daytime	Daily, whole day long	Dull, oppressive	None	Fear, phobia of tumor, sleep disturbances

Note. Based on information from Black & Wen, 1995; Forsyth & Posner, 1993; Ryan, 1996.

Figure 135-1. Etiology of Selected Headaches

Migraine
- Genetic predisposition
- Exposure to triggers (e.g., alcohol, hunger, hormone changes)
- Inhibition of cortical neuronal activity
- Reduction of cerebral blood flow
- Vasodilation of dural arteries
- Release of vasoactive substances (e.g., substance P, prostaglandins)

Cluster
- No generally accepted pathophysiology

Tension
- Proposed pathophysiology:
  - Hypersensitivity to incoming C fiber input from trigeminal nerve
  - Tonic contraction of jaw muscles
  - Depression, anxiety
  - Physiologic relation to migraine

---

    4. Located in occipital or bifrontal region

    5. Associated with morning nausea and vomiting and possibly papilledema and seizures

D. Physical exam

    1. Neurologic exam: Evaluate mental status, patient's awareness, cognitive abilities, and affect.

        a) Confusion

        b) Decreased attention span

        c) Memory loss

        d) Drowsiness

        e) Ataxia

    2. Change in vital signs: Could indicate late signs of increased intracranial pressure.

        a) Widening pulse pressure (i.e., increased systolic, decreased diastolic pressures)

        b) Bradycardia

        c) Severe hypertension

    3. HEENT exam

        a) Evidence of trauma

        b) Skull tenderness (i.e., subdural hematoma)

        c) Poor dentition, teeth grinding (i.e., bruxism), or jaw grinding

        d) Bogginess of sinuses with sinus headache (check by palpating)

        e) Pupil reactivity

        f) Assess for papilledema

        g) Limitation of motion and crepitus of temporomandibular joint

        h) Otitis media: Acute and chronic

        i) Mastoiditis

    4. Neck exam

        a) Meningeal signs, nuchal rigidity, or anterior flexion

        b) Tenderness to palpation of shoulders, neck, and occiput (with tension headache)

        c) Decrease in range of motion (with tension headaches)

IV. Diagnostic tests
  A. Laboratory: Blood evaluation—According to history
    1. CBC
      a) Infection
      b) Marked leukocytosis associated with acute leukemia, which may present with headache
      c) Anemia
    2. Chemistries
      a) Renal failure (can cause headache)
      b) Underlying systemic disease
    3. Prothrombin and partial thromboplastin: Risk of intracranial bleeding leads to headache.
    4. Blood gas: Hypoxia results in headache.
    5. Drug screen: Cocaine and amphetamines cause intracranial hemorrhage; opioids can cause rebound headache.
  B. Radiology
    1. CT scans
      a) Identify location of tumor, metastasis, or edema.
      b) CT is most widely used and can detect 90% of brain tumors.
    2. MRI
      a) Identify location of tumor, metastasis, or edema.
      b) MRI better detects small tumors (< 0.5 cm), tumors adjacent to bone (i.e., pituitary adenomas, acoustic neuromas), brain stem tumors, and low-grade astrocytomas.
  C. Other: LP performed if CT or MRI can not confirm diagnosis.
    1. Infection (e.g., meningitis, encephalitis)
    2. Pseudotumor cerebri
    3. Meningeal cancer

V. Differential diagnosis
  A. Migraine
  B. Subarachnoid hemorrhage
  C. Meningitis (see Chapter 136)
  D. Subdural hematoma with history of closed head trauma
  E. Stroke
  F. Arteriovenous malformation
  G. Dental abscess
  H. Sinusitis (see Chapter 10)
  I. Acute glaucoma
  J. Hypertension (see Chapter 45)
  K. Systemic lupus erythematosus
  L. Trigeminal neuralgia
  M. Meningeal carcinoma
  N. Malignancy-related conditions

1. Brain metastasis (see Chapter 134)
2. Primary brain tumor

VI. Treatment
   A. Treatment of headache will be determined by its etiology.
      1. A combination of analgesics may be necessary for migraine and tension headaches.
      2. Some patients benefit from alternative therapies (e.g., biofeedback, acupuncture).
      3. Table 135-2 identifies selected pharmacologic interventions for migraine and tension headaches. Table 135-3 identifies agents for possible prophylactic use in treating prodromal symptoms.

Table 135-2. Selected Pharmacologic Management of Migraine and Tension Headaches

Drug	Dosing Regimen	Side Effects (Precautions)
Aspirin	325–650 mg po q 4 hr prn (some patients respond best to 1950 mg at onset)	Bleeding, gastrointestinal upset
Acetaminophen (Tylenol[a])	325–650 mg po q 4 hr prn	Liver toxicity
Naproxen (Naprosyn[b], Anaprox[c], Aleve[d])	500–750 mg po at onset, 250–375 q4 hour prn	Gastrointestinal toxicity, bleeding
Ibuprofen (Motrin[e], Advil[f], Nuprin[g])	400–800 mg po at onset, 300–800 q4 hour prn	
Indomethacin (Indocin[h])	25–50 mg po at onset, 25–50 q4 hour prn	
Ketorolac (Toradol[i])	10 mg po at onset, 10 mg q6 hour prn	
Ergotamine tartrate/caffeine (Cafergot[i], Wigraine[k]) Egotrmine tartrate sublingual (Ergomar[l]) Ergotamine tartrate/caffeine suppositories (Cafergot, Wigraine)	1–3 pills po at onset, 1 pill q 1/2 hr prn (maximum 5 pills/day, 12 pills/week)	Increase in nausea and vomiting, abdominal pain, muscle cramps (not to be used in pregnant women or patients with heart, liver, or kidney disease)
Sumatriptan (Imitrex[m])	6 mg SC (maximum 8 doses per month; each dose is $30)	Flushing, noncardiac chest pain, pain at injection site, paresthesia
Aspirin/butalbital/caffeine	1–2 pills po q 4 hr prn (maximum 6/day)	Dizziness, drowsiness (do not use if also taking monoamine oxidase [MAO] inhibitor)

[a] McNeil Consumer Healthcare, Fort Washington, PA; [b,c] Roche Pharmaceuticals Laboratories, Nutley, NJ; [d] Bayer Corporation, Consumer Care Division, Morristown, OH; [e] McNeil Consumer Healthcare, Fort Washington, PA; [f] Whitehall-Robins Healthcare, Madison, NJ; [g] Bristol-Myers Squibb Company, Princeton, NJ; [h] Merck & Co., Inc., West Point, PA; [i] Roche Pharmaceutical Laboratories, Nutley, NJ; [j] Novartis Pharmaceutical Corporation, East Hanover, NJ; [k] Organon Inc., West Orange, NJ; [l] Lotus Biochemical Corporation, Radford, VA; [m] Glaxo Wellcome, Philadelphia, PA

Note. Based on information from Carey, Lee, & Woeltje, 1998; DeGregorio & Barbier, 1998.

Table 135-3. Prophylactic Agents

Drug	Dosing Regimen	Side Effects
NSAIDs		
Naproxen (Naprosyn®a, Anaprox®b, Aleve®c)	250 mg po bid up to 375 mg tid	As previously indicated
Indomethacin (Indocin®d)	25 mg po tid up to 50 mg tid	
Beta-blockers		
Propranolol (Inderal®e)	20 mg po tid up to 80 mg qid	Fatigue, depression, impotence, gastrointestinal effects, decrease in blood pressure
Nadolol (Corgard®f)	40 mg po bid up to 80 mg qid	
Metoprolol (Lopressor®g)	50 mg po bid up to 100 mg qid	
Calcium channel blockers		
Verapamil (Calan®h, Isoptin®i)	80 mg po tid up to 160 mg tid	Constipation, fluid retention
Tricyclic antidepressants		
Amitriptyline (Elavil®j, Endep®k)	50 mg po q hs (start lower, **increase slowly**) up to 200 mg qhs	Weight gain, drowsiness, dry mouth, constipation
Nortriptyline (Pamelor®l)	50 mg po q hs (start lower, **increase slowly**) up to 150 mg qhs	Urinary retention
Serotonin agonists		
Sumatriptan (Imitrex®m)	6 mg SC or 25 mg po (two doses per 24 hours)	Dizziness, muscle weakness, neck pain, injection site reaction

[a,b] Roche Pharmaceuticals Laboratories, Nutley, NJ; [c] Procter & Gamble Pharm, Mason, Cincinnati, OH; [d] Merck & Co., Inc., West Point, PA; [e] Wyeth-Ayerst Pharmaceuticals, Philadelphia, PA; [f] Apothecon, Princeton, NJ; [g] Novartis Pharmaceutical Corporation, East Hanover, NJ; [h] G.D. Searle & Co., Chicago, IL; [i] Knoll Laboratories, Mount Olive, NJ; [j] AstraZeneca, Wilmington, DE; [k] Roche Pharmaceuticals Products, Inc., Manati, PR; [l] Novartis Pharmaceutical Corporation, East Hanover, NJ.

Note. Based on information from Carey, Lee & Woeltje, 1998; DeGregorio & Barbier, 1998.

B. Treatment of the underlying disease.
   1. If the etiology is a brain tumor, a combination of surgery, radiation therapy, and, perhaps, chemotherapy may be indicated.
   2. Metastatic disease to the brain often is treated with radiation therapy (see Chapter 134).
   3. Dexamethasone is used to decrease edema of the brain. The literature recommends various dosages but usually a bolus dose of 10 mg–100 mg IV followed by divided doses of 28 mg–50 mg/day.

VII. Follow-up
    A. Follow-up of brain tumors will require CT/MRI to assess the response to therapy.
    B. Some primary brain tumors (e.g., glioblastoma multiforme) have a poor prognosis and require frequent follow-up for symptom management. Survival in people with metastatic brain disease also is poor (median is three to six months).

VIII. Referrals
    A. Headache management requires a multidisciplinary approach, including referral to a pain service and headache center, if available.
    B. Brain tumor management requires the combined skills of medical and radiation oncology teams and neurosurgeons and, perhaps, physical and occupational therapists.

References

Black, P., & Wen, P. (1995). Clinical, imaging and laboratory diagnosis of brain tumors. In A. Kay & E. Law (Eds.), *Brain tumors* (pp. 199–214). Churchill, NY: Churchill Livingston.

Carey, C.F., Lee, H.H., & Woeltje, K.F. (1998). *The Washington manual of medical therapeutics* (29th ed.). Philadelphia: Lippencott-Raven.

DeGregorio, G.J., & Barbier, E.J. (1998). *Handbook of commonly prescribed drugs* (13th ed.). West Chester, PA: Medical Surveillance.

Diamond, S. (1995). The management of migraine and cluster headaches. *Comprehensive Therapeutics, 21,* 492–498.

Diener, H.C. (1999). Management of migraine: Tritons and beyond. *Current Opinions in Neurology, 12,* 2617.

Forsyth, P.A., & Posner, J.B. (1993). Headache in patients with brain tumors: A study of 111 patients. *Neurology, 43,* 1683–1693.

Gelb, D. (1995). *Introduction to clinical neurology.* Boston: Butterworth-Heinemann.

Ryan, W. (1996). Evaluation of patients with chronic headache. *American Family Physician, 54,* 1051–1057.

Shuyvan, G., Donglan, Z., & Yanguang, X. (1999). A comparative study on the treatment of migraine headache with combined distant and local acupuncture points versus conventional drug therapy. *American Journal of Acupuncture, 27,* 27–30.

Chapter

136.

Meningitis

Terri S. Armstrong, RN, MS, NP, CS

I. Definition: An inflammatory reaction involving any or all of the layers of the meninges surrounding the brain and spinal cord

II. Pathophysiology
   A. CSF flows through the pia and arachnoid layers; meningitis is a diffuse infection of these layers.
   B. Organisms, such as bacteria, fungi, or viruses, enter the CNS by various routes.
      1. Nasopharynx (most common site of entry in community-acquired meningitis)
      2. Ear canal
      3. Blood stream
      4. CNS
         a) Surgery
         b) Indwelling reservoirs and shunts
         c) LP
   C. Presence of bacterial cell wall fragments are thought to release cytokines (e.g., tumor necrosis factor, interleukin-1B).
      1. This causes an inflammatory reaction with an influx of leukocytes into the subarachnoid space, forming a purulent exudate.
      2. This thickened exudate leads to cerebral edema, raised intracranial pressure, and neuronal damage.

III. Clinical features: Mortality from meningitis is high. In addition, acute sequelae can include cranial nerve palsies, seizures, hydrocephalus, coma, and cerebral herniation. If the person survives the meningitis, chronic complications, including sensorineural deafness, epilepsy, ataxia, hydrocephalus, cortical blindness, and cognitive deficits, often occur.
   A. Etiology: The cause can be infection (e.g., viral, bacterial, fungal) or chemical irritation (i.e., aseptic meningitis).
      1. Neutropenic patients: Usual pathogens are Enterobacteriaceae, *Pseudomonas aeruginosa*, *Bacillus subtilis*, or *Listeria monocytogenes*.
         a) Aspergillosis or zygomycosis
         b) Patients with meningococcal meningitis should be placed in respiratory isolation for at least the first 24 hours of treatment.

2. Deficiency in cell-mediated immunity (i.e., HIV/AIDS, lymphoma, bone marrow transplant): *Listeria monocytogenes* and *Cryptococcus neoformans* are the most common causes.

B. History
1. History of cancer and cancer treatment
2. Current medications: Prescribed and over-the-counter
3. History of presenting symptom(s): Precipitating factors, location, and duration
4. Changes in activities of daily living
5. History of recent infection, LP, oropharyngral surgery
6. Recent foreign travel

C. Signs and symptoms
1. Minor changes in cognition to obtundation/coma
2. Fever
3. Seizures (30%)
4. Headache (often bifrontal and associated with photophobia, nausea, and vomiting) can be acute onset; excruciating pain may make raising the head difficult.
5. Neck stiffness
6. Rash
7. Nausea and vomiting (vomiting may be severe and projectile; movement may cause nausea)

D. Physical exam
1. Vital signs: Fever (101°F–104°F; 38.3°C–40°C), chills
2. Neurologic exam: Altered cognitive function (i.e., mental cloudiness, stupor, coma)
3. Eye exam
   a) Photophobia, diplopia
   b) Papilledema
4. Integument exam
   a) Petechiae and purpura lesions (with meningococcal meningitis)
   b) Nonblanching rash, indicating infection with meningococcal organism
   c) Dry, flushed skin, indicating fever
5. Musculoskeletal exam
   a) Kerning's test: Flex one of the patient's legs at the hip and knee, then straighten the knee; note resistance and pain (50% of patients with meningitis have positive test).
   b) Brudzinki's sign: With the patient recumbent, place your hands behind the patient's head and flex the neck forward; note resistance or pain and watch for flexion of the patient's hips and knees in reaction to the maneuver (50% of meningitis patients have positive test).
   c) Nuchal rigidity (i.e., resistance to forward neck flexion)
   d) Changes in strength/balance (e.g., hemiparesis, paraparesis) or balance changes (e.g., ataxia or apraxia)

IV. Diagnostic tests
A. Laboratory

1. Platelet count: To assess for thrombocytopenia prior to LP
   a) Spinal subdural hematoma can occur if thrombocytopenia is present and can potentially lead to permanent neurologic deficits, including paraplegia.
   b) Guidelines for performing LP in the presence of thrombocytopenia include
      (1) If the platelet count is 20,000/mm³ or rapidly dropping, transfuse platelets immediately prior to performing LP.
      (2) If disseminated intravascular coagulation (DIC) or prolonged PT/PTT is present, implement corrective measures (i.e., two units fresh frozen plasma) during LP.
      (3) Use a 22-gauge spinal needle to perform the tap; hold pressure over the LP site for at least five minutes after completion, and apply a pressure dressing.
      (4) Perform frequent neurologic evaluation after exam, concentrating on strength and sensation of the lower extremities and difficulty with urination; assess for low back pain.
      (5) Transfuse additional platelets if pain or neurologic signs develop.
2. LP: To completely evaluate for meningitis and to determine the causative organism CSF obtained via LP should be sent to the laboratory for (see Table 136-1)
   a) Cell count and differential
   b) Glucose
   c) Protein
   d) Gram stain and culture
   e) Fungal culture, India ink preparation, cryptococcal antigen
   f) Cytology

Table 136-1. Assessment of CSF Results From Lumbar Puncture

Parameter	Normal	Abnormalities Seen with Meningitis	Possible Cause
Opening pressure	100–180 mm Hg	>200 mm Hg	Block of CSF flow, hydrocephalus, mass, lesion
Color	Clear, colorless	Xanthochromic, yellow, cloudy	High protein, presence of red blood cells, increased cell count
Red blood cells	None	Blood tinged, grossly bloody	Traumatic tap, subarachnoid hemorrhage
White blood cells	0–6 mm³	>10	Bacterial infections, viral infections (may have predominantly lymphocytes), tuberculous meningitis, metastatic neoplastic process
Glucose	50–75 mg/dl (60% of blood glucose level)	< 40 mg/dl	Bacterial meningitis, tuberculous meningitis, carcinomatous meningitis
Protein	15–45 mg/dl (1% of serum protein)	> 60	Spinal block (accumulation of infectious material blocking CSF flow), carcinomatosis tumors located in proximity to the dura, meningitis

Note. Based on information from Chipps, Clanin, & Campbell, 1992.

    3. Blood culture: Positive in 40%–60% of patients with *Haemophilus influenzae* and meningococcal and pneumococcal meningitis.

  B. Radiology

    1. CT of the head: Complete prior to LP if patient exhibits focal neurologic symptoms (test is nondiagnostic but essential to rule out mass or lesion, which may cause herniation during LP).

    2. MRI of the head: Indicated when cerebral edema, abscess, or demyelinating encephalitis is suspected.

V. Differential diagnosis

  A. Septicemia

  B. Carcinomatous meningitis

  C. Brain abscess with parameningeal inflammation

  D. Spinal cord compression (see Chapter 138)

  E. Brain metastasis (see Chapter 134)

  F. Paraneoplastic syndromes (see Appendix 12)

VI. Treatment

  A. If meningitis is suspected, hospitalize patient to conduct diagnostic workup, initiate treatment; and monitor hemodynamic stability.

    1. If hemodynamically unstable, transfer patient to an intensive care unit.

    2. Patients with meningitis can develop alterations in cardiac function, impaired respiratory drive, and increased intracranial pressure.

    3. If acute bacterial meningitis is suspected, do not delay performing LP and administering antibiotics.

  B. Antibiotics

    1. The initial treatment for meningitis is empiric, with the first dose administered immediately after LP and before obtaining culture results.

    2. Third-generation cephalosporins are the mainstay of treatment because they effectively penetrate CSF (see Appendix 1).

      a) Cefotaxime: 2 g q 6 hours IV

      b) Ceftriaxone: 2 g q 12 hours IV

    3. Empiric treatment for immunocompromised patients should include

      a) Ampicillin (for possible Listeria): 2 g q 4 hours IV

      b) Broad-spectrum cephalosporin (e.g., ceftazidime) that has more inclusive activity against gram-negative organisms Note: Use clinical judgment when determining immune status; the practical definition of an ANC < 500 should serve as a guideline. Additional considerations include ANC < 500 when nadir has not been reached, hematologic malignancy, HIV status, and concurrent medications (e.g., corticosteroids).

    4. Use combination gram-negative and gram-positive activity (i.e., vancomycin 1–2 g IV q 12 hours, ceftazidime) for patients who have recently undergone a neurosurgical procedure or have indwelling shunts or reservoirs.

    5. Treat patients with fungal meningitis with one of the following.

      a) Amphotericin B: 0.5–1 mg/kg/day IV or 0.7 mg/kg/day for 10–14 days

      b) Fluconazole: 400 mg po qd for 8–10 weeks

6. Patients suspected of having a viral-induced meningitis should be treated with broad-spectrum antibiotics until a bacterial cause of meningitis has been excluded.
7. Empirically treat patients with suspected herpes simplex virus (HSV) meningitis with acyclovir IV 30 mg/kg per day in three divided doses.
   a) Continue therapy for 10–14 days.
   b) Treat arboviral and enteroviral meningitis with supportive care only.
8. When the results of CSF culture are obtained and antibiotic-susceptibility testing is available, direct antibiotic coverage toward the known pathogen.
   a) Optimal duration of therapy for bacterial meningitis is not known.
   b) Recommended duration of therapy is 10 days for *Haemophilus influenzae* and 10–14 days for *Streptococcus pneumoniae*.
   c) Treat Listeria for at least 14 days in the normal host and 21 days in the immunocompromised host.
C. Steroids
   1. The use of steroids in adult patients with meningitis is controversial.
      a) Steroids are thought to alter the permeability of the blood brain barrier, thus affecting an agent's ability to penetrate and treat the infection.
      b) The main positive effect has been decreased sensorineural hearing loss shown in children with *Haemophilus influenzae* meningitis.
   2. Steroids should be given with, or just before, the first dose of antimicrobial therapy.
      a) It is theorized that initially administering steroids without initiating treatment can lead to opening of the blood brain barrier, resulting in increased intracranial pressure.
      b) Patients exhibiting signs of increased intracranial pressure or cerebral edema should use steroids to help manage these effects.
   3. Recommended treatment
      a) Dexamethasone: 0.15 mg/kg IV every six hours for four days
      b) Continued dosing and appropriate tapering is controversial; should be based on the patient's clinical recovery.
      c) Do not stop steroids without taper.
D. Offending agent: Remove the offending agent in patients with indwelling reservoirs, evidence of surgical abscess, or bone flap infection to prevent recurrence of infection and neurologic symptoms.
E. Hyperthermia
   1. Hypothermia blankets or tepid baths
   2. Acetaminophen 325 mg orally or rectally every four hours prn
F. Life support: Mechanical ventilation may be required in instances of worsening cognitive functions, altered respiratory patterns, and increased intracranial pressure.

VII. Follow-up
   A. Assess for return of function and appropriately refer to supportive services.
   B. Closely observe during hospitalization and rehabilitation; depends on the severity of symptoms and time to recovery.

VIII. Referrals
   A. Neurologist/neurosurgeon: For invasive testing, surgery, or management of seizures

B. Infectious disease specialist: If uncommon organism is causative agent
C. Physical/occupational/speech therapist: Depends on degree of involvement

References

Adams, R., & Victor, M. (1993). Nonviral infections of the nervous system. *Principles of neurology* (5th ed.). New York: McGraw-Hill, Inc.

Chipps, E., Clanin, N., & Campbell, V. (1992). *Neurologic disorders.* St. Louis: Mosby.

Lambert, H. (1994). Meningitis. *Journal of Neurology, Neurosurgery, and Psychiatry, 57,* 405–415.

Quagliarello, V., & Scheld, W. (1997). Treatment of bacterial meningitis. *New England Journal of Medicine, 336*(10), 708–715.

Richardson, M. (1996). Bacterial meningitis. *British Journal of Hospital Medicine, 55,* 685–688.

Segreti, J., & Harris, A. (1996). Acute bacterial meningitis. *Infectious Disease Clinics of North America, 10,* 797–808.

Tunkel, A., & Scheld, W. (1995). Acute bacterial meningitis. *Lancet, 346,* 1675–1680.

Chapter

137. Neurotoxicity

Terri S. Armstrong, RN, MS, NP, CS

I. Definition: Neurotoxicity refers to the effects of cancer treatment on the various components of the CNS, peripheral nervous system, cranial nerves, or any combination.

II. Pathophysiology: Various chemotherapeutic agents are associated with specific neurotoxicity syndromes (see Table 137-1).
   A. The blood-brain barrier and blood-nerve barrier protect the central and peripheral nervous systems against potentially neurotoxic effects. Therefore, most chemotherapeutic agents do not harm these structures.
   B. Nerves damaged from chemotherapy have a decreased number of large-diameter myelinated nerve fibers and degenerating nerve fibers in the axon and myelin sheaths.
   C. The primary site of damage to the CNS, the brain and spinal cord, is the cerebellum.
   D. Biotherapy causes alterations in cognitive functioning and personality, often in the absence of neurologic signs.
      1. Cytokines may bypass the blood brain barrier by altering vascular permeability, permitting substances that are normally excluded to enter the brain or by acting at circumventricular organs, where the blood-brain barrier is normally leaky.
      2. Interleukin-2 (IL-2) alters cerebrovascular permeability (i.e., capillary leak syndrome).
      3. IL-2, tumor necrosis factor, and alpha interferon alter hypothalamic actions.
   E. The nervous system is thought to be relatively radioresistant; damage that occurs following radiation probably is related to vascular insufficiency.

III. Clinical features: Several neurotoxic syndromes have been identified, including encephalopathy, peripheral neuropathy, cerebellar toxicity, myelopathy, and cranial nerve palsies.
   A. Risk factors that influence toxic effects on the nervous system
      1. A drug's ability to pass through the blood-brain or blood-nerve barriers
      2. The nervous system's sensitivity to the treatment
      3. Pre-existing neurologic problem (i.e., history of transient ischemic attacks, stroke, brain metastasis, hereditary neuropathy)
      4. Concomitant neurotoxic agents (e.g., isoniazid)
      5. Age (i.e., children, the elderly)
      6. Impaired renal or hepatic function

Table 137-1. Neurotoxicity Syndromes

Syndrome	Associated Agents and Dosages	Risk Factors	Presenting Signs and Symptoms	Time Frame for Occurrence
Acute encephalopathy	5-fluorouracil (>15 mg/kg), ifosfamide, cyclophosphamide, carmustine (>275 mg/m²/cycle), procarbazine, interleukin-2, interferon	• Low serum albumin • High serum creatinine • Prior treatment with cisplatin (ifosfamide) • Presence of pelvic cancers (ifosfamide)	Confusion, hallucinations, aphasia, lethargy, somnolence, and, occasionally, seizures	During course of several-day regimen: Usually resolves in 10 days to 2 weeks; may be irreversible and lead to death
Chronic encephalopathy	Intrathecal cytarabine, thiotepa, methotrexate; intravenous methotrexate, cytarabine, ifosfamide; intraarterial carmustine, cisplatin	• Increased incidence with chemotherapy given immediately after or concomitantly with radiation therapy to the brain	Progressive loss of cognitive function (i.e., dementia) that may progress to coma or death	Two months to two years after treatment
Cerebellar toxicity	Cytarabine (doses > 1 g/m²), 5-fluorouracil (bolus > 15 mg/kg)	• Age over 50 years • Cumulative dose • Less than one hour infusion rate • Impaired renal function • Hepatic dysfunction • History of previous neurologic event • Receiving CNS radiation therapy or concomitant CNS toxic drugs	Global cerebellar dysfunction (e.g., truncal, limb, gait ataxia; dysarthria and ataxia)	During course of several-day regimen: Usually resolves in five to seven days; damage may be permanent, irreversible
Peripheral neuropathy	*Large fiber:* cisplatin *Small fiber:* vincristine, paclitaxel *Motor:* vincristine, cisplatin, paclitaxel *Autonomic:* vincristine	• Prior neuropathy (diabetic or congenital)	*Large fiber:* Stocking-glove distribution, loss of position and vibration sense *Small fiber:* Stocking-glove distribution, loss of pain and temperature sensation *Motor:* Loss of deep tendon reflexes, foot drop *Autonomic:* Constipation, obstipation, ileus, fluctuations in blood pressure	*Large fiber:* Delayed, usually beginning weeks to months after therapy initiated; may take up to one year to resolve *Small fiber/autonomic/motor:* Temporally related to administration of chemotherapy

(Continued on next page)

Table 137-1. Neurotoxicity Syndromes (Continued)

Syndrome	Associated Agents and Dosages	Risk Factors	Presenting Signs and Symptoms	Time Frame for Occurrence
Cranial nerve palsies	Vincristine		Usually involves the facial nerve (cranial nerve VII) or affects extraocular movements (cranial nerves III, V, VI)	Rare, usually temporally related to administration of drug
Myelopathy	Intrathecal cytarabine, methotrexate, spinal radiation		Sensory loss, upper and lower motor neuron dysfunction, radiating pain, bowel or bladder dysfunction	Hours to days after treatment; may be transient or progressive

Note. From "Neurologic, Pulmonary, and Cutaneous Toxicities of High-Dose Chemotherapy," by T. Armstrong, D. Rust, and J. Kohtz, 1997, *Oncology Nursing Forum, 24*(Suppl. 1), p. 25. Copyright 1997 by Oncology Nursing Press, Inc. Adapted with permission.

      7. Cranial irradiation (increased risk with concomitant intrathecal chemotherapy)

      8. Intrathecal/intraventricular chemotherapy

      9. High-dose chemotherapy or biotherapy

B. Etiology

    1. Chronic encephalopathy

      a) Chronic encephalopathy is most commonly associated with intrathecal/intra-ventricular administration of agents (e.g., cytarabine, methotrexate, thiotepa), particularly when followed by radiotherapy.

        (1) The effect generally occurs six months to two years after therapy.

        (2) Neurologic dysfunction can progress to severe impairment, coma, or death.

    2. Peripheral neuropathy

    3. Cerebellar toxicity

      a) Radiation directly to the cerebellum

      b) Chemotherapeutic agents (e.g., cytarabine, 5-flourouracil)

      c) Cytokines (e.g., alpha interferon, interleukin, tumor necrosis factor)

    4. Myelopathy

      a) Following direct instillation of chemotherapy to the spinal fluid

      b) Delayed radiation- induced damage to the spinal cord

    5. Cranial nerve palsies: Thought to be a direct effect of specific chemotherapeutic agents (e.g., vincristine)

C. History

    1. History of cancer and cancer treatment

    2. Current medications: Prescribed and over-the-counter

    3. History of presenting symptom(s): Precipitating events, location, and duration

    4. Changes in activities of daily living

    5. Past medical history: Stroke, brain aneurysm, head trauma, diabetes mellitus

D. Signs and symptoms

    1. Encephalopathy

      a) Poor memory

      b) Difficulty naming objects

      c) Difficulty completing tasks

      d) Loss of ability to read/write

      e) Agitation

      f) Somnolence

      g) Inability to perform activities of daily living

    2. Peripheral ncuropathy

      a) "Pins and needles" sensation in hands/feet

      b) Numbness in hands/feet

      c) Pain in hands/feet

      d) Abdominal pain

      e) Constipation

      f) Difficulty walking

      g) Weakness in ankles

      h) Impotence

      i) Urinary retention

3. Cerebellar toxicity
   a) Slurred speech
   b) Difficulty with tasks requiring fine motor control (e.g., buttoning buttons, writing)
   c) Unsteadiness when walking
   d) Confusion
4. Myelopathy
   a) Back pain from LP at site of chemotherapy injection
   b) Radiating pain, described as "electrical shock," with flexion of neck
   c) Weakness of legs
   d) Loss of sensation or paresthesias in legs
   e) Loss of control of bowel/bladder function
5. Cranial nerve palsies: Depends on which cranial nerve is affected
   a) Cranial nerve I: Decreased ability to smell
   b) Cranial nerve II: Decreased visual acuity
   c) Cranial nerves III, IV, VI: Extraocular eye movement abnormalities
   d) Cranial nerve V: Numbness of the face; jaw pain
   e) Cranial nerve VII: Weakness of the face
   f) Cranial nerve VIII: Hearing loss
   g) Cranial nerve IX, X: Difficulty swallowing
   h) Cranial nerve XII: Difficulty controlling tongue, chewing, or swallowing

E. Physical exam: Focus on neurologic exam.
1. Encephalopathy
   a) Mental status: Poor recall or short- or long-term memory
   b) Unable to follow simple commands
   c) Unable to read/write, button a shirt, use a zipper
   d) Agitation or somnolence
   e) Decreased cortical sensory function
      (1) Stereognosis: Place a familiar object in the patient's hand to determine if difficulty exists in identifying objects by touching.
      (2) Two-point discrimination: Simultaneously using the sides of two pens, touch the skin, alternating irregularly with a one-point touch; patient normally can discriminate about 2–3 mm.
      (3) Graphesthesia: Trace symbols, shapes, and numbers on the skin and have patient identify.
   f) Slowed rapid alternating movements
2. Peripheral neuropathy
   a) Loss of position/vibration sense (e.g., in great toe or finger), indicating large sensory fiber loss
   b) Loss of hot/cold and pain sensations, indicating small sensory fiber loss
   c) Loss of deep tendon reflexes
   d) Foot drop, indicating loss of strength
   e) "Slap gait" (i.e., steppage)
   f) Cardiac exam: Orthostatic hypotension
3. Cerebellar toxicity

        a) Truncal ataxia (i.e., inability to sit upright)

        b) Limb ataxia (i.e., unsteady gait)

        c) Dysarthria (i.e., slurred speech)

        d) Nystagmus noted with extraocular movement exam

        e) Altered mini-mental status exam (i.e., mental clouding or confusion)

        f) Uncoordinated writing or drawing

        g) Inability to perform rapid alternating movements

        h) Altered movement accuracy (i.e., dysmetria on finger-to-nose or heel-to-shin testing)

4. Myelopathy

        a) Sensory loss (often a discrete level)

        b) Radiating pain in radicular pattern (made worse with palpation)

        c) Decreased strength or muscle weakness in lower extremities

        d) Hyperactive or hypoactive deep tendon reflexes and Babinski reflex positive

        e) Abdominal exam

           (1) Distended bowel/bladder

           (2) Hypoactive or absent bowel sounds

        f) Rectal exam: Decreased anal sphincter tone

5. Cranial nerve palsies: Depends on which cranial nerve is affected (see Appendix 5).

        a) Cranial nerve II: Decreased visual acuity

        b) Cranial nerves III, IV, VI: Extraocular eye movement abnormalities

        c) Cranial nerve V: Numbness of the face

        d) Cranial nerve VII: Weakness of the face, fasciculation, facial asymmetry, and inability to raise eyebrows, squeeze eyes shut, or purse lips on one or both sides

        e) Cranial nerve VIII: Hearing loss

        f) Cranial nerves IX, X: Difficulty swallowing, uvula asymmetry, decreased soft palate movement, hoarseness

        g) Cranial nerve XII: Difficulty controlling tongue, chewing, or swallowing; decreased tongue strength; tongue deviation; fasciculation

IV. Diagnostic tests: Diagnostic tests are performed to confirm that no other cause of the presenting symptoms exists; order is based on physical exam findings.

  A. Laboratory

    1. Chemistry profile: Assess for electrolyte imbalance, liver function abnormalities to rule out other causes of symptoms.

    2. Ammonia level: If encephalopathy is suspected

    3. Thyroid function test: To rule out hypothyroidism and hyperthyroidism

    4. B_{12} level: To assess for deficiency (presents with peripheral neuropathy or encephalopathy)

  B. Radiology: CT or MRI of brain or spine: Indicated in patients with neurologic findings to rule out metastasis, tumor, radiation damage, cord compression, hematoma, or abscess.

    1. Cerebellar damage: May be normal or reveal atrophy months after symptoms present.

2. Myelopathy: MRI of spine may show edema of cord from chemotherapy or radiation-induced damage.
3. CT scan can evaluate skull metastasis.
4. MRI is used to rule out brain stem metastasis or vascular lesions.

C. Other
1. Electroencephalogram: To rule out ongoing seizures or pinpoint structural abnormalities.
2. LP
   a) To rule out carcinomatous meningitis.
   b) To evaluate for Guillain-Barré syndrome (especially indicated in patients with lymphoma with pure motor loss).
   c) Elevation of myelin basic protein in chemotherapy-induced myelopathy.
3. Nerve conduction tests and electromyography: May be helpful in determining extent and type of peripheral neuropathy.
   a) Demyelination dispersion
   b) Axonal neuropathy

V. Differential diagnosis
   A. Acute neurologic event (e.g., stroke, hemorrhage)
   B. Brain or spinal metastasis (see Chapter 134)
   C. Electrolyte imbalance (see Chapters 144–148)
   D. Syndrome of inappropriate antidiuretic hormone (see Chapter 94)
   E. Diabetes mellitus (see Chapter 143)
   F. Vitamin B_{12} deficit (see Chapter 114)
   G. Hereditary neuropathy (e.g., Charcot-Marie-Tooth disease)
   H. Paraneoplastic syndromes (see Appendix 12)

VI. Treatment: Effective treatment is not available for most neurotoxicities associated with chemotherapy, biotherapy, and radiation therapy; methods of prevention and careful monitoring are paramount to minimize the effects.
   A. Prevention
   1. Careful neurologic screening of patients with pre-existing neurologic deficits (e.g., a patient with Charcot-Marie-Tooth disease [hereditary motor-sensory neuropathy] or diabetic neuropathy is more likely to experience difficulty with peripheral neuropathy) allows for adequate assessment of patients during treatment by establishing their baseline functional status.
   2. Patients receiving intraventricular chemotherapy should undergo an Indium-111-DTPA CSF flow.
      a) This study assesses normal CSF flow by injecting tracer into the reservoir system and observing for flow of tracer out of the ventricles, around the spinal cord, and up over the convexities of the brain.
      b) Failure of tracer to flow indicates a communicating hydrocephalus and abnormal retention of fluid within the ventricular system.
      c) Injection of chemotherapy into the ventricular system when abnormal flow is demonstrated can lead to retention of the injected drug and rapid development of leukoencephalopathy.

3. Alterations in cognitive function and leukoencephalopathy are known to be more profound if intrathecal chemotherapy is administered concomitantly with radiation therapy, or if radiation therapy precedes the administration of chemotherapy. Careful treatment planning reduces the risk and/or severity of encephalopathy.

B. Monitoring

1. If an underlying neuropathy exists in a patient receiving an agent known to cause peripheral neuropathy (e.g., vincristine, cisplatin, paclitaxel, docetaxel), they should be carefully monitored for the development of decreased intestinal motility and placed on bowel regimen.

2. If evidence of neurotoxicity occurs during treatment, the treatment should be modified or stopped based on the severity of symptoms. Continued treatment with the offending agent often leads to worsening of effects and the potential for irreversibility.

C. Treatment: Most aimed at symptomatic improvement and supportive care.

1. Seizure precautions (see Chapter 139)

   a) Status, emergency management is indicated.

   b) Existence of seizures mandates further evaluation to determine whether they are chemotherapy-related.

   c) Most seizures associated with chemotherapy are self-limited and require little or no treatment.

   d) Phenytoin (Dilantin®, Parke-Davis, Morris Plains, NJ) is the most commonly used anticonvulsant if medication is required (see Chapter 134).

2. Encephalopathy: Most effectively treated by stopping treatment, limiting patient environmental stimuli, supporting nutrition, and maintaining fluid and electrolyte status.

   a) Prevention of self-injury during this period also limits permanent dysfunction.

   b) With chronic encephalopathy, patient may require assistance with basic needs and activities of daily living.

   c) The rate and extent of progression cannot be predicted and may require 24-hour supervision and assistance in some cases.

3. Cerebellar toxicity: Carefully monitor for occurrence; stop treatment when recognized.

   a) Utilization of physical, speech, and occupational therapists often can decrease the extent of dysfunction.

   b) Provision of emotional and physical support during recovery allows for enhanced coping mechanisms for deficits that may be permanent.

4. Peripheral neuropathy: Treatment modification or stopping the offending agent may be necessary if the neuropathy progresses (see Chapter 131 and Appendix 10a/b)

   a) Agents that have been shown to reduce pain include

      (1) Anticonvulsants

         (a) Phenytoin (Dilantin): Initial dose 100 mg po tid and titrate up or for more rapid relief; give 18 mg/kg over one day then 100 mg tid.

         (b) Carbamazepine (Tegretol®, Novartis Pharmaceuticals Corporation, East Hanover, NJ): Initial dose 200 mg po bid and titrate up.

        (c) Gabapentin (Neurontin®, Parke Davis, Morris Plains, NJ): Initial dose 300 mg po bid and titrate up.

        (d) All dosages are increased slowly to allow lowest dose possible for symptomatic improvement.

     (2) Tricyclic antidepressants (e.g., amitriptyline [Elavil®, AstraZeneca, Wilmington, DE])

     (3) Topical agent: Capsaicin cream

     (4) Zinc sulfate 220 mg po bid

  b) Provide a safe environment.

  c) Teach patient skills to avoid injury.

     (1) Loss of pain/temperature sensation: Instruct patient to use hot pads and gardening gloves; decrease water temperature setting.

     (2) Loss of vibration/position sense: Instruct patient to remove throw rugs and use nightlights; instruct on the use of visual clues.

VII. Follow-up

  A. Follow-up will depend on the specific neurotoxic effect, degree of dysfunction, and concomitant medical problems.

  B. All patients experiencing a neurotoxic syndrome will require collaborative care among the advance practice nurse, physician, and specific therapies.

  C. The extent of dysfunction and the patient's recovery will influence further cancer treatment.

VIII. Referrals

  A. Neurologist: For neurologic evaluation and diagnosis of symptoms

  B. Physical, occupational, or speech therapist: Depends on deficits

References

Armstrong, T., Rust, D., & Kohtz, J. (1997). Neurologic, pulmonary, and cutaneous toxicities of high-dose chemotherapy. *Oncology Nursing Forum, 24*(Suppl. 1), 23–33.

Berger, T., Malayeri, R., Doppelbauer, A., Krajnik, G., Huber, H., Durr, E., & Pirlcer, R. (1997). Neurological monitoring of neurotoxicity incuded by paclitaxel/cisplatin chemotherapy. *European Journal of Cancer, 33,* 1393–1399.

Gilbert, M.R., & Grossman, S.A. (1986). The incidence and nature of neurologic problems in patients with solid tumors. *American Journal of Medicine, 81,* 951–954.

Gilbert, M.R. (1995). Neurologic complications. In M. Abeloff, J.O. Armitage, & A.S. Lichter (Eds.), *Clinical oncology* (pp. 771–788). New York: Churchill Livingstone.

Gilbert, M.R., & Armstrong, T. (1995). Neurotoxicities. In M. Lotze, J. Kirkwood, & J. Yasko (Eds.), *Current cancer therapeutics, cancer medicine* (2nd ed.) (pp. 364–369). Philadelphia: Churchill Livingstone.

138. Spinal Cord Compression

Nancy C. Grandt, RN, CNP, MS, AOCN®

I. Definition: A condition in which pressure or impingement is exerted on the spinal cord

II. Pathophysiology
   A. Ninety-five percent of spinal cord compressions (SCCs) are caused by metastatic disease in the epidural space or outside of the spinal cord. The remaining 5% are caused by primary tumors arising from the vertebral column and supporting structures.
      1. Tumors usually invade the epidural space anterior to the cord.
      2. The vertebral body at the level of cord compression often is destroyed or extensively involved.
      3. Cord compression eventually infarcts the spinal cord.
   B. Tumor invades the epidural space by
      1. Direct extension of tumor into the space following bony erosion of vertebral body (i.e., with lung, breast, prostate cancers)
      2. Lymph node growth through intervertebral foramina (lymphoma)
      3. Hematogenous spread from an emboli
      4. Metastasizing to the epidural space without bone involvement.
   C. Neurologic deficits result from these mechanisms by
      1. Direct compression of spinal cord/cauda equina
      2. Interruption of vascular supply to the spinal cord
      3. Compression resulting from vertebral collapse secondary to pathologic bone involvement and dislocation of the vertebral bodies.

III. Clinical features: Manifestations vary with location of compression and degree of block, including pain, motor weakness, autonomic dysfunction, and sensory loss. Early recognition and diagnosis of SCC cannot be overemphasized. The single critical prognostic factor in SCC is the neurologic status at the time of diagnosis. The greatest likelihood of full ambulation, sensation, and bowel and bladder control after treatment correlates with the extent of injury to the cord. Therapy will not reverse fixed paralysis of more than 48 hours duration.
   A. Etiology
      1. The most common malignancies associated with SCC are lung, breast, prostate, and renal cell cancers; multiple myeloma; melanoma; neuroblastoma; sarcomas; lymphomas; and head and neck tumors.

2. Site of compression incidence
   a) Cervical region: 10%
   b) Thoracic region: 70%
   c) Lumbosacral region: 20% (cancers generally arise from the gastrointestinal tract)

B. History: A complete history will assist in noting classic signs and symptoms of SCC (e.g., pain). Be aware that the time interval between initial cancer diagnosis and development of SCC can be months to longer than 20 years.
   1. History of cancer and cancer treatment
   2. Current medications: Prescribed and over-the-counter
   3. History of presenting symptom(s): Precipitating factors, location, and duration. Associated symptoms are numbness, tingling, or coldness of the extremities or affected areas; urinary difficulties (e.g., hesitancy, frequency, incontinence), difficulty passing stool, and difficulty in walking.
   4. Changes in activities of daily living

C. Signs and symptoms
   1. Pain: Present in > 95% of patients; occurs in one or two vertebrae of the actual compression
      a) Can be persistent, focal, radicular, or referred
      b) May be acute in onset, or more commonly, develops insidiously over weeks to months and predates any other symptoms; most commonly bilateral if in legs
      c) Radicular pain: Usually follows a dermatome (see Appendix 18) of involved nerve roots and will increase with spinal movement
      d) Localized pain: Described as constant, dull, aching, and progressive
      e) Worsens with movement, coughing, and sneezing and may awaken patient at night
   2. Motor weakness: Seen in 75% of patients; usually follows course of a nerve
      a) Degree depends on level of compression .
      b) Varies from unsteadiness to foot drop to paralysis
      c) Described as a heaviness, spasticity, or stiffness
      d) Can progress to sexual dysfunction and paralysis
   3. Sensory loss: Seen in 50% of patients at diagnosis.
      a) Symptoms depend on the level and degree of compression.
      b) Usually starts as numbness and paresthesia but can progress to loss of sensation of light touch, pain, and heat.
   4. Autonomic dysfunction: Usually last symptom to occur.
      a) Bladder and bowel dysfunction is present in approximately 50% of patients at diagnosis.
      b) Urinary symptoms include urinary hesitancy, retention, overflow, and incontinence.
      c) Bowel problems begin as difficulty expelling stool and loss of feeling and progress to constipation or incontinence.
      d) Impotence

D. Physical exam
   1. Back exam: Percussion elicits tenderness at level of compression.

2. Musculoskeletal/neurological exam
   a) Increased radicular pain with straight leg raises with lumbar or thoracic compression
   b) Pain of cervical compression with neck flexion
   c) Decreased strength in affected extremities
   d) Loss of sensation for light touch, pain, or temperature in affected extremities
   e) Loss or decrease of positional sense (proprioceptive loss)
   f) Decreased deep tendon reflexes at level of compression and hyperactive below level of compression
   g) Decreased muscle coordination
   h) Unsteady gait
3. Absence of sweating below level of compression may be noted.
4. Autonomic dysfunction abdominal exam
   a) Distended colon
   b) Palpable bladder
   c) Large postvoid residual urine volume

IV. Diagnostic tests
   A. Laboratory: Not indicated
   B. Radiology
      1. Spine radiographs
         a) Shows vertebral body collapse, pedicle erosion, or vertebral lesions in > 85% of epidural metastases
         b) Detects 72% of epidural cord compressions
         c) May not show early SCC because 50% of bone must be destroyed before evident on films
         d) Not unusual to find multiple sites
      2. MRI: Replaced myelogram for detecting epidural SCC; entire spine readily imaged; is noninvasive, safe, more specific, and sensitive, particularly to extradural, intradural, intramedullary, or extravertebral lesion diagnoses; can detect paraspinal masses
      3. CT scan
         a) Superior to MRI for evaluating vertebral stability and bone destruction (perform before surgical management of epidural cord compression)
         b) Accurate in location of cord compression
         c) Used in planning radiation therapy fields
         d) Mandatory to use when
            (1) MRI is nondiagnostic or unavailable
            (2) Patient is obese (i.e., > 300 pounds)
            (3) Patient is unable to lie still
            (4) Patient has claustrophobia, severe pain, scoliosis, or a pacemaker.
      4. Bone scan: May identify vertebral bony metastases or fractures
         a) Useful for patient follow-up
         b) Not specific to epidural tumors or SCC
         c) Can have false results secondary to specific disease processes
      5. Myelogram: Accurately determines upper and lower extent of lesion
         a) Ascertains if more than one lesion is present

       b) Risk of further neurological deterioration from LP
       c) Reserved for patients who have poor CT or MRI results, cannot undergo CT or MRI procedures, or have uncontrolled pain
       d) Used to obtain CSF samples to rule out meningeal carcinomatosis

V. Differential diagnosis
  A. Transverse myelitis
  B. Ischemic myelomalacia
  C. Syphilis (see Chapter 93)
  D. Multiple sclerosis
  E. Subacute combined degeneration of the cord
  F. Motor neuron disease
  G. Epidural abscess
  H. Spinal epidural hemorrhage and hematomyelia
  I. Acute disk protrusion (pain relieved by sitting)
  J. Chronic compressive myelopathy
    1. Cervical spondylosis
    2. Lumbar stenosis
  K. Ankylosing spondylitis
  L. Rheumatoid arthritis (see Chapter 108)
  M. Paget's disease

VI. Treatment: Timely treatment is imperative to preserve maximal function. Therapy decisions are made depending on type of tumor, level of compression, rapidity of onset or duration of symptoms, and availability of clinical experience. Treatment outcomes are better for lesions on lower spine than upper spine.
  A. Glucocorticoids: To reduce vasogenic edema, pain, and oncolytic effects.
    1. Emergent compression: 100 mg bolus of dexamethasone IV, followed by 24 mg po every 6 hours for 48–72 hours; tapered through the course of radiation therapy
    2. Partial compression or metastasis: 5 mg po of dexamethasone every 6 hours; tapered through the course of radiation therapy
    3. Steroid taper can be safely managed with a 10% dose reduction every two days.
  B. Local radiation: With or without chemotherapy
    1. Radiosensitive tumors
    2. Total dose of radiation therapy 3,000–4,000 cGy.
  C. Surgery
    1. Nonradiosensitive tumors or following maximum dose of radiation therapy
      a) Usually last resort for patients with limited life expectancy
      b) Often patient is not a surgical candidate.
    2. Removal of neurofibroma, meningioma, or other extramedullary tumors
    3. Mandatory tissue diagnosis
      a) Unknown cause of SCC but possibility of abscess or hematoma
      b) Rarely can remove entire tumor
    4. Laminectomy: Relieves compression and stabilizes spine when patient has longer than two to three months anticipated survival

        a) Surgical decompression: Anterolateral resection is principle surgical treatment for epidural metastases arising from the vertebral body

        b) For removal of posterior lesions

        c) Treatment of pathological fractures caused by symptomatic spinal metastases

    D. Chemotherapy: Adjuvant treatment to radiation therapy or surgery

      1. Chemosensitive tumor (e.g., lymphoma, neuroblastoma, germ cell tumor)

      2. Recurrent tumor at previously treated radiation site

      3. Noncandidates for surgery

    E. Pain management

      1. Scheduled oral or parenteral opioids (see Appendices 8a/b and 10a/b).

      2. Epidural blocks

      3. Intrathecal opioids

      4. Trial of an anticonvulsant (e.g., gabapentin); (see Appendix 10a/b) may take four to six weeks for maximal effect.

      5. Steroids: Vasogenic edema; also can decrease pain secondary to the reduction of the mechanical compression of the cord.

VII. Follow-up: Most important prognostic factor in SCC is pretreatment neurological status

    A. Short-term

      1. Response to treatment, pain, sphincter control, and motor function

      2. Damage to urinary tract caused by urinary retention with bladder distention and injury to detrusor muscle

      3. Mechanical respiratory failure in high cervical cord lesions

      4. Severe hypertension and bradycardia in response to stimuli or bladder or bowel distention (see Chapters 43 and 45)

    B. Long-term

      1. Neurologic dysfunction

        a) Urinary tract infections

        b) Pressure sores

      2. Existing neurologic status

      3. Adjustment to existing motor and autonomic dysfunction

VIII. Referrals

    A. Radiologist: To confirm diagnosis

    B. Radiation oncologist/neurosurgeon/neurologist/oncologist: Depends on treatment regimen

    C. Homecare services (e.g., physical therapist, home health aid)

References

Bucholtz, J.D. (1999). Metastatic epidural spinal cord compression. *Seminars in Oncology Nursing, 15,* 150–159.

Bucholtz, J.D. (1998). Central nervous system metastases. *Seminars in Oncology Nursing, 14,* 61–72.

Helweg-Larsen, S. (1996). Clinical outcome in metastatic spinal cord compression. A prospective study of 153 patients. *Acta Neurologica Scandinavica, 94*, 268–275.

Kelly, K.M., & Lange, B. (1997). Oncologic emergencies. *Pediatric Clinics of North America, 14*(1), 61–72.

Labovich, T.M. (1994). Selected complications in the patient with cancer: Spinal cord compression, malignant bowel obstruction, malignant ascites, and gastrointestinal bleeding. *Seminars in Oncology Nursing, 10,* 189–197.

Makris, A., & Kunkler, I.H. (1995). Controversies in the management of metastatic spinal cord compression. *Clinical Oncology, 7*(77), 77–81.

Sundaresan, N., Sachdev, V.P., Holland, J.F., Moore, F., Sung, M., Paciucci, P.A., Wu, L., Kellingher, K., & Hough, L. (1995). Surgical treatment of spinal cord compression from epidural metastasis. *Journal of Clinical Oncology, 13,* 2330–2335.

Chapter

139. Seizures

Amy Crawford Minchin, RN, MSN, ANCC

I. Definition: An abrupt alteration of neurologic function caused by excessive activation of cerebral neurons in the limbic system or cerebral cortex

II. Physiology/Pathophysiology
   A. Normal
      1. Two cerebral hemispheres, each divided into lobes, form the cerebrum.
      2. The outer layer, the cerebral cortex, contains the higher mental functions and is responsible for general movement, visceral functions, perception, behavior, and the integration of these functions.
         a) Frontal lobe contains the motor cortex associated with voluntary skeletal movement and speech. Emotions, affect, and self-awareness also are located in this lobe.
         b) Parietal lobe processes sensory data (e.g., tactile, visual, olfactory, auditory sensations).
         c) Occipital lobe contains the vision center.
         d) Temporal lobe is responsible for perceiving and interpreting sounds and determining their source. Integration of taste, smell, balance, behavior, emotion, and personality occurs here.
         e) Limbic system mediates certain patterns of behavior that determine survival (e.g., mating, aggression, fear, affection). Memory functions, particularly short-term, depend on the limbic system.
   B. Pathophysiology: Seizure is a paroxysmal alteration in consciousness or other cerebral cortical function; results from a synchronous activation of neurons in one focal area or throughout the brain.
      1. Cerebral function is disturbed by abnormal and excessive electrical discharges (action potentials) that are synchronous.
      2. These discharges occur in groups of cortical neurons.
      3. There is often no discernible cause for seizures, particularly in adults with new onset.

III. Clinical features: A seizure disorder is characterized by episodic, sudden, violent, and involuntary contractions of a group of muscles, resulting from excessive discharge of cerebral neurons. Seizures are classified as generalized or partial (see Figure 139-1).

A. Etiology/classifications
  1. Neuronal loss or scarring from previous surgeries, head trauma, vascular malformations, or brain metastasis may promote conduction of abnormal electrical conduction and discharge.
  2. Generalized seizures involve abnormal symmetric activity in both hemispheres.
  3. Absence (formerly called petit mal) seizures, are brief and have no obvious motor symptoms.
  4. Partial seizures begin in a focused area of the cortex and often are preceded by abnormal sensations that are recognized as the earliest portion of the seizure.
      a) Simple partial seizure: Focal neurologic events with intact consciousness.
      b) Complex partial seizure: Causes loss of consciousness.
  5. Seizure disorders may result from a variety of diseases, genetics, or changes in the neuron's environment. Seizures can occur from
      a) Cerebral lesions (e.g., brain tumor, brain metastasis)
      b) Biochemical disorders (e.g., from alcohol, hypoglycemia)
      c) Cerebral trauma
      d) Idiopathic epilepsy.

Figure 139-1. The International Classification of Epileptic Seizures

I. Primary generalized seizures
   A. Generalized tonic-clonic
   B. Absence
   C. Myoclonic
   D. Atonic
II. Partial seizures
   A. Simple partial
   B. Complex partial
   C. Partial with secondary generalization
III. Unclassified epileptic seizures

B. History: The patient often cannot recall the seizure; thus, it may be necessary to direct questions to an observer of the event. Obtain a clear description of the event, including its surrounding circumstances.
  1. History of cancer and cancer treatment
  2. Current medications: Prescribed and over-the-counter
  3. History of presenting symptom(s): Precipitating factors, onset, and duration. Associated symptoms are loss of consciousness, loss of bowel or bladder control, confusion, movement of extremities, and insomnia.
  4. Changes in activities of daily living
  5. Past medical history: Mental retardation, head trauma, epilepsy, HIV infection
  6. Social history: Alcohol, illicit drug use
  7. Family history: Seizure disorders
  8. History of recent infection
C. Signs and symptoms: Clinical symptoms depend on the location of the affected groups of neurons.
  1. The episode is usually described as abrupt.
  2. Altered level of consciousness (except in focal seizures)
      a) Unconsciousness: Generalized seizures
      b) Impaired consciousness: Complex partial seizures
      c) No impairment: Simple partial seizures
  3. Changes in muscle tone, posture, and muscle movement: Generalized seizures (unconsciousness during these events is followed by a period of confusion)

    4. Involuntary activity: Motor, sensory, incontinence

    5. A postictal state, which may be characterized by somnolence or headache, following seizure

    6. Amnesia regarding event

    7. An unusual feeling, smell, or sensation of dissociation before the event

D. Physical exam

    1. Neurologic exam

       a) Automatism (i.e., repetitive movements, such as lip smacking, chewing, hand movements) may indicate ongoing seizure activity.

       b) Hyperreflexia

       c) Extensor response to plantar stimulation (e.g., positive Babinski)

       d) Focal neurologic deficits may be evaluated during complete neurological exam following the seizure; paralysis of one arm may suggest a focal onset.

    2. Vital signs: Orthostatic blood pressure changes

    3. Integument exam

       a) Needle track marks suggestive of IV drug abuse

       b) Lacerations, bruises, oral trauma, skeletal trauma

    4. Oral exam: Gum hyperplasia seen with chronic phenytoin therapy

IV. Diagnostic tests

A. Laboratory

    1. Chemical profile: To assess for metabolic imbalances that can cause seizures (e.g., hypoglycemia, hypernatremia) (see Chapters 144–148)

    2. Pregnancy test for women of childbearing age: Necessary before beginning anti-convulsants, as there are potentially harmful effects to the fetus

    3. Drug screen: Use of or withdrawal from substances (e.g., cocaine, crack cocaine, heroin) can cause seizure activity.

    4. Drug level of current anticonvulsant medication: For patients with previous seizure history

    5. CBC: To rule out thrombocytopenia, which could cause intracerebral bleed

    6. Alcohol blood level

B. Radiology: Head CT to evaluate for a source of cause (e.g., malignancy, head trauma); important to obtain in patients with a history of seizures or changes in seizure character.

C. Other

    1. Electroencephalogram is most helpful when obtained within 24 hours of the event.

       a) Obtain urgently if patient has persistent alterations in mental status.

       b) This helps to definitively differentiate seizure activity from psychogenic symptoms, motor activity due to neuromuscular conditions.

    2. LP: Consider if patient has existing malignancy or unresolved postictal state or is immunocompromised.

       a) Values can reveal CNS metastasis or CNS infections (e.g., toxoplasmosis in HIV).

       b) If increased intracranial pressure is suspected, CT must be reviewed prior to LP.

V. Differential diagnosis

A. Cerebrovascular event

B. Tumor

C. Trauma

D. Infection (e.g., meningitis, abscess) (see Chapter 136)

E. Migraine headache (see Chapter 135)

F. Alcohol withdrawal

G. Drug toxicity

H. Eclampsia

I. Chemotherapy side effect: High-dose 5-fluorouracil, intrathecal methotrexate, carmustine, ifosfamide

J. Brain metastasis (see Chapter 134)

K. Primary brain tumor

L. Psychiatric disorders

VI. Treatment: The major goals of treatment are identifying reversible etiologies of seizures and preventing further seizures.

A. Active seizure

1. Secure airway.

2. Insert IV access.

3. Protect from injury (i.e., use of a padded tongue blade may result in broken teeth).

4. Use supplemental oxygen if there is generalized seizure activity.

5. Determine blood glucose and treat as indicated. Hypoglycemia can increase risk of seizure activity.

6. If seizure lasts longer than several minutes, transport patient to nearest emergency department.

7. If patient has a known seizure disorder and experiences a typical event with recovery, evaluate as in sections III and IV.

   a) May require anticonvulsant adjustments, as reflected by serum levels and seizure activity.

   b) Anticonvulsants can be increased in nontoxic patients with normal or high normal anticonvulsant levels to control seizure activity.

   c) If seizure management is conducted by another provider, patient should be seen for follow-up.

B. Generalized seizures (see Table 139-1)

C. Partial seizures (see Table 139-2)

D. Elderly patients: Lower doses of drugs with a slower rate of titration often are necessary because of decreased liver metabolism and declining renal function.

E. Intractable epilepsy: Surgical treatment (lobectomy) may be indicated.

F. Patient education: Instruct patient as follows.

1. Do not drive or operate dangerous machinery until the workup is complete.

   a) Some states have laws requiring that physicians report people with seizures to the division of motor vehicles.

   b) States without reporting laws often require a seizure-free period of varying lengths before the patient can legally drive again.

2. Report symptoms of toxicity (e.g., blurred vision, ataxia, drowsiness) to healthcare provider.

Table 139-1. Medications for Generalized Seizures

Medication	Average Daily Dose	Maximum Daily Dose
Valproic acid (Depakote[a])	500 mg po qid	1,000 mg po qid
Carbamazepine (Tegretol[b])	200 mg po qid	400 mg po qid
Phenytoin (Dilantin[c]): Long half-life; patient may tolerate one bedtime dose	100 mg po tid	200 mg po tid
Ethosuximide (Zarontin[c])	250 mg bid	250 mg po qid
Clonazepam (Klonopin[d])	1 mg tid	5 mg po qid
Phenobarbital	60 mg qd	200 mg po qd

[a] Abbott Laboratories, Abbot Park, IL; [b] Novartis Pharmaceuticals Corporation, East Hanover, NJ; [c] Parke Davis, Morris Plains, NJ; [d] Roche Pharmaceuticals Laboratories, Nutley, NJ

Table 139-2. Medication for Partial Seizures

Medication	Average Daily Dose	Maximum Daily Dose
Valproic acid (Depakote[a])	500 mg po qid	1,000 mg po qid
Lamotrigine (Lamictal[b])	150 mg po bid	400 mg po bid
Carbamazepine (Tegretol[c])	200 mg qid	400 mg po qid
Gabapentin (Neurontin[d])	300 mg po tid as add-on therapy	1,200 mg po tid as add-on therapy

[a] Abbott Laboratories, Abbot Park, IL; [b] Glaxo Wellcome, Inc., Research Triangle Park, NC; [c] Novartis Pharmaceuticals Corporation, East Hanover, NJ; [d] Parke-Davis Pharmaceuticals, Morris Plains, NJ

3. Limit or avoid alcohol while taking anticonvulsants.
4. Report use of new prescriptions from other healthcare providers and over-the-counter drugs, as some drugs alter the metabolism of anticonvulsant.
5. Seizure medications are teratogenic.

VII. Follow-up
    A. Serum anticonvulsant levels are guides but should not be used alone to determine dosing. The patient's clinical status and seizure frequency are the most important factors to consider when determining the proper doses.
    B. Conduct CBC and serum chemistries with liver enzymes every three to four months to monitor renal and hepatic function and to assess for myelosuppression.
    C. Patients who experience multiple seizure types or have frequent generalized seizures are less likely to attain a prolonged seizure-free interval.
    D. Withdrawal of seizure medications can be considered for patients without risk factors (e.g., intracranial lesions, previous head trauma) for seizure recurrence after a two-year period without seizures; withdrawal for patients with risk factors can be considered after five seizure-free years. Withdrawal from seizure medication can precipitate a seizure.

VIII. Referrals
  A. Neurologist: Refer all patients experiencing a first seizure, particularly if
    1. Diagnosis of seizure is not certain
    2. Change in seizures exists
    3. Controlling seizures with medication is difficult
    4. Special testing is in question
    5. The patient is considering pregnancy.
    6. Abnormalities are found in the neurologic examination.
  B. Hospital: Evaluate patients experiencing a first seizure for
    1. Status epilepticus
    2. Primary illness requiring treatment
    3. Persistent postictal state
    4. Recent head trauma.
  C. Tertiary epilepsy center: Appropriate for patients who have had no satisfactory response after using two or three anticonvulsant medications.

References

Jagoda, A., & Richardson, L. (1997). The evaluation and treatment of seizures in the emergency department. *The Mount Sinai Journal of Medicine, 64*(4–5), 249–257.

Moore-Sledge, C. (1997). Evaluation and management of first seizure in adults. *American Family Physician, 56,* 1113–1120.

Mosewich, R., & So, E. (1996). A clinical approach to the classification of seizures and epileptic syndromes. *Mayo Clinic Proceedings, 71,* 405–414.

Sirven, J., & Liporace, J. (1997). New epileptic drugs: Overcoming the limitations of traditional therapy. *Postgraduate Medicine, 102*(1), 147–162.

Sperling, M., Bucurescu, M., & Kim, B. (1997). Epilepsy management: Advances in medical and surgical treatment. *Postgraduate Medicine, 102*(1), 102–119.

Yeh, K. (1997). High-dose 5-fluorouracil infusional therapy is associated with hyperammonaemia, lactic acidosis and encephalopathy. *Postgraduate Medicine, 75,* 464–465

Section XII. Metabolic

Symptoms

Medical Diagnosis

Chapter

140. Fever

Susan A. Ezzone, MS, RN, CNP

I. Definition
   A. An undiagnosed cause of temperature elevation equal to or greater than 38.3°C (101°F)
      1. For three or more weeks after at least a one-week hospitalization for evaluation
      2. For three outpatient days
      3. For three hospitalized days or two weeks with causes ruled out
   B. Neutropenic fever is a prolonged fever of greater than or equal to 38.3°C (101°F) in immunocompromised patients often associated with infection.
   C. The definition of fever in immunocompromised patients varies among authors, including a temperature above 38.5°, 38.3°, or 38°C (101.3°, 101°, 100.4°F).

II. Physiology/Pathophysiology
   A. Normal physiology
      1. Body temperature is normally controlled by the thermoregulatory center in the hypothalamus.
         a) The hypothalamus may be stimulated by pyrogens, including both endogenous and exogenous pathogens.
         b) During fevers, heat-loss mechanisms (e.g., vasodilation, sweating) assist in returning the temperature to normal levels.
   B. Pathophysiology
      1. Fever related to disease state superimposes the normal temperature cycle.
      2. Stimulus to the hypothalamus acting through somatic efferent nerves increases muscle tone to generate heat and raise the body temperature.
         a) Through a complex process, inflammatory cytokines stimulate cells to release prostaglandins.
         b) These prostaglandins travel to the hypothalamus, which increases muscle tone and raises the body set point temperature.
      3. Bacteremia or any stimuli that rapidly increases the hypothalamic set point can produce rigors.
         a) Cutaneous vasoconstriction occurs when the hypothalamus responds to a stimuli, thus the patient feels cold.
         b) Fever defervescence with fall in body temperature causes cutaneous vasodilation. Drenching sweat usually terminates an episode of fever.

4. Each degree of temperature results in a 7% increase in metabolic rate and increased demands on the heart.

   a) Extreme temperature (108°F, 42.1°C) causes direct cellular damage.

   b) Vascular endothelium seems particularly susceptible to such damage, thus disseminated intravascular coagulation (DIC [see Chapter 119]) usually results.

III. Clinical features: Fever may be caused by many different diseases and may be used as a marker of cancer progression. In patients with cancer, fever of unknown origin (FUO) may occur in the majority of cases without proven evidence of infection. Fever is generally increased in the evening and decreased in the morning.

   A. Risk factors

      1. Immunocompromised patients: Risk and type of infection vary depending on the disease status.

      2. Duration and severity of neutropenia

      3. Phagocytic and immune function

      4. Endogenous flora

      5. Exposure to pathogens

      6. Alteration in physical barriers (e.g., skin, oral mucosa)

      7. Invasive procedures (e.g., central venous catheters, surgery)

      8. Use of equipment (e.g., ventilators)

   B. Etiology

      1. Certain infectious pathogens have been reported to occur in immunocompromised patients (see Table 140-1).

      2. Immune mechanisms

         a) Connective tissue diseases

         b) Drug reactions

         c) Hemolytic anemia

      3. Vascular inflammation or thrombosis

      4. Inflammatory bowel disease

      5. Fever has been reported to occur during a course of chemotherapy in 40%–70% of cases and may be related to the antineoplastic agent used or tumor destruction.

      6. Neutropenic patients are at risk for infection because of immunosuppression induced by chemotherapy and/or radiation therapy, as well as alterations in physical barriers (e.g., splenectomy, central venous catheter placement, invasive procedures).

   C. History

      1. History of cancer and cancer treatment

      2. Current medications: Prescribed and over-the-counter

      3. History of presenting symptom(s): Precipitating factors, onset, and duration. Associated symptoms are headache; abdominal, back, and neck pain; and mental status changes.

      4. Changes in activities of daily living

      5. History of recent travel, insect bites, animal contact, toxic substance exposure, venipuncture, or injections

   D. Signs and symptoms: Refer to a reference on specific disease for further information.

Table 140-1. Host Defense Defects in the Immunocompromised Patient[a]: Relationship of Underlying Disease to Infectious Agents

Underlying Disease	Host Defense Defects[b]	Common Infectious Agents[c]
Acute nonlymphocytic leukemia	Neutropenia	Aerobic gram-negative bacilli • Enterobacteriaceae • *Pseudomonas aeruginosa* Fungi • Aspergillus • Candida
Chronic lymphocytic leukemia	Abnormal humoral immunity Abnormal cell-mediated immunity	Encapsulated bacteria • *Streptococcus pneumoniae* • *Haemophilus influenzae* • Neisseria
Hairy cell leukemia	Depressed cell-mediated immunity Abnormal monocyte function Leukopenia (monocytes, neutrophils)	Aerobic gram-negative bacilli • Enterobacteriaceae • *Pseudomonas aeruginosa* Herpes simplex • Mycobacterium (including tuberculosis and nontuberculous Mycobacteria) Fungi • Candida • *Cryptococcus neoformans*
Hodgkin's lymphoma	Depressed cell-mediated immunity	Herpes zoster
Myeloma	Abnormal humoral immunity	Encapsulated bacteria • *Streptococcus pneumoniae* • *Haemophilus influenzae* • Neisseria

[a] In each case, only host defects associated with the underlying diseases are noted.
[b] Only the major host defense defect(s) are listed; often, multiple defects are described.
[c] The most common organisms are noted.

Note. From "Fever in the Compromised Host" by G.R. Donowitz, 1996, *Infectious Disease Clinics of North America, 10*(1), pp. 132–133. Copyright 1996 by W.B. Saunders Company. Reprinted with permission.

1. Fever, diaphoresis
2. Chills or rigors: Uncontrolled violent shaking or trembling may precede or accompany fever.
3. Dyspnea, productive or nonproductive cough
4. Abdominal tenderness, nausea, vomiting, diarrhea
5. Weight loss
6. Lymphadenopathy
7. Arthralgia, myalgia

8. Skin rash, hyperpigmentation, edema, tenderness
9. Dry or watery eyes
10. Oral mucosal or tongue tenderness
11. Purulent drainage from wound or central venous catheter
12. Neutropenic patients: Unable to exhibit signs of infection (e.g., purulent drainage) except for fever

E. Physical exam
1. Vital signs: To monitor temperature elevation, tachycardia, tachypnea, hypotension; evaluate for signs of sepsis
2. General appearance
3. Integument exam: For rashes, altered integrity, petechiae, pustular or vesicular lesions, central venous catheter site for redness, swelling, drainage
4. HEENT exam
   a) Oral exam: For mucosal integrity, crythema, lesions, bleeding
   b) Ophthalmoscopic exam: To evaluate for infections in the eye
   c) Sinus exam: Tender or opacified sinuses, facial pain, nasal drainage
5. Pulmonary exam: Assess for abnormal lung sounds
6. Cardiac exam: For abnormal heart sounds (e.g., friction rubs, murmurs)
7. Abdominal exam: For masses or organomegaly, pain, rebound
8. Posterior thorax exam: For costovertebral tenderness
9. Musculoskeletal exam
   a) Muscle strength against gravity and resistance
   b) Joint exam: For range of motion, swelling, tenderness, erythema, warmth
10. Lymph exam: Lymph node enlargement and tenderness
11. Genital and perirectal exam: For rash, ulceration, lesions, induration, tenderness
12. Neurologic exam: For meningeal irritation, focal abnormalities, changes in mentation

IV. Diagnostic tests
A. Laboratory
1. CBC with differential
   a) Absolute neutrophil count (ANC)
   b) ANC < 500 cells/ul: Increases risk of infection
   c) ANC < 100 cells/ul: Increases risk of bacterial and fungal infection
   d) Increased bands or "shift to the left": Suggests bacterial infection
2. Liver function tests (LFTs): To evaluate hepatic function and liver disease
3. Uric acid: To evaluate kidney function and presence of gout
4. Blood cultures: For bacteria, fungi, viruses
5. Viral titers: For hepatitis, Epstein-Barr, cytomegalovirus, parvovirus
6. Urinalysis and urine culture
7. Stool cultures: For *Clostridium difficile*, ova, parasites, virus, fungus
8. Sputum cultures: For fungus, virus, legionella; acid-fast smear for tuberculosis
9. Wound culture
10. Rheumatoid factor: To evaluate for rheumatoid arthritis

11. Erythrocyte sedimentation rate (ESR): To evaluate inflammatory, autoimmune, or malignant disease
12. Antinuclear antibodies (ANA): To rule out systemic lupus erythematosus, poly-arthritis, lupoid hepatitis
13. Quantitative immunoglobulin (Ig) levels and subclasses: To evaluate for immune deficiency or allergies
14. Lyme disease titers: To rule out diagnosis of Lyme disease
15. Serum protein electrophoresis: To rule out protein deficiency and evaluate for renal, hepatic, gastrointestinal, and neoplastic diseases

B. Radiology
1. Chest radiography: To rule out pulmonary infiltrates, consolidation, or nodules
2. Radiographs of bones: Specific for diagnosis suspected
3. CT scans: High-resolution CT of the chest to evaluate Aspergillus pulmonary infection, presence of abscess or tumor
4. Echocardiogram or transesophageal echocardiogram (TEE): To evaluate for valvular disease
5. Bone scan: To detect infection or malignancy
6. Gallium scan: To evaluate benign or malignant neoplasms or inflammatory lesions
7. MRI: To evaluate for intracranial, spinal, or soft tissue abnormalities

C. Other
1. Bronchoscopy with lavage or biopsy: To evaluate for infection or malignant disease
2. Skin tests
   a) Tuberculin or purified protein derivative (PPD) may be done to evaluate for tuberculosis in patients who have been exposed or suspected of having the disease.
   b) Delayed hypersensitivity skin tests include six intradermal skin tests to evaluate a patient's cellular immune response.
      (1) May be done in patients with infections that are recurrent or caused by unusual organisms or who may have delayed hypersensitivity
      (2) Tests include Candida, staphage lysate, mixed respiratory, PPD, streptokinase-streptodornase, and trichophytin.
3. Bone marrow biopsy and aspirate: To evaluate for malignant disease or infection in the bone marrow
4. Other biopsies as indicated
   a) Open lung biopsy: To diagnose pulmonary disease as indicated
   b) Lymph node biopsy: To evaluate for malignant disease or infection
   c) Liver biopsy: To evaluate for hepatic disease, malignancy, or infection
   d) Skin biopsy: To evaluate for malignancy or infection

V. Differential diagnosis (see Table 140-2)
A. Tumor fever is common in the following diseases.
1. Lymphoma
2. Acute leukemia
3. Chronic leukemia
4. Multiple myeloma
5. Solid tumors

Table 140-2. Diseases Causing Fever of Unknown Origin

	Common	Uncommon	Rare
Malignancy	• Lymphoma • Metastases to liver/ CNS • Hypernephroma	• Hepatoma • Pancreatic carcinoma • Preleukemias • Colon carcinoma	• Atrial myxoma • CNS tumors • Myelodysplastic diseases

Infections	• Extrapulmonary tuberculosis (TB)
	• Renal TB
	• TB meningitis
	• Miliary TB
	• Intra-abdominal abscesses
	• Subdiaphragmatic abscesses
	  - Periappendiceal
	  - Pericolonic
	  - Hepatic
	• Pelvic abscesses
		• Subacute bacterial endocarditis
		• Cytomegalovirus
		• Toxoplasmosis
		• *Salmonella* enteric fevers
		• Intra/perinephric abscess
		• Splenic abscess
			• Periapical dental abscesses
			• Small brain abscesses
			• Chronic sinusitis
			• Subacute vertebral osteomyelitis
			• Chronic meningitis/encephalitis
			• Listeria
			• Yersinia
			• Brucellosis
			• Relapsing fever
			• Rat-bite fever
			• Chronic Q fever
			• Cat-scratch fever
			• HIV
			• Epstein-Barr virus mononucleosis (in the elderly)
			• Malaria
			• Leptospirosis
			• Blastomycosis
			• Histoplasmosis
			• Coccidioidomycosis
			• Cryptococcosis
			• Infected aortic aneurysm
			• Infected vascular grafts
			• Rocky Mountain spotted fever
			• Lyme disease
			• Leishmaniasis
			• Trypanosomiasis
			• Lymphogranuloma venereum
			• Permanently placed central IV line infections
			• Trichinosis
			• Prosthetic device infections
			• Relapsing mastoiditis

Rheumatologic	• Still's disease (adult, juvenile rheumatoid arthritis) • Temporal arteritis (elderly)	• Periarteritis nodosa • Rheumatoid arthritis (elderly)	• Septic jugular phlebitis • Systemic lupus erythematosus • Vasculitis (e.g., Takayasu's arteritis, hypersensitivity vasculitis) • Felty's syndrome • Pseudogout • Acute rheumatic fever • Sjögren's syndrome • Behcet's disease • Familial Mediterranean fever

(Continued on next page)

Table 140-2. Diseases Causing Fever of Unknown Origin *(Continued)*

	Common	Uncommon	Rare
Miscellaneous causes	• Drug fever • Cirrhosis • Alcoholic hepatitis	• Granulomatous hepatitis	• Regional enteritis • Whipple's disease • Fabry's disease • Hyperthyroidism • Hyperparathyroidism • Pheochromocytomas • Addison's disease • Subacute thyroiditis • Cyclic neutropenias • Polymyositis • Wegener's granulomatosis • Occult hematomas • Subacute aortic dissecting aneurysm • Weber-Christian disease • Sarcoidosis (e.g., basilar meningitis, hepatic granulomas) • Pulmonary emboli (multiple, recurrent) • Hypothalamic dysfunction • Habitual hyperthermia • Factitious fever • Giant hepatic hemangiomas • Mesenteric fibromatosis Pseudolymphomas • Idiopathic granulomatosis • Kikuchi's disease • Malakoplakia • Hyper IgD syndrome

Note. From "Fever of Unknown Origin (FUO)" (pp. 112–113), by B.A. Cunha in S.L. Gorbach, J.B. Bartlett, and N.R. Blacklow (Eds.), *Infectious Diseases* (2nd ed.), 1996, Philadelphia: W.B. Saunders. Copyright 1996 by W.B. Saunders Company. Reprinted with permission.

    B. Drug fevers that may occur at the start of therapy or one to two weeks later may be caused by antibiotics, diuretics, analgesics, antiarrhythmic and antiseizure medications, sedatives, and chemotherapy agents (see Figure 140-1).

    C. Nosocomial fever

    D. Early sign of septic shock

VI. Treatment

    A. Treatment of fever depends on etiology.

    B. Treat the underlying cause.

    C. Anti-infective therapy or prophylaxis (see Tables 140-3 and 140-4)

        1. Antibacterial therapy or prophylaxis using two drugs or monotherapy have been used in various combinations.

           a) Length of therapy is controversial.

           b) May be continued until neutropenia resolves.

Figure 140-1. Drugs Implicated in the Development of Fever

Common	Less Common	Rare
Atropine	Allopurinol	Salicylates (therapeutic doses)
Amphotericin B	Azathioprine	Corticosteroids
Asparaginase	Cimetidine	Aminoglycosides
Barbiturates	Hydralazine	Macrolides
Bleomycin	Iodides	Tetracyclines
Methyldopa	Isoniazid	Clindamycin
Penicillins	Rifampin	Chloramphenicol
Cephalosporins	Streptokinase	Vitamin preparations
Phenytoin	Imipenem	
Procainamide	Vancomycin	
Quinidine	Nifedipine	
Salicylates	NSAIDs	
Sulfonamides (including	Metoclopramide	
sulfa-containing laxatives)		
Interferon		

Note. From "Drug Fever" by D.H. Johnson & B.A. Cunha, 1996, *Infectious Disease Clinics of North America, 10*(1), p. 90. Copyright 1996 by W.B. Saunders Company. Reprinted with permission.

  c) Discontinue after resolution of fevers and other signs of infection.
 2. Antifungal therapy should be considered if fevers persist for four to seven days during neutropenia despite use of broad-spectrum antibiotics. Prophylactic use of antifungal agents (e.g., nystatin, clotrimazole, fluconazole, amphotericin-B) is common.
 3. Antiviral agents (e.g., acyclovir, ganciclovir) and various formulations of immunoglobulin are used to prevent and treat viral infections.
 4. In patients who remain febrile despite administration of anti-infective agents, consider discontinuing therapy because of potential drug fever.
 D. Antipyretics are often used to minimize the discomforts of fever (e.g., chills, seizures, delirium). Adverse effects may limit use of antipyretics.
  1. Acetaminophen: Preferred for patients with gastric ulcers and clotting disorders.
   a) Dosages of 325–650 mg orally every four hours may be used.
   b) Do not exceed 4,000 mg in a 24-hour period.
  2. Salicylate: May cause gastrointestinal, hepatic, and renal toxicity and alter blood coagulation.
   a) Dosages of 325–650 mg orally every four hours may be used.
   b) Doses may be alternated with acetaminophen.
  3. Nonsteroidal anti-inflammatory drugs (NSAIDs): Often used to treat fever caused by malignant disease (see Appendix 11)
  4. Corticosteriods: Side effects limit use for controlling fever; may be used for high fever unresponsive to other interventions.
 E. WBC growth factors (e.g., granulocyte colony-stimulating factor, [G-CSF], granulocyte macrophage colony-stimulating factor [GM-CSF]) are used to decrease the period of neutropenia and incidence of infection after administration of chemotherapy.

Table 140-3. Antibiotic Therapy in Patients With Neutropenia and Fever

Agent	Comments
Antibiotic	
Third-generation cephalosporins	Only ceftazidime and cefoperazone are appropriate for coverage of *Pseudomonas (P.) aeruginosa.*
Carbapenems	If *P. aeruginosa* is suspected or cultured, an amino-glycoside should be added.
Extended-spectrum penicillins	Because of the potential for resistance, piperacillin, azlocillin, or mezlocillin should be administered with either an aminoglycoside or a third-generation cephalosporin.
Monobactums	Aztreonam is an important alternative for patients allergic to beta-lactam antibiotics, but it should be combined with vancomycin for empirical therapy.
Quinolones	Important for gram-negative infection and possibly for use in low-risk patients with neutropenia; to avoid resistance, do not use for prophylaxis.
Vancomycin	Pathogen-directed therapy generally suffices. Empirical use can be restricted to centers with a high incidence of methicillin-resistant *Staphylococcus aureus.* Of concern, strains of vancomycin-resistant enterococci have been described.
Antifungal	
Amphotericin B	Still the best treatment. A dose of 0.6 mg per kilogram of body weight/day suffices for *Candida albicans* and cryptococcus; 1 mg/kg/day is preferred for *C. tropicalis* and 1 mg/kg/day is preferred for aspergillus. Premedication may be used to minimize side effects.
Ketoconazole	Not an alternative to amphotericin B for empirical therapy. Useful for thrush or esophagitis.
Fluconazole	Very effective for thrush or esophagitis. Value for systemic mycoses, including hepatosplenic candidiasis; requires additional study.
Antiviral	
Acyclovir	Oral therapy is not advised for severely immunocompromised patients with varicella-zoster infections. For such patients, parenteral therapy (1,500 mg/m^2/day in three divided doses) is indicated. For patients with herpes simplex, oral or parenteral therapy (750 mg/m^2/day in three divided doses) is satisfactory.
Ganciclovir	Used for cytomegalovirus retinitis and prevention of pneumonitis and is combined with an IV immunoglobulin for pneumonitis.
Antiparasitic	
Trimethoprim-sulfamethoxazole	Best drug for *Pneumocystis carinii* prophylaxis. Not required in all patients with cancer. Three times weekly is satisfactory (150 mg of trimethoprim/m^2/day in two divided doses).
Aerosolized pentamidine	Expensive and not as effective as trimethoprim-sulfamethoxazole in adults with HIV infection.

Note. From "Management of Fever in Patients With Cancer and Treatment-Induced Neutropenia," by P.A. Pizzo, 1993, *New England Journal of Medicine, 328*, p. 1326. Copyright 1993 by Massachusetts Medical Society. Reprinted with permission.

Table 140-4. Common Modifications or Additions to Initial Empirical Antibiotic Therapy in Patients With Neutropenia and Fever

Status of Symptoms	Modifications of Primary Regimen
Fever	
Persistent for > one week	Add empirical antifungal therapy with amphotericin B.
Recurrence after one week or later in patient with persistent neutropenia	Add empirical antifungal therapy.
Persistent or recurrent fever at time of recovery from neutropenia	Evaluate liver and spleen by CT, ultrasonography, or MRI for hepatosplenic candidiasis and evaluate need for antifungal therapy.
Blood stream cultures before antibiotic therapy	
Gram-positive organism	Add vancomycin pending further identification.
Gram-negative organism	Maintain regimen if patient is stable and isolate is sensitive. If *P. aeruginosa*, enterobacter, or citrobacter is isolated, add an aminoglycoside or an additional ß-lactam antibiotic.
Organism isolated during antibiotic therapy	
Gram-positive organism	Add vancomycin.
Gram-negative organism	Change to new combination regimen (e.g., imipenem plus gentamicin or vancomycin or gentamicin plus piperacillin).
Head, eyes, ears, nose, throat	
Necrotizing or marginal gingivitis	Add specific antianaerobic agent (e.g., clindamycin, metronidazole) to empirical therapy.
Vesicular or ulcerative lesions	Suspect herpes simplex infection; culture and begin acyclovir therapy.
Sinus tenderness or nasal ulcerative lesions	Suspect fungal infection with aspergillus or mucor.
Gastrointestinal tract	
Retrosternal burning pain	Suspect Candida, herpes simplex, or both. Add antifungal therapy; if no response, add acyclovir. Bacterial esophagitis also is a possibility. For patients who do not respond within 48 hours, consider endoscopy.
Acute abdominal pain	Suspect typhlitis and appendicitis if pain is in right lower quadrant. Add specific antianaerobic coverage to empirical regimen and monitor closely for need for surgical intervention.
Perianal tenderness	Add specific antianaerobic drug to empirical regimen and monitor need for surgical intervention, especially when patient is recovering from neutropenia.

(Continued on next page)

Table 140-4. Common Modifications or Additions to Initial Empirical Antibiotic Therapy in Patients With Neutropenia and Fever (Continued)

Status of Symptoms	Modifications of Primary Regimen
Respiratory tract	
New focal lesion in patient recovering from neutropenia	Observe carefully, as this may be a consequence of inflammatory response in concert with neutrophil recovery.
New focal lesion in patient with continuing neutropenia	Aspergillus is the chief concern. Perform appropriate cultures and consider biopsy. If patient is not a candidate for procedure, administer high-dose amphotericin B (1.5 mg/kg/day).
New interstitial pneumonitis	Attempt diagnosis by examining induced sputum or bronchoalveolar lavage. If not feasible, begin empirical treatment with trimethoprim-sulfa-methoxazole or pentamidine. Consider noninfectious causes and the need for open-lung biopsy if condition has not improved after four days of therapy.
Central venous catheters	
Positive culture for organisms other than bacillus species or Candida	Attempt to treat. Rotate antibiotic administration in patients with multiple-lumen catheters.
Positive culture for bacillus species or Candida	Remove catheter and treat appropriately.
Exit-safe infection in mycobacterium or aspergillus	Remove catheter and treat appropriately.
Tunnel infection	Remove catheter and treat appropriately.

Note. From "Management of Fever in Patients With Cancer and Treatment Induced Neutropenia" by P.A. Pizzo, 1993, *New England Journal of Medicine, 328,* p. 1326. Copyright 1993 by Massachusetts Medical Society. Reprinted with permission.

    1. Daily subcutaneous dosages are often used. G-CSF 5 mcg/kg ld; GM-CSF 250 mcg/m²/d
    2. Medication is discontinued when neutrophil recovery occurs (i.e., ANC > 5,000 cells/ul).
    3. May be instituted during febrile neutropenia; however, research does not support this use.
  F. Physical methods of controlling body temperature
    1. Tepid baths, sponging
    2. Ice packs, cooling blankets
    3. Air conditioning, fans

VII. Follow-up
  A. Frequent and repeated physical exams are imperative to evaluate FUO.
  B. Hospitalization may be required to evaluate FUO, especially in neutropenic patients whose ANC < 500 cells/ul.

VIII. Referrals: Referral may be necessary to assist in evaluating FUO. Variety of specialists (i.e., infectious disease, hematology, pulmonary, cardiology, gastroenterology, dermatology, rheumatology)

References

Cunha, B.A. (1996). Fever of unknown origin. *Infectious Disease Clinics of North America, 10,* 111–127.

Donowitz, G.R. (1996). Fever in the compromised host. *Infectious Disease Clinics of North America, 1,* 129–148.

Giamarellou, H. (1995). Empiric therapy for infections in the febrile, neutropenic, compromised host. *Medical Clinics of North America, 79,* 559–580.

Johnson, D.H., & Cunha, B.A. (1996). Drug fever. *Infectious Disease Clinics of North America, 1,* 985–991.

Klein, N.C., & Cunha, B.A. (1996). Treatment of fever. *Infectious Disease Clinics of North America, 10,* 211–216.

Knockaert, D.C., Vanneste, L.J., & Bobbaers, H.J. (1993). Fever of unknown origin in elderly patients. *Journal of Aging and Geriatrics Society, 41,* 1187–1192.

Miller, M.L., Szer, I., Yogez, R., & Bernstein, B. (1995). Fever of unknown origin. *Pediatric Rheumatology, 42,* 999–1015.

Pizzo, P.A. (1993). Management of fever in patients with cancer and treatment-induced neutropenia. *New England Journal of Medicine, 328,* 1323–1332.

Chapter

141.

Flu-Like Syndrome

Laura M. Stempkowski, RN, MS, CUNP, AOCN®

I. Definition: A cluster of constitutional symptoms that may include fever, chills, rigors, myalgia, and malaise

II. Physiology/Pathophysiology
   A. Normal
   1. The site for temperature control is the area in the brain termed the pre-optic anterior hypothalamus (PO/AH).
   2. Body temperature is controlled by the thermoregulatory set point, a narrow range of temperatures around 37°C (98.6°F).
      a) This is the optimal temperature for cellular metabolism and body functions.
      b) As body temperature rises above or below the set point, compensatory cooling or warming mechanisms are initiated to return the body temperature to the set point.
   B. Pathophysiology
   1. Flu-like syndrome results when exogenous (e.g., viruses, bacterial endotoxin, neoplastic cells, drugs) or endogenous (e.g., cytokines) pyrogens cause an increase in the thermoregulatory "set point."
   2. Although some exogenous pyrogens can directly affect the set point, most often their effects are mediated by cytokines (e.g., interleukin [IL] IL-1, IL-6, tumor necrosis factor) that cause the release of prostaglandins.
   3. Prostaglandin E can diffuse across the blood brain barrier into PO/AH, directly causing an increase in the set point.
   4. Chills and rigors result as muscle contractions generate heat to raise the body temperature to the new higher set point.
   5. When endogenous pyrogens blood levels fall or are blocked by an antipyretic (e.g., acetaminophen), the set point returns to normal and body temperature is lowered through sweating.
   6. This control mechanism may be suppressed in patients on steroids or anti-inflammatory agents.
   7. Fever caused by biological response modifiers are thought to be related to their role as endogenous pyrogens or to their ability to initiate other endogenous pyrogens (e.g., IL-1, IL-6). This would also explain the varying patterns among the different agents.

III. Clinical features: The onset, duration, and severity of symptoms is related to the etiology.
    A. History
        1. History of cancer and cancer treatment
        2. Current medications: Prescribed and over-the-counter
        3. History of presenting symptom(s): Precipitating factors, onset, and duration. Associated symptoms are elevated temperature, headache, myalgia, nausea/vomiting, diarrhea, sore throat, cough, and dysuria.
        4. Changes in activities of daily living
        5. Past medical history: Heart disease, lung disease, diabetes mellitus, anemia
    B. Signs and symptoms
        1. Rigors
        2. Fever
        3. Malaise
        4. Myalgia
        5. Arthralgia
        6. Anorexia
        7. Nausea/vomiting
        8. Diarrhea
        9. Headache
      10. Thirst
    C. Physical exam
        1. Vital signs
            a) Elevated temperature, pulse, and respirations
            b) Hypertension or hypotension
        2. Neurologic exam: Mental status—evaluate for somnolence, confusion, irritability, seizures, decreased performance status
        3. Integument exam: Hot, dry or diaphoretic
        4. Lymph exam: Adenopathy usually with infectious etiology
        5. Pulmonary exam: Crackles, rhonchi may indicate infection; pleural rub may indicate effusion.
        6. Abdominal exam: Increased bowel sounds and tenderness may indicate infection, especially rebound tenderness.

IV. Diagnostic tests
    A. Laboratory
        1. If flu-like syndrome is expected with current therapy, then no further workup is needed.
        2. If fever persists or does not respond to acetaminophen or nonsteroidal agent, a full culture work-up is indicated to rule out infection (see Chapter 140)
        3. CBC: If neutropenia or infection is suspected
    B. Radiology: Not indicated unless specific etiology is suspected

V. Differential diagnosis
    A. Infection
    B. Sepsis
    C. Toxic shock syndrome

    D. Febrile neutropenia (see Chapter 121)

    E. Drug-induced

        1. Chemotherapy (e.g., dacarbazine, bleomycin)

        2. Biotherapy (see Tables 141-1–141-6)

        3. Antibiotics (e.g., amphotericin B, vancomycin)

        4. Biophosphonates

    F. Influenza

    G. Common cold

VI. Treatment

    A. Implement measures to minimize discomfort from chills or rigors (i.e., additional blankets, clothing, heating pads, hot packs, hot water bottles)

    B. Painful rigors and chills

        1. Meperidine: 25 mg IV q 15 minutes, not to exceed 100 mg in one hour

        2. Morphine: 1–2 mg IV q 15 minutes, not to exceed 4 mg in one hour

        3. Monitor for hypotension

    C. Avoid using aspirin; provide pharmacologic comfort measures.

        1. Acetaminophen: 650–975 mg po every four hours

        2. Nonsteroidal anti-inflammatory drugs (NSAIDs [see Appendix 11])

    D. Nonpharmacological comfort measures

        1. Sponge bath, tepid shower

        2. Removal of extra blankets and clothing

        3. Cooling blanket

Table 141-1. Interferons

Symptom/Side Effect	Interferon-Alpha	Interferon-Beta	Interferon-Gamma
Fever	T_{max}^a in approximately six hours Duration is four to eight hours Dose-dependent Tolerance develops with daily doses	Fever pattern similar to that for IFN-alpha Frequently higher than 39.4°C	T_{max} in 10–12 hours Longer duration (up to 18 hours) Dose-dependent No tolerance develops with daily doses
Chills/rigors	Precede fevers	Precede fevers Dose-dependent	Within first hour Duration related to T_{max}
Myalgias	Occur with fevers	Common Mild to moderate in severity	Common Experienced by 30%–80% of all patients
Headache	Occurs with fevers	Common Generally mild to moderate	Common May be severe

ᵃ Peak temperature

Note. From "The Flu-Like Syndrome" (p. 244) by D.Haeuber in P.T. Rieger (Ed.), *Biotherapy: A Comprehensive Review*, 1995, Boston: Jones and Bartlett. Reprinted with permission.

Table 141-2. Hematopoietic Growth Factors

Symptom/Side Effect	Erythropoietin	Granulocyte-Colony-Stimulating Factor (G-CSF)	Granulocyte Macrophage-Colony-Stimulating Factor (GM-CSF)	Interleukin-3
Fever	None	None or low-grade Uncommon	Generally low-grade but may rise to 40°C	Nearly 100% of all patients have low-grade fever (≤ 40°C)
Chills/rigors	None		Absent or mild	Very common with fevers
Myalgias	None	Uncommon	Common General muscle aches, especially in the thighs May be severe enough to require analgesia	Not reported
Headache	None	Uncommon	Experienced by 50% of all patients Transient and mild	Common, especially at higher doses Usually mild but may require analgesia May be accompanied by neck stiffness

Note. From "The Flu-Like Syndrome" (p. 245) by D.Haeuber in P.T. Rieger (Ed.), *Biotherapy: A Comprehensive Review,* 1995, Boston: Jones and Bartlett. Reprinted with permission.

Table 141-3. Interleukin-2

Symptom/Side Effect	Interleukin-2 (IL-2)
Fever	Experienced by 80%–100% of all patients Dose-dependent T_{max} ᵃ Delayed onset (a) Bolus infusion: T_{max} in six hours with slow decline (b) Continuous IV infusion: Temperature elevated throughout, resolved two to three days after end of infusion
Chills/rigors	Common, precede fever May be more frequent and more severe when IL-2 is given with lymphokine activated killer cells and tumor-infiltrating lymphocyte cells
Myalgias	May accompany fever
Headache	May accompany fever

ᵃ Peak temperature
Note. From "The Flu-Like Syndrome" (p. 246) by D.Haeuber in P.T. Rieger (Ed.), *Biotherapy: A Comprehensive Review,* 1995, Boston: Jones and Bartlett. Reprinted with permission.

Table 141-4. Monoclonal Antibodies

Symptom/Side Effect	Monoclonal Antibodies
Fever	Common, experienced by 20%–100% of all patients Two patterns (a) During first hour of infusion (b) One to two hours after infusion
Chills/rigors	Occur with fever
Myalgias	Arthralgias are reported rather than myalgias
Headache	Not reported

Note. From "The Flu-Like Syndrome" (p. 246) by D. Haeuber in P.T. Rieger (Ed.), *Biotherapy: A Comprehensive review,* 1995, Boston: Jones and Bartlett. Reprinted with permission.

Table 141-5. Tumor Necrosis Factor

Symptom/Side Effect	Tumor Necrosis Factor (TNF)
Fever	Common, experienced by 40%–80% of all patients Dose-dependent severity Continuous IV infusion: Temperature elevated for 24 hours then returns to baseline 30-minute IV infusion: Fever peaks at one hour, returns to baseline after 4–6 hours Subcutaneous/IM injection: Temperature peaks at 2–10 hours, remains elevated for up to 20 hours
Chills/rigors	Common Appear within 15 minutes of start of IV infusion Follows fever pattern
Myalgias	Common
Headache	Common

Note. From "The Flu-Like Syndrome" (p. 247) by D. Haeuber in P.T. Rieger (Ed.), *Biotherapy: A Comprehensive review,* 1995, Boston: Jones and Bartlett. Reprinted with permission.

Table 141-6. Intravesical Bacillus Calmette-Guérin

Symptom/Side Effect	Intravesical Bacillus Calmette-Guérin (BCG)
Fever	Low-grade fever usually occurs at approximately the time of the third instillation and lasts 24 hours. Fever greater than 103°F (39.6°C) occurs in 3% of all patients and is usually limited to 48 hours or less.[a]
Chills/rigors	Uncommon
Malaise	More common at approximately the time of the third instillation and lasts 24 hours

[a] The main concern is the inability to distinguish an uncomplicated febrile reaction from the onset of a systemic BCG infection. Refer patient to physician (urologist). It is recommended that patients developing high fever be hospitalized for observation and treated with isoniazid 300 mg and rifampicin 600 mg po daily. Because BCG sepsis cannot be distinguished from gram-negative sepsis early on, it also is recommended that the patient be covered with broad-spectrum antibiotics.

Note. Based on information from Lamm, 1997.

E. Ensure adequate hydration for duration of fever.

F. Ensure periods of uninterrupted rest.

G. If gastrointestinal symptoms are present, give antiemetic and antidiarrheal agents.

H. Teach patient and family which symptoms to anticipate and which symptoms they should report.

I. If drug-related etiology, consider premediations
1. Tylenol® (McNeil-Consumer Healthcare, Fort Washington, PA) and Benadryl® (Warner-Lambert Consumer Healthcare, Morris Plains, NJ)
2. NSAIDs
3. Diazepam
4. Around-the-clock NSAIDs, Tylenol, or Benadryl

VII. Follow-up: Flu-like syndrome is self-limiting and does not require follow-up unless symptoms persist beyond the expected time frame.

VIII. Referrals: Not indicated

References

Bruce, J., & Grove, S. (1992). Fever: Pathology and treatment. *Critical Care Nurse, 12*(1), 40–49.

Haeuber, D. (1989). Recent advances in the management of biotherapy-related side effects: Flu-like syndrome. *Oncology Nursing Forum, 16*(Suppl. 6), 35–41.

Haeuber, D. (1995). The flu-like syndrome. In P.T. Rieger (Ed.), *Biotherapy: A comprehensive overview* (pp. 243–258.). Boston: Jones & Bartlett.

Lamm, D. (1997). Management of superficial bladder disease. In M.S. Ernstoff, J.A. Heaney, & R.E. Pechel (Eds.), *Urologic cancer* (pp. 255–271). Cambridge, MA: Blackwell Science, Inc.

Shelton, R., & Turnbough, L. (1999). Flulike syndrome. In C.H. Yarbro, M.H. Frogge, & M. Goodman (Eds.), *Cancer symptom management* (2nd ed.) (pp. 77–94).Boston: Jones & Bartlett.

Witter, F., Woods, A., Griffin, M., Smith, C., Nadler, P., & Lietman, P. (1988). Effects of prednisone, aspirin, and acetaminophen on in vivo biological response to interferon in humans. *Clinical Pharmacology and Therapeutics, 44,* 239–243.

Chapter

142. Thirst

Kathleen Murphy-Ende, RN, PhD, CFNP

I. Definition: The conscious desire for water

II. Physiology/Pathophysiology
  A. Normal: The thirst center, located in the hypothalamus, consists of neuronal cells, which function as osmoreceptors.
  B. Pathophysiology
    1. An increase in osmotic pressure in the cerebrospinal fluid of the third ventricle or in the circulating extracellular fluid promotes thirst.
    2. Intracellular dehydration, present in hypernatremia and hypercalcemia, is a common cause of increased osmolar concentration of the extracellular fluid.
    3. Other stimuli causing thirst are an increased production of angiotensin II, decreased cardiac output, and dryness of the mouth.

III. Clinical features: Thirst is a subjective symptom that may be accompanied by dry lips and mouth, polydipsia, and polyuria.
  A. Etiology
    1. Decreased fluid intake
    2. Increased fluid output
    3. Poor fluid transport
    4. Medication-induced
    5. Mouth breathing
    6. Electrolyte imbalance
    7. Hypothalamic-pituitary pathologic conditions
    8. Head and neck radiation
    9. Anxiety
  B. History
    1. History of cancer and cancer treatment
    2. Current medications: Prescribed and over-the-counter
    3. History of presenting symptom(s): Precipitating factors, location, and duration. Associated symptoms are dry mouth, excessive appetite, anxiety, depression, fever, night sweats, headache, shortness of breath, and edema.
    4. Changes in activities of daily living

      5. History of intake and output
      6. Past medical history: Diabetes mellitus, heart disease, endocrine factors, kidney disease
      7. Family history: Diabetes mellitus, thyroid disease

C. Signs and symptoms
    1. Polydipsia
    2. Polyuria
    3. Polyphagia
    4. Weakness
    5. Headache
    6. Lightheadedness
    7. Fever
    8. Edema
    9. Weight loss
    10. Dry mouth

D. Physical exam
    1. Weight loss or gain
    2. Vital signs: Hypotension and orthostatic with dehydration
    3. Integument
       a) Dry skin
       b) Poor skin turgor, indicating dehydration, renal disease
    4. Oral cavity
       a) Dry
       b) Thick saliva
       c) Dry or cracked lips
    5. Eyes: Microaneurysm, papilledema, microhemorrhages
    6. Cardiac exam: Murmur and gallop may indicate anemia
    7. Pulmonary exam: Rales indicating CHF, bronchitis, pneumonia
    8. Extremities: Pitting edema may indicate CHF, third-spacing, renal disease, malnutrition.

IV. Diagnostic tests
  A. Laboratory
    1. CBC: To rule out anemia, renal disease, occult volume depletion
    2. Urinalysis and urine electrolytes: An increase in sodium excretion > 20 mEq/24 hours indicates syndrome of inappropriate antidiuretic hormone (SIADH)
    3. Glucose: Increase may indicate diabetes mellitus or thyroid disease
    4. BUN and creatinine: To determine prerenal, intrinsic, or postrenal diseases
    5. Electrolytes: Hyponatremia seen in SIADH, hypokalemia, hypernatremia, hypercalcemia
    6. TSH: Decreased in hyperthyroidism (< 2 μU/ml)
    7. Serum parathyroid hormone: Increased in hyperparathyroidism (> 1.5 mol/l)
    8. Serum osmolality: Decreased in excessive fluid intake, increased in dehydration
    9. Urine osmolality: Increased (> 400 mOsm/kg) in SIADH
  B. Radiology: Not indicated

V. Differential diagnosis
   A. Decreased fluid intake
      1. Anorexia (see Chapter 62)
      2. Dehydration (see Chapter 147)
      3. Nausea and vomiting (see Chapter 59)
      4. Inability to feed self or ask for assistance
      5. Small bowel obstruction (see Chapter 63)
   B. Increased fluid output
      1. Diuresis
      2. Vomiting (see Chapter 59)
      3. Diarrhea (see Chapter 53)
      4. Fever (see Chapter 140)
      5. Diaphoresis
   C. Poor fluid transport
      1. Hemorrhagic or vasomotor shock
      2. Hypoalbuminemia
      3. CHF (see Chapter 40)
   D. Medications
      1. Alcohol
      2. Antidepressants
      3. Cyclophosphamide (high dose can induce SIADH)
      4. Diuretics
      5. Lithium
      6. Opioids
      7. Parasympatholytics (e.g., Levsin®, Schwartz Pharma Inc., Mequon, WI; Bentyl®, Merrell Pharmaceuticals, Inc., Cincinnati, OH; Robinul®, A.H. Robins Company, Inc., Richmond, VA)
      8. Steroids
   E. Mouth breathing
      1. Nasal obstruction
      2. Positioning
   F. Electrolyte imbalance (see Chapter 141–148)
   G. Pathological conditions
      1. Aldosteronism
      2. Chronic glomerulonephritis
      3. Diabetes mellitus (see Chapter 143)
      4. Diabetes insipidus
      5. Hyperparathyroidism
      6. Hyperthyroidism (see Chapter 149)
      7. Multiple sclerosis
      8. SIADH (see Chapter 94)
      9. Primary polydipsia

VI. Treatment
   A. Treatment should be directed at the underlying cause of thirst; however, thirst may occur as a side effect of medications or during the terminal phase of life.

B. Measure intake and output to assess altered balance in dehydration; large volume output in SIADH.
C. Frequent sips of fluid or ice chips
D. Artificial saliva
   1. Glandosane® (Fresenius Alctiengesellschaft, Germany): Spray once or twice in mouth every hour as needed.
   2. Moi-stir® (Kingswood Laboratories, Inc., Indianapolis, IN) oral swabsticks: Swab to oral tissue every hour as needed.
   3. Moist plus™ (Sage Products, Crystal Lake, IL): Spray once or twice in mouth every hour as needed.
   4. MouthKote® (Parnell Pharmaceuticals, Inc., Larkspur, CA): Spray once or twice in mouth every hour as needed.
E. Cholinergic agonist increases secretion of exocrine glands: Pilocarpine hydrochloride (Salagen®, MGI Pharma, Inc., East Minneapolis, MN): Initial dose is five mg po tid; titrate up to 10 mg tid if not responding and if tolerating lower doses.
F. Mouth rinses
   1. One liter of water mixed with one-half tablespoon of salt and one-half tablespoon of baking soda. Gargle with solution as needed for dry mouth.
   2. Biotene® (Laclede Professional Products, Inc., Dominquez, CA) mouthwash: Gargle as needed.
G. Products to stimulate salivary flow
   1. Biotene® dental chewing gum
   2. Sugarless gum
H. Lubrication of the lips
   1. Petroleum-based or vitamin E-based ointment
   2. Neutrogena® (Neutrogena Corporation, Los Angeles, CA) lip moisturizer
   3. Carmex® (Carma Laboratories, Inc., Franklin, WI) lip moisturizer
 I. Oral hygiene products
   1. Dry mouth toothpaste used after meals and at bedtime
   2. Portable battery-powered hand piece that delivers oral irrigation or suction as needed for comfort (SurgiLav®, Stryker Corporation, Kalamazoo, MI)
   3. Soft-bristle toothbrush
   4. Oral irrigator (Water Pik®, Teledyne Industries, Los Angeles, CA) used with water or antibacterial rinses
J. Hypodermoclysis can provide hydration for patients who are terminally ill if the goal is to maintain cognitive status.
   1. Administer a mixture of normal saline or normal saline with 5% dextrose and 20 mEq of potassium at a rate of 500–1,500 ml/24 hours subcutaneously.
   2. If necessary to increase absorption of fluid from the subcutaneous site, add hyaluronidase 500 units to each liter.
   3. Contraindications to hypodermoclysis are anasarca (generalized edema along with ascites) and severe thrombocytopenia.
   4. IV fluids are medically unnecessary and have numerous disadvantages in end-stage disease (e.g., cough, pulmonary congestion, choking, edema).

K. Education for palliative treatment includes explaining that decreased oral intake is natural in the terminal phase and that most patients do not feel hunger or thirst. IV fluid may increase discomfort.

VII. Follow-up
   A. Depends upon cause of thirst
   B. Thirst induced by pathologic condition will require follow-up according to condition.

VIII. Referrals: Only needed if underlying condition warrants referral

References

Fainsinger, R., & Bruera, E. (1994). The management of dehydration in terminally ill patients. *Journal of Palliative Care, 10*(3), 55.

McCann, R.M., Hall, W.J., & Groth-Juncher, A. (1994). Comfort care for terminally ill patients. The appropriate use of nutrition and hydration. *JAMA, 272,* 1263.

Rothman, J. (1997). Paraneoplastic syndromes. *Hospital Physician, 33*(8), 29–41.

Waller, A., & Caroline, N. (1996). Handbook of palliative care in cancer. Boston: Butterworth-Heinemann.

Waller, A., Hershkowitz, M., & Adunsky, A. (1994). The effect of intravenous fluid infusion on blood and urine parameters of hydration and on the state of consciousness in terminal cancer patients. *American Journal of Hospice Palliative Care, 11*(6), 22.

Chapter

143.

Diabetes Mellitus, Types 1 and 2
Susan Baird-Powell, RN, MSN, CRNP

I. Definition: A metabolic disorder consisting of high blood glucose levels and disruptions in the metabolism of carbohydrate, fat, and protein

II. Pathophysiology: Secondary to the pancreas' inability to produce enough or any insulin or the impairment of insulin action at the target cell.
   A. Insulin-dependent diabetes mellitus (IDDM): Type 1—Destruction of pancreatic beta cells that cause a decrease in insulin-producing cells.
   B. Non-insulin-dependent diabetes mellitus (NIDDM): Type 2
      1. Insulin production may be impaired.
      2. Insulin resistance: Target cells have fewer receptors for insulin.

III. Clinical features
   A. Risk factors
      1. IDDM: Type 1
         a) Occurs most often in patients younger than age 20 and in patients with European heritage
         b) Accounts for 10%–15% of all diabetes mellitus
      2. NIDDM: Type 2
         a) Occurs most often in patients older than age 40
         b) Accounts for 80%–90% of all diabetes mellitus
         c) Familial: Trait is autosomal dominant.
         d) Approximately 60%–80% of patients are overweight.
   B. History
      1. History of cancer and cancer treatment
      2. Current medications: Prescribed and over-the-counter
      3. History of presenting symptom(s): Precipitating factors, onset, and duration
      4. Changes in activities of daily living
      5. History of weight change, diet recall for 24 hours, exercise
      6. Past medical history of infections, hypertension, increased triglyceride or cholesterol levels
      7. Family history: Diabetes mellitus, cardiovascular disease
      8. Women: History of gestational diabetes

C. Signs and symptoms
1. IDDM (Type 1): Classic presentation is abrupt and severe.
    a) Early signs and symptoms
        (1) Polydipsia
        (2) Polyphagia
        (3) Polyuria
        (4) Weight loss
        (5) Fatigue
        (6) Weakness
        (7) Blurred vision
        (8) Abdominal pain
        (9) Nausea
        (10) Vomiting
        (11) Vaginal itching
        (12) Frequent infections
        (13) Skin rashes
    b) Later signs and symptoms/long-term problems
        (1) Decreased appetite
        (2) Bloating
        (3) Dehydration
        (4) Decreased level of consciousness
        (5) Microvascular and neurogenic complications: Extremities cold with de-creased or absent pedal pulses, paresthesia, decreased vision, constipation with nocturnal diarrhea, neurogenic bladder, nocturia, impotence
2. NIDDM (Type 2): Classic presentation is slow and gradual and often discovered as an incidental finding.
    a) Patient may exhibit no signs or symptoms.
    b) Early signs and symptoms
        (1) Polydipsia
        (2) Polyphagia
        (3) Polyuria
        (4) Fatigue
        (5) Blurred vision
        (6) Decreased healing
        (7) Frequent infections: Vaginal, urinary, skin
D. Physical exam
1. IDDM (Type 1)
    a) General appearance: Ill
    b) Vital signs: Tachycardia, orthostatic blood pressure
    c) Height and weight: Thin, recent weight loss
    d) HEENT exam
        (1) Eyes: Complete ophthalmic exam to rule out retinopathy and blurred vision
        (2) Mouth: Complete mouth and dental exam
        (3) Neck: Thyroid enlargement
    e) Integument exam: Loose skin folds, rashes, infections; check feet carefully for any current or possible future source of infection

  f) Cardiac exam: Flat neck veins (supine) indicate dehydration; check all peripheral pulses, decreased capillary refill to assess for vascular insufficiency

  g) Extremities: Cool, pretibial edema, weakness with decreased strength

  h) Neurologic exam: Decreased vibratory/position sense of peripheral nerves, decreased extraocular movements

 2. NIDDM (Type 2)

  a) Complete physical examination: May be normal

  b) Vital signs: Hypertension

  c) Weight: Usually overweight

  d) As disease progresses, may have similar clinical findings to IDDM (Type 1).

IV. Diagnostic tests

 A. Laboratory

  1. Serum glucose: To confirm diagnosis

   a) Fasting serum glucose > 126 mg/dl on two separate occasions

   b) Apparent signs and symptoms (e.g., polydipsia, polyphagia, polyuria, weight loss) and a random serum glucose > 200 mg/dl

  2. Oral glucose tolerance test: Usually not needed for diagnosis

  3. Urinalysis: Positive for glucose and ketones

  4. Hemoglobin A_{1c} (i.e., glycosylated hemoglobin)

   a) Blood test used to assess the degree of glucose control

   b) May be abbreviated as HbA_1 or HbA_{1c}

   c) Reflects the average blood glucose level for the past two months

   d) Adult value ranges

    (1) 4.0–6.0%: Normal

    (2) 7.0–9.0%: Well-controlled diabetic

    (3) > 9%: Poorly-controlled diabetic

 B. Radiology: Not indicated

 C. Other tests

  1. Cytoplasmic islet cell antibodies (ICAs): Positive serum test confirms the diagnosis of IDDM (Type 1).

  2. Serum C-peptide: Low indicates low levels of endogenous insulin.

V. Differential diagnosis

 A. Medications: Secondary effects, including hyperglycemia

  1. Oral contraceptives

  2. Corticosteroids

  3. Thiazides

  4. Phenytoins

  5. Beta-adrenergic blocking agents

  6. Calcium channel blockers

  7. Clonidine

  8. Nicotinic acid

  9. Pentamidine

  10. Cyclosporine

        11. Tricyclic antidepressants

        12. Phenothiazines

        13. Streptozocin chemotherapy

  B. Diseases

      1. Benign renal glucosuria

      2. Renal tubular disease

      3. Diabetes insipidus

      4. Cushing's disease

      5. Pheochromocytoma

      6. Acromegaly

      7. Severe stress secondary to trauma, burns, or infection

      8. Pancreatitis (see Chapter 72)

      9. Pancreatic cancers

         a) Glucagonoma (malignant)

         b) Malignant insulinoma

      10. Cirrhosis (see Chapter 64)

      11. Paraneoplastic syndrome (see Appendix 12)

VI. Treatment

  A. Patient education, nutrition counseling, exercise recommendations

      1. Should be part of plan for all diabetics

      2. May be only treatment plan needed for Type 2 diabetics with a mild or moderately elevated fasting blood glucose of < 300 mg/dl

  B. Patient education

      1. Teach basic pathophysiology of the disease.

      2. Discuss long-term problems associated with diabetes mellitus; stress importance of how good blood sugar control can prevent or delay complications.

      3. Teach signs and symptoms of diabetes mellitus that patient should be aware of and when it is appropriate to call the clinician.

      4. Provide a telephone number for patient to call to voice concerns or ask questions.

      5. Teach caregiver appropriate actions in case of emergency. It is important to note that infections can cause hyperglycemia as well as hypoglycemia, depending on the type of infection and how the patient responds.

         a) Hyperglycemia: Symptoms evolve over several hours to several days.

           (1) Signs and symptoms

              (a) Increased thirst

              (b) Increased urination

              (c) Increased blood glucose

              (d) Ketones present in the urine

              (e) Stomach pain

              (f) Body aches

              (g) Weakness, fatigue

              (h) Labored breathing

              (i) Anorexia

              (j) Nausea

              (k) Vomiting

        (2) Patient/caregiver actions
            (a) Call physician immediately
            (b) If able to swallow, drink fluids without sugar
            (c) Check blood sugar: Type 1, every hour; Type 2, before every meal and at bedtime
            (d) Check urine for ketones
        (3) Causes of hyperglycemia
            (a) Insufficient insulin
            (b) Oversufficient food intake
            (c) Infection
            (d) Emotional stressors
            (e) Medications (see "Differential Diagnosis," pp. 839–840)
     b) Hypoglycemia: Symptoms evolve over minutes to hours.
        (1) Signs and symptoms
            (a) Cold sweats
            (b) Fainting sensation
            (c) Dizziness
            (d) Headache
            (e) Heart pounding
            (f) Trembling
            (g) Nervousness
            (h) Vision blurred
            (i) Hunger
            (j) Personality changes
            (k) Unconsciousness
        (2) Patient/caregiver actions
            (a) Take two to three glucose tablets or liquids or foods containing sugar (e.g., regular soda, fruit juice) followed by a protein source.
            (b) Check blood sugar level every 15 minutes until blood sugar increases to normal range, then once an hour for two hours.
            (c) Do not give insulin.
            (d) If unconscious, do not give anything by mouth and seek immediate emergency care.
            (e) If unconscious, give glucagon per directions on the package and seek immediate emergency care.
        (3) Causes of hypoglycemia
            (a) Oversufficient insulin
            (b) Insufficient food intake
            (c) Overexercising
            (d) Delayed or missed meal
            (e) Infection
  6. Teach how to check blood sugar by glucometer and how to draw and administer insulin.
  7. "Sick day" rules
     a) Weigh patient three times a day; weight loss may indicate dehydration, so advise patient to drink more liquids and salty fluids (e.g., soup).

b) Check urine ketones every three to four hours. If positive, more insulin is needed.
c) Extra insulin is 10%–20% of total daily insulin dose, using 100 as a baseline blood glucose. This extra dose is given every three hours around the clock.
   (1) Administer 10% extra dose if glucose > 240 and ketones are negative.
   (2) Administer 20% extra dose if glucose > 240 and ketones are positive.
d) Call physician if
   (1) Unsure what to do
   (2) Vomiting/diarrhea does not stop
   (3) Weight loss continues
   (4) Overall symptoms do not improve
   (5) Blood sugar stays above normal, despite extra insulin
   (6) Ketones do not clear from urine.
e) Rarely does insulin ever need to be decreased; even with decreased intake, illness affects how insulin works so extra is needed until resolution.

8. Foot care
   a) Inspect feet daily, including between toes. Carefully check for any open areas of breakdown, cuts, scratches, blisters, or bruises.
   b) Wash feet daily with lukewarm water and a mild soap. After patting dry, especially between the toes, apply lanolin except to nails and between toes. If feet perspire excessively, use talcum powder, not cornstarch.
   c) Use clothing (e.g., thermal or wool socks) to keep feet warm. Never use external sources (e.g., heating pads, hot water bottles).
   d) Pressure points in shoes may cause corns and calluses on the feet. Do not use home remedies or razor blades to remove them. If they persist, see a podiatrist for removal. Inserts may be made to specially fit the foot and relieve the pressure caused by shoes.
   e) Inspect shoes daily for foreign objects or sharp inside edges.
   f) Cut toenails straight across; do not cut down into the corners, only file corners with an emery board. If thick nails or ingrown toenails are a problem, consult a podiatrist.
   g) Change socks daily. Wear properly fitting stockings.
   h) Wear comfortable shoes that fit properly. Leather soles with leather heels are best because they will breathe, allowing moisture to escape. Break in new shoes slowly, checking feet carefully for sore or reddened areas. Avoid pointed-toe or open-toe shoes.
   i) Never walk barefoot, including inside the house.

C. Nutrition counseling
   1. IDDM (Type 1): Plan meals to correlate with the calories and nutrients that the amount of insulin given is expected to metabolize.
   2. Patient should eat meals at the same time each day; the amount of calories and nutrients also should be consistent.
   3. NIDDM (Type 2): Calorie reduction in the diet can decrease weight, leading to
      a) Decreased morbidity and mortality
      b) Decreased hyperlipidemia, hyperglycemia, and hypertension.
   4. Nutrition recommendations: IDDM (Type 1) and NIDDM (Type 2)

    a) Carbohydrates should comprise 50%–60% of total calories, preferably unrefined carbohydrates and fiber.

    b) Protein should comprise < 0.8 g/kg/day or < 20% of total calories.

    c) Fat and cholesterol should comprise 25%–30% of total calories.

        (1) < 300 mg of cholesterol per day

        (2) Fats should be unsaturated.

    d) Calculate ideal body weight and caloric requirements for each patient.

    e) Calories should be distributed as follows.

        (1) Breakfast: 20%

        (2) Lunch: 20%

        (3) Dinner: 30%

        (4) Midmorning snack: 10%

        (5) Midafternoon snack: 10%

        (6) Bedtime snack: 10%

D. Exercise recommendations: Exercise increases the patient's metabolism, has a positive effect on serum glucose levels, and, over time, can decrease insulin resistance.

    1. IDDM (Type 1)

        a) No standard guidelines developed.

        b) Patients should be taught to assess their blood sugar in relation to amount and intensity of exercise and make appropriate decreases in their insulin dose. This reduction will vary from patient to patient.

        c) Conduct cardiac examination before starting exercise program.

        d) Start slow and gradually increase intensity and length of time.

        e) Do not give insulin within one hour of exercising secondary to an increased rate of absorption.

        f) Give insulin at site away from those most affected by exercise (i.e., abdomen rather than thigh) secondary to an increased rate of absorption.

        g) Patient may need additional snack before and after exercise.

    2. NIDDM (Type 2)

        a) Patient should exercise at least three days a week for 20–45 minutes; daily exercise preferred.

        b) Include gradual warm-up and cool-down.

        c) Aerobic exercise is recommended at 50%–70% of patient's maximum O_2 uptake.

    3. IDDM (Type 1) and NIDDM (Type 2): If foot or eye problems are present, avoid strenuous exercise.

E. Oral hypoglycemics

    1. Used in NIDDM (Type 2) that cannot be controlled with diet and exercise.

    2. Comparison (see Table 143-1)

    3. Of those patients with NIDDM (Type 2) placed on oral agents, 30%–40% will not respond.

    4. Patients with NIDDM (Type 2) who should not be placed on oral agents

        a) Patients with sulfa allergy (no sulfonylureas)

        b) Patients with liver damage

        c) Patients with renal damage

        d) Alcohol abusers

Table 143-1. Comparison of Oral Hypoglycemics

Drug	Dose Range/Day	Maintenance Dose/Day
First-Generation Sulfonylureas		
Chlorpropamide (Diabinese[a])	Before breakfast: 100–750 mg	Once before breakfast or divided doses before meals: 100–500 mg
Tolazamide (Tolinase[b])	With meals: 100–1,000 mg	With meals: 100–1,000 mg
Tolbutamide (Orinase[b])	Before breakfast: 1–3 g	Once before breakfast or divided doses before meals: 0.25–3 g
Second-Generation Sulfonylureas		
Glimepiride (Amaryl[c])	Once daily with first main meal: 1–8 mg	Once daily with meal: 1–4 mg
Glipizide (Glucotrol[a])[e]	Before breakfast: 5–40 mg	Once before breakfast or divided doses before meals: 5–40 mg
Glyburide (Glynase[d])	With meal: 1.5–12 mg	Once with meal or divided doses: 0.75–12 mg
Biguanide		
Metformin (Glucophage[e])	With meal: 850–2550 mg	With meals: 850 mg bid with maximum 850 mg tid
Alpha-Glucosidase Inhibitor		
Acarbose (Precose[f])	With meals: 75–300 mg	With meals: 50–100 mg tid

[a] Pfizer Inc., New York, NY; [b] The Upjohn Company, Kalmazoo, MI; [c] Hoechst Marion Roussel, Kansas City, MO; [d] Pharmacia & Upjohn, Peapack, NJ; [e] Bristol-Myers Squibb, Princeton, NJ; [f] Bayer Corporation, West Haven, CT

    5. Possible side effects of oral hypoglycemics
      a) Hypoglycemia
      b) Gastrointestinal problems
        (1) Nausea
        (2) Diarrhea
        (3) Constipation
        (4) Cholestatic jaundice
      c) Dermatologic reaction (i.e., allergic reaction)
      d) Goitrogenic
    6. General rules and considerations for oral agents
      a) Start treatment with low doses.
      b) Using self-monitoring as a guide, increase the dose every one to two weeks until
        (1) Glucose is in the acceptable range (70–120)
        (2) Maximum dose does not control glucose.
      c) Prescribe once a day if a low dose controls blood glucose.

  d) Increase frequency when higher doses are needed to control blood glucose; amount of each dose will depend on when patient's blood sugar runs the highest (i.e., am or pm).

  e) Allow one month for therapy to succeed before attempting a change.

  f) If blood glucose does not respond

   (1) Change oral agents

   (2) Change to insulin

   (3) Add insulin to current oral agent.

F. Insulin

 1. Types

  a) Prescribe human insulin for new patients with IDDM (Type 1): Decreased insulin allergies, decreased resistance, decreased lipoatrophy

  b) If patient is already using pork or beef insulin and blood glucoses are acceptable, do not change regimen.

  c) Four types: Regular, intermediate, long-acting, mixed

  d) Comparison (see Table 143-2)

 2. General rules and considerations for patients requiring insulin

  a) Initially: 0.5–1.0 units/kg/day

  b) Divide total daily dose: 2/3 before breakfast, 1/3 before supper

  c) Before breakfast: 2/3 intermediate-acting and 1/3 short-acting

Table 143-2. Comparison of Insulin Types

Action and Type	Onset (Hours)	Peak (Hours)	Duration (Hours)
Short-Acting			
Insulin-analog injection Insulin lispro injection (Humalog® [a])	0.25	0.5–1.5	6–8
Regular	0.1–1.0	1–5	5–7
Semilente	0.5–2.0	1–6	12–16
Intermediate-Acting			
Insulin zinc suspention (Lente® [b])	1–2	2–14	18–48
NPH	1–2	2–14	18–48
NPH (70%) mixed with regular (30%) (Mixtard®[b], Novolin® 70/30[b])	0.5	4–8	24
Long-Acting			
Protamine zinc (PZI)	2–8	8–24	36–38
Insulin zinc suspention, extended (Ultralente® [b])	2–6	8–26	36+

[a] Eli Lilly & Company, Indianapolis, IN; [b] Novo Nordisk Pharmaceuticals, Inc., Bagsvaerd, Denmark

d) Before supper: 1/2 intermediate-acting and 1/2 short-acting

e) Patient should monitor blood glucose five times/day initially (i.e., before each meal, before bed, and between 2–4 am) for three days and record. If a blood glucose control of < 170 mg/dl is not achieved, increase insulin by 2–5 units.

f) When looking at a patient's home glucose monitoring record to make dosage changes, think carefully about what type and amount of insulin is affecting the blood sugar at a given time.

g) Patient education is extremely important regarding storage and mixing of insulin, site selection and administration, disposal of medical waste, and correct self-monitoring technique and timing.

h) Review patient's other medications for those causing increased or decreased action of insulin or oral agent.

i) Drug interactions (see Figure 143-1)

VII. Complications of diabetes mellitus and therapy
    A. Hyperglycemic episodes
    B. Hypoglycemic episodes
    C. Diabetic ketoacidosis (DKA): Occurs in IDDM (Type 1)
        1. Signs and symptoms: Marked hyperglycemia, ketonuria, and electrolyte, fluid, and pH imbalances that can result in coma and death
        2. Cause: Severe stressors (e.g., trauma, infection, heart attack); also can occur as a result of noncompliance with insulin therapy
        3. Treatment: Administer fluids and insulin, correct metabolic acidosis, monitor labs.
    D. Hyperosmolar nonketotic syndrome: Occurs in patients on oral agents, the elderly, and patients with undiagnosed NIDDM (Type 2)
        1. Signs and symptoms: Marked hyperglycemia, dehydration, and hyperosmolarity without ketoacidosis; can result in coma

---

Figure 143-1. Drug Interactions in the Treatment of Diabetes

Drugs That Intensify Hypoglycemia		Drugs That Counteract Hypoglycemia	
With oral agents	**With insulin**	**With oral agents**	**With insulin**
Nonsteroidal anti-inflammatory drugs	Ethanol	Calcium channel blockers	Corticosteroids
Sulfonamide antibiotics	Alpha-blockers	Combination oral contraceptives	Diltiazem
Ethanol (used acutely)	Anabolic steroids	Glucocorticoids	Dobutamine
Ranitidine	Beta-blockers	Phenothiazines	Epinephrine
Cimetidine	Clofibrate	Thiazide diuretics	Oral contraceptives
Beta-blockers (with tolbutamide)	Fenfluramine		Smoking
	Guanethidine		Thiazide diuretics
	MAO inhibitors		Thyroid hormone
	Pentamidine		Niacin
	Phenylbutazone		
	Salicylates		
	Sulfinpyrazone		
	Tetracycline		

    2. Cause: Medications (e.g., calcium channel blockers, phenytoin, propranolol, thiazide diuretics, corticosteriods)

    3. Treatment: More fluids and less insulin than DKA

  E. Retinopathy

  F. Nephropathy

  G. Cardiovascular disease/hypertension

  H. Neuropathy

  I. Autonomic nervous system conditions

  J. Foot ulcers/peripheral vascular disease

  K. Poor wound healing

VIII. Special considerations for diabetic patients with cancer

  A. Stop Glucophage® (Bristol-Myers Squibb Co., Princeton, NJ) 72 hours prior to using contrast material with CT scans, as Glucophage may increase nephrotoxicity.

  B. Hospitalized patients being treated with chemotherapy or for acute illness may need a sliding scale of regular insulin regimen to meet their needs.

    1. Blood sugar: < 200: No insulin

    2. 201–250: 2 units of insulin

    3. 251–300: 4 units of insulin

    4. 301–350: 6 units of insulin

    5. 351–400: 8 units of insulin

    6. > 400: Call physician.

  C. Corticosteroids used in antiemetic regimens will increase glucose levels; avoid using or support patient with insulin. Monitor serum glucose levels.

  D. If hyperglycemia is incidentally found during cancer treatment, begin assessing patient's needs with pattern blood glucose levels.

  E. Unless the oncologist will regulate the patient's insulin or oral-agent needs, the primary physician should evaluate the patient when uncontrolled glucose levels are detected.

  F. Prior to a surgical procedure, the patient should reduce insulin by 1/3–1/2 the morning of surgery.

  G. Avoid using dextrose solutions for hydration fluids or admixtures.

  H. Admit patients with protracted nausea and vomiting for management.

IX. Follow-up

  A. Newly diagnosed diabetics on insulin need access to a clinician to report blood glucose levels and receive instructions regarding changes in insulin dose.

  B. Patients starting oral agents or with substantial changes in their insulin therapy should be seen in one week.

  C. When a desirable blood glucose level is achieved, see patient every three to four months; conduct skin, lower extremities, foot, and fundoscopic exam at each visit.

  D. Ophthalmologic exam: Yearly to assess for retinopathy

  E. Chest x-ray and EKG: Yearly to assess for cardiomegaly and cardiovascular disease

  F. Full physical exam: Yearly, including neurologic exams; labs include lipid profile, BUN and creatinine, and urinalysis.

  G. Assess fasting blood glucose level or postprandial blood glucose at each visit.

H. Measure hemoglobin A$_{1c}$ two to four times/year, depending on control of blood sugars.

X. Referrals
  A. Support groups: Educate all diabetic patients on available resources.
  B. Diabetes educator to teach regarding medication and self-care measures
  C. Dietician for diet education
  D. Endocrinologist: For
    1. Diagnosis
    2. Initial treatment plan
    3. Diabetic ketoacidosis, hyperosmolar nonketotic syndrome
    4. Failed response to therapy
  E. Nephrologist: Diabetic renal disease
  F. Cardiologist: Cardiovascular disease, hypertension
  G. Urologist: Impotence, incontinence
  H. Podiatrist: Foot care
  I. Ophthalmologist: Retinopathy

References

Brietzke, S.A. (1996). Diabetes mellitus, Type I. In R.E. Rakel (Ed.), *Saunders manual of medical practice* (pp. 626–628). Philadelphia: Saunders.

Davidoff, F. (1997). Blood sugar, disease, and nondisease. *Annals of Internal Medicine, 127*(3), 235–237.

Gallichan, M. (1997). Self-monitoring of glucose by people with diabetes: Evidence-based practice. *British Medical Journal, 314*(7085), 964–967.

Macready, M. (1997). American Diabetes Association calls for testing all those over 45. *British Medical Journal, 315*(7099), 11.

Parke-Davis. (1997). Oral hypoglycemic agents in Type II diabetes mellitus. *Rezulin (troglitazone).* Morris Plains, NJ: Warner-Lambert Company.

Wilson, B.E. (1996). Diabetes mellitus, Type II. In R.E. Rakel (Ed.), *Saunders manual of medical practice* (pp. 629 631). Philadelphia: Saunders.

144. Hypocalcemia/Hypercalcemia

Wendy J. Smith, RN, MSN, ACNP, AOCN®

I. Definition
   A. Normal serum calcium (Ca⁺⁺) is 8.5–10.5 mg/dl (4.5–5.5 mEq/l). The normal level for ionized serum calcium is 4.6–5.3 mg/dl (2.2–2.5 mEq/l).
   B. Hypocalcemia exists when the serum calcium is < 8.5 mg/dl or the ionized calcium level is < 4.6 mg/dl.
   C. Hypercalcemia exists when the serum calcium is > 10.5 mg/dl or the ionized calcium level is > 5.3 mg/dl.

II. Physiology/Pathophysiology
   A. Normal physiology
       1. Majority of body's calcium (99%) is deposited in the bones in an inorganic compound termed hydroxyapatite.
           a) Only 1% is in the extracellular fluid.
           b) Of this 1%, half is bound to protein, primarily albumin, and the remaining half is in an ionized (i.e., free) form.
           c) Ionized calcium is the form needed for calcium physiologic functions.
           d) Calcium and phosphorus (PO$_4$) are stored in the bone and are regulated by the kidneys, yet they have opposite effects. When the serum Ca⁺⁺ decreases, PO$_4$ increases; when Ca⁺⁺ increases, PO$_4$ decreases.
       2. Normal calcium function
           a) Major cation involved in the formation of bone and teeth
           b) Cofactor in blood coagulation, converting prothrombin to thrombin
           c) Ionized calcium: Necessary for neuromuscular function, nerve impulse transmission, and skeletal muscle contraction
           d) Maintenance of cellular membrane permeability
               (1) Increased calcium levels decrease cellular permeability.
               (2) Decreased calcium levels increase cellular permeability.
       3. Hormone regulators of calcium balance
           a) Calcitriol (1,25-dihydroxycholecalciferol), the most active metabolite of vitamin D (Vit D$_3$), promotes absorption of calcium from the intestines.
               (1) Vitamin D is synthesized by the skin in response to exposure to ultraviolet rays.

    (2) Calciferol (Vit D_2) is obtained from oral supplements and fortified milk.

    (3) Both are transferred to the liver and metabolized to form calcifediol, which is then transferred to the kidneys and converted to calcitriol.

   b) Parathyroid hormone (PTH) is released in response to low serum calcium and increases reabsorption of calcium via the kidney and removal of calcium from the bone.

   c) Calcitonin, which is secreted from the thyroid gland, inhibits calcium resorption and increases renal excretion (i.e., calcitonin opposes the action of PTH when calcium levels are elevated).

 B. Hypocalcemia pathophysiology

  1. Condition is caused by the inability to metabolize calcitriol, which is needed to absorb calcium from the small intestines, and phosphorus retention by the kidneys.

  2. A large volume of cells are injured or destroyed, resulting in the release of cellular contents (e.g., potassium and phosphorus) into the blood, overwhelming the kidneys (e.g., tumor lysis syndrome).

  3. Rapid administration of blood transfusions can lead to hypocalcemia because the citrate solution, used to store whole blood, binds with calcium, decreasing the amount of ionized (free) calcium.

  4. Alkalosis also increases the binding of calcium to proteins, thereby decreasing the amount of ionized calcium available.

 C. Hypercalcemia pathophysiology

  1. Paraneoplastic syndromes in ovarian, kidney, or lung cancer can secrete an ectopic source of PTH, referred to as parathyroid-related protein (PTHrP). This promotes the release of calcium and phosphate from the bone, reabsorption of calcium and magnesium via the kidney, and increased indirect absorption from the intestine through its role in converting vitamin D to calcitriol.

  2. Granulomatous diseases (e.g., TB, sarcoidosis) are thought to increase Ca^{++} as a result of macrophages present in granulomatous tissue producing calcitriol (elevated serum levels of this active metabolite have been found).

III. Clinical features

 A. Etiologies

  1. Hypocalcemia

   a) Absence of PTH

    (1) Hereditary hypoparathyroidism

    (2) Acquired hypoparathyroidism

    (3) Hypomagnesemia

   b) Ineffective PTH

    (1) Chronic renal failure

    (2) Lack of vitamin D

     (a) Decreased intake

     (b) Decreased sunlight

     (c) Defective metabolism

      i) Anticonvulsant therapy

      ii) Intestinal malabsorption

       c) PTH overwhelmed: Acute hyperphosphatemia
          (1) Tumor lysis syndrome
          (2) Acute renal failure
       d) Medication-induced: Loop diuretics, plicamycin, phosphate preparation, aminoglycosides, cholestyramine, pamidronate

  2. Hypercalcemia
       a) Parathyroid-related
          (1) Hyperparathyroidism
          (2) Lithium therapy
       b) Malignancy-related (see Appendix 12)
       c) Vitamin-related
          (1) Vitamins D and A intoxication
          (2) Sarcoidosis or other granulomatous disease
       d) Immobilization: Generally elevates Ca^{++} only in combination with another process
       e) Medication-induced: Thiazides (decreases Ca^{++} excretion by the kidneys), steroids, calcium supplements)
       f) Renal failure

B. History
  1. History of cancer and cancer treatment
  2. Current medications: Prescribed and over-the-counter
  3. History of presenting symptom(s): Precipitating factors, location, and duration. Associated symptoms are nausea, vomiting, diarrhea, constipation, twitching, tingling, or numbness (especially around mouth or fingers), muscle spasms, and abdominal cramps.
  4. Changes in activities of daily living
  5. Past medical history: Surgery of the thyroid gland, neck surgery, kidney stones
  6. Family history of glandular cancers (e.g., multiple endocrine neoplasia) or hypocalcemia

C. Signs and symptoms
  1. Hypocalcemia
       a) Symptoms and signs vary with rate of onset and acuity; with mild or chronic hypocalcemia, patients may be asymptomatic.
       b) Anxiety or irritability
       c) Tetany: Intermittent tonic/spasmodic muscle contractions
          (1) Twitching
          (2) Paresthesia
          (3) Carpopedal spasm
          (4) Laryngeal spasm
          (5) Seizures/convulsions
       d) Abdominal cramps
       e) Lethargy
       f) Depression
       g) Stupor/coma
  2. Hypercalcemia

    a) Fatigue

    b) Weakness (i.e., muscles become flaccid)

    c) Lethargy

    d) Depression

    e) Anorexia

    f) Nausea

    g) Constipation

    h) Polyuria, polydipsia

    i) Stupor/coma

    j) Flank pain may develop if precipitates of calcium salts form renal calculi.

  D. Physical exam

    1. Hypocalcemia

     a) Special tests (see Appendix 13)

      (1) Positive Chvostek's sign: Tapping on the facial nerve just below the temple in front of the ear will elicit twitching or contractions of the facial muscle.

      (2) Positive Trousseau's sign: Applying a blood pressure cuff to occlude the brachial artery for three to five minutes elicits contraction of the hand and fingers.

     b) Cardiac exam: Evaluate blood pressure and heart rate and rhythm, looking for evidence of weak contractions, dysrhythmia, hypotension, CHF.

     c) Pulmonary exam: Listen for evidence of laryngospasm, presence of stridor.

     d) Abdominal exam: Assess for hyperactive bowel sounds.

     e) Musculoskeletal: Evaluate muscle strength and assess for spasms/contractions.

    2. Hypercalcemia

     a) Assess mental status.

     b) Cardiac exam

      (1) Evaluate heart rate and rhythm, looking for bradycardia/dysrhythmia.

      (2) Check orthostatic pressures, and assess for dehydration.

     c) Abdominal

      (1) Assess bowel sounds, which may be decreasing.

      (2) Check for costovertebral tenderness/flank pain.

     d) Neurologic: Observe for delayed deep tendon reflexes.

     e) Musculoskeletal exam: Evaluate muscle strength and tone.

 IV. Diagnostic tests

  A. Laboratory tests for hypo/hypercalcemia (see Table 144-1)

  B. Radiology: Plain films and/or bone scans may be indicated, depending on the etiology

  C. Other: EKG not a diagnostic tool but may be indicated to evaluate for conduction abnormalities in severe hypo/hypercalcemia

    1. Hypocalcemia: Evaluate for lengthened ST segment, prolonged QT interval, blocks.

    2. Hypercalcemia: Evaluate for shortened ST segment, shortened QT interval, dysrhythmia, evidence of digitalis toxicity.

 V. Differential diagnosis

  A. Hypocalcemia

Table 144-1. Laboratory Tests for Evaluating Calcium Imbalances

Test	Hypocalcemia	Hypercalcemia	Comments
Serum Ca^{++}	< 8.5 mg/dl (4.5 mEq/l)	> 10.5 mg/dl (5.5 mEq/l)	
Ionized Ca^{++}	< 4.6 mg/dl (2.2 mEq/l)	> 5.3 mg/dl (2.5 mEq/l)	More expensive/not readily available
Serum PO$_4$	Normal in vitamin D deficiency	Decrease or normal (variable in bone metastases)	Ca^{++} and PO$_4$ usually have inverse relationship (increase PTH decrease PO$_4$)
Mg^{++}	Decrease or normal	Decrease or normal	Looking for potential causes of decrease Ca^{++}
			Decrease Mg^{++} decrease Ca^{++}
			Mg^{++} may also be low in hypophosphatemia because of increased renal excretion.
BUN/Creatinine	Increase, decrease, or normal	Decrease, increase, or normal	Looking for renal dysfunction.
Serum albumin	Decrease or normal	Increase or normal	Hypoalbuminemia is most common cause of decreased Ca^{++}. When albumin is low, calculate corrected calcium.*
Parathyroid hormone (PTH)	Decrease or normal, increase	Increase, decrease, or normal	Hypercalcemia of malignancy may cause increased Ca^{++} and decreased PTH.
Urine PO$_4$	Decrease in PTH deficiency	Increase or normal	
Urine Ca^{++}	Decrease	Increase or normal	

* Corrected Ca^{++}= {serum Ca^{++}(mg/dl)} + [4–serum albumin (g/dl)] x 0.8

1. Malabsorption (e.g., chronic diarrhea, small bowel resection, pelvic radiation)
2. Renal failure/insufficiency (most common cause) (see Chapter 83)
3. Hypoparathyroidism
4. Alkalosis
5. Hypoalbuminemia
6. Vitamin D deficiency
7. Hyperphosphatemia
8. Medullary carcinoma of the thyroid
9. Malnutrition/total parenteral nutrition (see Chapter 158)
10. Pancreatitis: Release of lipase, causing fatty acids to bind to Ca^{++} (see Chapter 72)
11. Tumor lysis syndrome
   B. Hypercalcemia

1. Hyperparathyroidism (primary or secondary)
2. Adrenal insufficiency: Addison's disease
3. Thyrotoxicosis
4. Malignancy: Paraneoplastic syndrome (see Appendix 12) or bone metastasis
5. Hypophosphatemia
6. Granulomatous disease (e.g., TB, sarcoidosis)
7. Immobility
8. Other: Familial hypocalciuric hypercalcemia, Paget's disease

VI. Treatment: The goal is to restore normal serum calcium.
   A. Hypocalcemia
      1. Mild/asymptomatic
         a) No oral PTH replacement available; therefore calcium supplements (e.g., calcium carbonate) are an effective alternative. Calcium carbonate is the recommended source for replacement.
         b) One to two grams of elemental calcium/day is recommended in two to four divided doses.
         c) Calcium carbonate products and elemental calcium content
            (1) Oscal® (SmithKline Beecham Consumer Healthcare L.P.): 250–500 mg/tablet (most expensive form)
            (2) Tums® (SmithKline Beecham Consumer Healthcare L.P.): 200 mg/tablet (least expensive form)
            (3) Caltrate® (American Cyanamid Company, Wayne, NJ): 600 mg/tablet
            (4) Calcimax® (Slim-Fast Foods Company, West Palm Beach, FL): 325 mg/tablet
         d) Constipation is a potential side effect of calcium supplementation.
         e) Oral calcium supplements should be administered an hour before meals and at bedtime to improve absorption. In achlorhydric patients (i.e., those using H_2 antagonists or proton pump inhibitors) food improves absorption.
         f) Vitamin D is often given with calcium to enhance intestinal absorption of calcium. Products providing a combination of calcium and vitamin D are available.
            (1) In over-the-counter combination form, the daily dose of vitamin D is 400–1,000 IU/day.
            (2) If separate supplementation is utilized, vitamin D_2 (e.g., ergocalciferol) is the recommended replacement form; daily dosage range is 200–400 units.
            (3) Calcitriol (Rocaltrol®, Hoffman-La Roche Pharmaceuticals, Nutley, NJ) is another option; usual starting dose is 0.25 µg/day.
         g) Hypercalcemia is a possible side effect but usually can be treated with hydration. Because it is a slow-acting replacement, side effects may not appear for one to four months after initiating therapy.
         h) Correct hypomagnesemia (see Chapter 146).
         i) Phosphate binds (in hyperphosphatemia) with aluminum hydroxide (see Chapter 148).

2. Severe/symptomatic hypocalcemia (associated with tetany, seizures, arrhythmia)
   a) Calcium gluconate 10% (93 mg of elemental calcium in 10 ml): One to two ampules IV is administered over 10–15 minutes.
      (1) Caution in administration is necessary to avoid hypotension or dysrhythmia; administer no faster than 30–60 mg of elemental calcium per minute.
      (2) Onset of action is immediate; however, duration of effect is short.
      (3) If symptoms recur after initial IV calcium replacement, continuous infusion is usually recommended until patient is stabilized.
      (4) Recommended infusion is 15 mg calcium/kg of body weight in one liter of D_5W or NS IV over four to six hours.
   b) Calcium chloride 10% is another source, which actually renders more ionized calcium. Calcium chloride infiltration results in tissue injury and sloughing, making it a less-desirable choice.
B. Hypercalcemia: Treatment is individualized based on serum calcium levels, presenting symptoms, renal function, and underlying cause/prognosis (i.e., in situations in which malignancy is refractory to treatment, aggressive interventions to correct hypercalcemia may be seen as less beneficial to the patient considering poor prognosis/terminal state).
   1. Mild hypercalcemia (10.5–12 mg/dl)
      a) Hydration is the gold standard. Oral hydration may be possible.
         (1) Recommended that the patient consume 2–4 l/day.
         (2) This may be difficult for patients who are anorexic, or this volume may precipitate or aggravate nausea.
      b) For the majority of cases, IV hydration with isotonic saline (0.9%) is recommended.
         (1) Dehydration, increased Ca^{++}-induced nausea/vomiting, and/or polyuria must be corrected to restore intravascular volume and to promote diuresis.
         (2) Amount of fluid and rate of administration depend on the patient's cardiovascular and renal status.
         (3) Initiate hydration with normal saline at a rate of 250–500 cc/hour or two to four liters/day.
      c) Replace electrolytes as needed (to correct hypokalemia and hypomagnesemia).
   2. Chronic hypercalcemia: Oral neutral phosphates are rarely used since the advent of biphosphonates. Though they are not the first choice, they may have a role in managing chronic hypercalcemia
      a) Fleet Phospho-Soda® (C.B. Fleet Company, Lynchburg, VA) is the most common form used (contains 815 mg PO_4, 33 mEq sodium/5 cc).
      b) The usual starting dose 1 g/d in divided doses.
      c) Risk of diarrhea increases with dosage.
      d) An additional concern is the risk of extraskeletal precipitation of calcium phosphate, primarily in the soft tissue.
      e) Contraindicated in renal failure or when serum $PO_4 > 3.8$ mg/dl.
      f) Do not use with aluminum-containing antacids, as PO_4 binds with aluminum.
   3. Severe hypercalcemia (> 12 mg/dl)
      a) Rehydration and electrolyte replacement, as noted above, are the first and most important interventions.

b) Correct underlying cause of hypercalcemia (e.g., hyperparathyroidism, malignancy, TB).

c) Loop diuretics:

    (1) Once volume deficits are restored, IV furosemide may be administered 20–80 mg every four hours to enhance calciuresis and prevent fluid volume overload. Furosemide may exacerbate hypercalcemia if given before the patient is completely hydrated.

    (2) Thiazide diuretics can impair calcium excretion and should be avoided.

d) Calcitonin

    (1) Very useful in reducing the serum calcium quickly.

    (2) Effects may be seen within a few hours.

    (3) Disadvantage is that it is not effective for long-term control because tachyphylaxis (i.e., loss of efficacy) develops within 24–72 hours.

    (4) May be used initially until other interventions (e.g., biphosphonates) have time to take effect.

    (5) Average dose is four units/kg IM or SC every 12 hours.

    (6) Side effects are generally mild and infrequent and include inflammatory reactions at the site of injection, nausea and vomiting, abdominal cramping, increased urinary frequency, and fever.

e) Corticosteroids: Concomitant use may prolong the effectiveness of calcitonin, or they may have a calcium-lowering effect when used alone.

    (1) Prednisone: 40–60 mg/day po or the equivalent hydrocortisone 100–150 mg IV every 12 hours

    (2) Not as effective in primary hyperparathyroidism or when used as a single agent

f) Plicamycin (Mithramycin®, Bayer Corporation Pharmaceutical Division, West Haven, CT): 25 µg/kg/day IV over four to six hours, daily for two to four days

    (1) One of the oldest medications used for hypercalcemia

    (2) Inhibits bone resorption

    (3) Though effective in lowering serum calcium, duration of effect is short, and retreatment is often necessary within three to eight days.

    (4) Plicamycin is excreted via the kidneys and is also nephrotoxic; therefore, it is not recommended in patients who are dehydrated or whose renal function is compromised.

    (5) Possible side effects: Nausea, vomiting, myelosuppression; toxicities are seen more often with repeated doses.

    (6) Plicamycin is a vesicant.

    (7) Although it is one of the least-expensive agents, it has a short length of effectiveness, must be repeated sooner, and may have cumulative adverse effects with additional doses (e.g., increased morbidity). Thus, it may not be the most cost-effective approach.

g) Gallium nitrate: 100–200 mg/m^2/day by continuous IV infusion over five days

    (1) Inhibits bone resorption

    (2) Length of treatment prohibits management on an outpatient basis.

      (3) Possible side effects: Nephrotoxicity (contraindicated with impaired renal function and with other nephrotoxic agents), hypophosphatemia, nausea, vomiting, pain at injection site

      (4) When considering cost of treatment, also consider cost of hospitalization.

      (5) Duration of effect is 8–11 days.

   h) Biphosphonates: Pamidronate (Aredia®, Novartis Pharmaceutical Corporation, East Hanover, NJ) is the most potent biphosphonate.

      (1) Most conducive to outpatient management, most favorable side-effect profile (i.e., safe, nontoxic)

      (2) Effective > 95% of the time with long duration of effect (up to 4 weeks) and has become the mainstay of treatment for moderate to severe hypercalcemia

      (3) May be used monthly in managing chronic hypercalcemia of malignancy

      (4) Inhibits bone resorption with normalization of serum calcium within one week

      (5) Apparent dose-response effect enables more accurate dosing specific to severity of calcium level (i.e., doses of 30–60 mg may be given for serum calcium levels between 12–16 mg/dl; dose of 90 mg for serum calcium > 16 mg/dl).

      (6) Given as an IV infusion over two to four hours in 500–1,000 ml of normal saline, 0.45% normal saline, or 5% dextrose in water (D_5W)

      (7) Minimal side effects: Fever, phlebitis, hypocalcemia, hypophosphatemia

      (8) Calcitonin and pamidronate may be used together initially until Ca^{++} normalizes.

VII. Follow-up

  A. Hypocalcemia

    1. Mild/asymptomatic

      a) Patient may be followed on an outpatient basis.

      b) Frequency of serum calcium level depends on patient's condition and compliance, but every one to three months is probably adequate.

      c) Instruct patient on the signs and symptoms of hypocalcemia and management with oral supplements, as well as when to notify a healthcare provider.

    2. Severe hypocalcemia

      a) Serum calcium level should be monitored every four to six hours until stable. Once stable and IV replacement is discontinued, frequency is reduced.

      b) If patient is discharged on oral supplements, follow serum calcium weekly for one to two weeks, then decrease frequency with evidence of stable, asymptomatic condition.

  B. Hypercalcemia

    1. Mild/asymptomatic

      a) Patient may be followed on an outpatient basis.

      b) Frequency of serum calcium level depends on patient's overall condition; if stable, every one to three months may be adequate.

      c) Instruct patient on the signs and symptoms of hypercalcemia and when to notify a healthcare provider.

2. Severe
   a) Monitor serum calcium level daily until stable.
   b) Instruct patient on the signs and symptoms of hypercalcemia.
   c) If pamidronate is used for initial treatment and patient is stable, serum calcium level may be followed monthly after discharge.
   d) Other interventions have a shorter duration of effectiveness; therefore, weekly monitoring of serum calcium may be needed.
   e) Frequency of follow-up varies depending on patient's overall condition and recurrence of symptoms.

VIII. Referrals
   A. Management of mild hypo/hypercalcemia may only necessitate oral supplements or hydration; the level of physician collaboration or referrals depend on the underlying cause and response to treatment.
   B. Specialists: Referral based on underlying cause (i.e., suspected thyroid malignancy may require referral to surgeon for biopsy and/or neck surgery).
   C. Endocrinologist: If unable to determine underlying cause or if patient inadequately responds to treatment.

References

See pages 888-889.

145.

Hypokalemia/Hyperkalemia

Wendy J. Smith, RN, MSN, ACNP, AOCN®

I. Definition
- A. Normal serum potassium (K^+) ranges from 3.5–5.5 mEq/l.
- B. Hypokalemia exists when the K^+ is < 3.5 mEq/l
- C. Hyperkalemia exists when the K^+ is > 5.5 mEq/l.

II. Physiology/Pathophysiology
- A. Normal physiology
  1. Potassium is the most abundant intracellular cation. Only a small portion (approximately 2%–3%) is found in the extracellular fluids.
  2. Potassium has a critical role in cellular function, neuromuscular activity, and cardiac conduction.
     - a) Maintains intracellular osmolality and a balance (i.e., electrical neutrality) between hydrogen (H^+) and sodium (Na^+) within the cell
     - b) Maintains a stable resting membrane potential for transmitting and conducting nerve impulses
     - c) Plays a role in depositing glycogen in skeletal and liver cells in response to insulin
  3. The body does not store potassium; therefore, the body requires a minimum intake of 40–60 mEq/day.
  4. Several internal factors help to regulate potassium excretion/balance.
     - a) 80% is excreted by the kidneys in response to hyperkalemia and/or aldosterone hormone.
     - b) 15% is excreted through the gastrointestinal tract.
     - c) 5% is lost through the skin.
- B. Hypokalemia pathophysiology
  1. Can occur without actual loss of total body K^+ through processes that result in a shift of potassium from the extracellular fluid into the cell (i.e., intracellular)
  2. In acidosis, K^+ moves out of the cell in exchange for H^+.
     - a) There may be a normal or high serum K^+ when, in actuality, the total body K^+ may be depleted.
     - b) Kidneys continue to excrete potassium; hypokalemia becomes more evident.
     - c) In diabetic ketoacidosis, if the total body potassium is low and insulin is administered, a shift of K^+ back into the cells and severe hypokalemia occur.

3. In metabolic alkalosis, loss of K^+ occurs from severe K^+ depletion caused by an increase in bicarbonate reabsorption.
4. Hypovolemia stimulates the renin-angiotensin system, which, in turn, leads to secretion of aldosterone and K^+ excretion via the kidneys.
5. Anabolic cellular activity increases the demand for intracellular potassium, which can cause K^+ depletion, such as in cellular repair following trauma or injury.
6. Pseudohypokalemia may occur with leukocytosis because of an increased uptake of K^+ by WBCs after blood specimen has been drawn.

C. Hyperkalemia pathophysiology: K^+ excess in extracellular fluid results from increased intake, decreased output, or redistribution of K^+ from the intracellular to the extracellular fluid compartment.

III. Clinical features
A. Etiologies
  1. Hypokalemia: Decreased intake of K^+
    a) Malnutrition
    b) Cachexia
  2. Excessive loss of K^+
    a) Diarrhea
    b) Laxative abuse
    c) Vomiting
    d) Suctioning
    e) Intestinal fistula
    f) Diuretics
    g) Excessive mineralocorticoid effects
      (1) Primary aldosteronism
      (2) Secondary aldosteronism
    h) Excessive glucocorticoid effects
      (1) Cushing's syndrome
      (2) Exogenous steroids
      (3) Ectopic adrenocorticotropic hormone production
    i) Renal tubular disease
      (1) Renal tubular acidosis
      (2) Antibiotics
    j) Magnesium depletion
  3. Internal imbalance
    a) Alkalosis
    b) Insulin effect
    c) Increased RBC production following administration of vitamin B_{12} or erythropoietin
    d) Increased WBC production following administration of colony-stimulating factors
    e) Diabetic ketoacidosis
  4. Hyperkalemia
    a) Excessive oral K^+ intake

       b) Impaired K$^+$ excretion

          (1) Acute and chronic renal failure

          (2) K$^+$-sparing diuretics

   5. Internal imbalance

       a) Severe cellular injury: Tumor lysis syndrome

          (1) Most common cancers: Leukemia, lymphoma (especially Burkitt's)

          (2) Rare in solid tumors

       b) Acidosis

       c) Marked thrombocytosis or leukocytosis

   6. Incorrect handling of blood specimen

       a) Tight tourniquet application

       b) Blood sample from arm where K$^+$ infusing

   7. Hemolysis of aging donated RBCs

B. History

   1. History of cancer and cancer treatment

   2. Current medications: Prescribed and over-the-counter

   3. History of present symptom(s): Precipitating factors, location, and duration. Associated symptoms are history of nausea/vomiting, diarrhea, constipation, abdominal distention, abdominal cramping, muscle weakness, numbness or tingling, and palpitations.

   4. Changes in activities of daily living

   5. Past medical history: Diabetes mellitus, kidney disease, hypertension

C. Signs and symptoms

   1. Clinical manifestations possible in hypokalemia and hyperkalemia

       a) Nausea

       b) Vertigo

       c) Diarrhea

       d) Muscular weakness

       e) Flaccid paralysis

       f) Paresthesia

   2. Hypokalemia

       a) Anorexia

       b) Constipation

       c) Polyuria

       d) Fatigue

       e) Alteration in mental status (e.g., depression, drowsiness, confusion)

       f) Leg cramps

       g) Diaphoresis

   3. Hyperkalemia

       a) Abdominal cramps

       b) Tachycardia initially, then progresses to bradycardia and, in severe cases, cardiac arrest

       c) Oliguria or anuria

       d) Restlessness

       e) Irritability

D. Physical exam
   1. Mental status: Assess alertness/responsiveness, orientation, mood and behavior; drowsiness, malaise, mental depression, and confusion are seen in hypokalemia.
   2. Cardiac exam: Note heart rate and rhythm. Dysrhythmia can be seen in hypo/hyperkalemia; pulse tends to be weak in hypokalemia.
   3. Abdominal exam: Observe for abdominal distention and character of bowel sounds; decreased bowel sounds present with decreased K^+.
   4. Musculoskeletal exam: Note appearance and test strength in muscle groups; muscles are soft and flabby in hypokalemia; flaccid paralysis and respiratory paralysis can occur in severe imbalances but are more often associated with severe hypokalemia.
   5. Neurologic exam: Assess deep tendon reflexes; decreased in hypokalemia.

IV. Diagnostic tests
   A. Laboratory
      1. Electrolytes: To identify electrolyte imbalances and possible causes, it is important to draw a serum Na^+, K^+, Cl^-, CO_2, and Mg^{++}.
         a) Magnesium decreases: Potassium decreases.
         b) Magnesium increases: Potassium increases.
         c) Carbon dioxide: Could indicate metabolic acidosis (e.g., as in severe dehydration), potassium increases.
         d) Carbon dioxide increases: Indicates metabolic alkalosis, potassium increases; if $CO_2 > 55$, superimposed respiratory acidosis results, complicating true picture of electrolyte balance.
         e) Sodium decreases: Potassium increases (i.e., where adrenocortical hormones are deficient).
         f) Sodium decreases: Potassium decreases (e.g., in some cases of GI losses or with extensive use of diuretics).
      2. BUN and creatinine increases: Hyperkalemia results.
      3. If tumor lysis syndrome is suspected, include serum uric acid, calcium, and phosphorous in labs; hyperuricemia, hyperphosphatemia, hyperkalemia, hypocalcemia, along with abnormal renal function (increased creatinine), are the metabolic abnormalities seen.
      4. Urine potassium: May help to determine if potassium loss is extrarenal (urine $K^+ < 20$ mEq) or the result of excess renal excretion (urine $K^+ > 40$ mEq)
      5. Digoxin level: For individuals with hypokalemia (low K^+ increases the risk of digitalis toxicity)
      6. Glucose: Hyperglycemia can occur with hypo/hyperkalemia.
   B. Radiology: Not indicated
   C. Other
      1. EKG: While not useful as a diagnostic tool, may be necessary to evaluate for impaired conduction or dysrhythmias; the greatest danger in hyperkalemia is cardiac toxicity.
         a) Hypokalemia: Flat or inverted T-wave, ST-T changes, prolonged QT interval, evidence of digitalis toxicity

       b) Hyperkalemia: Peaked T-waves, prolonged PR wave interval and widening of QRS complex, tachycardia, bradycardia, cardiac arrest

V. Differential diagnosis
  A. Hypokalemia
     1. Malnutrition
     2. Laxative abuse
     3. Hypomagnesemia (see Chapter 146)
     4. Renal failure or renal tubular acidosis (see Chapter 83)
     5. Primary or secondary hyperaldosteronism
     6. Metabolic alkalosis
     7. Paraneoplastic syndrome (e.g., ACTH-producing bronchogenic tumor) (see Appendix 12)
     8. Gastrointestinal loss (e.g., diarrhea, vomiting, fistula, nasogastric suctioning) (see Chapters 53 and 59)
     9. Anabolic state (e.g., rapidly proliferating tumor, secondary to granulocyte stimulating factor administration)
     10. Pseudohyperkalemia
     11. Iatrogenic/medication-induced
  B. Hyperkalemia
     1. Iatrogenic/medication-induced
     2. Renal failure (see Chapter 83)
     3. Dehydration (see Chapter 147)
     4. Metabolic acidosis
     5. Diabetes/insulin deficiency (see Chapter 143)
     6. Primary (e.g., Addison's disease) or secondary (e.g., adrenal metastases [see Chapter 89], angiotensin-converting enzyme [ACE] inhibitors) hypoaldosteronism
     7. Laboratory/sampling error

VI. Treatment: The goal of treatment is to restore potassium balance, evidenced by serum K^+ of 3.5–5.5 mEq/l.
  A. Hypokalemia
     1. Treat the underlying cause (e.g., alkalosis, bronchogenic carcinoma, leukemia, hyperaldosteronism).
     2. Dietary replacement is sometimes preferred for mildly depressed/asymptomatic serum potassium levels (3–3.5 mEq/l).
        a) Not always possible if patient is anorexic, nauseous, or simply unable to consume an adequate amount of potassium-rich foods.
        b) Encourage patients to eat foods rich in potassium (e.g., fresh or dried fruits, fruit juice, vegetables, meats, nuts).
     3. Adjust medications as needed (i.e., change loop diuretic to a potassium-sparing diuretic, such as spironolactone, triamterene, or amiloride).
     4. For moderate hypokalemia (3 mEq/l), especially in patients at risk for cardiac dysrhythmias, oral supplements are recommended (refer to Table 145-1).

Table 145-1. Examples of Oral Potassium Supplements

Tablets	mEq/tablet	Liquids	mEq/ml	Powders	mEq/pack
Kaon-CL®ᵃ	6.7 mEq	Kaochlor®ʰ, Kay Ciel®ⁱ, Klorvess®ⁱ, Kaon®ʰ	20 mEq	K-Lor®ˡ	15 mEq
Klor-Con®ᵇ, Micro-K®ᶜ, Slow-K®ᵈ	8 mEq			Kay Ciel®ⁱ, K-Lor®ᶠ, Klor-Con®ᵇ, Klorvess®ⁱ	20 mEq
Kaon-CL®ᵃ, Klotrix®ᵉ, K-Tab®ᶠ, K-Dur®ᵍ, Micro-K®ᶜ	10 mEq	Kaon-CL®ᵃ	40 mEq		
				K-Lyte-CL®ᵉ, Klor-Con®ᵇ	25 mEq
K-Dur®ᵍ	20 mEq				

ᵃErbamont Inc., Columbus, OH; ᵇUpsher-Smith Laboratories, Inc., Minneapolis, MN; ᶜA.H. Robins Company Incorporated, Richmond, VA; ᵈCiba-Geigy Corporation, New York, NY; ᵉMead Johnson & Company, Evansville, IN; ᶠAbbott Laboratories, North Chicago, IL; ᵍKey Pharmaceuticals Inc., Kenilworth, NJ; ʰWarren-Teed Pharmaceuticals, Inc., Columbus, OH; ⁱCooper Laboratories, Inc., Bedford Hills, NY; ʲSandoz-Wander, Inc., Hanover, NJ

a) Potassium chloride (KCl) is the preferred form because it separates easily and enhances the reabsorption of K^+ and Cl^- in exchange for Na^+ and HCO_3. This enables a more rapid correction of hypokalemia. It is also beneficial in correcting metabolic alkalosis.

b) For correction of deficiency: Average dose of KCl is 20–40 mEq bid to qid, depending on the severity of hypokalemia.

c) For prophylaxis: Average dose is 16–24 mEq daily.

d) KCl also comes in a slow-release form (e.g., Slow-K®, Ciba-Geigy Corporation, New York, NY), which contains 8 mEq of potassium; usually administered in dosages of 2–4 tablets/day.

e) Potassium bicarbonate contains 25 mEq/tablet and is usually given in doses of one tablet bid or tid (e.g., K-Lyte®, Mead Johnson & Company, Evansville, IN).

f) Potassium bicarbonate or potassium citrate are more-appropriate choices for patients with metabolic acidosis, as they tend to alkalinize. KCl is more appropriate for patients on thiazide diuretics because they lose chloride.

g) Potassium supplements can irritate the GI tract and should be administered with or close to meals.

   (1) The slow-release preparations are to be taken with a full glass of water.

   (2) These supplements can cause a bitter aftertaste, indigestion, and nausea, interfering with patient compliance.

   (3) Instruct the patient regarding potential side effects and properly taking supplements.

   (4) Find the supplement that the patient prefers and best tolerates to enhance compliance.

5. IV replacement is indicated when (see Table 145-2)

   a. Patients are unable to take oral supplements (i.e., patients with severe nausea/vomiting, GI upset)

Table 145-2. General Guidelines for IV Serum Potassium (K⁺) Replacement

Serum Potassium (K⁺) Level	Dose	Considerations
> 2.5 mEq/l	20–40 mEq/l at 125 cc/hour	May be administered in smaller volumes (e.g., 50–100 cc). Normally, rate exceeding 10 mEq/hour is not required unless EKG changes are present.
< 2.5 mEq/l (severe)	40–60 mEq/l	Dose should not exceed 40 mEq/hour.

Note. For life-threatening dysrhythmia or paralysis, patients must be admitted for cardiac monitoring; patients may need more concentrated doses of K⁺ (e.g., 40–100 mEq/hour), which requires close physician collaboration.

      b. Severe hypokalemia (< 2.5 mEq/l) exists
      c. Cardiac dysrhythmia occurs
      d. Severe myopathy exists.
    6. Potassium is very irritating to the veins.
      a. It must be diluted (preferably < 40 mEq/l) and administered slowly (usual rate of 10 mEq/hour in adults).
      b. Concentrations > 40 mEq/l must be administered through a central line.
    7. Never give potassium IV push.
    8. Normal saline is recommended diluent with KCl, because dextrose may initially worsen hypokalemia (i.e., dextrose stimulates insulin production, which causes K⁺ to shift intracellularly).
  B. Hyperkalemia
    1. Treat underlying cause (e.g., acidosis, adrenocortical insufficiency).
    2. Verify that K⁺ is truly elevated (e.g., repeat serum K⁺, measure plasma K⁺; avoid treating pseudohyperkalemia).
    3. Review and adjust medications as needed (e.g., discontinue potassium supplements, salt substitutes, ACE inhibitors, NSAIDs, potassium-sparing diuretics).
    4. Loop diuretics (e.g., furosemide) will increase K⁺ excretion.
    5. Mild to moderate hyperkalemia (5.5–6 mEq/l) may only require dietary restrictions or medication adjustment if patient's condition is stable (if symptomatic, refer to Table 145-3).

VII. Follow-up: Depends on the severity of the imbalance, the aggressiveness of the intervention, and the patient's overall condition. Following are general guidelines.
  A. Hypokalemia
    1. Oral replacement: Adequate renal function is necessary because kidneys maintain normal potassium balance. In situations where inadequate renal function exists, there is a risk of developing an iatrogenic hyperkalemia with potassium supplementation.
      a) Patient should respond within 72 hours. If serum K⁺ does not respond notably within 72–96 hours, suspect hypomagnesemia and obtain/recheck a serum Mg⁺⁺ level.
      b) When serum potassium level stabilizes, monitor K⁺ weekly for one to three weeks. If stable, follow-up may be extended to every one to three months, depending on patient's overall condition.

Table 145-3. Guidelines for Treatment of Hyperkalemia

Serum Potassium (K⁺) Level	Drug	Dose	Considerations
5.5–6	Furosemide	40–160 mg IV or po daily	
5.5–6.5	Sodium polystyrene sulfonate (Kayexalate®ᵃ)	Oral: Usually 15 g 1–4 times/day	Combined with 20% sorbitol (50–100 cc) to prevent constipation.
		Rectal: 30–50 g every six hours (contraindicated in diarrhea)	With 20% sorbitol as retention enema (retain 30 minutes minimum).
			When K⁺ normalizes, maintenance dose of 15 g/day may be needed.ᶜ
			Monitor Ca⁺⁺ and Mg⁺⁺ because they are removed with sodium polystyrene.ᶜ
6.5–7mEq/l (severe, life-threatening)	Sodium bicarbonate	1–2 ampules (44–88 mEq) IV over 2–5 minutes	These are all *temporary* measures with a duration of only 1–2 hours. These measures do not clear K⁺ from the body but rather promote shift of K⁺ into cells.
	Calcium gluconate	10 ml of 10% solution IV over 5–10 minutes	
	Regular insulin	5–10 units with 50% glucose (or 1 unit per 3–5 g dextrose) (not recommended in diabetics)	
	Nebulizer (Albuterol®ᵇ)	10–20 mg in 4 ml of normal saline nebulized over 10 minutes	

ᵃ Sterling Drug, Inc., New York, NY; ᵇ Dura Pharmaceuticals, Inc., San Diego, CA
ᶜ Hemodialysis is a very rapid and effective way to lower potassium; may be the most effective choice in life-threatening situations.

    2. IV replacement
        a) In severe hypokalemia, initially monitor serum K⁺ every three to six hours.
        b) For moderate hypokalemia, daily monitoring of serum K⁺ may be adequate.
        c) When patient's condition improves and potassium level stabilizes, reduce frequency.
        d) Convert to oral replacement when feasible, and follow guidelines above.
  B. Hyperkalemia
    1. For mild to moderate asymptomatic hyperkalemia, consider overall status. If patient is stable, has good renal function, is followed as an outpatient, and acute changes are unlikely, or if management is accomplished through diet or adjustment of medications, checking serum K⁺ weekly for one to three weeks is reasonable.

2. If potassium is stable or improved, extend follow-up to every one to three weeks.
3. In patients with severe hyperkalemia, and/or when sodium polystyrene is used, monitor K^+ levels every three to six hours until stabilized.
4. As condition improves, gradually extend frequency.

VIII. Referrals
   A. Hospital/critical-care unit physician: In cases of severe potassium imbalance ($K^+ < 2.5$ or > 6.5–7 mEq), the emergent situation requires admission to a hospital/critical care unit for cardiac monitoring and more aggressive interventions (e.g., dialysis).
   B. Consider complexity of cause of imbalance: Some causes (e.g., diet, dehydration, medication) may be relatively simple to correct. However, in individuals with complex medical problems (e.g., unstable diabetes mellitus, bronchogenic carcinoma with adrenal metastasis, acid-base imbalance, AIDS), consultation and close collaboration with a physician is needed. Referral to a specialist (e.g., endocrinologist, nephrologist) also may be indicated.

References

See pages 888-889.

146. Hypomagnesemia/ Hypermagnesemia

Wendy J. Smith, RN, MSN, ACNP, AOCN®

I. Definition
   A. Normal serum magnesium (Mg^{++}) is 1.5–2.5 mEq/l.
   B. Hypomagnesemia exists when the serum level is < 1.5 mEq/l.
   C. Hypermagnesemia exists when the serum level is > 2.5 mEq/l.

II. Physiology/Pathophysiology
   A. Normal physiology
      1. Approximately 45%–49% of the body's Mg^{++} is intracellular.
         a) It is the second major intracellular cation and is important in many enzymatic interactions.
         b) Approximately 50% is stored within the bone.
         c) The remaining 1%–5% is in the extracellular fluid.
         d) One-third of the extracellular magnesium is protein-bound; the remaining 2/3 is ionized (i.e., free).
      2. Like calcium and potassium, Mg^{++} is very important in transmission of nerve impulses and normal neuromuscular activity, as well as in normal cardiac contraction.
      3. Magnesium is absorbed via the small intestine.
         a) A little more than half of the nonabsorbed magnesium is excreted in the feces.
         b) Kidneys excrete approximately 40%.
      4. Magnesium homeostasis is influenced by parathyroid hormone (PTH), adrenocortical hormones, and vitamin D.
      5. The daily requirement is at least 200–300 mg.
      6. Magnesium imbalances rarely occur as an isolated electrolyte imbalance; usually accompanied by imbalances in potassium, calcium, and phosphate.
   B. Hypomagnesemia pathophysiology
      1. If serum potassium (K^+) or phosphorus (PO_4) is depleted, Mg^{++} loss will follow.
      2. Hypomagnesemia causes the release of PTH, as does hypocalcemia. A decrease in Mg^{++} interferes with the peripheral action of PTH on bone, resulting in hypocalcemia
      3. Aldosterone excess causes renal loss of Mg^{++}.
   C. Hypermagnesemia
      1. Inhibits the secretion of PTH
      2. Deficiency of adrenal cortical hormone will result in increased Mg^{++}.

III. Clinical features: The most common cause of hypermagnesemia is end-stage renal disease.
A. Etiology
1. Hypomagnesemia
    a) Primary nutritional deficiencies (i.e., chronic alcoholism)
    b) Drug-induced conditions (i.e., from platinum compounds, aminoglycosides, amphotericin B, diuretics, theophylline, colony-stimulating factors)
    c) Decreased gastrointestinal absorption
        (1) Malnutrition
        (2) Malabsorption
        (3) Diarrhea
    d) Endocrine disorders also may cause hypomagnesemia in relation to other resultant electrolyte imbalances or as a result of the effect on renal function.
        (1) Hyperparathyroidism
        (2) Hypo/hyperthyroidism
        (3) Diabetic ketoacidosis
        (4) Syndrome of inappropriate antidiuretic hormone
2. Hypermagnesemia: Adrenal insufficiency is another possible cause (e.g., hypo-aldosterone decreases excretion).
    a) Addison's disease
    b) End-stage renal disease
B. History
1. History of cancer and cancer treatment
2. Current medications: Prescribed and over-the-counter
3. History of presenting symptom(s): Precipitating factors, location, and duration
4. Changes in activities of daily living
5. Past medical history: Hypoparathyroidism, hypocalcemia, hypokalemia, kidney disease or failure, chronic diarrhea
C. Signs and symptoms
1. Hypomagnesemia: May take several weeks for symptoms to develop
    a) Similar to signs and symptoms of hypocalcemia (e.g., tetany-like symptoms)
    b) Anorexia
    c) Nausea/vomiting
    d) Lethargy
    e) Mental confusion
    f) Paresthesia
2. Hypermagnesemia: Symptomatic hypermagnesemia is rare.
    a) Muscle weakness
    b) Nausea
    c) Vomiting
    d) Diaphoresis
    e) Flaccid paralysis (may develop respiratory paralysis)
    f) CNS depression (e.g., drowsiness, confusion)
D. Physical exam
1. Hypomagnesemia
    a) Assess mental status: Confusion

        b) Vital signs: Hypertension

        c) Cardiac exam: Rate and rhythm; dysrhythmia (e.g., premature ventricular contractions)

        d) Musculoskeletal exam: Assess for hyperactive deep tendon reflexes.

        e) Special tests (see Appendix 13)

            (1) Observe for evidence of tetany.

            (2) Check for positive Chvostek's or Trousseau's signs.

  2. Hypermagnesemia

        a) Assess mental status: Drowsiness

        b) Vital signs: Hypotension

        c) Musculoskeletal exam

            (1) Evaluate for decreased muscle strength.

            (2) Assess for decreased loss in deep tendon reflexes.

IV. Diagnostic tests

  A. Laboratory

    1. Serum magnesium: < 1.5 or > 2.5 mEq/l

    2. Electrolytes: K^+ may be decreased

    3. Serum calcium: May be decreased

    4. BUN and creatinine: Increase may indicate renal insufficiency/failure.

    5. Urine magnesium in hypomagnesemia may help to determine if deficiency is from renal losses.

    6. Digoxin level may be indicated for patients who are taking digoxin, as hypomagnesemia increases the risk of digoxin toxicity.

  B. Radiology: Not indicated

  C. Other: EKG may be indicated to assess cardiac dysrhythmias (e.g., premature ventricular contractions, ventricular tachycardia; flat or inverted T-waves, depressed ST segment).

V. Differential diagnosis

  A. Hypomagnesemia

    1. Malabsorption

    2. Malnutrition

    3. Hyperparathyroidism

    4. Iatrogenic/medications

        a) Parenteral alimentation

        b) Loop or osmotic diuretics

        c) Cisplatin

        d) Amphotericin B

        e) Aminoglycosides

    5. Hypocalcemia (see Chapter 144)

    6. Hypokalemia (see Chapter 145)

    7. Hyperthyroidism (see Chapter 149)

    8. Hyperaldosteronism

  B. Hypermagnesemia

    1. Renal insufficiency/failure (see Chapter 83)

2. Excess intake (e.g., magnesium-containing antacids/laxatives)
3. Diabetic ketoacidosis (severe dehydration)
4. Adrenal insufficiency

VI. Treatment: To restore normal serum magnesium
  A. Hypomagnesemia
    1. Treat underlying cause.
    2. Replacement of magnesium in patients with renal failure must be done with extreme caution to avoid hypermagnesemia.
    3. For mild or chronic hypomagnesemia, oral replacement is preferred.
        a) Magnesium oxide (e.g., Mag-Ox or Uro-Mag, Blaine Company, Erlanger, NY) in doses of 250–500 mg (12.55–25 mEq) may be administered 2–4 times a day.
        b) Diarrhea is the major side effect of magnesium supplements.
        c) In patients with normal renal function, little chance of overcorrecting and causing hypermagnesemia exists because the kidneys normally excrete Mg^{++} without difficulty.
    4. Severe/symptomatic hypomagnesemia may be corrected using IV magnesium sulfate.
        a) Initially, 1–2 g of magnesium sulfate in 100 cc normal saline infused IV over one hour.
        b) After this initial bolus, a continuous infusion is recommended at a rate of 240–1,200 mg/day during the critical period (until symptoms resolve).
        c) It is recommended that IV magnesium replacement be continued over several days to replace intracellular magnesium.
            (1) 1 mEq/kg of magnesium sulfate 10% solution IV can be given with half of this amount in the first three hours
            (2) The remaining half should be administered over the last 21 hours.
        d) Mg^{++} content in this maintenance infusion may be reduced to 120 mg/day.
        e) Adjust the rate of the infusion to maintain serum Mg^{++} below 2.5 mEq/l.
  B. Hypermagnesemia
    1. Correct underlying cause (e.g., renal insufficiency/failure).
    2. Prevent hypermagnesemia in patients with renal failure by reducing dietary intake and avoiding magnesium-containing antacids/laxatives.
    3. Dialysis may be necessary, as renal function is almost always impaired in patients with hypermagnesemia.
    4. In the absence of renal failure, 0.45% normal saline infused at 150–200 ml/hr and furosemide 20–80 mg daily in divided doses may enhance renal excretion; consider patient's overall cardiovascular status in determining appropriate fluid volume, rate, and dose of furosemide.
    5. Calcium is an antagonist to magnesium.
        a) Temporary/immediate treatment in severe/symptomatic hypermagnesemia: 10–20 ml of 10% calcium gluconate (100–200 mg of elemental calcium) may be given IV over 10 minutes.
        b) For less-severe deficiencies or for maintenance: 20 ml of 10% calcium gluconate in one liter of normal saline, infused at 150–200 ml/hour (for patients with normal renal function).
        c) Collaboration with physician is needed in this situation.

VII. Follow-up
 A. In severe/symptomatic hypo/hypermagnesemia, follow serum magnesium at least daily. Patient's overall condition and other medical problems must be considered in determining the frequency of laboratory studies.
 B. In mild to moderate imbalances, serum magnesium may be followed less frequently. In stable patients, Mg^{++} may initially be monitored weekly as body stores are replenished.
 C. If hypomagnesemia is chronic, follow-up may be extended to every one to three months based on stability of serum Mg^{++}; replacement dose, based on individual patient's condition.
 D. Patients on renal dialysis will probably need close monitoring of electrolytes and Mg^{++}; frequency usually is coordinated with dialysis unit and nephrologist.

VIII. Referrals
 A. Dietician: Consultation may be of benefit for patients who need to restrict dietary intake.
 B. Nephrologist: Indicated for patients with renal failure and treatment of severe/symptomatic hypo/hypermagnesemia.
 C. Endocrinologist: For consultation with patients with an underlying endocrine disorder.

References

See pages 888-889.

147.

Hyponatremia/Hypernatremia

Wendy Smith, RN, MSN, ACNP, AOCN®,
and Susan Baird-Powell, RN, MSN, CRNP

I. Definition
   A. Normal serum sodium (Na) level ranges from 135–146 mEq/l.
   B. Hyponatremia exists when the serum sodium level is < 130 mEq/l.
   C. Hypernatremia exists when the serum sodium level is > 146 mEq/l.

II. Physiology/Pathophysiology
   A. Normal physiology
      1. Sodium is the primary extracellular cation with the principle role in maintaining serum osmolality and maintenance of the balance in body fluids.
      2. Functions of sodium
         a) Neuromuscular activity: On the cellular level, the sodium-pump controls influx and efflux of sodium and potassium, thereby aiding in depolarization and repolarization during transmission/conduction of nerve impulses.
         b) Maintains acid-base balance, as it readily links with transport of bicarbonate or chloride.
      3. Water balance is regulated by vasopressin (i.e., antidiuretic hormone [ADH]).
         a) Release of ADH, in response to a decrease in blood volume or an increase in serum osmolality, results in an increase in the permeability of cells lining the renal tubules.
         b) This leads to increased reabsorption of water, restoration of blood volume, increased concentration of urine, and normalization of osmolality.
      4. Aldosterone is a mineralocorticoid produced by the adrenal cortex.
         a) When blood volume is low, the juxtaglomerular cells of the kidney release renin.
         b) Renin spurs the synthesis of angiotensin I, which is then converted to angiotensin II. Angiotensin II in turn stimulates the secretion of aldosterone, which then promotes the reabsorption of sodium and water.
   B. Hyponatremia pathophysiology: Occurs in a three-step process
      1. Osmotic pressure decreases in the extracellular fluid.
      2. Osmotic pressure is higher inside the cells, so water moves into the cell cytoplasm.
      3. This results in a decrease in overall plasma volume, and the patient may exhibit signs and symptoms of hypovolemia.
   C. Hypernatremia pathophysiology

1. Most prominent cause of hypernatremia is free water deficit, which leads to hypovolemia and increased plasma osmolarity (i.e., water loss > than Na^+).
2. A hyperosmolar state draws fluid from the intracellular to the extracellular compartment.

III. Clinical features
  A. Etiologies
    1. Hyponatremia etiologies
      a) Hypovolemic: Loss of water in excess of sodium or loss of sodium and water with water replacement (intake)
        (1) Vomiting
        (2) Diarrhea
        (3) Burns
        (4) GI suctioning
        (5) Addison's disease (hypoaldosteronism or adrenal insufficiency)
        (6) Diuretics
        (7) Osmotic diuresis
      b) Hypervolemic: Increase in total body water exceeds increase of sodium
        (1) Severe CHF
        (2) Cirrhosis
        (3) Nephrotic syndrome
        (4) Administration of D_5W, resulting in rapidly metabolized dextrose
        (5) Renal failure (acute and chronic)
      c) Euvolemic: Excessive inappropriate vasopressin (AVP) secretion, impaired excretion of free water, or excessive water intake
        (1) SIADH
          (a) Pulmonary disease (e.g., pneumonia, tuberculosis)
          (b) CNS disorders (e.g., tumors, meningitis, stroke, trauma)
          (c) Stressful conditions
          (d) Drug-induced conditions
            i) Morphine
            ii) Tricyclic antidepressants
            iii) Cyclophosphamide, cicplatin, vincristine
            iv) Nicotine
            v) Sulfonylurea
            vi) Interleukin-2
        (2) Hypothyroidism
        (3) Cortisol deficiency
        (4) Water intoxication
      d) Pseudohyponatremia: Conditions reflect a measurement phenomena rather than an abnormality of the relative amounts of water and saline in the body.
        (1) Hyperlipidemia
        (2) Hyperglycemia
        (3) Hyperproteinemia
    2. Hypernatremia: High water loss in relation to sodium

       a) Diarrhea
       b) Profuse sweating
       c) Burns
       d) Respiratory infections
       e) Diabetes insipidus
       f) Diabetes mellitus
       g) Vomiting
       h) Medication-induced: Lithium, lactulose, hypertonic saline, sodium bicarbonate

B. History
   1. History of cancer and cancer treatment
   2. Current medications: Prescribed and over-the-counter
   3. History of presenting symptom(s): Precipitating factors, location, and duration. Associated symptoms are nausea, vomiting, and diarrhea.
   4. Changes in activities of daily living
   5. History of urine output and fluid intake
   6. Past medical history of headaches, use of tap water enemas

C. Signs and symptoms: Severity depends on acuity and extent of imbalance.
   1. Hyponatremia and hypernatremia
       a) Nausea
       b) Lethargy
       c) Confusion
       d) Vomiting
       e) Anorexia
       f) Tachycardia
       g) Dry skin/mucous membrane
       h) Convulsions
       i) Coma
   2. Hyponatremia
       a) Diarrhea
       b) Abdominal cramps
       c) Lethargy/weakness
       d) Generalized muscle weakness
       e) Headaches
       f) Confusion
       g) Evidence of fluid retention may be observed with dilutional hyponatremia (e.g., weight gain, edema).
       h) Salt craving (with hypovolemia, especially adrenal insuffiency)
       i) Postural dizziness
       j) Seizures
       k) Thirst
       l) Decreased urine output
   3. Hypernatremia
       a) Polyuria
       b) Restlessness
       c) Fever

        d) Muscle twitches/tremors/weakness

        e) Unsteady gait

        f) Flushed, dry skin

  D. Physical exam

    1. Observe behavior and evaluate mental status (i.e., confusion, lethargy versus restlessness).

    2. Vital signs

      a) Pulse: Weak, normal, or fast

      b) Blood pressure

        (1) Hyponatremia: Hypotension and orthostatic hypotension

        (2) Hypernatremia: Hypertension

      c) Temperature: Low-grade may occur with hypernatremia.

      d) Weight loss: May occur in hyponatremia

    3. HEENT exam: Dry mouth (hyponatremia)

    4. Integument exam: Edema or decreased skin turgor depends on etiology of hyponatremia.

    5. Cardiac exam

      a) Tachycardia (hyponatremia)

      b) Decreased neck veins or jugular vein distention, depending on etiology of hyponatremia

    6. Neurologic exam

      a) Assess muscle strength, and observe for twitching, tremors, and weakness (hyper/hyponatremia).

      b) Observe gait for ataxia (hypernatremia).

      c) Assess mental status for confusion and speech changes (hyponatremia).

      d) Assess for decreased deep tendon reflexes (hyponatremia); hyperactive reflexes (hypernatremia).

IV. Diagnostic tests

  A. Laboratory

    1. Serum electrolytes (Na^+, K^+, Cl^-, CO_2): Look for electrolyte imbalance; CO_2 an indicator of acid/base status).

    2. Serum glucose

      a) Hyperglycemia may cause pseudohyponatremia by shifting water from intracellular fluid to extracellular fluid (ECF), diluting Na^+.

      b) In diabetic ketoacidosis, Na^+ can be increased, decreased, or normal.

    3. BUN and creatinine: Increase in renal insufficiency and dehydration

    4. Serum osmolality (normal 280–295 mOsm/kg): A rough estimate of serum osmolality can be measured by doubling the serum sodium. To calculate serum osmolality, use the following formula: 2 x Serum sodium + BUN/3 + glucose/18 = serum osmolality

    5. Urine sodium

      a) Elevated in SIADH or in hypernatremia where there is a net sodium gain

      b) May be low in hypovolemia in the presence of normal renal function

      c) Low when there is extrarenal sodium loss, as in vomiting/diarrhea *d)* Elevated with renal loss of sodium, as in nephropathy

    6. Urine specific gravity: < 1.010 can indicate hyponatremia; > 1.025 can indicate hypernatremia.

    7. Thyroid-stimulating hormone: If clinical picture warrants (hypothyroidism associated with decreased Na^+)

    8. Arterial blood gases: Consider to better assess acid/base balance in patients who are critically ill.

    9. Adrenocorticotropic hormone (ACTH) stimulation test: If adrenal insufficiency is suspected

  B. Radiology: Not indicated

V. Differential diagnosis

  A. Hyponatremia

    1. Pseudohyponatremia (e.g., hyperproteinemia, hyperlipidemia)

    2. SIADH (see Chapter 94)

    3. Gastrointestinal loss: Nausea, vomiting, diarrhea, suctioning (see Chapters 53 and 59)

    4. Dilutional hyponatremia/increased extracellular volume (e.g., CHF, renal failure) (see Chapters 40 and 83)

        a) Water intoxication secondary to increased consumption of beer or water

        b) Hydration with D_5W

    5. Hypoaldosteronism (primary or secondary)

    6. Adrenal insufficiency

    7. Severe burns

    8. Hypothyroidism (see Chapter 150)

    9. Nephrotic syndrome

    10. Low Na^+ diet (usually gradual onset)

  B. Hypernatremia

    1. Dehydration (secondary to renal and nonrenal losses or inadequate fluid intake)

    2. Nephrogenic diabetes insipidus

    3. CNS malignancy/metastasis (CNS diabetes insipidus)

    4. Hyperaldosteronism (primary or secondary)

VI. Treatment: The goal of therapy is directed toward restoring Na^+ balance, as well as volume status.

  A. Hyponatremia: Sodium replacement must be done cautiously. If sodium is replaced too rapidly, acute and potentially severe neurologic complications may occur as a result of osmotic demyelination.

    1. Treat underlying condition (e.g., SIADH, hyperglycemia, hypothryoidism, hypoaldosteronism/adrenal insufficiency).

    2. Patients with hypotonic hyponatremia from excess extracellular fluid (ECF) are usually asymptomatic.

        a) Restrict water and sodium intake.

        b) Average daily requirement of sodium is 2–4 g; however, the average amount consumed is 8–15 g.

        c) A cautious restriction would be 1–3 g of sodium and 0.5–1.5 liters of water per day; degree of restriction depends on severity of hyponatremia and extent of ECF excess.

       d) Serum sodium will gradually increase over several days.

       e) Comfort measures for dry mouth include ice chips, sips of water, mouth care, lip moisturizer.

3. Patients with CHF may benefit more from loop diuretics and an angiotensin-converting enzyme (ACE) inhibitor.

       a) Diuretics are not a primary choice for treating dilutional hyponatremia and in some circumstances are contraindicated.

       b) In CHF (hypervolemic hyponatremia), the cardiac output is less effective, leading to decreased glomerular filtration rate (GFR).

       c) The combination of decreased GFR and low sodium are stimuli for the secretion of ADH and aldosterone, causing further retention of water and salt.

       d) This could further compromise renal blood flow, which, in turn, prohibits deliverance of sodium to the distal tubules for excretion, thereby causing a further rise in sodium.

4. When the sodium loss is out of proportion to water loss (e.g., vomiting, diarrhea), treatment involves restoring the extracellular volume. This is usually accomplished with isotonic saline (0.9%). The rate of replacement depends on the severity of symptoms.

       a) A reasonable, recommended rate of increasing serum sodium concentration is 0.5–1 mEq/l/hour until serum sodium reaches 120 mEq/l, then reduce rate to 0.5 mEq/l/hour.

       b) Incremental sodium increase over 24 hours should not exceed 12 mEq/l.

5. Severe/symptomatic (<120 mEq/l) hyponatremia may necessitate administration of hypertonic (3%) saline approximately 25 ml/hour for correction rate of <0.5 mEq/l/hour.

       a) Requires close monitoring of urinary and serum sodium; consider ICU monitoring.

       b) Furosemide is indicated to increase the net loss of free water.

B. Hypernatremia: Avoid rapid correction because the patient may develop neurologic complications from cerebral edema.

1. Correct underlying cause of water loss.

2. Replace fluids and electrolytes.

       a) Restore severely hypovolemic patients (i.e., with evidence of orthostatic hypotension or oliguria) to euvolemia with isotonic saline (0.9%) followed by 0.45% saline or D₅W.

       b) Rate of replacement depends on severity of volume depletion, as well as cardiac and renal status.

       c) Clinical parameters for adequate volume replacement are stabilization of blood pressure and heart rate and restoration of adequate urine output (<25 ml/hour indicates inadequate renal perfusion).

       d) The desired incremental decrease in serum sodium is 0.5 mEq/l/hour in asymptomatic patients or 1 mEq/l/hour in symptomatic patients.

       e) In patients with mild hypovolemia and hypernatremia, oral hydration to replace free water is preferred. Otherwise, use 0.45% saline followed by D₅W.

       f) Encourage euvolemic patients with hypernatremia to drink water, or give D₅W IV to help enhance excretion of excess sodium.

g) Hypernatremia associated with hypervolemia may require loop diuretics to promote excretion of excess sodium. If renal failure exists, dialysis may be indicated.

VII. Follow-up: Hyponatremia and hypernatremia
   A. Follow-up varies depending on severity of imbalance and patient's overall medical condition.
   B. For severe/symptomatic hypo/hypernatremia, monitor serum sodium, serum osmolality, urine sodium, and specific gravity or urine osmolality every four hours until stable.
   C. Stable/asymptomatic imbalances may be monitored less frequently (i.e., daily or every other day until cause is corrected or stable safe level is maintained for inpatients; weekly or monthly for stable outpatients).

VIII. Referrals: Hyponatremia and hypernatremia
   A. Physician: For treatment of severe/symptomatic imbalances, collaborate with the physician.
   B. Endocrinologist: Referral to or consultation with an endocrinologist may be necessary for sodium imbalances that result from hypo/hyperaldosteronism or hypo/hyperadrenalism.
   C. Nephrologist: Referral to or consultation with a nephrologist is recommended for patients with renal failure or nephrotic syndrome or for patients in need of dialysis.

References

See pages 888-889.

Chapter

148. Hypophosphatemia/ Hyperphosphatemia

Wendy J. Smith, RN, MSN, ACNP, AOCN®

I. Definition

  A. Normal serum phosphorous (PO_4) ranges from 2.5–4.5 mg/dl (1.7–2.6 mEq/l).

  B. Hypophosphatemia exists when the serum phosphorous is < 2.5 mg/dl.

  C. Hyperphosphatemia exists when the serum phosphorous is > 4.5 mg/dl.

II. Physiology/Pathophysiology

  A. Normal physiology

    1. PO_4 is the major intracellular anion.

    2. Approximately 80%–85% of PO_4 is found in the bones and teeth. The remaining 15%–20% is in the intracellular fluids.

    3. Functions of PO_4

      a) Vital part of an enzyme, 2,3-diphosphoglycerate (2,3-DPG), which facilitates the release of oxygen from hemoglobin within the RBCs.

      b) Involved in maintaining normal neuromuscular activity.

      c) Involved in metabolism of proteins, fats, and carbohydrates and in maintaining acid-base balance.

    4. Calcium and phosphorus have an inverse relationship (i.e., when one goes up the other goes down, as in hyperparathyroidism, when calcium increases, phosphorus decreases).

    5. Two hormones that influence phosphorus balance are parathyroid hormone (PTH) and the active form of vitamin D (calcitriol).

      a) PTH increases the excretion of phosphorus by the renal tubules.

      b) PTH stimulates the formation of calcitriol, which, in turn, enhances absorption of phosphorus from the GI tract.

    6. About 90% of phosphorus is excreted by the kidneys; the remaining is excreted via the GI tract.

  B. Hypophosphatemia pathophysiology

    1. Phosphorous is efficiently/readily absorbed from the GI tract. Therefore, anything that might affect the intake or absorption of PO_4 could lead to a deficiency.

    2. Alkalosis causes an intracellular shift of PO_4, decreasing serum levels.

  C. Hyperphosphatemia pathophysiology

    1. Cell destruction following chemotherapy can lead to release of substantial amounts of phosphate, potassium, uric acid, and other intracellular products into the blood.

Because of the high amounts of these substances, the kidneys' ability to clear these intracellular constituents can be compromised, leading to hyperphosphatemia, hyperkalemia, hyperuricemia, and hypocalcemia (tumor lysis syndrome).

2. In conditions such as hypoparathyroidism, a decrease in PTH causes a decrease in osteoclastic activity within the bone resulting in decreased Ca^{++} in the blood and increased absorption of PO_4 and bicarbonate in the renal tubules.

III. Clinical features
  A. History
    1. History of cancer and cancer treatment
    2. Current medications: Prescribed and over-the-counter
    3. History of presenting symptom(s): Precipitating factors, location, and duration
    4. Changes in activities of daily living
    5. Hypophosphatemia
       a) Social history of alcohol intake
       b) Past medical history: Hypercalcemia, hyperparathyroidism, poorly controlled diabetes mellitus, kidney failure
    6. Hyperphosphatemia: History of hypoparathyroidism, kidney failure
  B. Signs and symptoms
    1. Hypophosphatemia
       a) Confusion
       b) Irritability
       c) Seizures
       d) Muscle weakness
       e) Paresthesia
       f) Tremors
       g) Anorexia
       h) Bone or muscle pain
    2. Hyperphosphatemia
       a) Tachycardia
       b) Nausea
       c) Diarrhea
  C. Physical exam
    1. Hypophosphatemia
       a) Vital signs (e.g., decreased heart rate with hypophosphatemia, increased blood pressure with hypophosphatemia with CHF)
       b) Assess for change in mental status (e.g., confusion).
       c) Integument exam
          (1) Observe for signs of tissue hypoxia (e.g., cyanosis).
          (2) Observe for evidence of platelet dysfunction (e.g., petechial hemorrhages).
       d) Cardiac and pulmonary exam: Assess for signs of CHF, crackles, edema, jugular vein distention.
       e) Musculoskeletal exam
          (1) Test reflexes (decreased in hypophosphatemia).

        (2) Assess muscle strength (decreased in hypophosphatemia; may have difficulty speaking or with hand grasp).

    2. Hyperphosphatemia

      a) Vital signs: Tachycardia

      b) Assess mental status.

      c) Musculoskeletal exam

        (1) Test reflexes: Hyperreactivity

        (2) Evaluate muscle strength: Assess for spasms/contractions.

      d) Special tests (see Appendix 13)

        (1) Positive Chvostek's sign: Tapping on the facial nerve just below the temple in front of the ear will elicit twitching or contractions of the facial muscle.

        (2) Positive Trousseau's sign: Applying a blood pressure cuff to occlude the brachial artery for three to five minutes elicits contraction of the hand and fingers.

IV. Diagnostic tests

  A. Hypophosphatemia: Laboratory

    1. CBC: If anemia is present (especially with phosphate < 1 mg/dl), look for evidence of hemolytic process

      a) LDH—elevated

      b) Bilirubin—elevated

      c) Haptoglobin—decreased

      d) Peripheral smear—presence of schisocytes

    2. Serum PO_4: Decreased

    3. Alkaline phosphatase: Increase may indicate increased osteoblastic activity.

    4. Arterial blood gases (ABGs) may be helpful, as alkalosis (especially respiratory) moves PO_4 into cells, which leads to decreased serum PO_4.

    5. PTH level: Increased in hyperparathyroidism.

    6. Serum calcium increased

    7. Serum magnesium: May be decreased because of increased renal excretion in hypophosphatemia

    8. Urine phosphorus: > 100 mg/day indicates renal loss. If less, consider decreased intake or malabsorption process.

    9. In severe deficiency (< 1 mg/dl), check urine for evidence of myoglobin (rhabdomyolysis can occur at this level).

  B. Hyperphosphatemia: Laboratory

    1. Serum PO_4 increased

    2. Serum calcium: Inverse relationship, usually decreased

    3. BUN and creatinine: Increase indicates renal insufficiency (decreased PO_4 excretion).

    4. If potassium and phosphate are elevated and calcium is decreased, suspect tumor lysis syndrome. Uric acid level is usually increased.

    5. ABGs may be helpful, as acidosis (especially respiratory) may cause PO_4 shift out of cells, which leads to increased serum PO_4.

    6. Serum calcium decreased

  C. Radiology: Not indicated

V. Differential diagnosis
  A. Hypophosphatemia
      1. Malnutrition
      2. Malabsorption
      3. Hyperparathyroidism
      4. Hypercalcemia (see Chapter 144)
      5. Hypomagnesemia (see Chapter 146)
      6. Alkalosis
      7. Vitamin D deficiency
      8. Inadequate PO_4 replacement in total parenteral nutrition
      9. Poorly controlled diabetes mellitus (see Chapter 143)
     10. Iatrogenic (e.g., diuretics, phosphate-binding antacids)
  B. Hyperphosphatemia
      1. Renal insufficiency/failure: Most common cause (see Chapter 83)
      2. Iatrogenic (e.g., oral phosphate supplements, phosphate laxatives)
      3. Hypoparathyroidism
      4. Tumor lysis syndrome
      5. Rhabdomyolysis: Acute breakdown of skeletal muscle

VI. Treatment: To restore normal phosphorus levels
  A. Hypophosphatemia
      1. Treating the underlying cause is usually the only intervention needed for moderate/
          asymptomatic hypophosphatemia (1.0–2.5 mg/dl).
      2. If moderate hypophosphatemia persists, oral supplementation is needed. A recom-
          mended dose is 0.5–1 g of elemental phosphorus/day in divided doses.
          a) Oral supplements may contain sodium and/or potassium, as well.
              (1) Neutra-Phos® (Willen Drug Company, Baltimore, MD): 250 mg elemental
                   phosphorus, 7 mEq sodium, 7 mEq potassium/capsule
              (2) Neutra-Phos K®: 250 mg elemental phosphorus, 14 mEq potassium/
                   capsule
              (3) Fleet Phospho-Soda® (C.B. Fleet Company, Inc., Lynchburg, VA): 815 mg
                   phosphorus, 33 mEq sodium/5 ml
          b) Diarrhea is the most common side effect of oral replacement.
      3. Precautions with phosphate replacement therapy (these are of greater concern with
          IV replacement)
          a) If replacement is too rapid, calcium-phosphate precipitates can form within the
              soft tissues, especially if hyperphosphatemia develops from overcorrection.
          b) Serum calcium and creatinine should be monitored, as hypocalcemia and/or renal
              failure can also occur with overcorrection.
      4. Patients receiving parenteral alimentation require phosphorus replacement. The
          average daily requirement varies from 620 mg–1,240 mg (see Chapter 158).
      5. Contraindications of administering phosphate salts
          a) Diabetic ketoacidosis: One exception might be pre-existing hypophosphatemia;
              however, the physician must decide how to treat hypophosphatemia in this
              situation.

           b) Renal failure/insufficiency

           c) Hypoparathyroidism

           d) Hypercalcemia: Correct hypercalcemia to normalize phosphorus.

      6. Severe/symptomatic hypophosphatemia (< 1 mg/dl): May necessitate IV replacement

           a) Patients often have complex electrolyte imbalances (e.g., hypomagnesemia/ hypokalemia).

           b) Serious problems can result from overcorrection and the development of hyperphosphatemia; close physician collaboration is required.

           c) IV replacement may be accomplished with 0.08–0.16 mmol/kg in 500 cc of 0.45% saline over 4–12 hours.

  B. Hyperphosphatemia

      1. Treat underlying cause (e.g., tumor lysis syndrome).

      2. Treat hypocalcemia if present (see Chapter 144).

      3. Restrict dietary phosphate

           a) Limit to 0.6–0.9 g/day.

           b) Food sources with high content of phosphorus include peanuts, dry beans, meat, fish, poultry, whole-grain cereals, and dairy products.

      4. Decrease absorption from the GI tract by administering oral phosphorus-binding antacids (e.g., Amphojel®, Wyeth-Ayerst Pharmaceuticals, Philadelphia, PA; Maalox®, Rhône-Poulenc Rorer Pharmaceuticals Inc., Collegeville, PA; Mylanta®, Johnson & Johnson-Merck Consumer Pharmaceutical Company, Fort Washington, PA) or calcium carbonate.

           a) Calcium carbonate is generally recommended to avoid the risk of aluminum toxicity, especially in patients with renal failure.

           b) The recommended dose is 0.5–1.5 g po tid with meals.

      5. In renal failure, dialysis may be required.

VII. Follow-up

  A. Hypophosphatemia

      1. When oral replacement is needed, daily monitoring of serum phosphorus, calcium, and creatinine are required until hypophosphatemia is corrected and dose is established.

      2. Frequency of monitoring thereafter depends on patient's overall condition and other health problems.

      3. Patients receiving phosphate in parenteral alimentation require daily monitoring of serum phosphorus and calcium initially. Decrease monitoring when the total parenteral formula and patient are stable.

      4. In severe/symptomatic hypophosphatemia, monitor serum phosphorus, calcium, and creatinine every six hours and adjust replacement interventions based on these labs and the patient's symptoms.

  B. Hyperphosphatemia

      1. When initiating calcium carbonate or phosphate-binders, monitor serum phosphorus and calcium daily until hyperphosphatemia is corrected and dose is established.

2. Frequency of monitoring thereafter depends on patient's overall condition and other health problems.
3. In patients with renal failure on dialysis, close monitoring of serum phosphorus and calcium is required. Frequency varies based on patient's overall condition and the physician's recommendations.

VIII. Referrals
   A. Physician: If cause cannot be determined and/or imbalance cannot be corrected in mild to moderate/asymptomatic hypophosphatemia or hyperphosphatemia
   B. Specialists: Referral/consultation may be needed to correct underlying causes (e.g., consult a nephrologist for renal failure, dialysis).
   C. Pharmacist/dietitian: If patients are receiving parenteral alimentation
   D. Dietitian: When dietary restrictions are necessary
   E. Close physician collaboration: For management of severe/symptomatic hypophosphatemia or hyperphosphatemia

References

Bari, Y.M., & Knochel, J.P. (1996). Hypercalcemia and electrolyte disturbances in malignancy. *Hematology/Oncology Clinics of North America, 10,* 775–790.

Berghmans, T. (1996). Hyponatremia related to medical anticancer treatment. *Supportive Cancer Care, 4,* 341–350.

Camp-Sorrell, D. (1998). Clinical focus: Hypercalcemia. *Clinical Journal of Oncology Nursing, 2,* 73–74.

Dagogo-Jack, S. (1998). Mineral and metabolic bone disease. In C.F. Carey, H.H. Lee, & K.F. Woeltje (Eds.), *The Washington manual: Manual of medical therapeutics* (29th ed.) (pp. 441–455). Philadelphia: Lippincott-Raven.

Dipiro, J.T., Talbert, R.L., Yee, G.Y., Matzke, G.R., Wells, B.G., & Posey, L.M. (1997). Pharmacotherapy: A pathophysiologic approach. Norwalk, CT: Appleton & Lange.

Edelson, G.W., & Kleeve-Koper, M. (1995). Hypercalcemic crisis. *Medical Clinics of North America, 79,* 79–92.

Holick, M.F., Krane, S.M., & Potts, J.T. (1998). Calcium, phosphorus, and bone metabolism: Calcium-regulating hormones. In A.S. Fauci, E. Braunwald, K.J. Isselbacher, J.D. Wilson, J.B. Martin, D.L. Kasper, S.L. Hauser, & D.L. Longo (Eds.), *Harrison's principles of internal medicine* (14th ed.) (pp. 2214–2227). New York: McGraw-Hill.

Hoffman, V. (1996). Tumor lysis syndrome: Implications for nursing. *Home Healthcare Nurse, 14,* 595–602.

Kaye, T. (1995). Hypercalcemia: How to pinpoint the cause and customize treatment. *Postgraduate Medicine, 97*(1), 153–160.

Mahon, S.M., & Casperson, D.S. (1993). Pathophysiology of hypokalemia in patients with cancer: Implications for nurses. *Oncology Nursing Forum, 20,* 937–946.

Mandal, A.K. (1997). Hypokalemia and hyperkalemia. *Medical Clinics of North America, 81,* 611–639.

Mundy, G.R., & Guise, T.A. (1997). Hypercalcemia of malignancy. *American Journal of Medicine, 103,* 134–145.

Okuda, T., Kurokawa, K., & Papdakis, M.A. (1998). Fluids and electrolyte disorders. In L.M. Tierney, S.J. McPhee, & M.A. Papdakis (Eds.), *Current medical diagnosis and treatment* (37th ed.). Stamford, CT: Appleton & Lange.

Ooi, S.B., Koh-Tai, B.C., Aw, T.C., Lau, T.C., & Chan, S.T. (1997). Assessment of dehydration in adults using hematologic biochemical tests. *Academia Emergency Medicine, 4,* 840–844.

Potts, J.T. (1998). Diseases of the parathyroid gland and other hyper- and hypocalcemic disorders. In A.S. Fauci, E. Braunwald, K.J. Isselbacher, J.D. Wilson, J.B. Martin, D.L. Kasper, S.L. Hauser, & D.L. Longo (Eds.), *Harrison's principles of internal medicine* (14th ed.) (pp. 2227–2247). New York: McGraw-Hill.

Rohaly-Davis, J., & Johnston, K. (1996). Hematologic emergencies in the intensive care unit. *Critical Care Quarterly, 18*(4), 35–43.

Rugo, H.S. (1998). Cancer. In L.M. Tierney, S.J. McPhee, & M.A. Papdakis (Eds.), *Current medical diagnosis and treatment* (37th ed.). Stamford, CT: Appleton & Lange.

Shapiro, J., & Richardson, G.E. (1995). Hyponatremia of malignancy. *Critical Reviews in Oncology/ Hematology, 18,* 129–135.

Singer, F.R., & Minoofar, P.N. (1995). Biphosphonates in the treatment of disorders of mineral metabolism. *Advances in Endocrinology Metabolism, 6,* 259–288.

Singer, G.G. (1998). Fluid and electrolyte management. In C.F. Carey, H.H. Lee, & K.F. Woeltje (Eds.), *The Washington manual: Manual of medical therapeutics* (29th ed.) (pp. 39–60). Philadelphia: Lippincott-Raven.

Singer, G.G., & Brenner, B.M. (1998). Fluid and electrolyte disturbances. In A.S. Fauci, E. Braunwald, K.J. Isselbacher, J.D. Wilson, J.B. Martin, D.L. Kasper, S.L. Hauser, & D.L. Longo (Eds.), *Harrison's principles of internal medicine* (14th ed.) (pp. 265–277). New York: McGraw-Hill.

Chapter

149.

Hyperthyroidism

Susan Baird-Powell, RN, MSN, CRNP

I. Definition
   A. Hyperthyroidism: An elevated concentration of thyroxine (T_4) or triiodothyronine (T_3) with or without symptoms of thyrotoxicosis
   B. Thyrotoxicosis: The clinical manifestations of hyperthyroidism
   C. Graves' disease: An autoimmune disease causing hyperthyroidism and frequently hypertrophy of the extraocular muscles with ophthalopathy

II. Pathophysiology
   A. An increase in the synthesis and release of T_4 and/or T_3 by the thyroid gland or ingestion of excessive amounts of exogenous thyroid hormone
   B. In Graves' disease, the usual regulatory pathways are disrupted by a mechanism that overstimulates the thyroid.
      1. Substances termed thyroid receptor antibodies (i.e., thyroid-stimulating immunoglobulin) adhere to the thyroid-stimulating hormone (TSH) receptors causing thyroid gland enlargement, increased vascularity, and increased amounts of thyroid hormone secretion.
      2. This newly formed hyperthyroid state causes suppression of TSH and thyrotropin-releasing hormone (TRH).
      3. A feedback loop between the thyroid and pituitary is lost. The increase in thyroid metabolism, iodine uptake, vascularity, and size are all caused by the TSH receptor antibodies.
      4. This continual overstimulation of the thyroid gland is evidenced by the rise in T_4 and T_3 levels. Occasionally T_3 will be elevated in isolation with normal T_4 levels.
      5. The increased levels of thyroid hormone circulating in the blood lead to many of the signs and symptoms of hyperthyroidism.
   C. Thyroid hormone stimulates calorigenesis and catabolism and enhances sensitivity to catecholamines.

III. Clinical features: Hyperthyroidism is common, with an estimated prevalence of 2.7% in the United States; most often occurs in women with Graves' disease, accounting for 85% of all cases. The prognosis for patients with hyperthyroidism is excellent if the correct treatment is implemented.

A. Etiologies
   1. Increased production of TSH by pituitary tumors (rare)
   2. Stimulation of thyroid TSH receptors by immunoglobulin: Graves' disease
   3. Autonomous thyroid production by thyroid nodules
   4. Increased release of thyroid hormone without increased production, typically occurring with thyroiditis
   5. Intake of exogenous hormone
B. History
   1. History of cancer and cancer treatment
   2. Current medications: Prescribed and over-the-counter
   3. History of presenting symptom(s): Precipitating factors, onset, and duration
   4. Changes in activities of daily living
   5. Past medical history of vision changes, neck swelling
   6. History of supplemental iodine intake
C. Signs and symptoms
   1. Nervousness
   2. Irritability
   3. Hyperactivity
   4. Fatigue
   5. Weight loss
   6. Palpitations
   7. Shortness of breath with exertion
   8. Excessive sweating
   9. Heat intolerance
   10. Increased appetite
   11. Frequent bowel movements (i.e., diarrhea)
   12. Weakness
   13. Tremor
   14. Menstrual changes (i.e., decreased flow)
   15. Insomnia
   16. Visual complaints
   17. Enlarging thyroid gland
   18. Lower extremity edema
   19. Depression
D. Physical exam: Hyperthyroidism may present with clinical disease but can present with subclinical disease.
   1. General appearance: Observe for nervousness, hyperactivity.
   2. Vital signs
      a) Blood pressure: Assess for systolic hypertension.
      b) Resting pulse: Note rate and regularity; assess for tachycardia.
      c) Temperature: Assess for signs of fever, indicating thyroid storm.
      d) Weight: Assess for recent weight loss.
   3. HEENT exam
      a) Hair: Assess for fine, silky, and/or thinning hair, indicating thyrotoxicosis.
      b) Eyes: Assess for exophthalmos, lid lag, lid retraction, extraoccular movements for stare, indicating thyrotoxicosis.

       c) Thyroid: Note enlargement, firmness, nodules, tenderness, indicating thyrotoxi-
          cosis. Graves' disease: Note nontender thyroid; may have bruits of the thyroid
          gland.

    4. Integument exam: Note if warm, moist, smooth; may have hyperpigmentation and
       dermopathy, indicating thyrotoxicosis.

    5. Cardiac exam: For angina, sinus tachycardia, paroxysmal supraventricular tachycar-
       dia, atrial fibrillation, systolic murmurs; congestive heart failure may be present
       during thyrotoxicosis.

    6. Lymph exam: Lymphadenopathy may be present, indicating an inflammatory
       response to increased thyroxine release (very unusual).

    7. Neurologic exam: Fine tremors of hands, tongue, or closed eyelids; hyperreflexia
       and proximal muscle weakness may be manifested in thyrotoxicosis.

IV. Diagnostic tests (see Table 149-1)

    A. Laboratory

        1. TSH

           a) Most important to evaluate because it is a very sensitive measure and may be
              detectable even before the T_4 and T_3 levels are elevated.

           b) Determines the pituitary response to circulating thyroid hormones

           c) Normal adult value range: 0.2–5.4 µU/ml

        2. T_4 and free thyroxine index (FT$_4$I)

           a) Predominant hormone produced by the thyroid gland

           b) In hyperthyroidism, values will be higher than the normal range.

              (1) Normal adult value range: T_4 per radioimmunoassay (RIA), 5–12 mg/dl;
                    FT$_4$I, 0.9–2.2 ng/dl

              (2) T_4 can be altered (increased or decreased) in conditions (e.g., chronic
                    disease) that involve plasma protein changes.

        3. T_3, RIA

           a) If T_4 level is normal (5% of patients with hyperthyroidism), order T_3; otherwise
              not necessary.

           b) Good indicator of T_3: Thyroid hormone

           c) Normal adult value range: 80–200 ng/dl

Table 149-1. Hyperthyroid Laboratory Values

Test	Findings	Normal Adult Value Range
Thyroid-stimulating hormone (TSH)	Decreased or undetectable	0.2–5.4 µU/ml
Thyroxine (T$_4$)	Increased	5–12 mg/dl (per radioimmunoassay)
Free thyroxine index (FT$_4$I)	Increased	0.9–2.2 ng/dl
If T$_4$ is normal, order T$_3$; otherwise not necessary.		
Triiodothyronine (T$_3$)	Increased	80–200 ng/dl

   4. WBC count: Should be measured if treatment with methimazole or propylthiouracil is planned, as both of these drugs can cause leukopenia (rare).
B. Radiology
   1. Thyroid scan:
      a) Useful test to evaluate nodular thyroid disease and to determine whether hyperthyroidism is a result of autonomously functioning nodules.
      b) Useful in patients with nodular goiter and hyperthyroidism to differentiate between
         (1) Multiple nodules concentrating radioiodine
         (2) If the nodules present are cold and the hyperfunctioning tissue is between nodules.
   2. Radioactive iodine uptake: Useful for diagnosing Graves' disease (i.e., high uptake) and thyroiditis (i.e., low uptake).

V. Differential diagnosis
   A. Graves' disease
   B. Multinodular goiter
   C. Solitary toxic nodule
   D. Thyroiditis
   E. TSH-secreting pituitary adenoma
   F. Choriocarcinoma
   G. Dermoid malignancy of ovary
   H. Other conditions that can mimic hyperthyroidism
      1. Panic disorder (see Chapter 152)
      2. Pheochromocytoma
      3. Uncontrolled diabetes mellitus (see Chapter 143)
      4. Myasthenia gravis
      5. Orbital tumors

VI. Treatment: If patients are undertreated or overtreated, hypothyroidism or hyperthyroidism may occur.
   A. Beta-adrenergic blockers
      1. First-line drug to stabilize hyperthyroidism induced palpitations, tachycardia, tremor, and diaphoresis.
      2. Propranolol (Inderal® LA, Wyeth-Ayerst Pharmaceuticals, Philadelphia, PA): 160–720 (maximum) mg po daily
      3. Atenolol (Tenormin®, AstraZeneca, Wilmington, DE): 50–200 mg (maximum) po daily
      4. Discontinue when euthyroid state is achieved.
   B. Antithyroid drugs (ATDs)
      1. Propylthiouracil
         a) Obstructs biosynthesis of thyroid hormone and inhibits peripheral conversion of T_4 to T_3.
         b) Used as primary therapy or secondary therapy to decrease thyroid hormone levels before and, possibly, after radioactive iodine therapy or thyroidectomy

    c) Rapid onset with euthyroid achieved in two to four weeks
    d) Initial adult dose is 50–300 mg po every six to eight hours (50 mg tablets).
    e) When euthyroid, maintenance dose is 50–100 mg bid.
    f) Treatment usually required for one to two years but can be long-term
  2. Methimazole (Tapazole®, Jones Pharma Inc., St. Louis, MO)
    a) Obstructs biosynthesis of thyroid hormone.
    b) Used as primary or secondary therapy to decrease thyroid hormone levels before and, possibly, after radioactive iodine therapy or thyroidectomy.
    c) Long-acting; euthyroid achieved in two to four weeks.
    d) Initial adult dose is 5–30 mg po every 12 hours (5 and 10 mg tablets).
    e) When euthyroid, maintenance dose is 5–10 mg qd or bid.
    f) Treatment usually required for one to two years.
  3. Both medications can be administered in increased amounts if patient is extremely ill.
  4. Agranulocytosis develops in approximately 0.3% of patients on either drug; therefore, baseline WBC count should be checked. Patients on ATDs should have WBC if fever or sore throat occurs.
C. Radioactive iodine therapy
  1. Most common therapy for hyperthyroidism in the United States
  2. Sodium iodide, I$_{131}$, Iodotope® (Olin Mathieson Chemical Corporation, New York, NY)
  3. Dose determined by radioactive iodine uptake test.
  4. Often causes hypothyroidism after therapy, necessitating lifelong thyroid hormone replacement.
  5. Contraindicated for females who are pregnant; always order human chorionic gonadotropin (serum beta HCG) on premenopausal females before initiating therapy.
  6. Females should use reliable birth control method for six months after therapy.
D. Surgery
  1. Seldom recommended unless patient failed other treatment or patient is poor candidate for medical treatment.
  2. Complications
    a) Hypoparathyroidism
    b) Laryngeal nerve damage
  3. Hypothyroid after surgery

VII. Follow-up: Goal is to maintain euthyroid state.
A. ß-adrenergic antagonists
  1. Evaluate, initially, every one to three months
  2. Then periodically, based on symptoms
B. ATDs
  1. Draw T$_4$ level and WBC count (after one month of therapy).
  2. After first month, draw T$_4$ level every two to three months.
  3. After three to four weeks, draw WBC with any dose changes.
  4. Draw liver enzymes every three to six months while on therapy.
C. Radioactive iodine

   1. Draw T_4 every 30 days after treatment.
   2. When euthyroid, draw TSH level every three to six months to assess if hypothyroid.
   D. Surgery
   1. Follow as needed for postoperative assessment.
   2. Follow two months after surgery to determine thyroid status.
   3. Follow as needed to maintain euthyroid state.

VIII. Referrals
   A. Endocrinologist: Consult for diagnosis and initiation of treatment.
   B. Ophthalmologist: Refer patients with more than mild ophthalmic signs and symptoms.
   C. Admission: If thyroid storm occurs, which is life-threatening medical emergency.
   1. Magnified signs and symptoms of hyperthyroidism, fever, and change in mental status.
   2. Usually occurs in conjunction with another illness or injury.
   3. Can occur spontaneously after withdrawal of medications for hyperthyroidism or after radioactive iodine treatment.
   4. Treatment
      a) Treat underlying cause.
      b) Use supportive treatments (e.g., proper fluid intake and nutrition, correct electrolytes)
      c) Implement pharmacologic support.

References

Lazarus, J.H. (1997). Hyperthyroidism. *Lancet, 349*(9048), 339–343.

Ludwig-Beymer, P., Huether, S.E., & Gray, D.P. (1994). Alterations of hormonal regulation. In K.L. McCance & S.E. Huether (Eds.), *Pathophysiology* (pp. 656–710). St. Louis: Mosby.

Singer, P.A., Cooper, D.S., Levy, E.G., Ladenson, P.W., Braverman, L.E., Daniels, G., Greenspan, F.S., McDougall, I.R., & Nikolai, T.F. (1995). Treatment guidelines for patients with hyperthyroidism and hypothyroidism. *JAMA, 273,* 808–812.

Surks, M.I., & Ocampo, E. (1996). Subclinical thyroid disease. *American Journal of Medicine, 100*(2), 217–223.

Vanderpump, M.P., Ahlquist, J.A., Franklyn, J.A., & Clayton, R.N. (1996). Consensus statement for good practice and audit measures in the management of hypothyroidism and hyperthyroidism. *British Medical Journal, 313,* 539–544.

Watts, R.S. (1996). Hyperthyroidism. In R.E. Rakel (Ed.), *Saunders manual of medical practice* (pp. 638–641). Philadelphia: Saunders.

Chapter

150.

Hypothyroidism

Rebecca A. Hawkins, RN, MSN, ANP, AOCN®

I. Definition: A decrease in the function of the thyroid gland, causing a reduced production of thyroid hormone, altering the body's natural function

II. Physiology/Pathophysiology
   A. Normal physiology
      1. The thyroid secretes predominantly thyroxine (T_4); triiodothyronine (T_3) results from the conversion of T_4 to T_3 by nonthyroidal tissues.
      2. Thyroid hormones (T_4 and T_3) are released under the control of the pituitary, which releases thyroid-stimulating hormone (TSH).
      3. The pituitary is under a classic negative feedback regulation by thyroid hormone circulation.
      4. The hypothalamus regulates pituitary release of TSH by secreting thyrotropin-releasing hormone (TRH).
   B. Pathophysiology
      1. Primary hypothyroidism
         a) Caused by impaired thyroid function.
         b) Hypothalamus responds with increased output of TRH, which triggers primary thyrotropin (TSH) secretion, stimulating thyroid gland enlargement, goiter formation, and synthesis of T_3 instead of T_4.
      2. Secondary hypothyroidism
         a) Caused by hypothalamic-pituitary dysfunction.
         b) TSH response is inadequate.
         c) Gland remains normal or reduced in size.
         d) T_3 and T_4 synthesis are equally reduced.

III. Clinical features
   A. Etiology can be from cancer, cancer treatments, or other conditions.
      1. Primary
         a) Idiopathic
         b) Radioactive iodine treatment for hyperthyroidism
         c) Thyroiditis (autoimmune or subacute)
         d) Iodine deficiency (rare in the United States)

    e) Drug-induced (antithyroid drugs and lithium)
    f) Cancer of the thyroid with thyroidectomy
    g) Infiltrative disorders of the thyroid
    h) Radiation to the neck
   2. Secondary
    a) Hypothalamic dysfunction
    b) Pituitary dysfunction
  B. History
   1. History of cancer and cancer treatment
   2. Current medications: Prescribed and over-the-counter
   3. History of presenting symptom(s): Precipitating factors, onset, and duration
   4. Changes in activities of daily living
  C. Signs and symptoms
   1. Fatigue, lethargy
   2. Cold intolerance
   3. Constipation
   4. Depressed appetite
   5. Slight weight gain (late symptom)
   6. Muscle cramps
   7. Mental sluggishness
   8. Heavy menstrual periods or abnormal bleeding
   9. Hoarseness
   10. Dyspnea on exertion
   11. Angina
  D. Physical exam
   1. Vital signs: Hypertension
   2. Integument exam
    a) Dry, brittle hair
    b) Dry, rough skin
   3. HEENT exam
    a) Periorbital edema
    b) Thyroid not palpable, unless goiter is present
   4. Cardiac exam
    a) Abnormal sounds: S_3, S_4 to muffled sounds of pericardial effusion
    b) Decreased capillary refill, indicating poor perfusion
   5. Pulmonary exam: Rales or rhonchi, indicating heart failure
   6. Neurologic exam: Hyporeflexia

IV. Diagnostic tests
  A. Laboratory (see Table 150-1)
   1. TSH
    a) Normal range: 0.3–5 µU/ml
    b) Recommended as first-line screening
    c) Can detect low levels of the normal range and is highly sensitive

Table 150-1. Diagnosis and Management of Hypothyroidism Disorders

Thyroid-Stimulating Hormone (TSH)	Thyroxine (T₄)	Diagnosis
High: >10 μU/ml	Low	Primary hypothyroidism
Borderline: 5.1–10 μU/ml	Low or borderline	Questionable subclinical hypothyroidism versus normal variant hypothyroidism
Normal: 0.3–5 μU/ml	Low	°Euthyroid sick syndrome

°Alterations in thyroid function tests in patients who have nonthyroidal disease.

    d) A rise in the TSH will precede other abnormalities in thyroid function tests when diagnosing primary hypothyroidism.
    e) Also recommended for monitoring of thyroid hormone replacement
  2. Total T_4 (serum T_4)
    a) Measures all T_4 that is bound to protein
    b) Can be affected by alterations in plasma proteins (i.e., from liver disease, malnutrition, chronic illness)
    c) More expensive test for monitoring or screening hypothyroidism
    d) Can be used to confirm hypothyroidism, although not as sensitive as TSH
    e) Less helpful in monitoring patients on replacement therapy
  3. Free T_4 (FT_4)
    a) Measures the metabolically active form of T_4, which is a better indicator of thyroid status than total T_4
    b) Traditionally used as first-line screening test, now used to confirm TSH assay
    c) Use FT_4 when diagnosing secondary hypothyroidism (TSH = low or normal; FT_4 = low), which is caused by TSH deficiency from hypothalamus. Thus, TSH assay not a sensitive diagnostic test.
  4. Serum T_3: Not a useful test for diagnosis or monitoring
  5. If secondary hypothyroidism is suspected, check other pituitary axis (e.g., gonadotropin/sex steroid, ACTH/cortisol).
  6. Hemoglobin and hematocrit: To rule out anemia, which is common with hypothyroidism
  7. Cholesterol level: Increased value associated with hypothyroidism
 B. Radiology: To rule out pituitary-hypothalamic pathology
  1. CT scan or MRI of sella/pituitary: May be indicated to rule out pituitary or hypothalamic etiology
  2. Chest x-ray: To rule out CHF and cardiomegaly, which is associated with hypothyroidism

V. Differential diagnosis
 A. Treatment-related
  1. Radioactive iodine (I^{131})

       2. Surgery: Total or subtotal thyroidectomy

       3. Propylthiouracil

       4. External beam radiation: Mantle field or thyroid field

   B. Autoimmune

       1. Primary disease: Atrophic thyroiditis (no goiter)

       2. Hashimoto's thyroiditis (goiter present)

   C. Idiopathic thyroid failure

   D. Congenital thyroid failure

   E. Iodine insufficiency (rare)

   F. Secondary hypothyroidism (from pituitary or hypothalamic dysfunction)

   G. Drug induced (lithium, iodine compounds, antithyroid drugs)

   H. Fluid overload

VI. Treatment: Patients may exhibit symptoms of hyperthyroidism if overtreated and symptoms of hypothyroidism if undertreated. Patients with adequate treatment are euthyroid.

   A. Continuous replacement therapy, adjust dose according to clinical response and laboratory findings

   B. Thyroid replacement medications

       1. Levothyroxine (Synthroid®, Knoll Pharmaceutical Company, Mount Olive, NJ): Most commonly used.

          a) Maintenance dose: 0.1–0.2 mg po qd

          b) Start at 0.05 mg daily and increase by 0.025–0.05 mg at six-week intervals until TSH is normalized.

          c) Elderly clients or those with coronary artery disease start on 0.025 mg qd, increasing dose every two to four weeks.

          d) Younger clients can begin at full dose.

       2. Sodium liothyronine (Cytomel®, Jones Medical Industries, St. Louis, MO): Rarely used because of short half-life.

          a) Maintenance dose: 25–75µg qd

          b) Start at 25 µg and increase by 12.5–25 µg every one to two weeks.

       3. Desiccated thyroid (Armour thyroid): Rarely recommended because contents are variable; more difficult to be precise with dosing

          a) Maintenance dose: 60–120 mg qd

          b) Start at 30 mg qd and increase by 15 mg every two to three weeks.

          c) Previously ordered in grains; 1 gr = 60 mg.

   C. If hypoadrenalism is diagnosed, give cortisone acetate prior to initiating replacement therapy.

VII. Follow-up

   A. The half-life of thyroxine is 7–10 days. It takes approximately five half-lives (35–50 days or five to seven weeks) to reach steady state. Check TSH blood level every two to four weeks of thyroid replacement therapy until TSH levels normalize as well as with each dose adjustment.

   B. Symptoms should improve within two weeks and resolve within three to six months.

VIII.   Referrals: Endocrinologist: May require referral for diagnosis and initiation of therapy; must refer patients who have uncontrolled levels of TSH

References

Bunevicius, R., Kazanavicius, G., Zalinkevicius, R., & Prange, A.J. (1999). Effects of thyroxine as compared with thyroxine plus triiodothyronine in patients with hypothyroidism. *New England Journal of Medicine, 340,* 424–429.

Cushing, G.W. (1993). Subclinical hypothyroidism. *Postgraduate Medicine, 94*(1), 95–107.

Grebe, S.K., Cooke, R.R., Ford, H.C., Fagertrom, J.N., Cordwell, D.P., Lever, N.A., Purdie, G.L., & Feek, C.M. (1997). Treatment of hypothyroidism with once weekly thyroxine. *Journal of Clinical Endocrinology Metabolism, 82,* 870–875.

Heitman, B., & Irizarry, A. (1995). Hypothyroidism: Common complaints, perplexing diagnosis. *Nurse Practitioner, 20*(3), 54–60.

Hershman, J.M., Ladenson, P.W., & Paulshock, B.Z. (1992). A savvy approach to thyroid testing. *Patient Care, 26*(3), 134–151.

Johnson, J.L., & Fellcetta, J.V. (1992). Hypothyroidism: A comprehensive review. *Journal of the American Academy of Nurse Practitioners, 4*(4), 131–138.

Kaplan, M.M. (1993). Thyroid hormone therapy. *Postgraduate Medicine, 93*(1), 249–262.

Kaye, T.B. (1993). Thyroid function tests. *Postgraduate Medicine, 93*(1), 81–90.

Mazzaferri, E.L., & Surks, M.I. (1999). Recognizing the faces of hypothyroidism. *Hospital Practice,* 34, 93–96, 101–105, 109–110.

Tell, R., Sjodin, H., Lundell, G., Lewin, F., & Lewenshohn, R. (1997). Hypothyroidism after external radiotherapy for head and neck cancer. *International Journal of Radiation Oncology, Biology, Physics, 39,* 303–308.

Chapter

151. Menopausal Symptoms and Menopause

Aurelie C. Cormier, RN, MS, AOCN®

I. Definition: The end of menstruation for at least 12 months as the result of the loss of ovarian function

II. Normal physiology
   A. The hypothalamus releases gonadotrophic-releasing hormone (GnRH) to stimulate the anterior pituitary to release follicle-stimulating hormone (FSH) and luteinizing hormone (LH).
   B. Premenopausal, the ovary is composed of eggs surrounded by granulosa cells in a sac or follicle.
   C. The follicle responds to FSH and LH by developing and producing estrogen, and ovulation occurs.
   D. At menopause, the ovary contains no follicles and does not respond.
   E. The follicular granulosa cells also produce diminishing levels of inhibin (a hormone that inhibits the synthesis and release of FSH), which then allows the anterior pituitary to release more FSH.
   F. The ovaries and adrenal glands also synthesize androstenedione (an androgen), which is converted to estrone (a weak estrogen) in peripheral tissue, liver, fat, and hypothalamic nuclei.

III. Clinical features: Typically, women may start to experience perimenopausal symptoms in their early to mid-forties and go through menopause at an average age of 51. However, women undergoing cancer treatment may develop premature menopause at any age. Menopause is a natural physiological process, and as such, is described as a normal stage of life.
   A. Risk factors for early menopause
      1. Chemotherapy agents
         a) Degree of occurrence is based on age, drug dose, and duration of treatment.
         b) Women over age 40 are at greater risk.
      2. Pelvic radiation
      3. Oophorectomy
   B. History
      1. History of cancer and cancer treatment
      2. Current medications: Prescribed and over-the-counter

3. History of presenting symptom(s): Precipitating factors, onset, and duration. Associated symptoms are hot flashes, night sweats, and insomnia.
4. Changes in activities of daily living
5. Menstrual and obstetrical history
    a) Menarche
    b) Time between periods
        (1) Flow
        (2) Length
        (3) Changes in menses
    c) Character of menses
    d) History of pregnancies, miscarriages, or abortions
        (1) Stillbirths
        (2) Premature births
        (3) Complications
    e) Use of hormonal therapy, including birth control pills, or gynecologic and obstetric procedures
6. Past medical history: Heart disease, overweight, hypertension, congenital or acquired hyperlipidemia, diabetes mellitus, osteoporosis, depression
7. Family history: Osteoporosis, heart disease

C. Signs and symptoms
1. No menstruation for 12 months; may be less in patients with cancer
2. Hot flashes
3. Night sweats
4. Insomnia
5. Fatigue
6. Anxiety
7. Depression
8. Irritability
9. Headache
10. Joint pains
11. Stomach upset
12. Decreased cognition
13. Forgetfulness
14. Dysuria, frequency, stress incontinence
15. Vaginal dryness, pruritis, dyspareunia

D. Physical exam
1. Vital signs and height: Assess for high blood pressure and decreased height, which may be present with estrogen deficiency.
2. Neck exam: Palpate thyroid to rule out hypothyroidism or hyperthyroidism. Symptoms with these conditions are similar to menopausal symptoms.
3. Breast exam: Assess for atrophy present with long-term estrogen deficiency.
4. Musculoskeletal exam: Assess for signs/symptoms of weakness or discomfort to evaluate for osteoporosis.
5. Pelvic exam: Assess for prolapse of the vagina, bladder, or rectum; vaginal atrophy with dyspareunia and/or mucosal dryness may be seen with prolonged low estrogen levels.

IV. Diagnostic studies: Usually not necessary to diagnose menopause. Symptoms and clinical manifestations will direct diagnosis.
  A. Laboratory
    1. To confirm diagnosis of menopause, check FSH and estradiol levels.
      a) FSH > 50 mIU/ml
      b) Estradiol < 50 pg/ml
    2. To rule out other medical causes of symptoms, check
      a) CBC: To rule out anemia
      b) Electrolytes: To rule out hypokalemia
      c) Serum glucose: To rule out diabetes mellitus
      d) Liver function tests: To rule out liver disease
      e) Thyroid function tests: To rule out thyroid disease
      f) Beta HCG: To rule out pregnancy in selected patients
    3. Lipid profile and cholesterol are important screening tools at the start of menopause.
      a) Low-density lipoprotein (LDL) rises (LDL < 130 = within normal limits [WNL])
      b) Total high-density lipoprotein (HDL) to LDL cholesterol ratio rises (total HDL: LDL cholesterol ratio < 7.5 = WNL)
      c) HDL becomes lower (HDL > 70 = WNL)
      d) Total cholesterol (< 200 = WNL); triglycerides 50–250 = WNL
  B. Radiology
    1. Mammogram: To rule out any breast lesions or abnormalities, especially if hormone therapy will be initiated
    2. Dual energy x-ray absorptiometry (DEXA): To measure bone density to assist patients in making informed decisions regarding initiation of hormone therapy.
      a) DEXA can be used to measure whole-body bone mass. Typically, it measures the bone density in the radius, hip, and spine.
      b) Bone mineral density (BMD) is reported in g/cm squared; bone mineral content (BMC) is reported in grams. Results are determined in comparison with those of age, sex, and race-matched controls.
      c) Reports indicate whether the BMD is normal or above or below levels of the comparison group. Results help to predict risk of fracture by estimating the standard deviation from the matched-controls.
        (1) Results > 2.5 indicate osteoporosis and require treatment.
        (2) Results between 1.5–2.5 may be treated or may be observed at regular intervals.
    3. Transvaginal ultrasound and a CA-125 are used to exclude ovarian pathology in patients with an abnormal adnexal mass or suspicious clinical features (e.g., gastrointestinal distress, abdominal pain, abnormal vaginal bleeding).
    4. Transvaginal ultrasound can be used to exclude endometrial pathology in patients taking tamoxifen.
  C. Other: Endometrial biopsy: To rule out malignancy if any abnormal bleeding

V. Differential diagnosis
  A. Estrogen excess or deficiency, perimenopausal condition
  B. Metabolic

        1. Hyperthyroidism (see Chapter 149)

        2. Pheochromocytoma

        3. Carcinoid syndrome

    C. Pregnancy or postpartum

    D. Panic attacks

    E. Drug-induced

        1. Endocrine drug therapy (e.g., levothyroxine sodium, liothyronine sodium, liotrix, thyroid, corticotropin, cosyntropin, desmopressin acetate, calcitonin)

        2. Sympathomimetic drugs (e.g., mephentermine sulfate, metaraminol, norepinephrine bitartrate)

        3. Tamoxifen

        4. Birth control pills

        5. Nicotinic acid

        6. Chemotherapy

    F. Lymphoma

    G. Metastatic disease

    H. Retroperitoneal radiation

    I. Radical hysterectomy

VI. Treatment

    A. When counseling women about treatment options, consider patient's medical history; risk assessment for cardiovascular disease, osteoporosis, and breast cancer; frequency and intensity of symptoms; and benefits and risks of treatments. Symptoms can be treated with or without hormone therapy.

    B. Treatment with hormone therapy must be individualized; patient should take the lowest possible dose to relieve symptoms in one to two weeks. Hormone therapy may be natural, conjugated equine, or synthetic and may be taken in pill, cream, ring, or patch form.

        1. Estrogen only

            a) Titrate to keep serum estradiol level between 50 pg/ml–150 pg/ml to treat symptoms and minimize side effects.

            b) Unopposed estrogen regimens may only be prescribed for women without a uterus.

            c) Women with a uterus require estrogen plus progesterone to avoid a 20% increase in the risk of endometrial cancer.

            d) If hormonal treatment is discontinued, it is best to taper over a three-month period.

            e) Estrogen pills or tablet formulation (see Table 151-1)

                (1) Estrogen alone has been shown to improve bone mass and reduce cardiovascular risk in postmenopausal women.

                (2) Estrogen increases HDLs and triglycerides, lowers LDLs and clotting factors, and dilates blood vessels; it does not raise blood pressure.

                (3) Estrogens that are nonnaturally occurring in humans (e.g., conjugated equine estrogen, ethinyl estradiol) have elevated potency in the liver relative to their estrogen potential.

Table 151-1. Estrogen Pills

Drugs	Dose	Comments
Premarin®ª	0.3 mg, 0.625 mg, 0.9 mg, 1.25 mg, 2.5 mg	Conjugated equine estrogen
Estrace®ᵇ	0.5 mg, 1 mg, 2 mg (scored)	Micronized estradiol
Estratab®ᶜ	0.3, 0.625 mg, 1.25 mg, 2.5 mg	Esterified estrogen
Estinyl®ᵈ	0.02 mg, 0.05 mg	Ethinyl estradiol
Ogen®ᵉ	0.625 mg, 1.25 mg, 2.5 mg, 5.0 mg	Estrone
Ortho-Est®ᶠ	0.625 mg (1.25 mg) (scored) 1.25 mg (2.5 mg) (scored)	Estrone
Menest®ᵍ	0.3 mg, 0.625 mg, 1.25 mg, 2.5 mg	Esterified estrogen

[a] Wyeth-Ayerst Pharmaceuticals, Philadelphia, PA; [b] Bristol-Myers Squibb Company, Princeton, NJ; [c] Solvay Pharmaceuticals, Inc., Marietta, GA; [d] Schering Corporation, Kenilworth, NJ; [e] Pharmacia & Upjohn, Peapack, NJ; [f] Woman First Healthcare, Inc., San Diego, CA; [g] Monarch Pharmaceuticals, Bristol, TN

(4) Side effects may include nausea, breast tenderness, weight gain, fluid retention, dizziness, headaches, breakthrough bleeding, gallbladder disease, or yeast infections.

(5) Less side effects are experienced with vaginal creams and rings.

(6) The addition of progesterone may negate some of the cardiovascular benefits of estrogen (see Tables 151-6 and 151-3).

f) Estrogen patches (see Table 151-2)

(1) Patches are applied to a clean, dry area of the trunk (e.g., lower abdomen, upper buttocks).

(2) Patches should not be applied to the breasts, waistline, or an area that receives direct sunlight. Rotate sites of application. Patients can shower, bathe, or swim with the patch.

(3) Patients with a uterus should have cyclic administration of the patch (i.e., three weeks on, one week off).

(4) In some patients, patches cause skin irritation and rashes; try a different patch if this occurs.

2. Estrogen with cyclic progesterone (see Table 151-3): Recommended regimens

a) Estrogen on days 1–25 and progesterone on days 16–25 of each month

b) Estrogen every day and progesterone on days 1–10 or 16–25 of each month

c) Patients may experience side effects of estrogen use, such as uterine cramping, nervousness, fatigue, and lower tolerance to glucose.

3. Estrogen + progesterone (see Table 151-3)

a) The disadvantage of these combinations is irregular and unpredictable menses in the first year of treatment.

Table 151-2. Estrogen Patches

Drugs	Dose	Comments
Estraderm®ᵃ	0.05 mg, 0.1 mg	Estradiol, apply twice/week
Vivelle®ᵃ	0.0375 mg, 0.05 mg	Estradiol, apply twice/week
	0.075 mg, 0.1 mg	
Climara®ᵇ	0.05 mg, 0.1 mg	Estradiol, apply once/week
Alora®ᶜ	0.05 mg, 0.075 mg, 0.1 mg	Estradiol, apply twice/week
Fempatch®ᵈ	0.025 mg	Estradiol, apply once/week It is recommended that women without a uterus take this drug on a continuous basis (was not studied in women with a uterus).

ᵃ Novartis Pharmaceuticals Corporation, East Hanover, NJ; ᵇ Berlex Laboratories, Richmond, CA; ᶜ Procter & Gamble Pharmaceuticals, Inc., Mason, OH; ᵈ Warner-Lambert Company, Morris Plains, NJ

Table 151-3. Estrogen/Progesterone Combination Pills

Drug	Dose	Comments
Premphase®ᵃ	0.625 mg + 5.0 mg	Conjugated estrogen with medroxyprogesterone acetate (MPA) involves two separate tablets: a maroon tablet containing 0.625 mg of premarin taken days 1–14 and a light blue tablet containing 0.625 mg of conjugated estrogen with 5 mg of MPA taken on days 15–28. Patients on this regimen will always have a monthly bleed.
Prempro™ᵃ	0.625 mg + 2.5–5.0 mg	Conjugated estrogen with MPA involves one tablet taken every day. The disadvantage of this regimen is irregular and unpredictable menses in the first year of treatment.

ᵃ Wyeth-Ayerst Pharmaceuticals, Philadelphia, PA

    b) Once the regimen is established, menses usually will disappear altogether.

    c) Side effects are the same as estrogen with cyclic progesterone.

  4. Estrogen with methyl testosterone (MeT) (see Table 151-4)

    a) Used for women who experience a lack of libido after menopause.

    b) MeT is a synthetic androgen and has been found to cause a dose-related elevation of high-density lipoprotein cholesterol.

    c) At this time, the effect on risk of heart disease is unknown.

    d) These drugs are to be administered cyclically on a short-term basis.

    e) Side effects of estrogen use plus testosterone can cause deepening of the voice, weight gain, an increase in body hair, balding of scalp hair, and acne.

  5. Estrogen vaginal creams (see Table 151-5)

    a) Used for the treatment of only genitourinary symptoms.

Table 151-4. Estrogen With Methyl Testosterone

Drugs	Dose	Comments
Estratest®ᵃ H.S.	0.625 mg with MeT 1.25 mg	Esterified estrogen (with methyltestosterone (half-strength)
Estratest®ᵃ	1.25 mg with MeT 2.5 mg	Esterified estrogen with methyltestosterone
Premarin®ᵇ with methyltestosterone	0.625 mg with 5 mg 1.25 mg with 10 mg	Conjugated estrogen with methyltestosterone

ᵃ Solvay Pharmaceuticals, Inc., Marietta, GA; ᵇ Wyeth-Ayerst Pharmaceuticals, Philadelphia, PA

Table 151-5. Estrogen Creams

Drugs	Dose	Prescribing Information
Premarin®ᵃ vaginal cream	0.625 mg/g (1/2–2 g applicator)	42.5 g tube, conjugated estrogen, administer qd for three to four weeks, then one to three times/week
Estrace®ᵇ vaginal cream	0.01% (0.01 mg/g) (1–4 g applicator)	42.5 g tube, estradiol, administer qd/one to two weeks, then one to three times/week
Ogen®ᶜ vaginal cream	1.5 mg/g (1–4 g applicator)	42.5 g tube, estrone, administer qd for three to four weeks, then one to three times/week

ᵃ Wyeth-Ayerst Pharmaceuticals, Philadelphia, PA; ᵇ Bristol-Myers Squibb Company, Princeton, NJ;
ᶜ Pharmacia & Upjohn, Peapack, NJ

      b) Estrogen is absorbed in systemic circulation for about one month until the vaginal mucosa becomes cornified; then, systemic absorption is minimal.

      c) Creams do not have beneficial effects on the cardiovascular system or bones.

      d) Women with a uterus must take progesterone when using vaginal cream, as it causes a build-up of the endometrial lining.

      e) The woman's partner can absorb estrogen during intercourse; men can develop breast tissue if a sufficient amount enters their blood stream on a regular basis.

      f) Creams have less side effects than oral or patch estrogens.

   6. Estrogen vaginal ring: Inserted into the upper third of the vagina once every three months (e.g., Estring® vaginal ring [Pharmacia & Upjohn, Peapack, NJ]: 2 mg [estradiol] every three months)

      a) Used to treat the genitourinary symptoms of vaginal dryness, pruritis, dyspareunia, and urinary urgency and dysuria.

      b) Progestin use is not necessary when using the vaginal ring.

      c) Ring does not interfere with sexual intercourse.

      d) If ring should fall out within a three-month time period, it can be washed with lukewarm water and reinserted.

      e) Less side effects than with oral or patch estrogens.

   7. Progestin (see Table 151-6)
      a) Some women who can not take estrogen to treat symptoms of hot flashes use progestin; may be useful in preventing osteoporosis.
      b) Natural micronized progesterone has not been found to alter the beneficial cardiovascular effects of estrogen. It has been shown to have less side effects (e.g., fluid retention, weight gain, depression, breast tenderness) than those associated with synthetic progestin.
      c) Synthetic progestin has variable effects on the lipoproteins.
         (1) Norethindrone and norethindrone acetate increase low-density lipoproteins and decrease high-density lipoprotein cholesterol, therefore negating some of the beneficial cardiovascular effects of estrogen.
         (2) Medroxyprogesterone acetate has a similar but less-dramatic effect.
         (3) Possible side effects are fluid retention, weight gain, uterine cramps, bloating, breast tenderness, depression, headache, nervousness, dizziness, weakness, and lower tolerance to glucose.
   8. Progesterone vaginal creams: Micronize natural progesterone
C. Symptom management without hormonal therapy
   1. Hormonal therapy usually is contraindicated in women with a history of breast or endometrial cancer, undiagnosed vaginal bleeding, active liver disease, or active thrombolic disorders. This position is being reconsidered, and it may be prescribed in selected patients after full discussion of benefits and risks.
   2. Strategies for reducing menopausal symptoms without hormonal replacement therapy
      a) Hot flashes

Table 151-6. Progestins

Drugs	Dose	Comments
Prometrium[®a]	100 mg bid or 200–400 mg	Natural micronized progesterone
Provera[®b]	2.5 mg, 5 mg, 10 mg (scored)	Medroxyprogesterone acetate
Amen[®c]	10 mg (scored)	Medroxyprogesterone acetate
Cycrin[®d]	2.5 mg, 5 mg, 10 mg (scored)	Medroxyprogesterone acetate
Aygestin[®d]	5 mg (scored)	Norethindrone acetate (synthetic progesterone)
Norlutate[®e]	5 mg (scored)	Norethindrone acetate
Nor-QD[®f]	0.35 mg	Norethindrone
Micronor[®g]	0.35 mg	Norethindrone
Depo-Provera[®b]	150 mg	IM once every three months

[a] Solvay Pharmaceuticals, Inc., Marietta, GA; [b] Pharmacia & Upjohn, Peapack, NJ; [c] Carnrick Laboratories, Cedar Knolls, NJ; [d] ESI Lederle Inc., Philadelphia, PA; [e] Parke-Davis, Morris Plains, NJ; [f] Watson Laboratories, Inc., Corona, CA; [g] Ortho-McNeil Pharmaceuticals, Raritan, NJ

(1) Stress management techniques (e.g., meditation, yoga, visualization, biofeedback): Have been shown to reduce the number of hot flashes by 40%–70% and the intensity by 28%.

(2) Phytoestrogens: Found in soy products (e.g., tofu, miso, tempeh, soy milk), lentils, and beans; are being studied; no definitive conclusions on effectiveness.

(3) Regular aerobic exercise: 20–30 minutes five to seven times/week or one hour three times/week

(4) Vitamin E: 400–1,200 IU/day

(5) Acupuncture: Clinical research ongoing

(6) Bioflavonoids: Found in citrus fruits, especially the pulp and white rind; in pill form, take 250 mg five to six times/day.

(7) Folic acid

(8) Dressing in layers of clothing

(9) Drinking lots of cold water

(10) Avoiding hot, humid weather, confined spaces, stress, caffeine, alcohol, hot drinks, and spicy foods may reduce the intensity and frequency of hot flashes.

(11) Medications

   (a) Megestrol acetate: 20 mg bid po (Megace®, Bristol-Myers Squibb, Princeton, NJ)

   (b) Clonidine: Initially 0.1 mg qd or 0.1 mg po bid

   (c) Catapres-TTS®-1 (clonidine 0.1 mg/day transdermal therapeutic system [Boehringer-Ingleheim Pharmaceuticals, Inc., Ridgefield, CT]): q seven days, apply to nonhairy skin on upper outer arm or chest

   (d) Catapres-TTS®-2 (clonidine 0.2 mg/day): q seven days

   (e) Methyldopa (Aldomet®, Merck & Co., Inc., West Point, PA): 250 mg po bid/48 hours, then 250–500 mg po qd or every night

   (f) Bellergal-S® (Sandoz Pharmaceuticals, East Hanover, NJ): Two tablets/day po; Bellergal (a combination of ergotamine tartrate, levorotatory belladonna alkaloids, and phenobarbital) must be used with caution, as it has addictive properties when used regularly.

b) Fatigue (see Chapter 155): Advise patient to

   (1) Determine most-energetic and least-energetic times of day; may be necessary to keep a journal for a week. Encourage patients to do the most important things when they feel the most energetic and the least important things when they are the least energetic.

   (2) Nap/rest at the time of the day when typically feeling the most tired. Several short periods of rest throughout the day may be the most beneficial.

   (3) Follow rest with exercise (e.g., power walking, swimming, low-impact aerobics, bike riding) for 20–30 minutes every day or one hour three to five times/week. These exercises can boost the energy level when performed on a regular basis.

   (4) Eat a nutritious diet, including fruits, vegetables, and low-fat foods.

   (5) Drink plenty of liquids, especially water, unless a cardiac problem exists.

   (6) Limit caffeine and alcohol, which, in some cases, can increase fatigue.

   (7) Set up a routine sleeping pattern.

      c) Vaginal dryness
        (1) Water-based vaginal moisture lubrication products
          (a) Astroglide® (Astro-Lube, Inc., North Hollywood, CA)
          (b) Replens® (Columbia Laboratories, Inc., Coconut Grove, FL) suppositories
          (c) Surgilube® (Day Chemical Company, New York, NY)
          (d) K-Y® Jelly (Johnson & Johnson, New Brunswick, NJ)
          (e) Lubrin® (Upsher-Smith Laboratories, Inc., Minneapolis, MN) vaginal lubricating suppositories
          (f) Lubafax® (Burroughs Wellcome & Co., Inc., New York, NY) suppositories
        (2) Oil-based vaginal moisture lubrication products
          (a) Creme de la femme® ("Especially" Products, Inc., Playa del Ray, CA)
          (b) Australian melaleuca oil (very beneficial for patients who have had chemotherapy or radiation therapy to the vaginal tissue)
          (c) Oil from vitamin E softgels or suppositories
        (3) Use of strategies that promote the flexibility of the vagina (e.g., regular intercourse, vaginal dilator [see Chapter 82]), improve muscle tone and circulation, decrease the chance of atrophy, and help to maintain the acidic pH of the vagina, thus reducing the risk of vaginal and bladder infections.
        (4) Use strategies that help to improve muscular and vascular tone of the vaginal tissue (e.g., regular Kegel exercises).
      d) Poor sleep
        (1) Do regular aerobic exercise.
        (2) Use of stress management techniques (e.g., meditation, yoga, visualization) that have been shown through research to improve sleep in women who are going through menopause or having difficulty sleeping.
        (3) Avoid alcohol.
        (4) Avoid or decrease intake of caffeine, especially late in the day.
        (5) Eat a light dinner.
  D. Insomnia, irritability, headache, anxiety, and memory problems: Hormone therapy (see Tables 151-1–151-6) and/or stress management techniques, regular aerobic exercise, and mental gymnastics strategies (e.g., crossword puzzles, word games).
  E. Dysphoric mood: Estrogen therapy, herbal therapy (e.g., St. John's wort 2–4 g/day); if no response in four to six weeks, switch to another therapy.
  F. Clinical depression: Antidepressant (e.g., fluoxetine hydrochloride, sertraline hydrochloride, amitriptyline pamoate, bupropion hydrochloride [see Appendix 2])
  G. Calcium supplementation
    1. Postmenopausal women: 1,500 mg/day
    2. Postmenopausal women taking hormone therapy: 1,000 mg/day
    3. Patient should take vitamin D 400 IU/day to promote calcium absorption.

VII. Follow-up
  A. Short-term: Reevaluate in one to three months for effectiveness of treatment, adequate hormonal serum levels, or any side effects.

    B. Long-term: Annual follow-up, including periodic Pap smears and/or endometrial biopsies to rule out pathology, or if any abnormal bleeding

VIII. Referrals
    A. Gynecologist or reproductive endocrinologist: For women who do not respond to initial treatment, have severe symptoms, have continued abnormal bleeding, or require a dilatation and curettage
    B. Internist or endocrinologist: For evaluation of medical conditions
    C. Psychiatric nurse, psychiatrist, or psychologist: To distinguish between mood disturbance, clinical depression, and psychiatric illness

References

Bluming, A. (1993). Hormone replacement therapy: Benefits and risks for the general postmenopausal female population and for women with a history of previously treated breast cancer. *Seminars in Oncology, 20,* 662–674.

Coldite, G. (1998). Relationship between estrogen levels, use of hormone replacement therapy, and breast cancer. *Journal of the National Cancer Institute, 90,* 814–823.

Glisson, J., Crawford, R., & Street, S. (1998). Review, critique, and guidelines for the use of herbs and homeopathy. *Nurse Practitioner, 24*(4), 44, 46, 53, 60, 65–67.

Hammond, C. (1997). Management of menopause. *American Family Physician, 55,* 1667–1674, 1679–1680.

Hargrove, J., & Eisenberg, E. (1995). Menopause. *Medical Clinics of North America, 79,* 1337–1356.

Knobf, M.T. (1998). Natural menopause and ovarian toxicity associated with breast cancer therapy. *Oncology Nursing Forum, 25,* 1519–1530.

Lockhart, J.S., & Mahon, S.M. (1998). Case in point… commentary: Counseling about hormone replacement therapy. *Oncology Nursing Forum, 25,* 663–664.

Love, S., & Lindsey, K. (1997). *Dr. Susan Love's hormone book.* New York: Random House.

Mayer, D., & Linscott, E. (1995). Information for women: Management of menopausal symptoms. *Oncology Nursing Forum, 22,* 1567–1570.

Myrkies, A., Wilcox, G., & Davis, S. (1998). Clinical review 92: Phytoestrogens. *Journal of Clinical Endocrinology and Metabolism, 83,* 297–303.

Snyder, G.M., Sielsch, E.C., & Reville, B. (1998). The controversy of hormone replacement therapy in breast cancer survivors. *Oncology Nursing Forum, 25,* 699–706.

Speroff, L., Glass, R., & Kase, N. (1994). *Clinical gynecologic endocrinology and infertility* (5th ed.). Baltimore: Williams & Wilkins.

Stone, A., & Pearlstein, T. (1994). Evaluation and treatment of changes in mood, sleep, and sexual functioning associated with menopause. *Obstetrics and Gynecology Clinics of North America, 21,* 391–398.

Wich, B., & Carnes, M. (1995). Menopause and the aging female reproductive system. *Endocrinology and Metabolism Clinics of North America, 24,* 273–295.

Woods, N. (1996). Cancer risk controversies: Women's exposure to exogenous ovarian hormones. *Oncology Nursing Updates Patient Treatment and Support, 3*(1), 1–16.

Section XIII. Miscellaneous

Symptoms

Medical Diagnosis

Chapter

152. Anxiety

Barbara St. Marie, RN, MA, CNP, ANP, GNP

I. Definition: Dominant psychophysiologic state of worry, autonomic hyperactivity, muscle tension, and hypervigilance

II. Pathophysiology: Anxiety is triggered by activation of the sympathetic nervous system, which involves
   A. The release of norepinephrine, creating a fight-or-flight response
   B. Serotonin interacting with numerous receptor subtypes on different types of neurons, creating various psychobiologic functions that can be disruptive.

III. Clinical features
   A. Etiology: Causes of release of norepinephrine are
      1. Situational and emotional stresses
      2. Medications
      3. Hereditary factors
      4. Substance use (e.g., cocaine, amphetamines, caffeine)
      5. Uncontrolled pain
      6. Metabolic dysfunction.
   B. History: Observations of the patient's presentation will guide the diagnosis.
      1. History of cancer and cancer treatment
      2. History of presenting symptom(s): Precipitating factors, onset, and duration. Associated symptoms are difficulty concentrating, irritability, and insomnia.
      3. Current medications: Prescribed and over-the-counter
      4. Changes in activities of daily living
      5. Past medical history: Anxiety, panic attacks, mental illness, hyperthyroidism, pheochromocytoma, diabetes mellitus
      6. Social history: Use of illicit drugs, alcohol, tobacco, and caffeine; quality of support systems
   C. Signs and symptoms of the most common anxiety disorders seen in primary care (see Figure 152-1)
   D. Physical exam
      1. Behavior observation
      2. Vital signs: To detect hypertension and tachycardia
      3. Neck exam: Palpate thyroid gland for nodules or enlargement

Figure 152-1. Signs and Symptoms of Anxiety Disorders

Generalized Anxiety Disorder	Panic Attack	Obsessive-Compulsive Disorder
• Excessive worry and anxiety about numerous events • Anxiety that occurs >50% of the time for at least six months • Difficulty in controlling worry • At least three of the following symptoms: - Restlessness - Fatigue - Difficulty concentrating - Irritability - Muscle tension - Sleep disturbance	• Brief episode of somatic complaints, including emotional discomfort and intense fear, that peaks within 10 minutes • At least four of the following symptoms: - Palpitations - Sweating - Trembling or shaking - Shortness of breath - Feeling of choking - Chest pain/discomfort - Nausea or abdominal distress - Dizziness, unsteadiness - Feelings of unreality or being detached from oneself - Fear of losing control - Fear of dying - Paresthesias - Chills or hot flashes	• Repeated, intrusive, and irrational thoughts • Repetitive behaviors or mental acts that consume much time such as - Constant tapping of fingers or feet - Obsessed with completing projects - Lip smacking

    4. Cardiac: To rule out dysrhythmia

    5. Pulmonary exam: To assess for abnormalities (e.g., decreased air exchange or dullness indicating pneumonia, plural effusion) or for other pulmonary diseases.

IV. Diagnostic studies: Review systems and physical exam findings to determine necessary laboratory testing.

    A. Laboratory

        1. Thyroid-stimulating hormone (TSH) test to detect hypothyroidism

        2. Glucose test to detect hypoglycemia

        3. Drug screens to detect substance abuse

    B. Radiology: Not indicated

V. Differential diagnosis

    A. Endocrine disease

        1. Hypoglycemia secondary to insulin reaction or pituitary dysfunction

        2. Hyperthyroidism (see Chapter 149)

    B. Cardiac dysrhythmia (see Chapter 43)

        1. Atrial fibrillation

        2. Premature ventricular contractions

    C. Pheochromocytoma: Rare occurrence

    D. Stress (situational or long-standing)

    E. Cardiopulmonary disease

    F. Abuse or withdrawal from substances (e.g., alcohol, caffeine, sedative-hypnotic drugs, tobacco)

G. Medications
  1. Decongestants
  2. Bronchodilators (e.g., theophylline, Ventolin® [Glaxo Wellcome Inc., Research Triangle Park, NC])
  3. Thyroid hormone
  4. Steroids
  5. Xanthine-containing drugs
H. Uncontrolled symptoms
  1. Pain
  2. Insomnia
  3. Dyspnea (see Chapter 23)

VI. Treatment
  A. Pharmacologic treatment: Antidepressants and anxiolytic medications are used to treat anxiety disorders (see Table 152-1).
    1. Some depressed patients with symptoms of anxiety may benefit from coadministration of a benzodiazepine and a selective serotonin re-uptake inhibitor (SSRI) at the initiation of treatment. After three weeks, the benzodiazepine should be discontinued, while continuing the SSRI.
    2. Withdrawal from benzodiazepine can be prevented by slowly tapering drug doses. Abrupt withdrawal may cause insomnia, irritability, muscle spasms, and seizures. The withdrawal rate depends on the half life of the drug. Gradual taper is recommended for individuals who have been on therapeutic doses for several months.
    3. Tricyclic antidepressants and SSRIs must be taken for one to six weeks to achieve a therapeutic effect; anxiolytic agents require one to two weeks before reaching full therapeutic effect.
  B. Nonpharmacologic treatment
    1. Encourage support from family, friends, and significant others.

Table 152-1. Effectiveness of Drugs Used to Treat Anxiety Disorders

Anxiety Disorder	SSRIs[a]	TCAs[b]	Anxiolytics	Atypical Antidepressants
Depression with symptoms of anxiety	Strong	Strong	Limited	Moderate
Generalized anxiety disorder	None	Strong	Moderate	None
Panic disorder	Strong	Strong	Strong (e.g., benzodiazepine)	Limited
Obsessive compulsive disorder	Strong	Strong (e.g., clomipramine)	Strong (buspirone)	None

[a] SSRI: selective serotonin re-uptake inhibitor
[b] TCA: tricyclic antidepressant

2. Provide patient education.
3. Offer psychotherapy, counseling, or support groups to allow expression of feelings and to provide reassurance.

VII. Follow-up
   A. One week after initiation of medication, the patient should be assessed for compliance and side effects and to offer encouragement.
   B. The patient should be reassessed three weeks later to assess response to medication.
   C. If patient is suicidal, he or she should be immediately triaged into mental health care or admitted to the hospital for close observation.

VIII. Referrals: Refer patient to counselor, psychologist, or psychiatrist for psychotherapy.

References

Black, D.W., Wesner, R., Bowers, W., & Gabel, J.A. (1993). Comparison of fluvoxamine, cognitive therapy, and placebo in the treatment of panic disorder. *Archives of General Psychiatry, 50,* 44–50.

Clark, D.A., Beck, A.T., & Beck, J.S. (1994). Symptom differences in major depression, dysthymia, panic disorder, and generalized anxiety disorder. *American Journal of Psychiatry, 151,* 205–209.

Coplan, J.D., Gorman, J.M., & Klein, D.F. (1992). Serotonin related functions in panic-anxiety: A critical overview. *Neuropsychopharmacology, 6,* 189–200.

Oehrberg, S., Christiansen, P.E., Behnke, K., Borup, A.L., Severin, B., Soegaard, J., Calberg, H., Judge, R., Ohrstrom, J.K., & Mannicher, P.M. (1995). Paroxetine in the treatment of panic disorder: A randomised, double blind, placebo-controlled study. *British Journal of Psychiatry, 167,* 374–379.

Pasacreta, J.V., & Pickett, M. (1998). Psychosocial aspects of palliative care. *Seminars in Oncology Nursing, 14,* 110–120.

Segar, M.L., Katch, V.L., Roth, R.S., Garcia, A.W., Portner, T.I., Glickman, S.G., Haslanger, S., & Wilkins, E.G. (1998). The effect of aerobic exercise on self-esteem and depressive and anxiety symptoms among breast cancer survivors. *Oncology Nursing Forum, 25,* 107–113.

153. Breast Tenderness/Nipple Discharge/Swelling/Lumps

Joanne Lester, MSN, RNC, OCN®, CNP

I. Definition: Often termed fibrocystic disease, a normal pattern of breast tissue changes

II. Physiology/Pathophysiology
   A. Normal
      1. Normally, breasts are tear-shaped with breast tissue extending from the clavicle to the ribs (second to the sixth) below the breast and from the midsternal line across to the midaxillary line.
      2. Breasts are composed of glandular tissue with a complex ductal system, lobules, and acini, adipose tissue, and connective fibrous tissue with suspensory ligaments and underlying fascia support.
         a) The percentage and composition of these tissues vary across a woman's life span, nutritional status, hereditary tendencies, and hormonal influences.
         b) Variations in breast tissue are related to hormonal influences (exogenous and endogenous) and are linked to
            (1) Estradiol stimulating proliferation of epithelial cells and increasing periductal vascularity
            (2) Progesterone inducing development of acini and opposing mesenchymal action of estrogen.
   B. Pathophysiology: Physiologic responses occur in epithelial, ductal, mesenchymal, and parenchymal tissues from endogenous and exogenous hormonal influences.

III. Clinical features
   A. Etiology
      1. Breast tenderness or swelling is often related to stromal edema, engorged breast ductal and parenchymal tissue (from lactation or hormonal influences [e.g., pregnancy]), menstrual cycle changes, exogenous hormone therapy, inflammatory changes, and nerve ending irritation.
      2. Nipple discharge may be caused by endogenous or exogenous hormonal influences (e.g., breastfeeding, pregnancy), changes in pituitary regulation, trauma, malignancy, or irritating ductal papillomatosis.
      3. Breast lumps may be benign in nature, caused by fatty deposits (lipoma), proliferative epithelial or mesenchymal tissue (fibroadenoma), collections of fluid (cyst), injury

(scar tissue or hematoma), or infection; or may be malignant in nature, caused by cancerous changes in the ductal, epithelial, or lobular tissues.

4. Etiology of symptoms may be related to ingestion of caffeine products, foods containing methylxanthine, and certain medications (commonly exogenous hormones).

B. History
   1. History of cancer and cancer treatment
   2. History of presenting symptom(s): Precipitating event, location, and duration
   3. Current medications: Prescribed and over-the-counter
   4. Changes in activities of daily living
   5. History of menstrual cycle: Age of menarche, age of premenopausal symptoms, age of menopause, recent changes in timing and characteristics of cycle, current timing of cycle
   6. History of pregnancies: Age of first pregnancy and/or first term pregnancy, number of pregnancies, breastfeeding history
   7. History of exogenous hormones (e.g., birth control pills, estrogen replacement, progesterone, fertility drugs)
   8. Family history: Fibrocystic disease, breast or ovarian cancer (including age of onset, lineage, laterality), and endogenous hormonal history of mother and female siblings
   9. Social history: Caffeine intake (e.g., coffee, tea, chocolate, cola products), sodium intake, alcohol use, and current diet
   10. Past medical history: Breast biopsy, self-breast examination, mammography and clinical breast exam

C. Signs and symptoms
   1. Breast tenderness/mastalgia
   2. Breast lumps
   3. Breast discharge
   4. Breast swelling
   5. Erythema
   6. Dimpling

D. Physical exam
   1. Visual exam with patient in sitting position and hands on hips, noting symmetry and contours of breast, skin changes (e.g., dimpling, retraction, erythema, nipple scaling), venous patterns, scars, and nipple position
   2. Lymph node exam, including anterior, central, and posterior axillary nodes; and supraclavicular and infraclavicular nodes
   3. Complete breast exam with patient in supine position with arms extended overhead to evaluate for masses and nodules, noting location by quadrant, centimeters from nipple borders, size, shape, mobility, consistency, and tenderness

IV. Diagnostic studies
   A. Laboratory
      1. Prolactin serum level for bilateral nipple discharge of unknown etiology to rule out pituitary disorder
      2. Tissue sampling

a) Fine-needle aspiration (FNA): With cytological examination

b) Core-needle biopsy: With pathological examination

c) Excisional biopsy: With pathological examination; must be performed for a definitive diagnosis of malignancy if a less invasive method of tissue sampling is done (e.g., FNA, core needle biopsy) with negative results and a high clinical suspicion exists.

B. Radiology: Mammogram must be done prior to FNA, otherwise local edema will obscure view.

1. Mammography guidelines

a) Asymptomatic woman without personal or significant family history of breast cancer: Yearly age 40 and after

b) Asymptomatic woman with personal history of breast cancer: Yearly, regardless of age

c) Asymptomatic woman with significant family history of breast cancer: Yearly at 10 years within the age of an immediate premenopausal family member's breast cancer diagnosis or yearly at age 35–40 if familial onset of breast cancer was postmenopausal (e.g., if mother is diagnosed with breast cancer at age 30, daughters should begin having yearly mammograms at age 20.)

d) Symptomatic woman with/without palpable lump: If aspiration or biopsy results show significant symptoms, obtain baseline prior to age 40. If malignancy exists, obtain current bilateral mammogram regardless of age.

2. Ultrasound guidelines (used to differentiate solid versus cystic/fluid-filled masses)

a) Symptomatic woman with palpable lump or spontaneous, unilateral nipple discharge: Obtain focused ultrasound on area of concern.

b) Ultrasound indicating solid mass: Consider tissue biopsy (an excisional biopsy must be performed to rule out malignancy).

c) Ultrasound indicating cystic mass: Consider FNA (an excisional biopsy must be performed to rule out malignancy).

d) Asymptomatic woman: No study necessary.

3. Nuclear medicine studies (used after consultation with a breast surgeon to further differentiate breast abnormalities and to help identify potential areas to biopsy)

a) Sestamibi scan

b) MRI

C. Other

1. Blood in nipple discharge: Hemoccult study

2. Breast malignancy: Further workup indicated according to stage of disease and presence or absence of symptoms

V. Differential diagnosis

A. Breast tenderness/mastalgia

1. Fibrocystic breast tissue

2. Underlying mass or malignancy

3. Effects of intake of caffeine, methylxanthine foods, or sodium

4. Effects of endogenous or exogenous hormones

5. Trauma or injury

      6. Inflammation or infection
- B. Breast lumps/masses
  1. Fibrocystic changes
  2. Fibroadenoma
  3. Cyst
  4. Hematoma
  5. Scar formation
  6. Infection, abscess
  7. Pseudolump (e.g., a rib)
  8. Malignancy
- C. Nipple discharge
  1. Fibrocystic changes
  2. Intraductal papilloma
  3. Mechanical stimulation
  4. Lactational changes
  5. Hormonal imbalance
  6. Pituitary disorder
  7. Inflammation, infection
  8. Malignancy
  9. Duct ectasia
- D. Breast swelling
  1. Fibrocystic changes
  2. Trauma, injury
  3. Endogenous or exogenous hormonal influence
  4. Fluid or sodium retention
  5. Inflammation, infection
  6. Malignancy

VI. Treatment
- A. Breast tenderness/mastalgia
  1. Decrease or eliminate exogenous hormones; regulate endogenous hormones (e.g., oral contraceptives).
  2. Wear supportive or sports bra.
  3. Take 400 units of vitamin E twice daily.
  4. Decrease or eliminate caffeine products.
  5. Decrease or eliminate sodium intake.
  6. Use mild diuretic, especially when premenstrual.
  7. Use analgesics (e.g., NSAIDs) (see Appendix 11).
  8. Apply heat or ice.
- B. Breast lumps/masses
  1. Decrease or eliminate exogenous hormones; regulate endogenous hormones.
  2. Undergo aspiration of cystic masses to verify presence of fluid and relieve tenderness.
  3. Undergo surgical excision of solid mass (e.g., lipoma near the bra line) to relieve tenderness.

      4. Appropriate treatment of infection, if indicated.
         a) Apply moist heat to the area four times a day.
         b) Use broad-spectrum antibiotic to cover most common organism or staphylococci or streptococci (see Appendix 1).
         c) Continuously wear supportive or sports bra.

  C. Nipple discharge
      1. Decrease or eliminate exogenous hormones; regulate endogenous hormones.
      2. Continuously wear supportive or sports bra.
      3. Undergo surgical ductal excision.
      4. Eliminate mechanical stimulation.

  D. Breast swelling
      1. Decrease or eliminate exogenous hormones; regulate endogenous hormones.
      2. Continuously wear supportive or sports bra.
      3. Use mild, potassium-sparing diuretic, especially when premenopausal.
      4. Appropriately treat infection, if indicated.
      5. Apply heat or ice, depending on etiology.
      6. Decrease or eliminate sodium intake.

VII. Follow-up
  A. Short-term follow-up should be done within two to three months of initial contact, depending on etiology and severity of problem. Treatment for infectious processes should be followed within one to two weeks.
  B. Long-term follow-up depends on the etiology and severity of the problem. All patients should be examined on an annual basis and, depending on age, undergo a mammogram.

VIII. Referrals
  A. Patients who improve significantly or spontaneously resolve (without evidence of underlying disease) generally do not require a physician referral.
  B. Patients with persistent symptoms, palpable mass, bloody nipple discharge, persistent infection, skin changes, nipple retraction, or evidence of malignancy should be immediately referred to a surgeon.

References

Barton, M.B., Elmore, J.G., & Fletcher, S.W. (1999). Breast symptoms among women enrolled in a health maintenance organization: Frequency, evaluation, and outcome. *Annals of Internal Medicine, 130,* 651–657.

Cady, B., Steele, Jr., G.D., Morrow, M., Gardner, B., Smith, B.L., Lee, N.C., Lawson, H.W., & Winchester, D.P. (1998). Evaluation of common breast problems: Guidance for primary care providers. *CA: A Cancer Journal for Clinicians, 48*(1), 49–64.

Lee, C.H., Philpotts, L.E., Horvath, L.J., & Tocino, I. (1999). Follow-up of breast lesions diagnosed as benign with stereotactic core-needle biopsy: Frequency of mammographic change and false-negative rate. *Radiology, 212,* 189–194.

Shapiro, T.J., Clark, P.M. (1995). Breast cancer: What the primary care provider needs to know. *Nurse Practitioner, 20*(3), 36–53.

Chapter

154.

Depression
Barbara St. Marie, RN, MA, CNP, ANP, GNP

I. Definition
   A. Major depression: A sustained alteration in mood, self-attitude, and vital sense
   B. Dysthymic disorder: A nonmajor depressive disorder characterized by a depressed mood continuing for at least two years
   C. Atypical depression: Includes major and dysthymic depression
   D. Situational depression: A depressive disorder that occurs because of current circumstances

II. Pathophysiology: Theories suggest a diminished catecholaminergic and serotonergic neurotransmission.

III. Clinical features
   A. Etiologies: Causes of decreased neurotransmitters are
      1. Medications
      2. Hereditary factors
      3. Substance abuse
      4. Sedentary lifestyle
      5. Situational and emotional stresses
      6. Presence of pain or other symptoms
      7. Metabolic impairment
      8. Cancer or chronic disease diagnosis.
   B. History: Careful evaluation of the patient's history and observation of the patient's presentation will guide the diagnosis of depression.
      1. History of cancer and cancer treatment
      2. Current medications: Prescribed and over-the-counter
      3. History of presenting symptom(s): Precipitating factors, onset, and duration. Associated symptoms are sadness, teariness, insomnia, change in appetite, and suicidal tendencies.
      4. Changes in activities of daily living
      5. Social history: Use of tobacco, alcohol, illicit drugs
      6. Family history: Depression, psychiatric illness
      7. Past medical history: Depression, psychiatric illness, myocardial infarction, surgical procedures, recent body image changes, hypothyroidism, Cushing's disease, Addison's disease, diabetes mellitus

C. Signs and symptoms (see Figure 154-1)
D. Physical exam: Nonspecific and usually objective in nature; several validated depression scales (e.g., Beck Depression Inventory, Zung Self-Rating Depression Scale) are helpful
  1. General observation
    a) Depressed mood
    b) Slow or agitated movements
    c) Injuries through falls, self-infliction, or physical abuse
    d) Alcohol odor on breath
    e) Impaired senses (e.g., hearing, vision), especially in elderly patients
    f) Pain and impaired function
  2. Cardiac examination to rule out dysrhythmia or new onset coronary artery disease

IV. Diagnostic studies
  A. Laboratory
    1. Thyroid-stimulating hormone (TSH) for detection of hypothyroidism
    2. Glucose (random or fasting) for detection of diabetes mellitus
    3. Hemoglobin for detection of anemia
    4. Syphilis (in elderly) or HIV for detection of disease
  B. Radiology: Not indicated

V. Differential diagnosis
  A. Bipolar mood disorder
  B. Neurologic disorders
    1. Dementia

Figure 154-1. Symptoms of Depression

Major Depression	Dysthymic Disorder	Atypical Depression
• >5% change in body weight	• Low self-esteem or self-confidence; feelings of inadequacy	• Includes major and dysthymic depressive symptoms such as:
• Change in appetite	• Feelings of pessimism, despair, hopelessness	- Hypersomnia
• Insomnia or hypersomnia		- Overeating
• Psychomotor agitation or retardation	• General loss of interest or pleasure	- Lethargy
• Fatigue or loss of energy	• Social withdrawal	- Changes in self-attitude
• Feelings of worthlessness or inappropriate guilt	• Chronic fatigue or tiredness	- Fatigue
• Diminished concentration or indecisiveness	• Feelings of guilt, brooding about the past	- Emotional numbness
• Recurrent thoughts of death or suicide	• Subjective feelings or irritability; excessive anger	- Panic attacks during depressive episodes
• Multiple somatic complaints	• Decreased activity, effectiveness, or productivity	- Seasonal depression
• Unaffected reaction to environment	• Difficulty in thinking reflected by poor concentration, poor memory, or indecisiveness	- May be seen with bipolar disorders

      2. Cerebral vascular accident

      3. Parkinson's disease

      4. Multiple sclerosis

      5. Temporal lobe epilepsy

  C. Endocrine disease

      1. Diabetes mellitus (see Chapter 143)

      2. Hypothyroid disease (see Chapter 150)

      3. Cushing's disease

      4. Addison's disease

  D. Infectious or inflammatory illness

  E. Stress

  F. Cardiopulmonary disease

  G. Cancer

  H. Head injury

   I. Folate, B_{12}, or thiamine deficiency (see Chapter 114)

   J. Examples of medication-induced

      1. Antihypertensive drugs (e.g., clonidine, methyldopa, reserpine, beta-blockers, diltiazem)

      2. Steroids

      3. Digitalis

      4. H_2 blockers (e.g., cimetidine, ranitidine)

      5. Isoniazid

      6. Neuroleptic drugs

      7. Multiphasic oral contraceptives

      8. Sedative-hypnotic drugs

  K. Withdrawal from abused substances (i.e., alcohol, cocaine, sedatives, anxiolytics, hypnotics, amphetamines)

  L. Uncontrolled symptoms

      1. Pain

      2. Nausea (see Chapter 59)

      3. Insomnia

VI. Treatment

  A. Treatment considerations include pharmacologic and/or nonpharmacologic interventions (i.e., psychotherapy). Factors to consider in deciding treatment are severity of symptoms, presence of psychosocial stressors, and presence of comorbid conditions.

  B. Pharmacologic treatment (see Appendix 2)

      1. Selective serotonin reuptake inhibitors (SSRIs) and/or tricyclic antidepressants (TCAs) are 90% effective in treating major depression and are recommended as the first-line treatment for moderate-to-severe depression. Several categories of antidepressants can be used. Table 154-1 provides examples of these agents.

         a) TCAs have been in clinical use for four decades. Prototypical drugs are imipramine and amitriptyline as mixed norepinephrine and serotonin uptake inhibitors. These agents demonstrate varying degrees of selectivity for the reuptake pumps for norepinephrine and serotonin with numerous autonomic actions.

Table 154-1. Drug Examples Used in Antidepressant Therapy

SSRI/TCA	Half-Life	Starting Dose	Maximum Dose	Patients > 65 Starting Dose	Patients > 65 Maximum Dose
Paroxetine (Paxil[®a])	24 hours	20 mg	50 mg	10 mg	40 mg
Sertraline (Zoloft[®b])	22–35 hours	50 mg	200 mg	25 mg	50 mg
Fluoxetine (Prozac[®c])	1–3 days after acute adminis-tration; 4–6 days after chronic admin-istration	20 mg	80 mg	5 mg	20 mg
Trazodone (Desyrel[®d])	8 hours	150 mg	600 mg	50 mg	150 mg
Nortriptyline (Pamelor[®e])	18–93 hours	25 mg	150 mg	10 mg	75 mg
Amitriptyline (Elavil[®f])	31–46 hours	25 mg	200 mg	5 mg	100 mg
Desipramine (Norpramin[®g])	73–96 hours	50 mg	200 mg	10 mg	75 mg

[a] SmithKline Beecham Pharmaceuticals, Philadelphia, PA; [b] Pfizer Inc., New York, NY; [c] Dista Products Company, a division of Eli Lilly & Company, Indianapolis, IN; [d] Apothecon, a division of Bristol-Myers Squibb Company, Princeton, NJ, [e] Novartis Pharmaceuticals Corporation, East Hanover, NJ; [f] AstraZeneca, Wilmington, DE; [g] Hoechst Marion Roussel, Kansas City, MO.

b) Heterocyclics, second- and third-generation antidepressants, are similar to the tricyclic agents.

c) SSRIs are unlike the tricyclic and heterocyclic agents in mechanism of action, having fewer toxicities but possibly causing nausea, decreased libido, and decreased sexual function.

d) Monoamine oxidase (MAO) inhibitors: MAO-A is the amine oxidase primarily responsible for norepinephrine, serotonin, and tyramine metabolism. MAO-B is more selective for dopamine and, thus, is most useful in the treatment of Parkinson's disease.

2. Dosages: Usual daily dose ranges are determined by the patient's acceptance of adverse effects (see Table 154-2)

a) Starting doses are usually small and increased to a predetermined daily dose that produces relief of depression or to the maximum tolerated dose.

b) Tricyclics may vary from a starting dose of 10 mg to 75 mg, depending upon the patient's size and tolerance of acute effects. Hospitalized patients could begin around 100 mg. After two to three days at this level, doses may be increased in increments of 25 mg every two to three days until a maintenance daily dose of 150 mg is reached. For patients who do not respond, the maximum dose could be increased to 300 mg.

c) Heterocyclic drugs and SSRIs (e.g., bupropion, venlafaxine, nefazodone) require divided doses during the day for the first few weeks, beginning with a dosage of 20 mg per day.

Table 154-2. Managing Side Effects of Antidepressant Therapy

Side Effect	Methods of Managing Side Effects
Headache	Eliminate caffeine; reduce dose; take analgesics.
Nausea	Take with food and large glass of water; reduce dose.
Insomnia	Take in morning; reduce dose; add sleep aid.
Orthostatic hypotension	Rise slowly from reclining or seated position; sit down if light-headedness occurs; maintain ample fluid intake; reduce dose.
Constipation	Increase fluid intake, exercise, and fiber intake; use stool softeners and bulk-forming agents.
Dry mouth	Use sugar-free candy or gum; maintain fluid intake.
Appetite stimulation and weight gain	Exclude concurrent eating disorder or depressive relapse; prescribe exercise and nutritional counseling; reduce dose; switch medications.
Sedation	Take medication at night; reduce dose.
Activation or treatment of emergent anxiety	Reduce dose; switch medications.

     C. Nonpharmacologic treatment
        1. Family support
        2. Patient education, support, reassurance
        3. Psychotherapy

VII. Follow-up
    A. See patient one week after starting antidepressant to assess compliance and side effects and to offer encouragement. Monitoring plasma concentration of antidepressant agents has uncertain value.
    B. See patient again in three weeks to assess response to medication. The patient is asked to self-assess feelings of well-being and improvement in symptoms (e.g., insomnia, appetite, anxiety).
    C. If patient is suicidal, immediately triage into mental health care or admit to hospital for close observation.
    D. After dosage is stable, monthly follow-up is important to maintain contact and support.
    E. The majority of patients with one episode of depression will have a recurrence within five years. Studies show that one year of maintenance therapy helps to prevent recurrences and that risk of relapse is greatest in the first two months after discontinuing medication. Individuals treated less than four months after response to medication have a higher incidence of relapse.

VIII. Referrals
    A. For patients with moderate-to-severe depression, refer to a counselor, psychologist, or psychiatrist.

    B. For patients with suicidal intent, hospitalize and/or enforce involuntary commitment with psychiatric intervention to provide short-term protection.

    C. For patients who respond poorly to medication, refer to a psychiatrist.

References

Newport, D.J., & Nemeroff, C.B. (1998). Assessment and treatment of depression in the cancer patient. *Journal of Psychosomatic Research, 45,* 215–237.

Passik, S.D., Dugan, W., McDonald M.V., Rosenfeld, B., Theobald, D.E., & Edgerton, S. (1998). Oncologists' recognition of depression in their patients with cancer. *Journal of Clinical Oncology, 16,* 1594–1600.

Payne, D.K., Hoffman, R.G., Teodoulou, M., Dosik, M., & Massie, M.J. (1999). Screening for anxiety and depression in women with breast cancer. Psychiatry and medical oncology gear up for managed care. *Psychosomatics, 40*(1), 64–69.

Schwenk, T.L. (1998). Cancer and depression. *Primary Care, 25,* 505–513.

Twillman, R.K., & Manetto, C. (1998). Concurrent psychotherapy and pharmacotherapy in the treatment of depression and anxiety in cancer patients. *Psychooncology, 7*(4), 285–290.

Valente, S.M., & Saunders, J.M. (1997). Diagnosis and treatment of major depression among people with cancer. *Cancer Nursing, 20,* 168–177.

Visser, M.R., & Smets, E.M. (1998). Fatigue, depression, and quality of life in cancer patients: How are they related? *Supportive Care in Cancer, 6*(2), 101–108.

Chapter

155. Fatigue

Lillian M. Nail, PhD, RN, FAAN

I. Definition: Self-perceived sensation of tiredness

II. Pathophysiology: Exact pathophysiology not known

III. Clinical features: Patterns of fatigue must be correlated with symptoms, laboratory data, physical exam findings, and life demands/activities to diagnose cause.
  A. Etiology
    1. As a symptom or result of cancer
      a) Not present in all patients with advanced disease; not seen at presentation in most early-stage malignancies
      b) Multiple mechanisms suggested and multiple etiologies likely in patients with advanced disease
        (1) Cachexia
        (2) Endocrine effects when tumor secretes hormones or interferes with normal endocrine function
        (3) Hypoxia as a result of circulatory or respiratory impairment
        (4) Anemia
          (a) Vessel erosion (e.g., colon cancer, gastric cancer, cervical cancer)
          (b) Bone marrow involvement
          (c) Liver involvement
          (d) Inadequate intake or absorption of protein, iron, or folic acid
          (e) Induction of chemotherapy or radiation therapy
        (5) Renal involvement (may interfere with erythropoietin production)
        (6) CNS involvement
        (7) Fluid/electrolyte imbalance
        (8) Infection
        (9) Liver involvement
        (10) Pain
        (11) Heightened immune system activity in response to tumor
    2. As a side effect of cancer treatment (prevalence >70%)

       a) Bolus chemotherapy-induced fatigue: Peaks within a few days after treatment and gradually declines to lowest point occurring at the next treatment

       b) Chemotherapy-induced anemia

       c) Steroid-induced muscle mass loss (prednisone, dexamethasone)

       d) Muscle mass loss/deconditioning (as a result of decreased physical activity)

       e) Decreased endocrine function related to surgery, radiation, or chemotherapy

       f) Cytokines (e.g., interferon, interleukin)

       g) Sleep disruption

       h) Changes in neurotransmitters

       i) Fluid/electrolyte imbalance

       j) Inadequate nutrition

       k) Infection

       l) Neuropathy

       m) Radiation therapy-induced fatigue: Occurs during the second or third week of treatment, peaks near the end of treatment, and gradually declines, most dramatically in the first four weeks post-treatment

   3. Comorbid factors

       a) Cardiac disease

       b) Respiratory disease

       c) Neuromuscular disease (e.g., multiple sclerosis, post-polio syndrome)

       d) Disorders of the immune system (e.g., rheumatoid arthritis, lupus)

       e) Clinical depression or anxiety

       f) Chronic fatigue syndrome

       g) Pregnancy

       h) Anemia

       i) Bleeding unrelated to cancer or cancer treatment

       j) Hormone deficiencies unrelated to cancer or cancer treatment

       k) Hormone excesses unrelated to cancer or cancer treatment

       l) Side effects of medications (e.g., opioids, sedatives, hypnotics, histamine blockers)

       m) Acute or chronic renal failure

       n) Liver problems (e.g., cirrhosis, hepatitis)

       o) Infection unrelated to cancer or cancer treatment

B. History

   1. History of cancer and cancer treatment: Assess patient self-report adjusting timing to type and pattern of treatment; use as cornerstone

   2. Current medications: Prescribed and over-the-counter

   3. History of presenting symptom(s): Precipitating factors, onset, and duration. Associated symptoms are sleep disturbances, continual sadness, and loss of appetite. Direct questions to relevant time frames and assess usual and highest levels of fatigue, as experienced by the patient, using a scale of 1–10 (lowest to highest level of fatigue).

   4. Changes in activities of daily living: Focus on impact of rather than decrease in performing activities.

     5. Past medical history: Depression, comorbid diseases

     6. Family history: Depression or recent losses

C. Signs and symptoms

     1. Cognitive ability

        a) Difficulty concentrating and processing information

        b) Short-term memory loss

        c) Speech difficulty (e.g., problems with finding, combining words)

     2. Activity

        a) Change in activity resulting from cancer treatment

        b) Decrease in discretionary activities (e.g., recreation, pastimes) likely before activities of daily living. A cognitive process is involved in decisions about activity; fatigue does not necessarily result in decreased activity.

     3. Role function

        a) Change in work, play, or study habits

        b) Decline in family interaction

        c) Change in community volunteer activities

        d) Shift in social interaction (i.e., using telephone rather than visiting)

     4. Affect

        a) Normal transient sadness reflecting patient feeling "out of sorts"

        b) Normal grieving process triggered by patient feeling loss of function as a result of fatigue

        c) Use of synonymous terms (e.g., weary, sluggish, dragged-out, heavy limbs, slow, tired)

D. Physical exam: None specific to treatment-related fatigue, but focus on identifying abnormalities that point to specific etiologic factors

     1. Neurologic exam: Assess mental status, cranial nerves, balance, coordination, sensation, and reflexes to evaluate for brain metastases, brain tumor, spinal cord compression, or neuropathy.

     2. HEENT exam: Assess mouth or throat lesions, enlarged thyroid, unusual discharge from throat or sinuses, and fluid or discharge in ears to evaluate for hypothyroidism, sinusitis, and infection.

     3. Musculoskeletal exam: Evaluate for focal or generalized weakness, muscle mass loss, joint pain, warm or edematous joints, muscle pain, muscle twitching, new limitations in range of motion, bone pain indicating arthritis, bone metastases, or fibromyalgia.

     4. Respiratory exam: Evaluate for adventitious sounds that may indicate pulmonary edema, chronic obstructive disease, or pneumonia.

     5. Cardiac exam: Evaluate for abnormal heart sounds and jugular venous distention that may indicate congestive heart failure, anemia, pericarditis, or cardiac tamponade.

     6. Abdominal exam: Evaluate for hepatomegaly, ascites, pain, tenderness, abnormal bowel sounds that may indicate obstruction, venous congestion, hepatitis, or cirrhosis.

     7. Genitourinary exam: Evaluate for lesions, pain, unusual discharge, or pelvic mass that may indicate sexually transmitted disease, or pelvic inflammatory disease.

     8. Integument exam: Evaluate for jaundice, poor turgor, changes in hair, rash, scratch marks, and lesions that suggest cellulitis, liver disease, dehydration, and hypothyroidism.

IV. Diagnostic tests

  A. Laboratory

     1. Complete blood count: Evaluate for anemia, thrombocytopenia, neutropenia.

     2. TSH level: Rule out hypothyroidism.

     3. Electrolytes: Rule out hypo/hyper abnormalities.

     4. Other appropriate laboratories: Confirm or rule out diagnosis.

  B. Radiology: As appropriate

V. Differential diagnosis: Differentiate between cancer-related fatigue and chronic fatigue syndrome by recognizing that malignancy and side effects of cancer treatment exclude patients from receiving a diagnosis of chronic fatigue syndrome.

  A. Sepsis (see Chapter 121)

  B. Dehydration (see Chapter 147)

  C. Hypothyroidism (see Chapter 150)

  D. Electrolyte abnormality (see Chapters 144–148)

  E. Depression (see Chapter 154)

  F. Menopause (see Chapter 151)

  G. Respiratory insufficiency or disease

  H. Neurologic impairment (central and peripheral)

  I. Cardiac disease

VI. Treatment

  A. Detection and correction of underlying problems

     1. Treat infection.

     2. Treat chemotherapy-induced anemia (erythropoietin [see Chapter 112]).

     3. Correct fluid and electrolyte problems (see Chapters 144–148).

     4. Correct hormone imbalances

     5. Correct metabolic and nutritional problems (see Chapter 62).

     6. Treat clinical depression (see Chapter 154).

     7. Optimize management and minimize self-care burden.

  B. Preparatory information

     1. Provide information to patients beginning treatment to help them understand fatigue, interpret it appropriately (i.e., as a treatment side effect rather than a symptom of metastatic cancer), and plan for it, which will decrease disruption in their usual activities.

     2. Include specific information about patterns of fatigue.

  C. Exercise

        1. Base prescription on individual assessment of functional capacity and limitations (e.g., results of physical therapy, exercise physiology, cardiac or pulmonary rehabilitation program).

        2. Prescribe moderate level.

        3. Consistently helpful across multiple studies when instituted during or following treatment

  D. Energy conservation

        1. Patients base level of conservation on their individual knowledge of patterns of fatigue and activity.

        2. Patients set priorities for maintaining, transferring, changing, and abandoning activities.

        3. Involve physical or occupational therapist to help to identify alternate ways (e.g., use of assistive devices) of performing desired activities.

        4. Effectively manage other side effects and symptoms (e.g., pain, nausea).

  E. Promoting sleep

        1. Limit sleep disruptions (e.g., hospital noise, family interruptions, pain, medication administration).

        2. Avoid stimulants (e.g., caffeine-containing medications or foods) prior to sleep.

        3. Implement adequate hygiene (e.g., clean bed) and usual bedtime routine, dim lighting, and encourage patient to spend time out of bed prior to sleeping.

        4. Use hypnotics appropriately (e.g., short-term basis, lowest effective dose, avoidance of drug interactions, evaluation of side effects).

        5. Use appropriate behavioral techniques (e.g., relaxation, imagery).

VII. Follow-up

  A. Assess outcome of interventions.

        1. Compare current level of fatigue with previous levels.

        2. Assess target of intervention (e.g., sleep, exercise level, hemoglobin/hematocrit).

        3. Remember that complex problems (e.g., fatigue) will generate complex intervention plans.

  B. Prepare patients completing treatment for persistence of fatigue.

        1. Continue assessment in post-treatment visits.

        2. Assess high levels of post-treatment fatigue against emerging data on late effects of treatment (e.g., cardiomyopathy, declines in endocrine function, persistent symptoms disrupting sleep).

        3. Evaluate post-treatment fatigue in relation to patterns emerging by type of treatment.

VIII. Referrals: Select resources based on etiology of problem or desired result of intervention.

  A. Physical therapist, exercise physiologist, or rehabilitation program to encourage exercise

  B. Physical or occupational therapist, homecare organization that provides home evaluation, or occupational health discipline with expertise in workplace ergonomics to promote energy conservation

C. Mental health providers with knowledge of cancer and cancer treatment to provide emotional support
D. Sleep laboratory team to evaluate for sleep disorders or apnea
E. Pain/symptom management teams to help manage side effects
F. Endocrinologist to help manage adrenal gland or thyroid gland problems
G. Infectious disease team to help manage sepsis, cellulitis

References

Berger, A. (1998). Patterns of fatigue and activity and rest during adjuvant breast cancer chemotherapy. *Oncology Nursing Forum, 25,* 51–62.

Centers for Disease Control and Prevention. (1997). *CFS defined: Screening tests for detecting common exclusionary conditions.* Retrived from the World Wide Web: http://www.cdc.gov/ncidod/diseases/cfs/defined5.htm

Cimprich, B. (1995). Symptom management: Loss of concentration. *Seminars in Oncology Nursing, 11,* 279–288.

Dean, G.E., Spears, L., Ferrell, B.R., Quan, W.D.Y., Groshon, S., & Michell, M.S. (1995). Fatigue in patients with cancer receiving interferon alpha. *Cancer Practice, 3,* 164–172.

Ferrell, B.R., Grant, M., Dean, G.E., Funk, B., & Ly, J. (1996). "Bone tired": The experience of fatigue and its impact on quality of life. *Oncology Nursing Forum, 23,* 1539–1547.

Glaspy, J., Bukowski, R., Steinberg, D., Taylor, C., Tchekmedyian, S., & Vadhan-Raj, S. (1997). Impact of therapy with epoetin alfa on clinical outcomes in patients with nonmyeloid malignancies during cancer chemotherapy in community oncology practice. *Journal of Clinical Oncology, 15,* 1218–1234.

Miaskowski, C., & Lee, K.A. (1999). Pain, fatigue, and sleep disturbances in oncology outpatients receiving radiation therapy for bone metastases: A pilot study. *Journal of Pain and Symptom Management, 17,* 320–332.

Mock, V., Dow, K., Meares, C., Grimm, P., Dienemann, J., Haisfield-Wolfe, M., Quitasol, W., Mitchell, S., Chakravarthy, A., & Gage, I. (1997). Effects of exercise on fatigue, physical functioning, and emotional distress during radiation therapy for breast cancer. *Oncology Nursing Forum, 24,* 991–1000.

NIH Technology Assessment Panel. (1996). Integration of behavioral and relaxation approaches into the treatment of chronic pain and insomnia. *JAMA, 276,* 313–318.

Portenoy, R.K., & Miaskowski, C. (1998). Assessment and management of cancer-related fatigue. In A. Berger, R.K. Portenoy, & D.E. Weissman (Eds.), *Principles and practice of supportive oncology* (pp. 109–118). Philadelphia: Lippincott.

Richardson, A. (1995). Fatigue in cancer patients: A review of the literature. *European Journal of Cancer Care, 4,* 30–32.

Richardson, A., Ream, E., & Wilson-Barnett, J. (1998). Fatigue in patients receiving chemotherapy: Patterns of change. *Cancer Nursing, 21,* 17–30.

Visser, M.R.M., & Smets, E.M.A. (1998). Fatigue, depression and quality of life in cancer patients: How are they related? *Supportive Care in Cancer, 6,* 101–108.

Winningham, M.L., Nail, L.M., Burke, M.B., Brophy, L., Cimprich, B., Jones, L.S., Pickard-Holley, S., Rhodes, V., St. Pierre, B., Beck, S., Glass, E.C., Mock, V. L., Mooney, K. H., & Piper, B. (1994). Fatigue and the cancer experience: The state of the knowledge. *Oncology Nursing Forum, 21,* 23–36.

Chapter

156.
Human Immunodeficiency Virus
Julie D. Painter, RN, MSN,OCN®

I. Definition: Human immunodeficiency virus (HIV) is the retrovirus that leads to the development of AIDS.

II. Pathophysiology
   A. HIV attacks the immune defenses.
   B. Once the virus enters the body, it attaches to the surface of CD4 and T lymphocytes because of its affinity for the CD4 receptors.
      1. As HIV multiplies, CD4 numbers decrease and the immune system is unable to fight infections.
      2. Once the virus attaches, it enters the lymphocyte and uncoats, which causes the virus RNA to transcribe to DNA by reverse transcriptase.
         a) This DNA may remain in the cytoplasm or become integrated into the host cell genome until a stimulus triggers virus replication.
         b) The virus enters the body, targeting and attacking cells that carry CD4 receptors.
         c) The virus eventually disrupts and destroys CD4 cells, which can result in the development of opportunistic infections and malignancy, such as lymphoma or Kaposi's sarcoma.
            (1) Opportunistic infections are not seen in people who otherwise have a healthy immune system.
            (2) These infections often can be caused by pathogens that are normally in the body but now are able to cause disease and infection.

III. Clinical features: HIV is considered most infectious during early stages when the virus is rapidly multiplying and in end stages when the immune system has been destroyed.
   A. High-risk populations
      1. Homosexual men
      2. Bisexuals
      3. IV drug users
      4. Recipients of blood products prior to 1985
      5. Newborns of infected mothers
   B. Etiology: HIV is transmitted by contact with infected bodily secretions or tissue through sexual intercourse, inoculation of blood or blood products, and perinatal transmission from mother to baby.

C. History: It is critical to note that many people diagnosed with HIV may not have sought healthcare attention until later after their diagnosis. Many people may have self-treated, discontinued treatment, or could not access medical care.
1. History of cancer and cancer treatment
2. Current medications: Prescribed and over-the-counter
3. History of presenting symptom(s): Precipitating factors, onset, and duration. Associated symptoms are fever, night sweats, weight loss, diarrhea, skin changes, sores, vaginitis, thrush, lymphadenopathy, attention deficits, headaches, blurred vision, nausea, and dysphagia.
4. Changes in activities of daily living
5. Past medical history: HIV, sexually transmitted diseases, blood or blood product transfusion, tuberculosis (TB)
6. Social history: Illicit drug, tobacco, and alcohol uses; sexual practices; and travel outside the United States.

D. Signs and symptoms
1. Acute viral syndrome: Occurs about two to eight weeks after exposure; Centers for Disease Control (CDC) category A, CD4 T cell count of 500 mm^3 or greater
   a) Anorexia
   b) Flu-like syndrome with fever, malaise, pharyngitis, headache, rash, lymphadenopathy
   c) Photophobia
   d) Arthralgia
2. Symptomatic HIV infection or AIDS-related complex (ARC): CDC category B, CD4 T cell count of 200–499/mm^3
   a) Weight loss greater than 10% of body weight
   b) Retro-orbital pain
   c) Diarrhea, nausea, dehydration
   d) Maculopapular rash
   e) Meningoencephalitis
   f) Peripheral neuropathy
   g) Fever
3. AIDS: CDC category C, CD4 T cell count of 200 mm^3 or less
   a) Generalized lymphadenopathy
   b) Fever or night sweats
   c) Symptoms of opportunistic infection (e.g., productive cough, fever, dysuria, shortness of breath)
   d) Dementia

E. Physical exam
1. Integument exam: Assess for Kaposi's sarcoma (lesion, nodule, or papule that appears on the skin, mucous membranes, and viscera as a dark brown or purple lesion), warts, molluscum contagiosum, fungal infection, skin turgor.
2. Assess weight.
3. HEENT exam
   a) Assess oral mucosa for lesions indicative of thrush, Kaposi's sarcoma, infections, or bleeding.

      b) Assess sinus for tenderness, failure to transilluminate, purulent drainage.

      c) Assess fundus for retinal hemorrhage or exudate or cotton wool spots indicative of cytomegalovirus.

4. Lymph node exam: Assess for lymphadenopathy and tenderness indicative of infection or malignancy.
5. Cardiovascular exam: Assess for murmurs or rubs that may indicate congestive heart failure or endocarditis.
6. Pulmonary exam: Rule out consolidation, effusion, or abnormal sounds indicative of HIV.
7. Abdominal exam: Assess for hepatomegaly and splenomegaly.
8. Neurologic exam: Evaluate mental status changes, neuropathy, or cerebellar changes indicative of HIV.
9. Genital exam: Assess perianal and perineal areas for lesions and signs of sexually transmitted diseases (e.g., drainage, ulcerations, erythema).

      a) Perform pelvic examination and Pap smear on women.

      b) Perform rectal exam to assess for tears, fissures, and signs of infection.

IV. Diagnostic studies

  A. Laboratory

    1. CBC: Evaluate for thrombocytopenia, leukopenia, anemia.
    2. Hepatic, renal, cardiac panels: Obtain baselines to monitor changes in liver, renal, and other systems related to drug therapy.
    3. Urinalysis: Conduct to rule out infection, depending on symptomatology (proteinuria seen in HIV nephropathy).
    4. Blood cultures: Obtain depending on suspected infection.
    5. Stool cultures: If diarrhea, rule out *Clostridium difficile* and other parasitic causes of diarrhea.
    6. Skin test for purified protein derivative: Conduct if TB exposure has occurred.
    7. Hepatitis B serology: Conduct to evaluate for positive result (approximately 90% of people with HIV have been exposed).
    8. Venereal Disease Research Laboratory test (VDRL) or rapid plasma reagin test (RPR): Conduct to evaluate for positive result (incidence of syphilis is significant in the HIV population).
    9. Serology studies for toxoplasmosis and cytomegalovirus: Conduct to evaluate symptomatology for possible encephalopathy.
   10. CD4 count, T4, T8 (helper/suppressor cell ratio): Conduct to evaluate infection risk.
   11. Viral load test: Perform prior to starting highly active antiretroviral therapies.
   12. Western blot: Perform to confirm diagnosis if enzyme-linked immunosorbent assay (ELISA) test is positive.

  B. Radiology: Chest x-ray is recommended if patient does not demonstrate TB antibody production with skin test; conduct to rule out infection (e.g., pneumonia, TB).

V. Differential diagnosis

  A. Hematologic disorders

  B. Lymphoma

C. Sexually transmitted diseases (see Chapters 86, 87, 89, 90, 95–98)

VI. Treatment
A. Diagnosed opportunistic infections: Treat as appropriate.
B. Antiretroviral therapy: See current guidelines and recommendations, as they are rapidly changing; dosing is based on the CD4 levels and viral load.
C. Prophylactic trimethoprim/sulfamethoxazole: Indicated for patients with CD4 levels less than 100/ mm^3; administer double-strength tablet per day (some studies show that dosage of three times weekly may be just as effective).
D. Prescribe vaccinations: Pneumococcal, hemophilus influenza, hepatitis

VII. Follow-up: Patient should be seen at least every three months to evaluate response to medications, monitor side effects, and assess for opportunistic infections.

VIII. Referrals: Patient should be referred to an infectious disease physician or a physician who is competent in the care of people with HIV.

References

Agency for Health Care Policy and Research, Public Health Service, U.S. Department of Health and Human Services. (1994). *Evaluation and management of early HIV infection. AHCPR Publication #94-0572*. Rockville, MD: U.S. Government Printing Office.

Dykeman, M., Fugate, K., & Lau, S. (1997). Human immunodeficiency virus: Early steps in management. *Nurse Practitioner, 22,* 94–96, 99–100.

Katsufrakis, P.J., & Daar, E.S. (1997). HIV/AIDS. Assessment, testing, and natural history. *Primary Care, 24,* 479–496.

McMahon-Casey, K., Cohen, F., & Hughes, A. (1996). *ANAC's core curriculum for HIV/AIDS nursing.* Philadelphia: Nursecom, Inc.

Minkoff, H.L., Eisenberger-Matityahu, D., Feldman, J., Burk, R., & Clarke, L. (1999). Prevalence and incidence of gynecologic disorders among women infected with human immunodeficiency virus. *American Journal of Obstetrics and Gynecology, 180,* 824–836.

Phair, J.P. (1999). Determinants of the natural history of human immunodeficiency virus type 1 infection. *Journal of Infectious Diseases, 179*(Suppl. 2), S384–386.

Phair, J.P., & Murphy, R.L. (1997). *Contemporary diagnosis and management of HIV/AIDS infections.* Newtown, PA: Handbooks in Health Care Company.

Schacker, T., Collier, A.C., Hughes, J., Shea, T., & Corey, L. (1996). Clinical and epidemiologic features of primary HIV infection. *Annals of Internal Medicine, 125,* 257–264.

USPHS/IDSA Prevention of Opportunistic Infections Working Group. (1997). *USPHS/IDSA guidelines for the prevention of opportunistic infections in persons infected with human immunodeficiency virus. MMWR, 46*(#RR-12), 1–46.

Walsek, C., Zafonte, M., & Bowers, J.M. (1997). Nutritional issues and HIV/AIDS: Assessment and treatment strategies. *Journal of Associated Nurses in AIDS Care, 8*(6), 71–80.

Chapter

157. Phlebitis
Dawn Camp-Sorrell, RN, MSN, FNP, AOCN®

I. Definition: Inflammation of a vein
   A. Superficial thrombophlebitis: A clot in a superficial vein with inflammation of the vein wall
   B. Pylephlebitis: Inflammation of the portal vein, superior mesenteric vein, or other abdominal veins

II. Pathophysiology
   A. Superficial phlebitis: Occurs spontaneously or secondary to some form of irritant or trauma; dehydration may contribute because of increased blood viscosity.
   B. Pylephlebitis: Usually a result of an infection, ischemic bowel, or massive ascites, which results in venous stasis

III. Clinical features: Patients who have recurrent superficial phlebitis, especially at a young age, should be evaluated for inherited coagulation disorders.
   A. Etiology
      1. Venous peripheral catheters
      2. Peripherally inserted central catheters (PICCs)
      3. Irritant medications or solutions
   B. History
      1. History of cancer and cancer treatment
      2. Current medications: Prescribed and over-the-counter
      3. History of presenting symptom(s): Precipitating events, location, and duration. Associated symptoms are fever and pain.
      4. Changes in activities of daily living
      5. Recent history of IV therapy
   C. Symptoms/signs
      1. Warmth, erythema, tenderness, swelling along vein wall
      2. Hard cord-like area along the vein
      3. Purulent drainage
   D. Physical exam
      1. Palpate extremities: Inflammation of the vein and measurement of an area of induration

2. Obtain temperature: Rule out fever
3. Palpate abdomen: Tenderness or organomegaly

IV. Diagnostic tests
   A. Laboratory
      1. Cultures: Any purulent drainage
      2. CBC: Platelets and absolute neutrophil counts
   B. Radiology: CT scan of abdomen to rule out abscess, obstruction, or ascites

 V. Differential diagnosis
   A. Deep venous thrombosis (see Chapter 41)
   B. Extravasation from vesicant agents
   C. Bowel obstruction (see Chapter 63)
   D. Cutaneous granulomatous phlebitis
   E. Nodular granulomatous phlebitis

VI. Treatment
   A. Superficial phlebitis: Treat with warm soaks and elevate the affected area for 72 hours. If phlebitis from a PICC is not resolved within 72 hours, consider discontinuing line.
   B. Pain: Administer NSAIDs (see Appendix 11).
   C. Neutropenia: Order antibiotics (see Chapter 121).
   D. Pylephlebitis: Implement anticoagulation therapy if the patient has a hypercoagulable state; perform surgical resection for ischemic bowel.

VII. Follow-up: Assess the peripheral phlebitis in 48 to 72 hours to ensure healing.

VIII. Referral: Not indicated unless area fails to heal, then refer patient to a dermatologist or internist for consultation.

References

Hara, K., Tsuzuki, T., Takagi, N., & Shimokata, K. (1997). Nodular granulomatous phlebitis of the skin: A fourth type of tuberculid. *Histopathology, 30*(2), 129–134.

Lie, J.T. (1996). Primary cutaneous phlebitis with visceral involvement. Unmasking of a masked villain. *Modern Pathology, 9,* 719–724.

Maki, D.G., & Ringer, M. (1991). Risk factors for infusion-related phlebitis with small peripheral venous catheters. A randomized controlled trial. *Annals of Internal Medicine, 114,* 845–853.

Perucca, R., & Micek, J. (1993). Treatment of infusion-related phlebitis. *Journal of Intravenous Nursing, 16*(5), 282–285.

Simamora, P., Pinsuwan, S., Alvarez, J.M., Myrdal, P.B., & Yalkowsky, S.H. (1995). Effect of pH on injection phlebitis. *Journal of Pharmaceutical Science, 84,* 520–522.

Chapter

158. Total Parenteral Nutrition Ordering and Monitoring

Susan A. Ezzone, MS, RN, CNP, and
Jay M. Mirtallo, MS, RPh, BCNSP

I. Definition
   A. Total parenteral nutrition (TPN) is a hypertonic IV nutrient solution that provides daily requirements of essential nutrients.
      1. Administered through central venous catheters
      2. Contains proteins (amino acids), carbohydrates (dextrose), fats (lipid emulsions), electrolytes, vitamins, micronutrients, trace elements, water and select medications; the solution may have an osmolality of 1,800–2,400 mOsm/liter.
      3. Meets full nutritional needs
   B. Peripheral parenteral nutrition (PPN) is an isotonic or slightly hypertonic solution.
      1. Administered through peripheral veins
      2. Partial caloric and protein supplementation may be provided. To avoid phlebitis, the PPN solution may have an osmolality of 900–1,000 mOsm/liter.
      3. Cannot meet full nutritional needs because additives are limited by the hypertonicity of the solution

II. Indications (see Figure 158-1)
   A. TPN may be used in patients who are malnourished or in highly catabolic states and unable to ingest adequate nourishment (> 50% of estimated calorie and protein needs) for seven days or more. Examples of conditions in which TPN may be used are listed in Figure 158-1.
   B. PPN may be used in patients who are unable to eat for 3–14 days.

Figure 158-1. Examples of Patient Conditions Requiring Total Parenteral Nutrition Administration

- Burns
- Cancer or cancer treatment (chemotherapy, radiation therapy)
- Crohn's disease
- Intestinal fistula or dysfunction
- Malnourishment
- Pancreatitis
- Short bowel syndrome
- Ulcerative colitis
- Gastrointestinal feeding contraindicated or ineffective
- Bone marrow/blood stem cell transplant (allogeneic or matched unrelated)

III. Ordering of TPN/PPN
   A. Standard formulas for parenteral nutrition are based on normal body functions and may be modified if hepatic or renal dysfunction occur (see Table 158-1).
   B. A 3-in-1 TPN solution that combines protein, carbohydrates, and fats may be ordered for long-term, cyclic, or home nutrition therapy (see Table 158-2).
   C. A 2-in-1 solution including protein and carbohydrates may be ordered for conditions intolerable to fat intake or administration of PPN solutions.
   D. Initial infusion rates are begun at one-third to one-half the goal rate required to meet the daily caloric requirement.
   E. The infusion rate may be increased by one liter per day until the goal rate is reached.
   F. Cyclic TPN is the preferred method of administration for home and long-term therapy and is most commonly given at night over 12–16 hours.
   G. Standard order forms are often used to ensure that parenteral solutions are ordered correctly and initial and ongoing monitoring is completed.
   H. Parenteral nutrition orders are based on actual body weight unless the patient is > 120% of their ideal body weight. Carbohydrate, protein, and fat requirements should be calculated in relation to the patient's condition or disease state.
   I. Special considerations may be necessary for specific patient conditions or diseases.
      1. Renal failure: Reduce protein, potassium, magnesium, phosphorus; restrict fluid.
      2. Liver failure: Reduce protein, potassium, magnesium, phosphorus; restrict fluid; monitor ammonia; monitor patient for encephalopathy.
      3. Pulmonary failure, diabetes mellitus, glucose intolerance: Reduce carbohydrate; increase fat calories to maximum of 30% of calories provided.
      4. Pancreatitis, critically ill patient: Reduce or eliminate fat.

Table 158-1. Characteristics of Parenteral Nutrition Formulas

Sample Formula			Formula Provides		Usual Caloric Density	Patient Condition
Dextrose g/l	Amino Acids g/l	Fat g/l	Calories/kg	Protein/kg (g)	Calories per ml	
150	40	30	30–33	1.0–1.3	1.0	Normal renal and liver function
150	50	30	28–30	1.5–2.0	1.0	Stress or sepsis
210	40	40	30–33	0.8–1.2*	1.2-1.3	Renal or liver failure
110	60	40	20–23	1.5	1.0	Obesity 120%–165% of ideal weight
70	60	20	15–18	2.0	0.7	>165% of ideal weight

* The protein dose is based on severity of renal and liver disease with adjustment to the highest dose tolerated.

Table 158-2. Daily Nutritional Requirements for Adult Total Parenteral Nutrition

Component	Standard Intake	Sample Formula
Nutrients		
Protein (amino acid)	1.0–1.3 g/kg	40 g/l (4% final concentration)
Carbohydrate (dextrose)	70%–85% of calories	150 g/l (15% final concentration)
Fat (lipid emulsion)	15%–30% of calories	30 g/l (3% final concentration)
Electrolytes		
Calcium	10–15 mEq	Sodium chloride 60 mEq/l
Magnesium	8–20 mEq	Sodium acetate 20 mEq/l
Phosphorus	20–40 mmol	Potassium chloride 20 mEq/l
Potassium	1–2 mEq/kg	Potassium phosphate 20 mEq of K+/l (provides 13.5 mmol phosphorus)
Sodium	1–2 mEq/kg	Calcium gluconate 1 g/l (11 mEq Ca)
Acetate	As needed for acid-base balance	Magnesium sulphate 1 g/l (19 mEq Mg)
Chloride	As needed for acid-base balance	
Multivitamins*	B complex with A, D,E and folic acid	MVI-12®, 10 ml
Trace elements		
Chromium	10–15 mg	Multiple trace elements 3 ml (contains zinc, copper, chromium and manganese)
Copper	0.3–0.5 mg	
Manganese	60–100 mg	
Zinc	2.5–5 mg	
Medications		
H_2 antagonists		
Cimetidine	300–600 mg	
Famotidine	20–40 mg	40 mg
Ranitidine	75–150 mg	
Heparin	3,000–5,000 units	
Insulin	10–60 U/l	Based on sliding scale usage
Iron	1–3 mg (not to be admixed with lipids)	
Volume	20–40 ml/kg	2,400 ml@100 ml/hr
Rate	Infuse over 24 hours or cycle as appropriate	Infuse over 24 hours

* Standard vitamin requirements for parenteral administration were established by the American Medical Association National Advisory Group in 1978. MVI-12® (Astra Pharmaceuticals, Wayne, PA) is formulated to provide the daily requirement of 12 vitamins with the exclusion of vitamin K, which should be administered in a dose of 2–4 mg/week unless contraindicated. Other parenteral vitamin products are available in similar but not equivalent doses as MVI-12.

IV. Assessment and ongoing monitoring
    A. Criteria for initiation of TPN/PPN
        1. Indications for TPN/PPN
        2. Nutritional assessment
        3. Evaluation of concurrent drug therapy
        4. Availability of central venous access for TPN
        5. Laboratory data (see Table 158-3)
    B. Ongoing monitoring of patient response to TPN/PPN
        1. Laboratory data (see Table 158-3)
        2. Central venous catheter (CVC) care
            a) Dedicate one lumen for the administration of TPN in multiple port catheters. Avoid blood draws from this lumen to minimize abnormal results caused by specimen contamination with TPN solution.
            b) Use sterile technique for dressing changes to CVC exit site and accessing CVC lumens.
            c) Assess for signs of exit site infection or sepsis.
        3. Monitor infusion of parenteral solution.
            a) Ensure correct volume of solution is infused at the prescribed rate.

Table 158-3. Monitoring of Laboratory Data

Initial and weekly laboratory data	Complete blood count with differential
	Blood urea nitrogen (BUN)
	Creatinine
	Electrolytes
	Glucose
	Calcium
	Magnesium
	Phosphate
	Liver function tests
	Cholesterol
	Triglycerides
	Coagulation studies
	Osmolality
	Transferrin
	Prealbumin
Daily monitoring of laboratory data for hospitalized patients	Complete blood count with differential
	BUN
	Creatinine
	Electrolytes
	Glucose
	Calcium
	Magnesium
	Phosphate
24-hour urine prior to initiation and weekly	Urine urea nitrogenn (UUN)
	Creatinine

  b) Document solution, volume, and rate infused.
  c) IV tubing with a 1.2 micron in-line filter should be changed every 24 hours.
  d) Check compatibility charts for administration of drugs with parenteral solutions as needed because of limited venous access.
4. Patient monitoring should include daily weight, intake and output, and blood glucose levels.

V. Complications of parenteral nutrition
  A. Mechanical complications
  B. Venous thrombosis
  C. Catheter occlusion
  D. Phlebitis
  E. Catheter-related sepsis
  F. Metabolic complications
  G. Hepatic dysfunction
  H. Renal dysfunction
   I. Biliary disease
  J. Gastric atrophy
  K. Refeeding syndrome
  L. Micronutrient deficiencies

References

ASPEN Board of Directors. (1998). Safe practices for parenteral nutrition formulations. *Journal of Parenteral and Enteral Nutrition, 22*(2), 49–66.

Bickston, S.J. (1995) Nutritional therapy. In G.A. Ewald & C.R. McKenzie (Eds.), *Manual of medical therapeutics* (28th ed.) (pp. 34–40). Boston: Little, Brown, & Co.

Mirtallo, J.M. (1997). *Practice guidelines for Ohio State University medical center.* Columbus, OH: Ohio State University Medical Center.

Skipper, A., & Marian, M.J. (1993). Parenteral nutrition. In M.M. Gottschlich, L.E. Matarese, & E.P. Shronts (Eds.), *Nutrition support dietetics: Core curriculum* (2nd ed.) (pp. 105–123). Gaithersburg, MD: Aspen Publishers.

Appendices

Appendix 1. Antibiotics for Treatment of Selected Organisms

Site of Infection	Most Common Etiology	Primary Antibiotic	Alternative Antibiotic
Abdomen			
Peritonitis (spontaneous bacterial peritonitis)	Enterobacteriaceae enterococcus	Cefotaxime 2 g q 8 hr IV for 2 wk	Ceftriaxone 2 g q 24 hr IV or ofloxacin 400 mg po q 12 hr
Secondary (e.g., bowel perforation)	Enterobacteriaceae enterococcus	Ticarcillin/clavulanate 3.1 g q 6 hr IV or piperacillin/tazobactam 3.375 g q 6 hr IV	Imipenem 0.5 g q 6 hours IV
Breast			
Mastitis	Staphylococcus aureus	Dicloxacillin 500 mg q 6 hr po or cefazolin 1 g q 8 hr IV for 10–14 d	Clindamycin 300 mg q 6 hr po
Brain			
Meningitis, aseptic	Enterovirus	IV fluids and analgesics	–
Meningitis, bacterial	Streptococcus pneumoniae, meningococci	Cefotaxime 2 g q 4–6 hr IV or po for 7–14 d or ceftriaxone 2 g IV q 12 hr	Vancomycin + ceftriaxone
Meningitis with impaired immunity	Gram-negative bacilli	Ampicillin 2 g IV q 4 hr + ceftazidime 2 g q 8 hr IV	–
Ear			
External otitis	Staphylococcus aureus Pseudomonas enterobacterial	Ear drops: Polymyxin B + neomycin + hydrocortisone qid Acute: dicloxacillin 500 mg po qid	Ofloxacin 0.3% solution bid
Otitis media	Streptococcus pneumoniae, Haemophilus influenzae	Amoxicillin 90 mg/kg/d po q 12 hr or trimethoprim/ sulfamethoxazole (TMP/SMX) 8 mg/kg/d divided dose q 12 hr po or ceftriaxone 50 mg/kg IM for 1 dose	Azithromycin
Mastoiditis	Streptococcus pneumoniae	As above	–
	Staphylococcus aureus	Nafcillin or oxacillin	–
Eye			
Conjunctivitis	Staphylococcus aureus, Streptococcus pneumoniae, Haemophilus influenzae	Ophthalmic erythromycin or gentamicin	–
Gallbladder			
Cholecystitis, biliary sepsis, common duct obstruction	Enterobacteriaceae enterococcus	Ticarcillin 4 g q 6 hr IV + metronidazole or ticarcillin/ clavulanate 3.1 g q 6 hr IV	Aztreonam 2 g q 8 hr IV + clindamycin 450– 900 mg q 8 hr IV

(Continued on next page)

Appendix 1. Antibiotics for Treatment of Selected Organisms *(Continued)*

Site of Infection	Most Common Etiology	Primary Antibiotic	Alternative Antibiotic
Genitourinary Prostatitis	*Enterobacteriaceae*	Ciprofloxacin 500 mg po bid for 4 wk or ofloxacin 300 mg bid po for 6 wk	TMP/SMX double-strength bid po for 1–3 months
Urinary tract infection	*Escherichia coli*	TMP/SMX double-strength 1 bid po for 3 d or ciprofloxacin 250 mg bid po for 3 d	–
Heart Bacterial endocarditis	*Staphylococcus aureus*	Nafcillin 2 g IV q 4 hr or oxacillin IV or dicloxacillin po 500 mg q 6 hr	Vancomycin + gentamycin
Lung Community-acquired pneumonia	*Streptococci pneumoniae, Haemophilus influenzae,* Mycoplasma	Azithromycin 0.5 g po x 1, then 0.25 g/d for 5–21 d or clarithromycin 500 mg po bid	TMP/SMX
Pharynx Pharyngitis	Group A *streptococcus*	Penicillin V 500 mg bid or 250 mg po qid for 10 d	Erythromycin 500 mg po qid x 10 d
Sinuses Sinusitis	*Streptococcus pneumoniae, Haemophilus influenzae*	Amoxicillin 875 mg q 12 hr or TMP/SMX double-strength 1 bid po for 10–14 d	Clarithromycin 500 mg po for 10 d
Skin Cellulitis	Group A *streptococcus, Staphylococcus aureus*	Nafcillin or oxacillin 2 g IV q 4 hr or dicloxacillin 500 mg q 6 hr po for 3 d post inflammation resolution	Erythromycin 500 mg po qid
Systemic Sepsis, not neutropenic	Gram-positive cocci, aerobic bacilli	Ticarcillin/clavulanate 3.1 g q 6 hr IV or piperacillin/tazobactam 3.375 g q 4 hr IV or imipenem 0.5 g q 6 hr IV	–
Sepsis, neutropenic	Aerobic gram-negative bacilli, *Staphylococcus aureus*	Ceftazidime 2 g q 8 hr IV or imipenem 0.5 g q 6 hr IV dual therapy with an antipseudomonal B-lactamase susceptible penicillin (e.g., carbenicillin, ticarcillin, mezlocillin, azlocillin, and piperacillin) + ceftazidime. Add vancomycin 1 g q 12 hr IV if venous access device present.	–

(Continued on next page)

Appendix 1. Antibiotics for Treatment of Selected Organisms *(Continued)*

Site of Infection	Most Common Etiology	Primary Antibiotic	Alternative Antibiotic
Venous access device	*Staphylococcus aureus*	Vancomycin 1 g q 12 hr IV for 10 days	Pull the device.

Note. This table is not a comprehensive antibiotic listing and should only be used as a guide. Duration of therapy may exist for specific infections. In general, therapy is continued 7–10 days after the patient becomes afebrile.

Appendix 2. Antidepressant Agents

Classification/Drug	Dose	Side Effects	Comments
SNRIs*, tricyclics (primary serotonin, mixed norepinephrine and serotonin uptake)			
Amitriptyline (Elavil®c, Endep®b)	25–75 mg po qd up to 150–300 mg qd	High sedation, dry mouth, blurred vision, constipation, urinary hesitancy, confusion, orthostatic hypotension, seizures, weight gain, sexual disturbances	Time to steady state, 4–10 days; up to one month before beneficial effects are seen
Clomipramine (Anafranil®c)	25–75 mg po qd up to 150–240 mg qd	As above	Steady state 7–14 days
Doxepin (Sinequan®d)	25–75 mg po qd up to 150–300 mg qd	As above	Steady state 2–8 days; 2–3 weeks for maximum effect; available in cream and elixir; used for chronic urticaria
Imipramine (Tofranil®c)	25–75 mg po qd up to 150–300 mg qd	Moderate sedation as above	Used for panic disorder; steady state 2–6 days
Trimipramine (Surmontil®e)	25–75 mg po qd up to 150–300 mg qd	As above	Steady state 2–6 days
SNRIs, tricylics (secondary)			
Desipramine (Norpramin®f)	25–75 mg po q am	Slight sedation, bad taste, as above	Steady state 2–11 days; response in first week
Nortriptyline (Pamelor®c, Aventyl®g)	25–50 mg po qd up to 50–150 mg qd	As above	Steady state 4–19 days; available in elixir
Protriptyline (Vivactil®h)	15 mg po q am up to 15–60 mg qd	As above	Steady state 4–19 days

(Continued on next page)

Appendix 2. Antidepressant Agents (Continued)

Classification/Drug	Dose	Side Effects	Comments
SNRIs, nontricylic (third-generation heterocyclic) (serotonin and norepinephrine)			
Venlafaxine (Effexor®e)	75 mg po qd up to 150–225 mg/d in divided doses	Nausea, somnolence, sweating, dizziness, anxiety, sexual disturbances, hypertension	Available in extended release
MAO* inhibitors (serotonin, norepinephrine, dopamine)			
Phenazine (Nardil®¹)	15 mg po tid up to 45–90 mg qd in divided doses	Headache, drowsiness, dry mouth, weight gain, postural hypotension, sexual disturbances, neuropathy	Give vitamin B₆ 50 mg po qd to avoid neuropathy; interacts with tyramine found in fermented foods and beverages; steady state 3–4 weeks
Tranylcypromine (Parnate®¹)	10 mg po q am up to 10–40 mg/d in divided doses	As above	As above
SSRIs*			
Citalopram (Celexa®k)	20 mg po qd up to 60 mg po qd	Anxiety, insomnia, tremor, GI symptoms, rashes, decreased libido, sexual dysfunction, slight sedation	Avoid astemizole, sibutramine, and cisapride; steady state: 7–9 days
Fluoxetine (Prozac®g)	20 mg po q am up to 40 mg po qd	As above	Available in elixir
Fluvoxamine (Luvox®¹)	50 mg po q d up to 100–300 mg po in divided doses	As above	Avoid theophylline; increases caffeine half-life
Sertraline (Zoloft®d)	50 mg po qd up to 200 mg po qd	As above	—
Paroxetine (Paxil®¹)	20 mg po qd up to 50–200 mg po qd	As above	Available in elixir

(Continued on next page)

Appendix 2. Antidepressant Agents (Continued)

Classification/Drug	Dose	Side Effects	Comments
NDRIs* (norepinephrine, some dopamine) Bupropion (Wellbutrin[®m])	100 mg po bid; after 4–7 days, increase to tid	Dizziness, dry mouth, sweating, tremor, aggravation of psychosis; potential seizures at high doses	Contraindicated with seizures, bulimia, anorexia; steady state 7–10 days
SARIs* (serotonin, 5HT$_2$ antagonists) Nefazodone (Serzone[®n])	100 mg po bid up to 300–600 mg qd in divided doses	Nausea, drowsiness, dizziness, insomnia, agitation	Avoid concurrent use with astemizole or cisapride
Trazodone (Desyrel[®n])	50 mg po qd up to 400–600 mg qd in divided doses	As above; high sedation	—

*SNRIs—serotonin-norepinephrine reuptake inhibitors; MAO—monoamine oxidase; SSRIs—selective serotonin reuptake inhibitors; NDRIs—norepinephrine-dopamine reuptake inhibitors; SARIs—serotonin antagonist and reuptake inhibitors

[a] Zeneca Pharmaceuticals, Wilmington, DE; [b] Roche Products Inc., Nutley, NJ; [c] Novartis Pharmaceuticals Corp., East Hanover, NJ; [d] Pfizer Inc., New York, NY; [e] Wyeth-Ayerst Laboratories, Philadelphia, PA; [f] Hoechst Marion Roussel, Kansas City, MO; [g] Eli Lilly & Co., Indianapolis, IN; [h] Merck & Co., Inc., West Point, PA; [i] Parke-Davis, Morris Plains, NJ; [j] SmithKline Beecham Pharmaceuticals, Philadelphia, PA; [k] Forest Laboratories, Inc., New York, NY; [l] Solvay Pharmaceuticals, Inc., Marietta, GA; [m] Glaxo Wellcome Inc., Research Triangle Park, NC; [n] Bristol-Myers Squibb Co., Princeton, NJ

Appendix 3. Antiemetic Agents

Classification	Generic Name	Trade Name(s)	Route	Dose/Schedule	Duration of Action	Adverse Events
Serotonin antagonist	Ondansetron	Zofran[®a]	IV	0.15 mg/kg, Q4H x 3 doses or 32 mg, 30 min. prechemotherapy x 1	half life = 3–4 hours	Headache, diarrhea, constipation, fever, transient increases in serum SGOT/SGPT
			PO	8 mg BID x 3 days	PO bioavailability 60%	
	Granisetron	Kytril[®b]	IV	10 mcg/kg over 5 min., within 30 min. of chemotherapy	half life = 8–10 hours	Headache, asthenia, diarrhea, constipation, fever, somnolence
			PO	1 mg BID		
	Dolasetron	Anzemet[®c]	PO	100 mg, one hour prechemotherapy	Peak: 1 hour	Headache, diarrhea, dizziness, fatigue, abnormal liver functions
			IV	1.8 mg/kg, 30 min. prechemotherapy, or fixed doses of 100 mg	Peak: 30 min	
Substituted benzamide	Metoclopramide	Reglan[®d]	IV	2.0–4.0 mg/kg Q2H x 4	Onset: 1–30 min. half life = 8–10 hours Duration: 2 hours	Sedation, akathisia, acute dystonic reactions (increased incidence in patients < 30 years), diarrhea (high doses), dry mouth
			PO	0.5–2.0 mg/kg Q3–4H	Onset: 0.5–1 hour Duration: 1–2 hours	
Phenothiazines	Prochlorperazine	Compazine[®b]	IM	10 mg Q3–4H	Onset: 10–20 min. Duration: 3–12 hours	Sedation, akathisia, extrapyramidal reactions, dry mouth, orthostatic hypotension, blurred vision
			IV	10–40 mg Q3–4H	Onset: 10–20 min. Duration: 3–4 hours	
			PO	10 mg Q4–6H	Onset: 30–40 min. Duration: 3–4 hours	
			Spansule	15–30 mg Q12H	Onset: 30–40 min. Duration: 10–13 hours	
			PR	25 mg Q4–6H	Onset: 60 min. Duration: 3–4 hours	
	Chlorpromazine	Thorazine[®b]	IM	12.5–50 mg Q4–6H	Onset: 15–30 min. Duration: 12 hours	Sedation, hypotension, dizziness, akathisia, extrapyramidal reactions, dry mouth
			IV	12.5–50 mg Q4–6H	Onset: 5 min.	
			PR	12.5–50 mg Q4–6H	Onset: erratic	
	Perphenazine	Trilafon[®e]	PO	4 mg Q4–6H	Onset: erratic Peak: 2–4 hours	Sedation, constipation, extrapyramidal reactions, dry mouth, rash
			IM	5 mg Q4H	Onset: 10 min. Duration: 6 hours	
			IV	5 mg Q4H or 5mg IVB followed by an infusion at 1 mg/hr for 10 hours; maximum dose 30 mg (inpatients) and 15 mg (outpatients) in 24 hours	Onset: 10 min. Duration: 6–24 hours	
	Thiethylperazine maleate	Torecan[®f] Norzine[®g]	IM PO PR	10 mg QD-TID 10 mg QD-TID 10 mg QD-TID	— Onset: 30–60 min. Onset: 45–60 min.	Drowsiness, extrapyramidal side effects (dystonia, torticollis, akathisia, gait disturbances), hypotension	Duration 3–4 hours
Corticosteroids	Dexamethasone	Decadron[®h]	IV	4–20 mg (10–20 mg given x 1, otherwise Q4–6H)	half life = 3–4 hours	Dyspepsia, hiccoughs, increased appetite, euphoria, insomnia, fluid retention, hyperglycemia
		Hexadrol[®i]	PO	4–8 mg Q4H x 4 doses	Peak 1–2 hours Duration: 2 days	

(Continued on next page)

Appendix 3. Antiemetic Agents (Continued)

Classification	Generic Name	Trade Name(s)	Route	Dose/Schedule	Duration of Action		Adverse Events
Corticosteroids (cont.)	Prednisone		PO	2.5–15 mg Q4–12H	Peak 1–2 hours	Duration: 1–1.5 days	Dyspepsia, hiccoughs, increased appetite, euphoria, insomnia, fluid retention, hyperglycemia
Butyrophenones	Haloperidol	Haldol[e]	IM PO IV	2–5 mg Q2H x 3–4 doses 2–5 mg Q2H x 3–4 doses 2 mg x 1	Onset: 15–30 min. Onset: 40 min. Onset: 15–30 min.	Duration: 3–6 hours Duration: 4–6 hours Duration: 3–6 hours	Sedation, akathisia, extrapyramidal reactions, orthostatic hypotension
	Droperidol	Inapsine[e,k]	IM IV	2–5 mg Q4–6H 2–5 mg Q4–6H or drip	Onset: 3–10 min.	Duration: 3–6 hours	Sedation, akathisia, extrapyramidal reactions, hypotension
Cannabinoids	Dronabinol	Marinol[e,f]	PO	2.5–10 mg 1–3 hours before chemotherapy, then Q2H x 4–6 doses/day	—	—	Sedation, dry mouth, euphoria or dysphoria, dizziness, orthostatic hypotension
Drugs used to augment antiemetics	Diphenhydramine	Benadryl[e,l]	PO IM IV	25–50 mg Q4H PRN 25–50 mg Q4H PRN 25–50 mg Q4H PRN	Peak 1–3 hours Onset: 30 min. Onset: Immediate	Duration: 4–7 hours Duration: 4–7 hours Duration: 4–7 hours	Sedation, dizziness, blurred vision/diplopia, dry mouth
	Lorazepam	Ativan[e,m]	IV PO SL	1–2 mg/m², not exceeding 3 mg 0.5–2 mg 0.5–2 mg	Peak 1–3 hours	Duration: 4–8 hours Duration 3–6 hours	Sedation, anterograde amnesia, dizziness, weakness, unsteadiness, disorientation, hypotension

[a] Glaxo Wellcome Oncology/HIV, Inc., Research Triangle Park, NC; [b] SmithKline Beecham Pharmaceuticals, Philadelphia, PA; [c] Hoechst Marion Roussel, Kansas City, MO; [d] A.H. Robins Company, Inc., Richmond, VA; [e] Schering Corporation, Kenilworth, NJ; [f] Roxane Laboratories, Inc., Columbus, OH; [g] The Purdue Frederick Company, Norwalk, CT; [h] Merck & Co., Inc., West Point, PA; [i] Organon Inc., West Orange, NJ; [j] McNeil Pharmaceutical, Raritan, NJ; [k] Janssen Pharmaceutica, Titusville, NJ; [l] Warner Wellcome, Morris Plains, NJ; [m] Wyeth-Ayerst Laboratories, Philadelphia, PA

Note. From "Serotonin Antagonists: State of the Art Management of Chemotherapy-Induced Emesis," by L.B. Cleri, 1995, Oncology Nursing: Treatment and Support, 2(1), pp. 1–19. Copyright 1995 by Lippincott-Raven. Adapted with permission.

Appendix 4. Antihistamines

Action: Antihistamines are reversible, competitive H_1 receptor antagonists which reduce or prevent most of the physiologic effects of histamine. They do not prevent histamine release or bind with histamine that has already been released.

Indications: Antihistamines are used to relieve the manifestations of immediate-type hypersensitivity reactions. They may also be used as a sedative, antiemetic, antitussive, antiparkinson agent, adjuncts to pre- or postoperative analgesic therapy, and to combat motion sickness and allergic rhinitis (running nose, sneezing, itching nose and watery eyes).

Contraindications for first-generation antihistamines:
- Hypersensitivity to antihistamines
- Narrow-angle glaucoma
- Stenosing peptic ulcer
- Symptomatic prostatic hypertrophy
- Asthma
- Monoamine oxidase inhibitor use
- Elderly patients
- Debilitated patients
- Patients taking cisapride

Contraindication to second-generation antihistamines:
- Hypersensitivity to antihistamines

The use of astemizole and terfenadine is contraindicated in significant hepatic or heart dysfunction, and concomitant erythromycin, clarithromycin, troleandomycin, quinine, mibefradil, ketoconazole or itraconazole therapy.

Classification	Generic	Brand Name	Adult Dose
Ethanolamines	Diphenhydramine	Benadryl®ᵃ	25–50 mg q 4 hrs
	Clemastine	Tavist®ᵇ	1.34 mg bid; do not exceed 8.04 mg daily
Ethylenediamines	Tripelennamine	PBZ®ᶜ	25–50 mg q 4–6 hrs
Alkylamines	Chlorpheniramine	Chlor-Trimeton®ᵈ	4 mg q 4–6 hrs
	Dexchlorpheniramine	Polaramine®ᵈ	2 mg q 4–6 hrs
	Brompheniramine	Dimetapp®ᵉ	10 mg bid
Phenothiazines	Promethazine	Phenergan®ᶠ	25–50 mg bid
Piperazines	Hydroxyzine	Atarax®ᵍ Vistaril®ᵍ	25 mg tid–qid
Piperazines (peripherally selected)	Cetirizine	Zyrtec®ᵍ	5–10 mg qd
Piperidines	Cyproheptadine	Periactin®ʰ	4–20 mg qd
	Azatadine	Optimine®ᵈ	1–2 mg bid
	Astemizole	Hismanal®ˡ	10 mg qd
	Loratadine	Claritin®ᵈ	10 mg qd
	Fexofenadine	Allegra®ⁱ	60 mg bid

ᵃ Warner-Lambert Consumer Healthcare, Morris Plains, NJ; ᵇ Novartis Consumer Products, Summit, NJ; ᶜ Ciba-Geigy Corp., Summit NJ; ᵈ Schering Corp., Kenilworth, NJ; ᵉ A.H. Robins Co., Richmond, VA; ᶠ Wyeth-Ayerst Laboratories, Philadelphia, PA; ᵍ Pfizer, Inc., New York, NY; ʰ Merck & Co., West Point, PA; ˡ Janssen Pharmaceutica, Titusville, NY; ⁱ Hoechst Marion Roussel, Kansas City, MO

Appendix 5. Cranial Nerves

Cranial Nerve	Function	Exam Technique	Deficits
I. Olfactory	Sensory: Smell	Test ability to identify aromatic odors one nostril at a time. Patient must have eyes closed. Use substances such as tobacco, alcohol, peppermint, or lemon. Commercially prepared smell kit available.	Inflammation of the mucous membranes, allergic rhinitis, and excessive smoking may interfere with ability to smell. Abnormalities: trauma or olfactory tract lesion; viral infections
II. Optic	Sensory: Visual acuity and visual fields	Test acuity with Snellen chart and Rosenbaum near vision chart. Perform ophthalmoscopic examination of fundi. Test peripheral fields by confrontation. Cover one eye at a time and have patient look at your eye. Have patient point to the finger that is moving. Compare patient's response to the time you first noted the movement. Check pupillary reaction to light.	Decreased visual acuity from drugs or compression from tumor of nerve, eye, or optic radiation within the brain; retinal ischemia, cataracts, glaucoma, nystagmus
III. Oculomotor	Motor: Raise eyelids, extraocular movement	Pupillary reaction to accommodation; ability to follow moving objects	Inability to adduct, elevate, and depress the eye; ptosis and non-reactive pupil
IV. Trochlear	Motor: Eye movement	Observe extraocular movements (EOMs) in the six cardinal points of gaze.	Unable to perform EOMs; unilateral third-nerve palsy; Horner's syndrome as a result of bronchogenic carcinoma with superior cervical ganglion involvement
V. Trigeminal	Motor: Jaw Sensory: Ophthalmic branch, maxillary branch, mandibular branch	Inspect face for muscle atrophy and tremors. Palpate jaw for strength with jaw clenched. Test for superficial pain and touch sensation with patient's eyes closed. Test corneal reflex if above is abnormal.	Loss of corneal reflex with or without impaired sensation suggests cerebellopontine angle tumors. Numbness of face may indicate neuropathy or brain stem tumor. Trismus may indicate oral cavity/oropharyngeal tumor. Trismus or muscle spasm of mandible may indicate drug reaction, such as phenothiazine. Deviation of mandible can be related to paralysis after a stroke.
VI. Abducens	Motor: Lateral eye movement	Observe for lateral eye movement	Sixth nerve is the first function to be lost in the presence of increased intracranial pressure.

(Continued on next page)

Appendix 5. Cranial Nerves *(Continued)*

Cranial Nerve	Function	Exam Technique	Deficits
VII. Facial	Motor: Muscles of face Sensory: Anterior tongue, ear canal, postauricular area	Inspect symmetry of facial features: Smile wrinkles forehead, shows teeth, close eyes. Test ability to identify salt and sweet taste.	Weakness of face; fasciculation; facial asymmetry may indicate stroke, tumor condition, nerve compression, inflammatory paralysis; inability to raise eyebrows, squeeze eyes shut, purse lips may indicate peripheral facial palsy (lower motor neuron) and central facial palsy (upper motor neuron)
VIII. Acoustic 1. Vestibular 2. Cochlear or auditory	Sensory: Hearing acuity, equilibrium	Test hearing acuity with whisper test. Compare bone and air conduction (Rinne). Test sound lateralization (Weber).	Ototoxic drugs alter hearing acuity. Hearing loss or impairment can result from tumors in the external auditory canal, middle ear, inner ear, or central auditory pathways or secondary to chemotherapy, impaction, chronic infection, or radiation damage. Vertigo can result from lesions of the vestibular, visual, or somatosensory system or vestibular dysfunction. Weber: Sound heard best in nonaffected ear. Bone conduction greater than air conduction indicates organ damage.
IX. Glossopharyngeal	Motor: Swallowing Sensory: Gag, taste	Test ability to identify sour and bitter tastes. Test gag reflex.	Difficulty swallowing may indicate tumor obstruction, stroke. Neurologic impairments (ALS, NIS) also may affect swallowing.
X. Vagus	Motor: Phonation and swallowing Sensory: Sensation behind ear and external ear canal	Inspect palate and uvula for symmetry with speech sounds. Observe gag reflex. Evaluate speech quality.	Difficulty swallowing may indicate neurologic impairment, obstruction, or stroke. Asymmetry of the uvula may indicate stroke or severe mucositis. Hoarseness may indicate injury to the laryngeal nerve.
XI. Spinal accessory	Motor: Turn head and shrug shoulders	Test trapezius muscle strength. Test sternocleidomastoid muscle strength.	Decreased strength from tumor invasion, injury, surgery; unable to shrug shoulders
XII. Hypoglossal	Motor: Movement of tongue	Inspect tongue for symmetry, tremors, and atrophy. Inspect tongue movement. Test tongue strength.	Tongue deviating to side of weakness may indicate stroke or tumor. Difficulty controlling tongue, difficulty chewing and swallowing may indicate stroke, severe mucositis, or tumor invasion. Fasciculation of tongue indicates a lower motor neuron lesion.

Appendix 6. Decongestant/Antihistamine Combinations

Product	Decongestant	Antihistamine	Adult Dose
Bromfed[®a]	Pseudoephedrine 60 mg	Brompheniramine 4 mg	One tablet q 4 hrs
Bromfed SR[®a]	Pseudoephedrine 120 mg	Brompheniramine 12 mg	One tablet q 12 hrs
Deconamine[®b] Klerist-D[TMc]	Pseudoephedrine 60 mg	Chlorpheniramine 4 mg	One tablet tid or qid
Semprex[®]-D[d]	Pseudoephedrine 60 mg	Acrivastine 8 mg	One tablet q 4–6 hrs
Carbiset[TMc] Carbodec[TMe] Rondec[®f]	Pseudoephedrine 60 mg	Carbinoxamine 4 mg	One tablet qid
Hista-Vadrin[®g]	Phenylpropanolamine 40 mg and phenylephrine 10 mg	Chlorpheniramine 6 mg	One tablet q 6 hrs
Histalet Forte[®h]	Phenylpropanolamine 50 mg and phenylephrine 10 mg	Chlorpheniramine 4 mg, pyrilamine 25 mg	One tablet bid or tid
Comhist[®i]	Phenylephrine 10 mg	Chlorpheniramine 2 mg, phenyltoloxamine 25 mg	One to two tablets tid (q 8 hrs)
R-Tannate Rhinatate[TMj] R-Tannamine[TMk] Rynatan[®l] Tanoral[®m] Triotann Tritan[TMn] Tri-Tannate[TMe]	Phenylephrine 25 mg	Chlorpheniramine 8 mg, pyrilamine 25 mg	One to two tablets q 12 hrs
Histalet[®h] Syrup/5 ml	Pseudoephedrine 45 mg	Chlorpheniramine 3 mg	10 ml qid
Anamine[®o] Syrup/5 ml	Pseudoephedrine 30 mg	Chlorpheniramine 2 mg	10 ml q 4–6 hrs
Deconamine[®b] Syrup/5 ml	D-pseudoephedrine 30 mg	Chlorpheniramine 2 mg	5–10 ml tid or qid
Bromfed[®a] Elixir/5 ml	Pseudoephedrine 30 mg	Brompheniramine 4 mg	10 ml tid
Ed-A-Hist[TMp] Liquid/ 5 ml	Phenylephrine 10 mg	Chlorpheniramine 4 mg	5 ml tid or qid
Histor-D[®i] Syrup/5 ml	Phenylephrine 10 mg	Chlorpheniramine 2 mg	5–10 ml q 4–6 hrs
Phenergan[TMq] VC Syrup/5 ml	Phenylephrine 5 mg	Promethazine 6.25 mg	5ml q 4–6 hrs, up to 20 ml
Carbodec[TMe] Syrup/ 5 ml Rondec[®f] Syrup/5 ml	Pseudoephedrine 60 mg	Carbinoxamine 4 mg	5 ml qid

(Continued on next page)

Appendix 6. Decongestant/Antihistamine Combinations *(Continued)*

Product	Decongestant	Antihistamine	Adult Dose
Triprolidine with pseudoephedrine/ 5 ml	Pseudoephedrine 30 mg	Triprolidine 1.25 mg	10 ml q 4–6 hrs up to 40 ml/day
Poly-Histine-D®ʳ Elixir/5 ml	Phenylpropanolamine 12.5 mg	Pyrilamine 4 mg, phenyl-toloxamine, 4 mg, phen-iramine 4 mg	10 ml q 4 hrs
Naldelate Syrup/5 ml	Phenylpropanolamine 20 mg, phenylephrine 5 mg	Chlorpheniramine 2.5 mg, phenyltoloxamine 7.5 mg	5 ml q 3–4 hrs up to 20 ml/day

[a] Muro Pharmaceutical, Inc., Tweksbury, MA; [b] Berlex Laboratories, Inc., Wayne, NJ; [c] Glenwood, Tenafly, NJ; [d] Glaxo Wellcome, Inc., Research Triangle Park, NC; [e] Rugby Laboratories, Inc., Corona, CA; [f] Dura Pharmaceuticals, San Diego, CA; [g] Scherer Laboratories, Inc., Plano, TX; [h] Solvay Pharmaceuticals, Inc., Marietta, GA; [i] Roberts Laboratories, Inc., Eatontown, NJ; [j] Major Pharmaceuticals, Inc., Livonia, MI; [k] Qualitest Products, Huntsville, AL; [l] Wallace Laboratories, Cranbury, NJ; [m] Parmed Pharmaceuticals, Inc., Niagara Falls, NY; [n] Eon, Laurelton, NY; [o] Mayrand, Greensboro, NC; [p] Edwards, Ripley, MS; [q] Wyeth-Ayerst Laboratories, Philadelphia, PA; [r] Sanofi Pharmaceuticals, Inc., New York, NY

Appendix 7. Decongestant Agents

Action: Decongestants stimulate alpha-adrenergic receptors of vascular smooth muscle and some have a beta-adrenergic property. The alpha-adrenergic effects cause intense vasoconstriction when applied directly to the mucosal membrane. Systemically the products have similar muted effects and result in mucosal membrane shrinkage which promotes drainage and improves ventilation and the stuffy feeling.

Indications: For the temporary relief of nasal congestion. Topical nasal decongestants should be limited to three days of therapy to prevent rebound congestion.

Contraindications:
- Monoamine oxidase inhibitor (MAO) therapy
- Hypersensitivity or idiosyncrasy to sympathomimetic amines (insomnia, dizziness, weakness, tremor or dysrhythmias)
- Patients with severe hypertension and coronary artery disease (especially with oral preparation)

Special considerations: Administer with caution in the elderly and patients with
- Hyperthyroidism
- Diabetes mellitus
- Cardiovascular disease
- Coronary artery disease
- Ischemic heart disease
- Increased intraocular pressure
- Prostatic hypertrophy
- Hypertension

Topical Preparations

Generic	Brand Names	Adult Dose
Phenylephrine	Neo-Synephrine®ᵃ (0.125% and 1%) Alconefrin®ᵇ 12 (0.16%) Neo-Synephrine (0.25%) Nostrilla®ᶜ (0.5%) Rhinall®ᵈ (0.25%) Sinex®ᵉ (0.5%)	2–3 sprays or drops in each nostril. Repeat every 3–4 hours (0.25% and 0.5%). The 1% solution should be repeated no more than every 4 hours.
Epinephrine	Adrenalin Chlorideᶠ (0.1%)	Apply locally as drops or spray as required.
Ephedrine	Vicks Vatronol®ⁿ (0.5%) Pretz-D®ᵍ (0.25%)	Dosage is product-specific; see label.
Naphazoline	Privine®ᶜ (0.05%)	1–2 drops or sprays in each nostril as needed
Oxymetazoline	Afrin®ʰ (0.05%) Allerest®ᶜ 12 hour (0.05%) Dristan®ⁱ Long Lasting (0.05%) Neo-Synephrine® (0.05%) Sinexᵉ (0.05%)	2–3 sprays or drops of 0.05% solution in each nostril bid or every 10–12 hours
Tetrahydrozoline	Tyzine®ʲ (0.1%)	2–4 drops of 0.1% solution in each nostril every 3–4 hours as needed or 3–4 sprays every 4–6 hours prn
Xylometazoline	Otrivin®ᵏ (0.1%)	2–3 drops or sprays (0.1%) in each nostril every 8–10 hours

(Continued on next page)

Appendix 7. Decongestant Agents *(Continued)*

Oral Preparations

Generic	Brand Names	Adult Dose
Pseudoephedrine	Sudafed®l Sudafedl 12 hour caplets (120 mg) Allermed®m (60 mg) Novafed®n (120 mg)	60 mg every 4–6 hours (sustained release every 12 hours)
Phenylpropan-olamine	Entex®o LA Propagest®p (25 mg tablet)	25 mg every 4 hours not to exceed 150 mg/day or 75 mg sustained release every 12 hours

[a] Bayer Consumer Care Division, Morristown, NJ; [b] PolyMedica, Woburn, MA; [c] Heritage Consumer Products, Brookfield, CT; [d] Scherer, Plano, TX; [e] Richardson-Vicks, Cincinatti, OH; [f] Parke-Davis, Ann Arbor, MI; [g] Parnell, Larkspur, CA; [h] Schering-Plough, Kenilworth, NJ; [i] Whitehall International, Madison, NJ; [j] Kenwood-Bradley, Fairfield, NJ; [k] Novartis Consumer Healthcare, East Hanover, NJ; [l] Warner-Lambert Consumer Healthcare, Morris Plains, NJ; [m] Murdock, Springvale, UT; [n] Hoechst Marion Roussell, Kansas City, MO; [o] Dura Pharmaceuticals, San Diego, CA; [p] Carnrick Laboratories, Inc., Mequon, WI

Appendix 8a. Dose Equivalents for Opioid Analgesics in Opioid-Naïve Children and Adults Less Than 50 kg Body Weight[1]

Drug	Approximate Equianalgesic Dose		Usual Starting Dose for Moderate to Severe Pain	
	Oral	Parenteral	Oral	Parenteral
Opioid agonist[2]				
Morphine[3]	30 mg q 3–4 h (repeat around-the-clock dosing) 60 mg q 3–4 h (single dose or intermittent dosing)	10 mg q 3–4 h	0.3 mg/kg q 3–4 h	0.1 mg/kg q 3–4 h
Morphine, controlled-release[3, 4] (MS Contin®a, Oramorph®b)	90–120 mg q 12 h	N/A	N/A	N/A
Hydromorphone[3] (Dilaudid®c)	7.5 mg q 3–4 h	1.5 mg q 3–4 h	0.06 mg/kg q 3–4 h	0.015 mg/kg q 3–4 h
Levorphanol (Levo-Dromoran®d)	4 mg q 6–8 h	2 mg q 6–8 h	0.04 mg/kg q 6–8 h	0.02 mg/kg q 6–8 h
Meperidine (Demerol®e)	300 mg q 2–3 h	100 mg q 3 h	N/R	0.75 mg/kg q 2–3 h
Methadone	20 mg q 6–8 h	10 mg q 6–8 h	0.2 mg/kg q 6–8 h	0.1 mg/kg q 6–8 h
Combination opioid/NSAID preparations[5]				
Codeine[6] (with aspirin or acetaminophen)	180–200 mg q 3–4 h	130 mg q 3–4 h	0.5–1 mg/kg q 3–4 h	N/A
Hydrocodone (in Lorcet®f, Lortab®g, Vicodin®c, others)	30 mg q 3–4 h	N/A	0.2 mg/kg q 3–4 h	N/A
Oxycodone (roxicodone, also in Percocet®h, Percodan®h, Tylox®i, others)	30 mg q 3–4 h	N/A	0.2 mg/kg q 3–4 h	N/A

[1]Caution: Doses listed for patients with body weight less than 50 kg cannot be used as initial starting doses in babies less than six months of age.

[2]Caution: Recommended doses do not apply to patients with renal or hepatic insufficiency or other conditions affecting drug metabolism and kinetics.

[3]Caution: For morphine, hydromorphone, and oxymorphone, rectal administration is an alternate route for patients who are unable to take oral medications. Equianalgesic doses may differ from oral and parenteral doses because of pharmacokinetic differences.

[4]Transdermal fentanyl (Duragesic®j) is an alternative. Transdermal fentanyl dosage is not calculated as equianalgesic to a single morphine dosage. See the package insert for dosing calculations. Doses above 25 μg/h should not be used in opioid-naïve patients.

[5]Caution: Doses of aspirin and acetaminophen in combination opioid/NSAID preparations also must be adjusted to the patient's body weight. Aspirin is contraindicated in children in the presence of fever or other viral disease because of its association with Reye's syndrome.

[6]Caution: Some clinicians recommend not exceeding 1.5 mg/kg of codeine because of an increased incidence of side effects with higher doses.

(Continued on next page)

Appendix 8a. Dose Equivalent for Opioid Analgesics in Opioid-Naïve Children and Adults Less Than 50 kg Body Weight[1] *(Continued)*

[a] The Purdue Frederick Co., Norwalk, CT; [b] Roxane Laboratories, Inc., Columbus, OH; [c] Knoll Laboratories, Mount Olive, NJ; [d] ICN Pharmaceuticals, Inc., Costa Mesa, NJ; [e] Sanofi Pharmaceuticals, Inc., New York, NY; [f] Forest Pharmaceuticals, Inc., New York, NY; [g] UCB Pharma, Inc., Smyrna, GA; [h] Endo Pharmaceuticals Inc., Chadds Ford, PA; [i] Ortho-McNeil Pharmaceutical, Raritan, NJ; [j] Janssen Pharmaceutica Inc., Titusville, NJ

Note. Published tables vary in the suggested doses that are equianalgesic to morphine. Clinical response is the criterion that must be applied for each patient; titration to clinical responses is necessary. Because complete cross-tolerance among these drugs does not exist, it is usually necessary to use a lower than equianalgesic dose when changing drugs and to retitrate to response.

Abbreviations: N/A—not available; N/R—not recommended; q—every

Appendix 8b. Dose Equivalents for Opioid Analgesics in Opioid-Naïve Adults and Children Greater Than 50 kg Body Weight[1]

Drug	Approximate Equianalgesic Dose		Usual Starting Dose for Moderate to Severe Pain	
	Oral	Parenteral	Oral	Parenteral
Opioid agonist[2]				
Morphine[3]	30 mg q 3–4 h (repeat around-the-clock dosing) 60 mg q 3–4 h (single dose or intermittent dosing)	10 mg q 3–4 h	30 mg q 3–4 h	10 mg q 3–4 h
Morphine, controlled-release [3, 4] (MS Contin®ª, Oramorph®ᵇ)	90–120 mg q 12 h	N/A	90–120 mg q 12 h	N/A
Hydromorphone[3] (Dilaudid®ᶜ)	7.5 mg q 3–4 h	1.5 mg q 3–4 h	6 mg q 3–4 h	1.5 mg q 3–4 h
Levorphanol (Levo-Dromoran®ᵈ)	4 mg q 6–8 h	2 mg q 6–8 h	4 mg q 6–8 h	2 mg q 6–8 h
Meperidine (Demerol®ᵉ)	300 mg q 2–3 h	100 mg q 3 h	N/R	100 mg q 3 h
Methadone	20 mg q 6–8 h	10 mg q 6–8 h	20 mg q 6–8 h	10 mg q 6–8 h
Oxymorphone[3] (Numorphanᶠ)	N/A	1 mg q 3–4 h	N/A	1 mg q 3–4 h
Combination opioid/NSAID preparations[5]				
Codeine[6] (with aspirin or acetaminophen)	180–200 mg q 3–4 h	130 mg q 3–4 h	60 mg q 3–4 h	60 mg q 2 h (IM/SC)
Hydrocodone (in Lorcet®ᵍ, Lortab®ʰ, Vicodin®ᶜ, others)	30 mg q 3–4 h	N/A	10 mg q 3–4 h	N/A
Oxycodone (roxicodone, also in Percocet®ʰ, Percodan®ʰ, Tylox®ⁱ, others)	30 mg q 3–4 h	N/A	10 mg q 3–4 h	N/A

[1] Caution: Recommended doses do not apply for adult patients with body weight less than 50 kg. For recommended starting doses for children and adults less than 50 kg body weight, see Appendix 8a.

[2] Caution: Recommended doses do not apply to patients with renal or hepatic insufficiency or other conditions affecting drug metabolism and kinetics.

[3] Caution: For morphine, hydromorphone, and oxymorphone, rectal administration is an alternate route for patients unable to take oral medications. Equianalgesic doses may differ from oral and parenteral doses because of pharmacokinetic differences.

[4] Transdermal fentanyl (Duragesic®ⁱ) is an alternative. Transdermal fentanyl dosage is not calculated as equianalgesic to a single morphine dose. See the package insert for dosing calculations. Doses above 25 µg/h should not be used in opioid-naïve patients.

[5] Caution: Doses of aspirin and acetaminophen in combination opioid/NSAID preparations also must be adjusted to the patient's body weight. Aspirin is contraindicated in children in the presence of fever or other viral disease because of its association with Reye's syndrome.

[6] Caution: Codeine doses above 65 mg often are not appropriate because of diminishing incremental analgesia with increasing doses but continually increasing nausea, constipation, and other side effects.

(Continued on next page)

Appendix 8b. Dose Equivalents for Opioid Analgesics in Opioid-Naïve Adults and Children Greater Than 50 kg Body Weight[1] (Continued)

Note. Published tables vary in the suggested doses that are equianalgesic to morphine. Clinical response is the criterion that must be applied for each patient; titration to clinical responses is necessary. Because there is not complete cross-tolerance among these drugs, it is usually necessary to use a lower than equianalgesic dose when changing drugs and to retitrate to response.

[a] The Purdue Frederick Co., Norwalk, CT; [b] Roxane Laboratories, Inc., Columbus, OH; [c] Knoll Laboratories, Mount Olive, NJ; [d] ICN Pharmaceuticals, Inc., Costa Mesa, NJ; [e] Sanofi Pharmaceuticals, Inc., New York, NY; [f] Endo Pharmaceuticals Inc., Chadds Ford, PA; [g] Forest Pharmaceuticals, Inc., New York, NY; [h] UCB Pharma, Inc., Smyrna, GA; [i] Ortho-McNeil Pharmaceutical, Raritan, NJ; [j] Janssen Pharmaceutica Inc., Titusville, NJ

Abbreviations: IM— intramuscular; N/A—not available; N/R—not recommended; q—every; SC—subcutaneous

Appendix 9. National Cancer Institute Common Toxicity Criteria, Version 2.0

Adverse Event	0	Grade 1	Grade 2	Grade 3	Grade 4

ALLERGY/IMMUNOLOGY

Adverse Event	0	1	2	3	4
Allergic reaction/ hypersensitivity (including drug fever)	none	transient rash, drug fever < 38°C (< 100.4°F)	urticaria, drug fever ≥ 38°C (≥ 100.4°F), and/ or asymptomatic bronchospasm	symptomatic bronchospasm, requiring parenteral medication(s), with or without urticaria; allergy-related edema/ angioedema	anaphylaxis

Note: Isolated urticaria, in the absence of other manifestations of an allergic or hypersensitivity reaction, is graded in the DERMATOLOGY/ SKIN category.

Allergic rhinitis (including sneezing, nasal stuffiness, postnasal drip)	none	mild, not requiring treatment	moderate, requiring treatment	-	-
Autoimmune reaction	none	serologic or other evidence of autoim- mune reaction but patient is asymptom- atic (e.g., vitiligo), all organ function is normal, and no treatment is required	evidence of autoim- mune reaction involving a non- essential organ or function (e.g., hypothyroidism), requiring treatment other than immuno- suppressive drugs	reversible autoimmune reaction involving function of a major organ or other toxicity (e.g., transient colitis or anemia), requiring short-term immuno- suppressive treatment	autoimmune reaction causing major grade 4 organ dysfunction; progressive and irreversible reaction; long-term adminis- tration of high-dose immunosuppressive therapy required

Also consider Hypothyroidism, Colitis, Hemoglobin, Hemolysis.

Serum sickness	none	-	-	present	-

Urticaria is graded in the DERMATOLOGY/SKIN category if it occurs as an isolated symptom. If it occurs with other manifestations of allergic or hypersensitivity reaction, grade as Allergic reaction/hypersensitivity.

Vasculitis	none	mild, not requiring treatment	symptomatic, requiring medication	requiring steroids	ischemic changes or requiring amputation
Allergy/Immunology- Other (Specify, _____)	none	mild	moderate	severe	life-threatening or disabling

AUDITORY/HEARING

Conductive hearing loss is graded as Middle ear/hearing in the AUDITORY/HEARING category.

Earache is graded in the PAIN category.

External auditory canal	normal	external otitis with erythema or dry desquamation	external otitis with moist desquamation	external otitis with discharge, mastoiditis	necrosis of the canal, soft tissue, or bone

Note: Changes associated with radiation to external ear (pinnae) are graded under Radiation dermatitis in the DERMATOLOGY/SKIN category.

Inner ear/hearing	normal	hearing loss on audiometry only	tinnitus or hearing loss, not requiring hearing aid or treatment	tinnitus or hearing loss, correctable with hearing aid or treatment	severe unilateral or bilateral hearing loss (deafness), not correctable
Middle ear/hearing	normal	serous otitis without subjective decrease in hearing	serous otitis or infection requiring medical intervention; subjective decrease in hearing; rupture of tympanic membrane with discharge	otitis with discharge, mastoiditis, or conductive hearing loss	necrosis of the canal, soft tissue, or bone
Auditory/Hearing- Other (Specify, _____)	normal	mild	moderate	severe	life-threatening or disabling

(Continued on next page)

Appendix 9. National Cancer Institute Common Toxicity Criteria, Version 2.0 *(Continued)*

Adverse Event	0	Grade 1	Grade 2	Grade 3	Grade 4

BLOOD/BONE MARROW

Adverse Event	0	1	2	3	4
Bone marrow cellularity	normal for age	mildly hypocellular or ≤ 25% reduction from normal cellularity for age	moderately hypocellular or > 25–≤ 50% reduction from normal cellularity for age or > 2 but < 4 weeks to recovery of normal bone marrow cellularity	severely hypocellular or > 50–≤ 75% reduction in cellularity for age or 4–6 weeks to recovery of normal bone marrow cellularity	aplasia or >6 weeks to recovery of normal bone marrow cellularity

Normal ranges:
children (≤ 18 years)	*90% cellularity average*				
younger adults (19–59)	60–70% cellularity average				
older adults (≥ 60 years)	50% cellularity average				

Note: Grade Bone marrow cellularity only for changes related to treatment not disease.

Adverse Event	0	1	2	3	4
CD4 count	WNL	< LLN–500/mm³	200–< 500/mm³	50–< 200/mm³	< 50/mm³
Haptoglobin	normal	decreased	-	absent	-
Hemoglobin (Hgb)	WNL	< LLN–10.0 g/dl < LLN–100 g/L < LLN–6.2 mmol/L	8.0–< 10.0 g/dl 80–< 100 g/L 4.9–< 6.2 mmol/L	65–< 80 g/L 65–80 g/L 4.0–< 4.9 mmol/L	< 6.5 g/dl < 65 g/L < 4.0 mmol/L
For leukemia studies or bone marrow infiltrative/myelophthisic processes, if specified in the protocol.	WNL	10–< 25% decrease from pretreatment	25–< 50% decrease from pretreatment	50–< 75% decrease from pretreatment	≥ 75% decrease from pretreatment
Hemolysis (e.g., immune hemolytic anemia, drug-related hemolysis, other)	none	only laboratory evidence of hemolysis [e.g., direct antiglobulin test (DAT, Coombs') schistocytes]	evidence of red cell destruction and ≥ 2g decrease in hemoglobin, no transfusion	requiring transfusion and/or medical intervention (e.g., steroids)	catastrophic consequences of hemolysis (e.g., renal failure, hypotension, bronchospasm, emergency splenectomy)

Also consider Haptoglobin, Hemoglobin

Adverse Event	0	1	2	3	4
Leukocytes (total WBC)	WNL	< LLN–3.0 x 10⁹/L < LLN–3,000/mm³	≥ 2.0–< 3.0 x 10⁹/L ≥ 2,000–< 3,000/mm³	≥ 1.0–< 2.0 x 10⁹/L ≥ 1,000–< 2,000/mm³	< 1.0 x 10⁹/L < 1,000/mm³
For BMT studies, if specified in the protocol.	WNL	≥ 2.0–< 3.0 X 10⁹/L ≥ 2,000–< 3,000/mm³	≥ 1.0–< 2.0 x 10⁹/L ≥ 1,000–< 2,000/mm³	≥ 0.5–< 1.0 x 10⁹/L ≥ 500–< 1,000/mm³	< 0.5 x 10⁹/L < 500/mm³

For pediatric BMT studies (using age, race, and sex normal values), if specified in the protocol.
		≥ 75–< 100% LLN	≥ 50 - < 75% LLN	≥ 25 - 50% LLN	< 25% LLN

Adverse Event	0	1	2	3	4
Lymphopenia	WNL	< LLN–1.0 x 10⁹/L < LLN–1,000/mm³	≥ 0.5–< 1.0 x 10⁹/L ≥ 500–< 1,000/mm³	< 0.5 x 10⁹/L < 500/mm³	-

For pediatric BMT studies (using age, race, and sex normal values), if specified in the protocol.
		≥ 75–< 100%LLN	≥ 50–< 75%LLN	≥ 25–< 50%LLN	< 25%LLN

(Continued on next page)

Appendix 9. National Cancer Institute Common Toxicity Criteria, Version 2.0 *(Continued)*

Adverse Event	0	Grade 1	2	3	4
Neutrophils/ granulocytes (ANC/AGC)	WNL	$\geq$ 1.5–< 2.0 x 10⁹/L $\geq$ 1500–< 2,000/mm³	$\geq$ 1.0–< 1.5 x 10⁹/L $\geq$ 1,000–< 1,500/mm³	$\geq$ 0.5–< 1.0 x 10⁹/L $\geq$ 500–< 1,000/mm³	< 0.5 x 10⁹/L < 500/mm³
For BMT studies, if specified in the protocol.	WNL	$\geq$ 1.0–< 1.5 x 10⁹/L $\geq$ 1,000–< 1,500/mm³	$\geq$ 0.5–< 1.0 x 10⁹/L $\geq$ 500–< 1,000/mm³	$\geq$ 0.1–< 0.5 x 10⁹/L $\geq$ 100–< 500/mm³	< 0.1 x 10⁹/L < 100/mm³
For leukemia studies or bone marrow in-filtrative/myelophthi-sic process if speci-fied in the protocol.	WNL	10–< 25% decrease from baseline	25–< 50% decrease from baseline	50–< 75% decrease from baseline	$\geq$ 75% decrease from baseline
Platelets	WNL	< LLN–75.0 x 10⁹/L < LLN–7,5000/mm³	$\geq$ 50.0–< 75.0 x 10⁹/L $\geq$ 50,000–< 75,000/mm³	$\geq$ 10.0–< 50.0 x 10⁹/L $\geq$ 10,000–< 50,000/mm³	< 10.0 x 10⁹/L < 10,000/mm³
For BMT studies, if specified in the protocol.	WNL	$\geq$ 50.0–< 75.0 x 10⁹/L $\geq$ 50,000–< 75,000/mm³	$\geq$ 20.0–< 50.0 x 10⁹/L $\geq$ 20,000–< 50,000/mm³	$\geq$ 10.0–< 20.0 x 10⁹/L $\geq$ 10,000–< 20,000/mm³	< 10.0 x 10⁹/L < 10,000/mm³
For leukemia studies or bone marrow infil-trative/myelophthisic process, if specified in the protocol.	WNL	10–< 25% decrease from baseline	25–< 50% decrease from baseline	50–< 75% decrease from baseline	$\geq$ 75% decrease from baseline
Transfusion: Platelets	none	-	-	yes	platelet transfusions and other measures required to improve platelet increment; platelet transfusion refractoriness associated with life-threatening bleeding (e.g., HLA or cross matched platelet transfusions)
For BMT studies, if specified in the protocol.	none	1 platelet transfusion in 24 hours	2 platelet transfusions in 24 hours	$\geq$ 3 platelet transfu-sions in 24 hours	platelet transfusions and other measures required to improve platelet increment; platelet transfusion refractoriness associated with life-threatening bleeding (e.g., HLA or cross matched platelet transfusions)
Also consider Platelets.					
Transfusion: pRBCs	none	*	-	Yes	-
For BMT studies, if specified in the protocol.	none	$\leq$ 2 u pRBC ($\leq$ 15cc/ kg) in 24 hours elective or planned	3 u pRBC (> 15 $\leq$ 30cc/kg) in 24 hours elective or planned	$\geq$ 4 u pRBC (> 30cc/ kg) in 24 hours	hemorrhage or hemolysis associated with life-threatening anemia; medical in-tervention required to improve hemoglobin
For pediatric BMT studies, if specified in the protocol.	none	$\leq$15mL/kg in 24 hours elective or planned	>15–$\leq$ 30mL/kg in 24 hours elective or planned	> 30mL/kg in 24 hours	
Also consider Hemoglobin.					
Blood/bone marrow-other (Specify, ____)	none	mild	moderate	severe	life-threatening or disabling

(Continued on next page)

Appendix 9. National Cancer Institute Common Toxicity Criteria, Version 2.0 *(Continued)*

Adverse Event	0	1	2	3	4
			Grade		
CARDIOVASCULAR (ARRHYTHMIA)					
Conduction abnormality/ atrioventricular heart block	none	asymptomatic, not requiring treatment (e.g., Mobitz type I second-degree AV block, Wenckebach)	symptomatic, but not requiring treatment	symptomatic and requiring treatment (e.g., Mobitz type II second-degree AV block, third-degree AV block)	life-threatening (e.g., arrhythmia associated with CHF, hypotension, syncope, shock)
Nodal/junctional arrhythmia/ dysrhythmia	none	asymptomatic, not requiring treatment	symptomatic, but not requiring treatment	symptomatic and requiring treatment	life-threatening (e.g., arrhythmia associated with CHF, hypotension, syncope, shock)
Palpitations	none	present	-	-	-
Note: Grade palpitations <u>only</u> in the absence of a documented arrhythmia.					
Prolonged QTc interval (QTc > 0.48 seconds)	none	asymptomatic, not requiring treatment	symptomatic, but not requiring treatment	symptomatic and requiring treatment	life-threatening (e.g., arrhythmia associated with CHF, hypotension, syncope, shock)
Sinus bradycardia	none	asymptomatic, not requiring treatment	symptomatic, but not requiring treatment	symptomatic and requiring treatment	life-threatening (e.g., arrhythmia associated with CHF, hypotension, syncope, shock)
Sinus tachycardia	none	asymptomatic, not requiring treatment	symptomatic, but not requiring treatment	symptomatic and requiring treatment of underlying cause	
Supraventricular arrhythmias (SVT/ atrial fibrillation/ flutter)	none	asymptomatic, not requiring treatment	symptomatic, but not requiring treatment	symptomatic and requiring treatment	life-threatening (e.g., arrhythmia associated with CHF, hypotension, syncope, shock)
Syncope (fainting) is graded in the NEUROLOGY category.					
Vasovagal episode	none	-	present without loss of consciousness	present with loss of consciousness	-
Ventricular arrhythmia (PVCs/bigeminy/trigeminy/ ventricular tachycardia)	none	asymptomatic, not requiring treatment	symptomatic, but not requiring treatment	symptomatic and requiring treatment	life-threatening (e.g., arrhythmia associated with CHF, hypotension, syncope, shock)
Cardiovascular/ Arrhythmia-Other (Specify, _____)	none	asymptomatic, not requiring treatment	symptomatic, but not requiring treatment	symptomatic, and requiring treatment of underlying cause	life-threatening (e.g., arrhythmia associated with CHF, hypotension, syncope, shock)
CARDIOVASCULAR (GENERAL)					
Acute vascular leak syndrome	absent	-	symptomatic, but not requiring fluid support	respiratory compromise or requiring fluids	life-threatening; requiring pressor support and/or ventilatory support
Cardiac—ischemia/ infarction	none	non-specific T-wave flattening or changes	asymptomatic, ST- and T-wave changes suggesting ischemia	angina without evidence of infarction	acute myocardial infarction

(Continued on next page)

Appendix 9. National Cancer Institute Common Toxicity Criteria, Version 2.0 *(Continued)*

Adverse Event	0	1	2	3	4
			Grade		
Cardiac left ventricular function	normal	asymptomatic decline of resting ejection fraction of ≥ 10% but < 20% of baseline value; shortening fraction ≥ 24% but < 30%	asymptomatic but resting ejection fraction below LLN for laboratory or decline of resting ejection fraction ≥ 20% of baseline value; < 24% shortening fraction	CHF responsive to treatment	severe or refractory CHF or requiring intubation

CNS cerebrovascular ischemia is graded in the NEUROLOGY category.

Adverse Event	0	1	2	3	4
Cardiac troponin I (cTnI)	normal	-	-	levels consistent with unstable angina as defined by the manufacturer	levels consistent with myocardial infarction as defined by the manufacturer
Cardiac troponin T (cTnT)	normal	≥ 0.03–< 0.05 ng/ml	≥ 0.05–< 0.1 ng/ml	≥ 0.1–< 0.2 ng/ml	≥ 0.2 ng/ml
Edema	none	asymptomatic, not requiring therapy	symptomatic, requiring therapy	symptomatic edema limiting function and unresponsive to therapy or requiring drug discontinuation	anasarca (severe generalized edema)
Hypertension	none	asymptomatic, transient increase by > 20 mmHg (diastolic) or to > 150/100* if previously WNL; not requiring treatment	recurrent or persistent or symptomatic increase by > 20 mmHg (diastolic) or to > 150/100* if previously WNL; not requiring treatment	requiring therapy or more intensive therapy than previously	hypertensive crisis

Note: For pediatric patients, use age-and sex-appropriate normal values > 95th percentile ULN.

Adverse Event	0	1	2	3	4
Hypotension	none	changes, but not requiring therapy (including transient orthostatic hypotension)	requiring brief fluid replacement or other therapy but not hospitalization; no physiologic consequences	requiring therapy and sustained medical attention, but resolves without persisting physiologic consequences	shock (associated with acidemia and impairing vital organ function due to tissue hypoperfusion)

Also consider Syncope (fainting).

Notes: Angina or MI is graded as Cardiac-ischemia/infarction in the CARDIOVASCULAR (GENERAL) category.

For pediatric patients, systolic BP 65 mmHg or less in infants up to 1 year old and 70 mmHg or less in children older than 1 year of age, use two successive or three measurements in 24 hours.

Adverse Event	0	1	2	3	4
Myocarditis	none	-	-	CHF responsive to treatment	severe or refractory CHF
Operative injury of vein/artery	none	primary suture repair for injury, but not requiring transfusion	primary suture repair for injury, requiring transfusion	vascular occlusion requiring surgery or bypass for injury	myocardial infarction; resection of organ (e.g., bowel, limb)
Pericardial effusion/ pericarditis	none	asymptomatic effusion, not requiring treatment	pericarditis (rub, ECG changes, and/or chest pain)	with physiologic consequences	tamponade (drainage or pericardial window required)
Peripheral arterial ischemia	none	-	brief episode of ischemia managed non-surgically and without permanent deficit	requiring surgical intervention	life-threatening or with permanent functional deficit (e.g., amputation)
Phlebitis (superficial)	none	-	present	-	-

Notes: Injection site reaction is graded in the DERMATOLOGY/SKIN category.

Thrombosis/embolism is graded in the CARDIOVASCULAR (GENERAL) category.

(Continued on next page)

Appendix 9. National Cancer Institute Common Toxicity Criteria, Version 2.0 *(Continued)*

Adverse Event	0	1	Grade 2	3	4
Syncope (fainting) is graded in the NEUROLOGY category.					
Thrombosis/ embolism	none	-	deep vein thrombosis, not requiring antico-agulant therapy	deep vein thrombosis, requiring anticoagu-lant therapy	embolic event including pulmonary embolism
Vein/artery operative injury is graded as Operative injury of vein/artery in the CARDIOVASCULAR (GENERAL) category.					
Visceral arterial ischemia (non-myocardial)	none	-	brief episode of ischemia managed nonsurgically and without permanent deficit	requiring surgical intervention	life-threatening or with permanent functional deficit (e.g., resection of ileum)
Cardiovascular/ General-Other (Specify, _____)	none	mild	moderate	severe	life-threatening or disabling
COAGULATION					
Note: See the HEMORRHAGE category for grading the severity of bleeding events.					
DIC (dissem-inated intravascular coagulation)	absent	-	-	laboratory findings present with <u>no</u> bleeding	laboratory findings <u>and</u> bleeding
Also consider Platelets.					
Note: Must have increased fibrin split products or D-dimer in order to grade as DIC.					
Fibrinogen	WNL	≥ 0.75–< 1.0 x LLN	≥ 0.5–< 0.75 x LLN	≥ 0.25–< 0.5 x LLN	< 0.25 x LLN
For leukemia studies or bone marrow infiltrative/myeloph-thisic process, if specified in the protocol.	WNL	< 20% decrease from pretreatment value or LLN	≥ 20–< 40% decrease from pretreatment value or LLN	≥ 40–< 70% decrease from pretreatment value or LLN	< 50 mg
Partial thromboplas-tin time (PTT)	WNL	> ULN–≤ 1.5 x ULN	> 1.5–≤ 2 x ULN	> 2 x ULN	-
Phlebitis is graded in the CARDIOVASCULAR (GENERAL) category.					
Prothrombin time (PT)	WNL	> ULN–≤ 1.5 x ULN	> 1.5–≤ 2 x ULN	> 2 x ULN	
Thrombosis/embolism is graded in the CARDIOVASCULAR (GENERAL) category.					
Thrombotic microangiopathy (e.g., thrombotic thrombocytopenic purpura/TTP or hemolytic uremic syndrome/HUS)	absent	-	-	laboratory findings present without clinical consequences	laboratory findings and clinical conse-quences, (e.g., CNS hemorrhage/bleed-ing or thrombosis/ embolism or renal failure) requiring ther-apeutic intervention
For BMT studies, if specified in the protocol.	-	evidence of RBC destruction (schistocy-tosis) without clinical consequences	evidence of RBC destruction with elevated creatinine (≤ 3 x ULN)	evidence of RBC destruction with creatinine (> 3 x ULN) not requiring dialysis	evidence of RBC destruction with renal failure requiring dialysis and/or encephalopathy
Also consider Hemoglobin (Hgb), Platelets, Creatinine.					
Note: Must have microangiopathic changes on blood smear (e.g., schistocytes, helmet cells, red cell fragments).					
Coagulation-Other (Specify, _____)	none	mild	moderate	severe	life-threatening or disabling

(Continued on next page)

Appendix 9. National Cancer Institute Common Toxicity Criteria, Version 2.0 *(Continued)*

Adverse Event	0	1	2	3	4
			Grade		
CONSTITUTIONAL SYMPTOMS					
Fatigue (lethargy, malaise, asthenia)	none	increased fatigue over baseline, but not altering normal activities	moderate (e.g., decrease in performance status by 1 ECOG level or 20% Karnofsky or *Lansky*) or causing difficulty performing some activities	severe (e.g., decrease in performance status by ≥ 2 ECOG levels or 40% Karnofsky or *Lansky*) or loss of ability to perform some activities	bedridden or disabling
Fever (in the absence of neutro-penia, where neutropenia is defined as AGC < 1.0 x 10⁹/L)	none	38.0–39.0°C (100.4–102.2°F)	39.1–40.0°C (102.3–104.0°F)	> 40.0°C (> 104.0°F) for < 24hrs	> 40.0°C (> 104.0°F) for > 24hrs
Also consider Allergic reaction/hypersensitivity.					
Note: The temperature measurements listed above are oral or tympanic.					
Hot flashes/flushes are graded in the ENDOCRINE category.					
Rigors, chills	none	mild, requiring symptomatic treatment (e.g., blanket) or non-narcotic medication	severe and/or prolonged, requiring narcotic medication	not responsive to narcotic medication	-
Sweating (diaphoresis)	none	mild and occasional	frequent or drenching	-	-
Weight gain	< 5%	5–< 10%	10–< 20%	≥ 20%	-
Also consider Ascites, Edema, Pleural effusion (non-malignant).					
Weight gain associated with Veno-Occlusive Disease (VOD), for BMT studies, if specified in the protocol.	< 2%	≥ 2–< 5%	≥ 5–< 10%	≥ 10% or as ascites	≥ 10% or fluid retention resulting in pulmonary failure
Also consider Ascites, Edema Pleural effusion (non-malignant).					
Weight loss	< 5%	5–< 10%	10–< 20%	≥ 20%	-
Also consider Vomiting, Dehydration, Diarrhea.					
Constitutional Symptoms-Other (Specify, _____)	none	mild	moderate	severe	life-threatening or disabling
DERMATOLOGY/SKIN					
Alopecia	normal	mild hair loss	pronounced hair loss	-	-
Bruising (in absence of grade 3 or 4 thrombocytopenia)	none	localized or in dependent area	generalized	-	-
Note: Bruising resulting from grade 3 or 4 thrombocytopenia is graded as Petechiae/purpura and Hemorrhage/bleeding with grade 3 or 4 thrombocytopenia in the HEMORRHAGE category, not in the DERMATOLOGY/SKIN category.					
Dry skin	normal	controlled with emollients	not controlled with emollients	-	-
Erythema multiforme (e.g., Stevens-Johnson syndrome, toxic epidermal necrolysis)	absent	-	scattered, but not generalized eruption	severe or requiring IV fluids (e.g., generalized rash or painful stomatitis)	life-threatening (e.g., exfoliative or ulcerating dermatitis or requiring enteral or parenteral nutritional support)

(Continued on next page)

Appendix 9. National Cancer Institute Common Toxicity Criteria, Version 2.0 *(Continued)*

Adverse Event	0	1	2	3	4
Flushing	absent	present	-	-	-
Hand-foot skin reaction	none	skin changes or dermatitis without pain (e.g., erythema, peeling)	skin changes with pain, not interfering with function	skin changes with pain, interfering with function	-
Injection site reaction	none	pain or itching or erythema	pain or swelling, with inflammation or phlebitis	ulceration or necrosis that is severe or prolonged, or requiring surgery	-
Nail changes	normal	discoloration or ridging (koilonychia) or pitting partial or complete	loss of nail(s) or pain in nailbeds	-	-
Petechiae is graded in the HEMORRHAGE category.					
Photosensitivity	none	painless erythema	painful erythema	erythema with desquamation	-
Pigmentation changes (e.g., vitiligo)	none	localized pigmentation changes	generalized pigmentation changes	-	-
Pruritus	none	mild or localized, relieved spontaneously or by local measures	intense or widespread, relieved spontaneously or by systemic measures	intense or widespread and poorly controlled despite treatment	-
Purpura is graded in the HEMORRHAGE category.					
Radiation dermatitis	none	faint erythema or dry desquamation	moderate to brisk erythema or a patchy moist desquamation, mostly confined to skin folds and creases; moderate edema	confluent moist desquamation, ≥ 1.5 cm diameter, not confined to skin folds; pitting edema	skin necrosis or ulceration of full thickness dermis; may include bleeding not induced by minor trauma or abrasion
Note: Pain associated with radiation dermatitis is graded separately in the PAIN category as Pain due to radiation.					
Radiation recall reaction (reaction following chemotherapy in the absence of additional radiation therapy that occurs in a previous radiation port)	none	faint erythema or dry desquamation	moderate to brisk erythema or a patchy moist desquamation, mostly confined to skin folds and creases; moderate edema	confluent moist desquamation, ≥ 1.5 cm diameter, not confined to skin folds; pitting edema	skin necrosis or ulceration of full thickness dermis; may include bleeding not induced by minor trauma or abrasion
Rash/desquamation	none	macular or papular eruption or erythema without associated symptoms	macular or papular eruption or erythema with pruritus or other associated symptoms covering < 50% of body surface or localized desquamation or other lesions covering < 50% of body surface area	symptomatic generalized erythroderma or macular, papular, or vesicular eruption or desquamation covering $\geq 50\%$ of body surface area	generalized exfoliative dermatitis or ulcerative dermatitis
Also consider Allergic reaction/hypersensitivity.					
Note: Stevens-Johnson syndrome is graded separatley as Erythema multiforme in DERMATOLOGY/SKIN category.					
Rash/Dermatitis, focal (associated with high-dose chemotherapy and bone marrow transplant)	none	faint erythema or dry desquamation	moderate to brisk erythema or a patchy moist desquamation, mostly confined to skin folds and creases; moderate edema	confluent moist desquamation, ≥ 1.5 cm diameter, not confined to skin folds; pitting edema	skin necrosis or ulceration of full thickness dermis; may include spontaneous bleeding not induced by minor trauma or abrasion

(Continued on next page)

Appendix 9. National Cancer Institute Common Toxicity Criteria, Version 2.0 *(Continued)*

Adverse Event	0	Grade 1	2	3	4
Rash/dermatitis associated with high dose chemotherapy or BMT studies. Rash/desquamation associated with graft versus host disease (GVHD) for BMT studies is specified in the protocol.	none	macular or papular eruption or erythema covering < 25% of body surface area without associated symptoms	macular or papular eruption or erythema with pruritus or other associated symptoms covering ≥ 25–< 50% of body surface or localized desquamation or other lesions covering ≥ 25–< 50% of body surface area	symptomatic generalized erythroderma or symptomatic macular, papular, or vesicular eruption, with bullous formation, or desquamation covering ≥ 50% of body surface area	generalized exfoliative dermatitis or ulcerative dermatitis or bullous formation

Also consider Allergic reaction/hypersensitivity.
Note: Stevens-Johnson syndrome is graded separately as Erythema multiforme in the DERMATOLOGY/SKIN category.

Adverse Event	0	1	2	3	4
Urticaria (hives, welts, wheals)	none	requiring no medication	requiring PO or topical treatment or IV medication or steroids for < 24 hours	requiring IV medication or steroids for ≥24 hours	-
Wound-infectious	none	cellulitis	superficial infection	infection requiring IV antibiotics	necrotizing fasciitis
Wound-non-infectious	none	incisional separation	incisional hernia	fascial disruption without evisceration	fascial disruption with evisceration
Dermatology/Skin-Other (Specify, _____)	none	mild	moderate	severe	life-threatening or disabling

		ENDOCRINE			
Cushingoid appearance (e.g., moon face, buffalo hump, centripetal obesity, cutaneous striae)	absent	-	present	-	-

Also consider Hyperglycemia, Hypokalemia.

Adverse Event	0	1	2	3	4
Feminization of male	absent	-	-	present	-
Gynecomastia	none	mild	pronounced or painful	pronounced or painful and requiring surgery	-
Hot flashes/flushes	none	mild or no more than 1 per day	moderate and greater than 1 per day	-	-
Hypothyroidism	absent	asymptomatic, TSH elevated, no therapy given	symptomatic or thyroid replacement treatment given	patient hospitalized for manifestations of hypothyroidism	myxedema coma
Masculinization of female	absent	-	-	present	-
SIADH (syndrome of inappropriate anti-diuretic hormone)	absent	-	-	present	-
Endocrine-Other (Specify, _____)	none	mild	moderate	severe	life-threatening or disabling

		GASTROINTESTINAL			

Amylase is graded in the METABOLIC/LABORATORY category.

Adverse Event	0	1	2	3	4
Anorexia	none	loss of appetite	oral intake significantly decreased	requiring IV fluids	requiring feeding tube or parenteral nutrition

(Continued on next page)

Appendix 9. National Cancer Institute Common Toxicity Criteria, Version 2.0 *(Continued)*

Adverse Event	0	1	2	3	4
			Grade		
Ascites (non-malignant)	none	asymptomatic	symptomatic, requiring diuretics	symptomatic, requiring therapeutic paracentesis	life-threatening physiologic consequences
Colitis	none	-	abdominal pain with mucus and/or blood in stool	abdominal pain, fever, change in bowel habits with ileus or peritoneal signs, and radiographic or biopsy documentation	perforation or requiring surgery or toxic megacolon

Also consider Hemorrhage/bleeding with grade 3 or 4 thrombocytopenia, Hemorrhage/bleeding without grade 3 or 4 thrombocytopenia, Melena/GI bleeding, Rectal bleeding/hematochezia, Hypotension.

Adverse Event	0	1	2	3	4
Constipation	none	requiring stool softener or dietary modification	requiring laxatives	obstipation requiring manual evacuation or enema	obstruction or toxic megacolon
Dehydration	none	dry mucous membranes and/or diminished skin turgor	requiring IV fluid replacement (brief)	requiring IV fluid replacement (sustained)	physiologic consequences requiring intensive care; hemodynamic collapse

Also consider Diarrhea, Vomiting, Stomatitis/pharyngitis (oral/pharyngeal mucositis) Hypotension.

Adverse Event	0	1	2	3	4
Diarrhea Patients without colostomy:	none	increase of < 4 stools/day over pre-treatment	increase of 4–6 stools/day, or nocturnal stools	increase of ≥ 7 stools/day or incontinence; or need for parenteral support for dehydration	physiologic consequences requiring intensive care; or hemodynamic collapse
Patients with colostomy:	none	mild increase in loose, watery colostomy output compared with pretreatment	moderate increase in loose, watery colostomy output compared with pre-treatment, but not interfering with normal activity	severe increase in loose, watery colostomy output compared with pre-treatment, interfering with normal activity	physiologic consequences, requiring intensive care; or hemodynamic collapse
For BMT diarrhea associated with GVHD studies, if specified in the protocol.	none	> 500–≤ 1,000 ml of diarrhea/day	> 1,000–≤ 1,500 ml of diarrhea/day	> 1,500 ml of diarrhea/day	severe abdominal pain with or without ileus
For Pediatric BMT studies, if specified in the protocol.		*> 5–< 10 ml/kg of diarrhea/day*	*> 10–< 15 ml/kg of diarrhea/day*	*> 15 ml/kg of diarrhea/day*	*-*

Also consider Hemorrhage/bleeding with grade 3 or 4 thrombocytopenia, Hemorrhage/bleeding without grade 3 or 4 thrombocytopenia, Pain, Dehydration, Hypotension.

Adverse Event	0	1	2	3	4
Duodenal ulcer (requires radiographic or endoscopic documentation)	none	-	requiring medical management or non-surgical treatment	uncontrolled by outpatient medical management; requiring hospitalization	perforation or bleeding, requiring emergency surgery
Dyspepsia/heartburn	none	mild	moderate	severe	-
Dysphagia, esophagitis, odynophagia (painful swallowing)	none	mild dysphagia, but can eat regular diet	dysphagia, requiring predominantly pureed, soft, or liquid diet	dysphagia, requiring IV hydration	complete obstruction (cannot swallow saliva) requiring enteral or parenteral nutritional support, or perforation

Note: If the adverse event is radiation-related, grade <u>either</u> under Dysphagia—esophageal related to radiation <u>or</u> Dysphagia—pharyngeal related to radiation.

(Continued on next page)

Appendix 9. National Cancer Institute Common Toxicity Criteria, Version 2.0 *(Continued)*

Adverse Event	0	1	2	3	4
			Grade		
Dysphagia—esophageal related to radiation	none	mild dysphagia, but can eat regular diet	dysphagia, requiring predominantly liquid, pureed, or soft diet	dysphagia requiring feeding tube, IV hydration, or hyper-alimentation	complete obstruction (cannot swallow saliva); ulceration with bleeding not induced by minor trauma or abrasion or perforation

Also consider Pain due to radiation, Mucositis due to radiation.

Note: Fistula is graded separately as Fistula—esophageal.

Adverse Event	0	1	2	3	4
Dysphagia—pharyngeal related to radiation	none	mild dysphagia, but can eat regular diet	dysphagia, requiring predominantly pureed, soft, or liquid diet	dysphagia, requiring feeding tube, IV hydration or hyper-alimentation	complete obstruction (cannot swallow saliva); ulceration with bleeding not induced by minor trauma or abrasion or perforation

Also consider Pain due to radiation, Mucositis due to radiation.

Note: Fistula is graded separately as Fistula—pharyngeal.

Adverse Event	0	1	2	3	4
Fistula—esophageal	none	-	-	present	requiring surgery
Fistula—intestinal	none	-	-	present	requiring surgery
Fistula—pharyngeal	none	-	-	present	requiring surgery
Fistula—rectal/anal	none	-	-	present	requiring surgery
Flatulence	none	mild	moderate	-	-
Gastric ulcer (requires radio-graphic or endo-scopic documenta-tion)	none	-	requiring medical management or non-surgical treatment	bleeding without perforation, uncon-trolled by outpatient medical management, requiring hospitaliza-tion or surgery	perforation or bleeding, requiring emergency surgery

Also consider Hemorrhage/bleeding with grade 3 or 4 thrombocytopenia, Hemorrhage/bleeding without grade 3 or 4 thrombocytopenia.

Adverse Event	0	1	2	3	4
Gastritis	none	-	requiring medical management or non-surgical treatment	uncontrolled by out-patient medical management, requiring hospitaliza-tion or surgery	life-threatening bleeding, requiring emergency surgery

Also consider Hemorrhage/bleeding with grade 3 or 4 thrombocytopenia, Hemorrhage/bleeding without grade 3 or 4 thrombocytopenia.

Hematemesis is graded in the HEMORRHAGE category.

Hematochezia is graded in the HEMORRHAGE category as Rectal bleeding/hematochezia.

Adverse Event	0	1	2	3	4
Ileus (or neuro-constipation)	none	-	intermittent, not requiring intervention	requiring non-surgical intervention	requiring surgery
Mouth dryness	normal	mild	moderate	-	-

Mucositis

Note: Mucositis not due to radiation is graded in the GASTROINTESTINAL category for specific sites: Colitis, Esophagitis, Gastritis, Stomatitis/pharyngitis (oral/pharyngeal mucositis), and Typhlitis; or the RENAL/GENITOURINARY category for Vaginitis.

Radiation-related mucositis is graded as Mucositis due to radiation.

(Continued on next page)

Appendix 9. National Cancer Institute Common Toxicity Criteria, Version 2.0 *(Continued)*

Adverse Event	0	1	Grade 2	3	4
Mucositis due to radiation	none	erythema of the mucosa	patchy pseudomembranous reaction (patches generally ≤ 1.5 cm in diameter and non-contiguous)	confluent pseudo-membranous reaction (contiguous patches generally > 1.5 cm in diameter)	necrosis or deep ulceration; may include bleeding not induced by minor trauma or abrasion

Also consider Pain due to radiation.

Notes: Grade radiation mucositis of the larynx here.

　　　Dysphagia related to radiation is also graded as <u>either</u> Dysphagia—esophageal related to radiation <u>or</u> Dysphagia—pharyngeal related to radiation, depending on the site of treatment.

Nausea	none	able to eat	oral intake significantly decreased	no significant intake, requiring IV fluids	-
Pancreatitis	none	-	-	abdominal pain with pancreatic enzyme elevation	complicated by shock (acute circulatory failure)

Also consider Hypotension.

Note: Amylase is graded in the METABOLIC/LABORATORY category.

Pharyngitis is graded in the GASTROINTESTINAL category as Stomatitis/pharyngitis (oral/pharyngeal mucositis).

Proctitis	none	increased stool frequency, occasional blood-streaked stools, or rectal discomfort (including hemorrhoids), not requiring medication	increased stool frequency, bleeding, mucus discharge, or rectal discomfort requiring medication; anal fissure	increased stool frequency/diarrhea, requiring parenteral support; rectal bleeding, requiring transfusion; or persistent mucus discharge, necessitating pads	perforation, bleeding or necrosis or other life-threatening complication requiring surgical intervention (e.g., colostomy)

Also consider Hemorrhage/bleeding with grade 3 or 4 thrombocytopenia, Hemorrhage/bleeding without grade 3 or 4 thrombocytopenia, Pain due to radiation.

Notes: Fistula is graded separately as Fistula—rectal/anal.

　　　Proctitis occurring more than 90 days after the start of radiation therapy is graded in the RTOG/EORTC Late Radiation Morbidity Scoring Scheme.

Salivary gland changes	none	slightly thickened saliva/may have slightly altered taste (e.g., metallic); additional fluids may be required	thick, ropy, sticky saliva; markedly altered taste; alteration in diet required	-	acute salivary gland necrosis
Sense of smell	normal	slightly altered	markedly altered	-	-
Stomatitis/pharyngitis (oral/pharyngeal mucositis)	none	painless ulcers, erythema, or mild soreness in the absence of lesions	painful erythema, edema, or ulcers but can eat or swallow	painful erythema, edema, or ulcers requiring IV hydration	severe ulceration or requires parenteral or enteral nutritional support or prophylactic intubation
For BMT studies, if specified in the protocol.	none	painless ulcers, erythema, or mild soreness in the absence of lesions	painful erythema, edema, or ulcers but can swallow	painful erythema, edema, or ulcers preventing swallowing or requiring hydration or parenteral (or enteral) nutritional support	severe ulceration requiring prophylactic intubation or resulting in documented aspiration pneumonia

Note: Radiation-related mucositis is graded as Mucositis due to radiation.

Taste disturbance (dysgeusia)	normal	slightly altered	markedly altered	-	-

(Continued on next page)

Appendix 9. National Cancer Institute Common Toxicity Criteria, Version 2.0 *(Continued)*

Adverse Event	0	1	2	3	4
			Grade		
Typhlitis (inflammation of the cecum)	none	-	-	abdominal pain, diarrhea, fever, and radiographic or biopsy documentation	perforation, bleeding or necrosis or other life-threatening complication requiring surgical intervention (e.g., colostomy)

Also consider Hemorrhage/bleeding with grade 3 or 4 thrombocytopenia, Hemorrhage/bleeding without grade 3 or 4 thrombocytopenia, Hypotension, Febrile neutropenia.

Adverse Event	0	1	2	3	4
Vomiting	none	1 episode in 24 hours over pretreatment	2–5 episodes in 24 hours over pretreatment	≥ 6 episodes in 24 hours over pretreatment; or need for IV fluids	Requiring parenteral nutrition; or physiologic consequences requiring intensive care; hemodynamic collapse

Also consider Dehydration.

Weight gain is graded in the CONSTITUTIONAL SYMPTOMS category.

Weight loss is graded in the CONSTITUTIONAL SYMPTOMS category.

Adverse Event	0	1	2	3	4
Gastrointestinal-Other (Specify, _____)	none	mild	moderate	severe	life-threatening or disabling

HEMORRHAGE

Notes: Transfusion in this section refers to pRBC infusion.

For _any_ bleeding with grade 3 or 4 platelets (< 50,000), _always_ grade Hemorrhage/bleeding with grade 3 or 4 thrombocytopenia. Also consider platelets, transfusion-pRBC, and transfusion-platelets in addition by grading the site or type of bleeding.

If the site or type of hemorrhage/bleeding is listed, also use the grading that incorporates the site of bleeding: CNS hemorrhage/bleeding, Hematuria, Hematemesis, Hemoptysis, Hemorrhage/bleeding with surgery, Melena/lower GI bleeding, Petechiae/purpura (Hemorrhage/bleeding into skin), Rectal bleeding/hematochezia, Vaginal bleeding.

If the platelet count is ≥ 50,000 and the site or type of bleeding is listed, grade the specific site. If the site or type is _not_ listed and the platelet count is ≥ 50,000, grade Hemorrhage/bleeding without grade 3 or 4 thrombocytopenia and specify the site or type in the OTHER category.

Adverse Event	0	1	2	3	4
Hemorrhage/bleeding with grade 3 or 4 thrombocytopenia	none	mild without transfusion	-	requiring transfusion	catastrophic bleeding, requiring major non-elective intervention

Also consider Platelets, Hemoglobin, Transfusion-platelet, Transfusion-pRBCs or type of bleeding. If the site is not listed, grade as Hemorrhage-Other (Specify site,_____)

Note: This adverse event must be graded for any bleeding with grade 3 or 4 thrombocytopenia.

Adverse Event	0	1	2	3	4
Hemorrhage/bleeding without grade 3 or 4 thrombocytopenia	none	mild without transfusion	-	requiring transfusion	catastrophic bleeding requiring major non-elective intervention

Also consider Platelets, Hemoglobin, Transfusion-platelet, Transfusion-pRBCs. Hemorrhage-Other (Specify site,_____)

Note: Bleeding in the absence of grade 3 or 4 thrombocytopenia is graded here only if the specific site or type of bleeding is not listed elsewhere in the HEMORRHAGE category.

Adverse Event	0	1	2	3	4
CNS hemorrhage/bleeding	none	-	-	bleeding noted on CT or other scan with no clinical consequences	hemorrhagic stroke or hemorrhagic vascular event (CVA) with neurologic signs and symptoms
Epistaxis	none	mild without transfusion	-	requiring transfusion	catastrophic bleeding, requiring major non-elective intervention

(Continued on next page)

Appendix 9. National Cancer Institute Common Toxicity Criteria, Version 2.0 *(Continued)*

Adverse Event	0	1	2	3	4
			Grade		
Hematemesis	none	mild without transfusion	-	requiring transfusion	catastrophic bleeding, requiring major non-elective intervention
Hematuria (in the absence of vaginal bleeding)	none	microscopic only	intermittent gross bleeding, no clots	persistent gross bleeding or clots; may require catheterization or instrumentation, or transfusion	open surgery or necrosis or deep bladder ulceration
Hemoptysis	none	mild without transfusion	-	requiring transfusion	catastrophic bleeding, requiring major non-elective intervention
Hemorrhage/ bleeding associated with surgery	none	mild without transfusion	-	requiring transfusion	catastrophic bleeding, requiring major non-elective intervention

Note: Expected blood loss at the time of surgery is not graded as an adverse event.

Adverse Event	0	1	2	3	4
Melena/GI bleeding	none	mild without transfusion	-	requiring transfusion	catastrophic bleeding, requiring major non-elective intervention
Petechiae/purpura (hemorrhage/ bleeding into skin or mucosa)	none	rare petechiae of skin	petechiae or purpura in dependent areas of skin	generalized petechiae or purpura of skin or petechiae of any mucosal site	-
Rectal bleeding/ hematochezia	none	mild without transfusion or medication	persistent, requiring medication (e.g., steroid suppositories) and/or break from radiation treatment	requiring transfusion	catastrophic bleeding, requiring major non-elective intervention
Vaginal bleeding	none	spotting, requiring < 2 pads per day	requiring ≥ 2 pads per day, but not requiring transfusion	requiring transfusion	catastrophic bleeding, requiring major non-elective intervention
Hemorrhage-Other (Specify site, ...)	none	mild without transfusion	-	requiring transfusion	catastrophic bleeding, requiring major non-elective intervention

			HEPATIC		
Alkaline phosphatase	WNL	> ULN–2.5 x ULN	> 2.5–5.0 x ULN	> 5.0–20.0 x ULN	> 20.0 x ULN
Bilirubin	WNL	> ULN–1.5 x ULN	> 1.5–3.0 x ULN	> 3.0–10.0 x ULN	> 10.0 x ULN

Bilirubin associated with graft versus host disease (GVHD) for BMT studies, if specified in the protocol.
Note: The following criteria are used only for bilirubin associated with graft versus host disease.

	normal	≥ 2–< 3 mg/100 ml	≥ 3–< 6 mg/100 ml	≥ 6–< 15 mg/100 ml	≥ 15 mg/100 ml
GGT (g-Glutamyl transpeptidase)	WNL	> ULN–2.5 x ULN	> 2.5–5.0 x ULN	> 5.0–20.0 x ULN	> 20.0 x ULN
Hepatic enlargement	absent	-	-	present	-

Note: Grade Hepatic enlargement only for changes related to adverse events including VOD.

Hypoalbuminemia	WNL	< LLN–3 g/dl	≥ 2–< 3 g/dl	< 2 g/dl	-

(Continued on next page)

Appendix 9. National Cancer Institute Common Toxicity Criteria, Version 2.0 *(Continued)*

Adverse Event	Grade 0	1	2	3	4
Liver dysfunction/ failure (clinical)	normal	-	-	asterixis	encephalopathy or coma
Portal vein flow	normal	-	decreased portal vein flow	reversal/retrograde portal vein flow	-
SGOT (AST) (serum glutamic oxaloacetic transaminase)	WNL	> ULN–2.5 x ULN	> 2.5–5.0 x ULN	> 5.0–20.0 x ULN	> 20.0 x ULN
SGPT (ALT) (serum glutamic pyruvic transami- nase)	WNL	> ULN–2.5 x ULN	> 2.5–5.0 x ULN	> 5.0–20.0 x ULN	> 20.0 x ULN
Hepatic-Other (Specify, _____)	none	mild	moderate	severe	life-threatening or disabling
INFECTION/FEBRILE NEUTROPENIA					
Catheter-related infection	none	mild, no active treatment	moderate, localized infection, requiring local or oral treatment	severe, systemic infection, requiring IV antibiotic or antifungal treatment or hospital- ization	life-threatening sepsis (e.g., septic shock)
Febrile neutropenia (fever of unknown origin without clinically or microbiologically documented infection) (ANC < 1.0 x 10⁹/L, fever ≥ 38.5°C)	none	-	-	present	life-threatening sepsis (e.g., septic shock)

Also consider Neutrophils.
Note: Hypothermia instead of fever may be associated with neutropenia and is graded here.

Adverse Event	0	1	2	3	4
Infection (docu- mented clinically or microbiologically) with grade 3 or 4 neutropenia (ANC < 1.0 x 10⁹/L)	none	-	-	present	life-threatening sepsis (e.g., septic shock)

Also consider infection.
Note: Hypothermia instead of fever may be associated with neutropenia and is graded here. In the absence of documented infection with grade 3 or 4 neutropenia, with fever is graded as Febrile neutropenia.

Adverse Event	0	1	2	3	4
Infection with unknown ANC	none	-	-	present	life-threatening sepsis (e.g., septic shock)

Note: This adverse event criterion is used in the rare case when ANC is unknown.

Adverse Event	0	1	2	3	4
Infection without neutropenia	none	mild, no active treatment	moderate, localized infection, requiring local or oral treatment	severe, systemic infection, requiring IV antibiotic or antifungal treatment, or hospital- ization	life-threatening sepsis (e.g., septic shock)

Also consider Neutrophils.

Wound infectious is graded in the DERMATOLOGY/SKIN category.

Adverse Event	0	1	2	3	4
Infection/Febrile Neutropenia-Other (Specify, _____)	none	mild	moderate	severe	life-threatening or disabling

(Continued on next page)

Appendix 9. National Cancer Institute Common Toxicity Criteria, Version 2.0 *(Continued)*

Adverse Event	0	1	2	3	4
			Grade		
LYMPHATICS					
Lymphatics	normal	mild lymphedema	moderate lymphedema requiring compression; lymphocyst	severe lymphedema limiting function; lymphocyst requiring surgery	severe lymphedema limiting function with ulceration
Lymphatics-Other (Specify, _____)	none	mild	moderate	severe	life-threatening or disabling
METABOLIC/LABORATORY					
Acidosis (metabolic or respiratory)	normal	pH < normal, but ≥ 7.3	-	pH < 7.3	pH < 7.3 with life-threatening physiologic consequences
Alkalosis (metabolic or respiratory)	normal	pH > normal, but ≤ 7.5	-	pH > 7.5	pH > 7.5 with life-threatening physiologic consequences
Amylase	WNL	> ULN–1.5 x ULN	> 1.5–2.0 x ULN	> 2.0–5.0 x ULN	> 5.0 x ULN
Bicarbonate	WNL	< LLN–16 mEq/dl	11–15 mEq/dl	8–10 mEq/dl	< 8 mEq/dl
CPK (creatine phosphokinase)	WNL	> ULN–2.5 x ULN	> 2.5–5 x ULN	> 5–10 x ULN	> 10 x ULN
Hypercalcemia	WNL	> ULN–11.5 mg/dl > ULN–2.9 mmol/L	> 11.5–12.5 mg/dl > 2.9–3.1 mmol/L	> 12.5–13.5 mg/dl > 3.1–3.4 mmol/L	> 13.5 mg/dl > 3.4 mmol/L
Hypercholesterolemia	WNL	> ULN–300 mg/dl > ULN–7.75 mmol/L	> 300–400 mg/dl > 7.75–10.34 mmol/L	> 400–500 mg/dl > 10.34–12.92 mmol/L	> 500 mg/dl > 12.92 mmol/L
Hyperglycemia	WNL	> ULN–160 mg/dl > ULN–8.9 mmol/L	> 160–250 mg/dl > 8.9–13.9 mmol/L	> 250–500 mg/dl > 13.9–27.8 mmol/L	> 500 mg/dl > 27.8 mmol/L or acidosis
Hyperkalemia	WNL	> ULN–5.5 mmol/L	> 5.5–6.0 mmol/L	> 6.0–7.0 mmol/L	> 7.0 mmol/L
Hypermagnesemia	WNL	> ULN–3.0 mg/dl > ULN–1.23 mmol/L	-	> 3.0–8.0 mg/dl > 1.23–3.30 mmol/L	> 8.0 mg/dl > 3.30 mmol/L
Hypernatremia	WNL	> ULN–150 mmol/L	> 150–155 mmol/L	> 155–160 mmol/L	> 160 mmol/L
Hypertriglyceridemia	WNL	> ULN–2.5 x ULN	> 2.5–5.0 x ULN	> 5.0–10 x ULN	> 10 x ULN
Hyperuricemia	WNL	> ULN–≤ 10 mg/dl ≤ 0.59 mmol/L without physiologic consequences	-	> ULN–≤ 10 mg/dl ≤ 0.59 mmol/L with physiologic consequences	> 10 mg/dl > 0.59 mmol/L
Also consider Tumor lysis syndrome, Renal failure, Creatinine, Hyperkalemia.					
Hypocalcemia	WNL	< LLN–8.0 mg/dl < LLN–2.0 mmol/L	7.0–< 8.0 mg/dl 1.75–< 2.0 mmol/L	6.0–< 7.0 mg/dl 1.5–< 1.75 mmol/L	< 6.0 mg/dl < 1.5 mmol/L
Hypoglycemia	WNL	< LLN–55 mg/dl < LLN–3.0 mmol/L	40–< 55 mg/dl 2.2–< 3.0 mmol/L	30–< 40 mg/dl 1.7–< 2.2 mmol/L	< 30 mg/dl < 1.7 mmol/L
Hypokalemia	WNL	< LLN–3.0 mmol/L	-	2.5–< 3.0 mmol/L	< 2.5 mmol/L
Hypomagnesemia	WNL	< LLN–1.2 mg/dl < LLN–0.5 mmol/L	0.9–< 1.2 mg/dl 0.4–< 0.5 mmol/L	0.7–< 0.9 mg/dl 0.3–< 0.4 mmol/L	< 0.7 mg/dl < 0.3 mmol/L
Hyponatremia	WNL	< LLN–130 mmol/L	-	120–< 130 mmol/L	< 120 mmol/L
Hypophosphatemia	WNL	< LLN–2.5 mg/dl < LLN–0.8 mmol/L	≥ 2.0–< 2.5 mg/dl ≥ 0.6–< 0.8 mmol/L	≥ 1.0–< 2.0 mg/dl ≥ 0.3–< 0.6 mmol/L	< 1.0 mg/dl < 0.3 mmol/L

(Continued on next page)

Appendix 9. National Cancer Institute Common Toxicity Criteria, Version 2.0 *(Continued)*

Adverse Event	0	1	Grade 2	3	4
Hypothyroidism is graded in the ENDOCRINE category.					
Lipase	WNL	> ULN–1.5 x ULN	> 1.5–2.0 x ULN	> 2.0–5.0 x ULN	> 5.0 x ULN
Metabolic/Laboratory-Other (Specify, _____)	none	mild	moderate	severe	life-threatening or disabling
MUSCULOSKELETAL					
Arthralgia is graded in the PAIN category.					
Arthritis	none	mild pain with inflammation, erythema or joint swelling but not interfering with function	moderate pain with inflammation, erythema, or joint swelling interfering with function, but not interfering with activities of daily living	severe pain with inflammation, erythema, or joint swelling and interfering with activities of daily living	disabling
Muscle weakness (not due to neuropathy)	normal	asymptomatic with weakness on physical exam	symptomatic and interfering with function, but not interfering with activities of daily living	symptomatic and interfering with activities of daily living	bedridden or disabling
Myalgia (tenderness or pain in muscles) is graded in the PAIN category.					
Myositis (inflammation/damage of muscle) Also consider CPK. Note: Myositis implies muscle damage (i.e., elevated CPK).	none	mild pain, not interfering with function	pain interfering with function, but not interfering with activities of daily living	pain interfering with function and interfering with activities of daily living	bedridden or disabling
Osteonecrosis (avascular necrosis)	none	asymptomatic and detected by imaging only	symptomatic and interfering with function, but not interfering with	activities of daily living symptomatic and interfering with	activities of daily living symptomatic; or disabling
Musculoskeletal-Other (Specify, _____)	none	mild	moderate	severe	life-threatening or disabling
NEUROLOGY					
Aphasia, receptive and/or expressive, is graded under Speech impairment in the NEUROLOGY category.					
Arachnoiditis/ meningismus/ radiculitis Also consider Headache, Vomiting, Fever.	absent	mild pain not interfering with function	moderate pain interfering with function but not interfering with activities of daily living	severe pain interfering with activities of daily living	unable to function or perform activities of daily living; bedridden; paraplegia
Ataxia (incoordination)	normal	asymptomatic but abnormal on physical exam, and not interfering with function	mild symptoms interfering with function but not interfering with activities of daily living	moderate symptoms interfering with activities of daily living	bedridden or disabling
CNS cerebrovascular ischemia	none	-	-	transient ischemic event or attack (TIA)	permanent event (e.g., cerebral vascular accident)
CNS hemorrhage/bleeding is graded in the HEMORRHAGE category.					
Cognitive disturbance/learning problems	none	*cognitive disability; not interfering with work/ school performance; preservation of intelligence*	*cognitive disability; interfering with work/ school performance; decline of 1 SD (Standard Deviation) or loss of developmental milestones*	*cognitive disability; resulting in significant impairment of work/ school performance; cognitive decline > 2 SD*	*inability to work/ frank mental retardation*

(Continued on next page)

Appendix 9. National Cancer Institute Common Toxicity Criteria, Version 2.0 *(Continued)*

Adverse Event	0	Grade 1	2	3	4
Confusion	normal	confusion or disorientation or attention deficit of brief duration; resolves spontaneously with no sequelae	confusion or disorientation or attention deficit interfering with function, but not interfering with activities of daily living	confusion or delirium interfering with activities of daily living	harmful to others or self; requiring hospitalization
Cranial neuropathy is graded in the NEUROLOGY category as Neuropathy-cranial.					
Delusions	normal	-	-	present	toxic psychosis
Depressed level of consciousness	normal	somnolence or sedation not interfering with function	somnolence or sedation interfering with function, but not interfering with activities of daily living	obtundation or stupor; difficult to arouse; interfering with activities of daily living	coma
Syncope (fainting) is graded in the NEUROLOGY category.					
Dizziness/ lightheadedness	none	not interfering with function	interfering with function, but not interfering with activities of daily living	interfering with activities of daily living	bedridden or disabling
Dysphasia, receptive and/or expressive, is graded under Speech impairment in the NEUROLOGY category.					
Extrapyramidal/ involuntary movement/ restlessness	none	mild involuntary movements not interfering with function	moderate involuntary movements interfering with function, but not interfering with activities of daily living	severe involuntary movements or torticollis interfering with activities of daily living	bedridden or disabling
Hallucinations	normal	-	-	present	toxic psychosis
Headache is graded in the PAIN category.					
Insomnia	normal	occasional difficulty sleeping not interfering with function	difficulty sleeping interfering with function, but not interfering with activities of daily living	frequent difficulty sleeping, interfering with activities of daily living	-
Note: This adverse event is graded when insomnia is related to treatment. If pain or other symptoms interfere with sleep, do NOT grade as insomnia.					
Irritability (children < 3 years of age)	*normal*	*mild; easily consolable*	*moderate; requiring increased attention*	*severe; inconsolable*	*-*
Leukoencephalopathy associated radiological findings	none	mild increase in SAS (subarachnoid space) and/or mild ventriculomegaly; and/or small (+/- multiple) focal T2 hyperintensities, involving periventricular white matter or < 1/3 of susceptible areas of cerebrum	moderate increase in SAS; and/or moderate ventriculomegaly; and/ or focal T2 hyperintensities extending into centrum ovale, or involving 1/3 to 2/3 of susceptible areas of cerebrum	severe increase in SAS; severe ventriculomegaly; near total white matter T2 hyperintensities or diffuse low attenuation (CT); focal white matter necrosis (cystic)	severe increase in SAS; severe ventriculomegaly; diffuse low attenuation with calcification (CT); diffuse white matter necrosis (MRI)
Memory loss	normal	memory loss not interfering with function	memory loss interfering with function, but not interfering with activities of daily living	memory loss interfering with activities of daily living	amnesia
Mood alteration— anxiety, agitation	normal		mild mood alteration not interfering with function moderate mood alteration interfering	with function, but not interfering with activities of daily living severe mood	alteration interfering with activities of daily living suicidal ideation or danger to self

(Continued on next page)

Appendix 9. National Cancer Institute Common Toxicity Criteria, Version 2.0 *(Continued)*

Adverse Event	0	1	2	3	4
			Grade		
Mood alteration—depression	normal	mild mood alteration not interfering with function	moderate mood alteration interfering with function, but not interfering with activities of daily living	severe mood alteration interfering with activities of daily living	suicidal ideation or danger to self
Mood alteration—euphoria	normal	mild mood alteration not interfering with function	moderate mood alteration interfering with function, but not interfering with activities of daily living	severe mood alteration interfering with activities of daily living	danger to self
Neuropathic pain is graded in the PAIN category.					
Neuropathy—cranial	absent	-	present, not interfering with activities of daily living	present, interfering with activities of daily living	life-threatening, disabling
Neuropathy—motor	normal	subjective weakness but no objective findings	mild objective weakness interfering with function, but not interfering with activities of daily living	objective weakness interfering with activities of daily living	paralysis
Neuropathy—sensory	normal	loss of deep tendon reflexes or paresthesia (including tingling), but not interfering with function	objective sensory loss or paresthesia (including tingling), interfering with function, but not interfering with activities of daily living	sensory loss or paresthesia interfering with activities of daily living permanent sensory	loss that interferes with function
Nystagmus	absent	present	-	-	-
Also consider Vision—double vision.					
Personality/behavioral	normal	change, but not disruptive to patient or family	disruptive to patient or family	disruptive to patient and family; requiring mental health intervention	harmful to others or self; requiring hospitalization
Pyramidal tract dysfunction (e.g., tone, hyperreflexia, positive Babinski, fine motor coordination)	normal	asymptomatic with abnormality on physical examination	symptomatic or interfering with function, but not interfering with activities of daily living	interfering with activities of daily living	bedridden or disabling; paralysis
Seizure(s)	none	-	seizure(s) self-limited and consciousness is preserved	seizure(s) in which consciousness is altered	seizures of any type that are prolonged, repetitive, or difficult to control (e.g., status epilepticus, intractable epilepsy)
Speech impairment (e.g., dysphasia or aphasia)	normal		awareness of receptive or expressive dysphasia, not impairing ability to communicate	receptive or expressive dysphasia, impairing ability to communicate	inability to communicate
Syncope (fainting)	absent	-	-	present	-
Also consider CARDIOVASCULAR (ARRHYTHMIA), Vasovagal episode, CNS cerebrovascular ischemia.					
Tremor	none	mild and brief or intermittent but not interfering with function	moderate tremor interfering with function, but not interfering with activities of daily living	severe tremor interfering with activities of daily living	-

(Continued on next page)

Appendix 9. National Cancer Institute Common Toxicity Criteria, Version 2.0 *(Continued)*

Adverse Event	0	Grade 1	Grade 2	Grade 3	Grade 4
Vertigo	none	not interfering with function	interfering with function, but not interfering with activities of daily living	interfering with activities of daily living	bedridden or disabling
Neurology-Other (Specify, _____)	none	mild	moderate	severe	life-threatening or disabling
OCULAR/VISUAL					
Cataract	none	asymptomatic	symptomatic, partial visual loss	symptomatic, visual loss requiring treatment or interfering with function	-
Conjunctivitis	none	abnormal ophthalmologic changes, but asymptomatic or symptomatic without visual impairment (i.e., pain and irritation)	symptomatic and interfering with function, but not interfering with activities of daily living	symptomatic and interfering with activities of daily living	-
Dry eye	none	mild, not requiring treatment	moderate or requiring artificial tears	-	-
Glaucoma	none	increase in intraocular pressure but no visual loss	increase in intraocular pressure with retinal changes	visual impairment	unilateral or bilateral loss of vision (blindness)
Keratitis (corneal inflammation/corneal ulceration)	none	abnormal ophthalmologic changes but asymptomatic or symptomatic without visual impairment (i.e., pain and irritation)	symptomatic and interfering with function, but not interfering with activities of daily living	symptomatic and interfering with activities of daily living	unilateral or bilateral loss of vision (blindness)
Tearing (watery eyes)	none	mild, not interfering with function	moderate: interfering with function, but not interfering with activities of daily living	interfering with activities of daily living	-
Vision—blurred vision	none	-	symptomatic and interfering with function, but not interfering with activities of daily living	symptomatic and interfering with activities of daily living	-
Vision—double vision (diplopia)	normal	-	symptomatic and interfering with function, but not interfering with activities of daily living	symptomatic and interfering with activities of daily living	-
Vision—flashing lights/floaters	normal	mild, not interfering with function	symptomatic and interfering with function, but not interfering with activities of daily living	symptomatic and interfering with activities of daily living	-
Vision—night blindness (nyctalopia)	normal	abnormal electro-retinography but asymptomatic	symptomatic and interfering with function, but not interfering with activities of daily living	symptomatic and interfering with activities of daily living	-
Vision—photophobia	normal	-	symptomatic and interfering with function, but not interfering with activities of daily living	symptomatic and interfering with activities of daily living	-
Ocular/Visual-Other (Specify, _____)	normal	mild	moderate	severe	unilateral or bilateral loss of vision (blindness)

(Continued on next page)

Appendix 9. National Cancer Institute Common Toxicity Criteria, Version 2.0 *(Continued)*

Adverse Event	0	1	2	3	4
			Grade		
			PAIN		
Abdominal pain or cramping	none	mild pain not interfering with function	moderate pain: pain or analgesics interfering with function, but not interfering with activities of daily living	severe pain: pain or analgesics severely interfering with activities of daily living	disabling
Arthralgia (joint pain)	none	mild pain not interfering with function	moderate pain: pain or analgesics interfering with function, but not interfering with activities of daily living	severe pain: pain or analgesics severely interfering with activities of daily living	disabling
Arthritis (joint pain with clinical signs of inflammation) is graded in the MUSCULOSKELETAL category.					
Bone pain	none	mild pain not interfering with function	moderate pain: pain or analgesics interfering with function, but not interfering with activities of daily living	severe pain: pain or analgesics severely interfering with activities of daily living	disabling
Chest pain (non-cardiac and non-pleuritic)	none	mild pain not interfering with function	moderate pain: pain or analgesics interfering with function, but not interfering with activities of daily living	severe pain: pain or analgesics severely interfering with activities of daily living	disabling
Dysmenorrhea	none	mild pain not interfering with function	moderate pain: pain or analgesics interfering with function, but not interfering with activities of daily living	severe pain: pain or analgesics severely interfering with activities of daily living	disabling
Dyspareunia	none	mild pain not interfering with function	moderate pain interfering with sexual activity	severe pain preventing sexual activity	–
Dysuria is graded in the RENAL/GENITOURINARY category.					
Earache (otalgia)	none	mild pain not interfering with function	moderate pain: pain or analgesics interfering with function, but not interfering with activities of daily living	severe pain: pain or analgesics severely interfering with activities of daily living	disabling
Headache	none	mild pain not interfering with function	moderate pain: pain or analgesics interfering with function, but not interfering with activities of daily living	severe pain: pain or analgesics severely interfering with activities of daily living	disabling
Hepatic pain	none	mild pain not interfering with function	moderate pain: pain or analgesics interfering with function, but not interfering with activities of daily living	severe pain: pain or analgesics severely interfering with activities of daily living	disabling
Myalgia (muscle pain)	none	mild pain not interfering with function	moderate pain: pain or analgesics interfering with function, but not interfering with activities of daily living	severe pain: pain or analgesics severely interfering with activities of daily living	disabling
Neuropathic pain (e.g., jaw pain, neurologic pain, phantom limb pain, post infectious neuralgia, or painful neuropathies)	none	mild pain not interfering with function	moderate pain: pain or analgesics interfering with function, but not interfering with activities of daily living	severe pain: pain or analgesics severely interfering with activities of daily living	disabling

(Continued on next page)

Appendix 9. National Cancer Institute Common Toxicity Criteria, Version 2.0 *(Continued)*

Adverse Event	0	1	2	3	4
			Grade		
Pain due to radiation	none	mild pain not interfering with function	moderate pain: pain or analgesics interfering with function, but not interfering with activities of daily living	severe pain: pain or analgesics severely interfering with activities of daily living	disabling
Pelvic pain	none	mild pain not interfering with function	moderate pain: pain or analgesics interfering with function, but not interfering with activities of daily living	severe pain: pain or analgesics severely interfering with activities of daily living	disabling
Pleuritic pain	none	mild pain not interfering with function	moderate pain: pain or analgesics interfering with function, but not interfering with activities of daily living	severe pain: pain or analgesics severely interfering with activities of daily living	disabling
Rectal or perirectal pain (proctalgia)	none	mild pain not interfering with function	moderate pain: pain or analgesics interfering with function, but not interfering with activities of daily living	severe pain: pain or analgesics severely interfering with activities of daily living	disabling
Tumor pain (onset or exacerbation of tumor pain due to treatment)	none	mild pain not interfering with function	moderate pain: pain or analgesics interfering with function, but not interfering with activities of daily living	severe pain: pain or analgesics severely interfering with activities of daily living	disabling

Tumor flare is graded in the SYNDROME category.

Adverse Event	0	1	2	3	4
Pain-Other (Specify, _____)	none	mild	moderate	severe	disabling

PULMONARY

Adverse Event	0	1	2	3	4
Adult Respiratory Distress Syndrome (ARDS)	absent	-	-	-	present
Apnea	none	-	-	present	requiring intubation
Carbon monoxide diffusion capacity (DL_{CO})	≥ 90% of pretreatment or normal value	≥ 75–< 90% of pretreatment or normal value	≥ 50–< 75% of pretreatment or normal value	≥ 25–< 50% of pretreatment or normal value	< 25% of pretreatment or normal value
Cough	absent	mild, relieved by non-prescription medication	requiring narcotic antitussive	severe cough or coughing spasms, poorly controlled or unresponsive to treatment	-
Dyspnea (shortness of breath)	normal	-	dyspnea on exertion	dyspnea at normal level of activity	dyspnea at rest or requiring ventilator support
Forced Expiratory Volume (FEV_1)	≥ 90% of pretreatment or normal value	≥ 75–< 90% of pretreatment or normal value	≥ 50–< 75% of pretreatment or normal value	≥ 25–< 50% of pretreatment or normal value	< 25% of pretreatment or normal value
Hiccoughs (hiccups, singultus)	none	mild, not requiring treatment	moderate, requiring treatment	severe, prolonged, and refractory to treatment	-

(Continued on next page)

Appendix 9. National Cancer Institute Common Toxicity Criteria, Version 2.0 *(Continued)*

Adverse Event	0	Grade 1	Grade 2	Grade 3	Grade 4
Hypoxia	normal	-	decreased O_2 saturation with exercise	decreased O_2 saturation at rest, requiring supplemental oxygen	decreased O_2 saturation, requiring pressure support (CPAP) or assisted ventilation
Pleural effusion (non-malignant)	none	asymptomatic and not requiring treatment	symptomatic, requiring diuretics	symptomatic, requiring O_2 or therapeutic thoracentesis	life-threatening (e.g., requiring intubation)
Pleuritic pain is graded in the PAIN category.					
Pneumonitis/pulmonary infiltrates	none	radiographic changes but asymptomatic or symptoms not requiring steroids	radiographic changes and requiring steroids or diuretics	radiographic changes and requiring oxygen	radiographic changes and requiring assisted ventilation
Pneumothorax	none	no intervention required	chest tube required	sclerosis or surgery required	life-threatening
Pulmonary embolism is graded as Thrombosis/embolism in the CARDIOVASCULAR (GENERAL) category.					
Pulmonary fibrosis	none	radiographic changes, but asymptomatic or symptoms not requiring steroids	requiring steroids or diuretics	requiring oxygen	requiring assisted ventilation
Radiation-related pulmonary fibrosis is graded in the RTOG/EORTC Late Radiation Morbidity Scoring Scheme—Lung.					
Voice changes/stridor/larynx (e.g., hoarseness, loss of voice, laryngitis)	normal	mild or intermittent hoarseness	persistent hoarseness, but able to vocalize; may have mild to moderate edema	whispered speech, not able to vocalize; may have marked edema	marked dyspnea/stridor requiring tracheostomy or intubation
Notes: Cough from radiation is graded as cough in the PULMONARY category. Radiation-related hemoptysis from larynx/pharynx is graded as Grade 4 Mucositis due to radiation in the GASTROINTESTINAL category. Radiation-related hemoptysis from the thoracic cavity is graded as Grade 4 Hemoptysis in the HEMORRHAGE category.					
Pulmonary-Other (Specify, _____)	none	mild	moderate	severe	life-threatening or disabling
RENAL/GENITOURINARY					
Bladder spasms	absent	mild symptoms, not requiring intervention	symptoms requiring antispasmodic	severe symptoms requiring narcotic	-
Creatinine	WNL	> ULN–1.5 x ULN	> 1.5–3.0 x ULN	> 3.0–6.0 x ULN	> 6.0 x ULN
Note: Adjust to age-appropriate levels for pediatric patients.					
Dysuria (painful urination)	none	mild symptoms requiring no intervention	symptoms relieved with therapy	symptoms not relieved despite therapy	-
Fistula or GU fistula (e.g., vaginal, vesico-vaginal)	none	-	-	requiring intervention	requiring surgery
Hemoglobinuria	-	present	-	-	-
Hematuria (in the absence of vaginal bleeding) is graded in the HEMORRHAGE category.					
Incontinence	none	with coughing, sneezing, etc.	spontaneous, some control	no control (in the absence of fistula)	-
Operative injury to bladder and/or ureter	none	-	injury of bladder with primary repair	sepsis, fistula, or obstruction requiring secondary surgery; loss of one kidney; injury requiring anastomosis or reimplantation	septic obstruction of both kidneys or vesicovaginal fistula requiring diversion

(Continued on next page)

Appendix 9. National Cancer Institute Common Toxicity Criteria, Version 2.0 *(Continued)*

Adverse Event	0	1	2	3	4
			Grade		
Proteinuria	normal or < 0.15 g/24 hours	1+ or 0.15–1.0 g/24 hours	2+ to 3+ or 1.0–3.5 g/ 24 hours	4+ or > 3.5 g/24 hours	nephrotic syndrome
Note: If there is an inconsistency between absolute value and dip stick reading, use the absolute value for grading.					
Renal failure	none	-	-	requiring dialysis, but reversible	requiring dialysis and irreversible
Ureteral obstruction	none	unilateral, not requiring surgery	-	bilateral, not requiring surgery	stent, nephrostomy tube, or surgery
Urinary electrolyte wasting (e.g., Fanconi's syndrome, renal tubular acidosis)	none	asymptomatic, not requiring treatment	mild, reversible, and manageable with oral replacement	reversible but requiring IV replace-ment	irreversible, requiring continued replacement
Also consider Acidosis, Bicarbonate, Hypocalcemia, Hypophosphatemia.					
Urinary frequency/ urgency	normal	increase in frequency or nocturia up to 2 x normal	increase > 2 x normal but < hourly	hourly or more with urgency, or requiring catheter	-
Urinary retention	normal	hesitancy or dribbling, but no significant re-sidual urine; retention occurring during the immediate postop-erative period	hesitancy requiring medication or occa-sional in/out catheter-ization (< 4 x per week), or operative bladder atony requiring indwelling catheter be-yond immediate post-operative period but for < 6 weeks	requiring frequent in/ out catheterization (≥ 4 x per week) or urological intervention (e.g., TURP, suprapu-bic tube, urethrotomy)	bladder rupture
Urine color change (not related to other dietary or physi-ologic cause e.g., bilirubin, concen-trated urine, hem-aturia)	normal	asymptomatic, change in urine color	-	-	-
Vaginal bleeding is graded in the HEMORRHAGE category.					
Vaginitis (not due to infection)	none	mild, not requiring treatment	moderate, relieved with treatment	severe, not relieved with treatment, or ulceration not requiring surgery	ulceration requiring surgery
Renal/Genitouri-nary-Other (Specify, _____)	none	mild	moderate	severe	life-threatening or disabling
SECONDARY MALIGNANCY					
Secondary Malignancy-Other (Specify type, _____) excludes metasta-sis from initial primary.	none	-	-	-	present
SEXUAL/REPRODUCTIVE FUNCTION					
Dyspareunia is graded in the PAIN category.					
Dysmenorrhea is graded in the PAIN category.					
Erectile impotence	normal	mild (erections impaired but satisfac-tory)	moderate (erections impaired, unsatisfac-tory for intercourse)	no erections	-

(Continued on next page)

Appendix 9. National Cancer Institute Common Toxicity Criteria, Version 2.0 *(Continued)*

Toxicity	0	1	2	3	4
			Grade		
Female sterility	normal	-	-	sterile	-
Feminization of male is graded in the ENDOCRINE category.					
Irregular menses (change from baseline)	normal	occasionally irregular or lengthened interval, but continuing menstrual cycles	very irregular, but continuing menstrual cycles	persistent amenorrhea	-
Libido	normal	decrease in interest	severe loss of interest	-	-
Male infertility	-	-	oligospermia (low sperm count)	azoospermia (no sperm)	-
Masculinization of female is graded in the ENDOCRINE category.					
Vaginal dryness	normal	mild	requiring treatment and/or interfering with sexual function, dyspareunia	-	-
Sexual/Reproductive Function-Other (Specify, _____)	none	mild	moderate	severe	disabling
SYNDROMES (not included in previous categories)					
Acute vascular leak syndrome is graded in the CARDIOVASCULAR (GENERAL) category.					
ARDS (Adult Respiratory Distress Syndrome) is graded in the PULMONARY category.					
Autoimmune reactions are graded in the ALLERGY/IMMUNOLOGY category.					
DIC (disseminated intravascular coagulation) is graded in the COAGULATION category.					
Fanconi's syndrome is graded as Urinary electrolyte wasting in the RENAL/GENITOURINARY category.					
Renal tubular acidosis is graded as Urinary electrolyte wasting in the RENAL/GENITOURINARY category.					
Stevens-Johnson syndrome (erythema multiforme) is graded in the DERMATOLOGY/SKIN category.					
SIADH (syndrome of inappropriate antidiuretic hormone) is graded in the ENDOCRINE category.					
Thrombotic microangiopathy (e.g., thrombotic thrombocytopenic purpura/TTP or hemolytic uremic syndrome/HUS) is graded in the COAGULATION category.					
Tumor flare	none	mild pain not interfering with function	moderate pain; pain or analgesics interfering with function, but not interfering with activities of daily living	severe pain; pain or analgesics interfering with function and interfering with activities of daily living	disabling
Also consider Hypercalcemia.					
Note: Tumor flare is characterized by a constellation of symptoms and signs in direct relation to initiation of therapy (e.g., antiestrogens/androgens or additional hormones). The symptoms/signs include tumor pain, inflammation of visible tumor, hypercalcemia, diffuse bone pain, and other electrolyte disturbances.					
Tumor lysis syndrome	absent	-	-	present	-
Also consider Hyperkalemia, Creatinine.					
Urinary electrolyte wasting (e.g., Fanconi's syndrome, renal tubular acidosis) is graded under the RENAL/GENITOURINARY category.					
Syndromes-Other (Specify, _____)	none	mild	moderate	severe	life-threatening or disabling

Note. From *National Cancer Institute Common Toxicity Criteria, Version 2.0* [Online], revised March 23, 1998. Available: http://ctep.info.nih.gov/CTC3/ctc.htm [1999, January 20].

Appendix 10a. Adjuvant Drugs for Neuropathic Cancer Pain

Category	Mechanism of Action	Specific Drugs	Dose	Side Effects	Indications
Antidepressants	Block the reuptake of serotonin and norepinephrine in the central nervous system	Tricyclic antidepressants: amitriptyline, doxepine, imipramine, clomipramine, desipramine, nortriptyline	10–25 mg at bedtime initially; titrate to maximum dose of 150 mg at bedtime	Sedation, dry mouth, orthostatic hypotension, constipation, agitation	First-line therapeutic approach for neuropathic pain, continuous or intermittent and lancinating dyesthesias, diabetic neuropathy, postherpetic neuralgia, facial pain, postmastectomy pain
Anticonvulsants	Membrane stabilizer altering sodium and calcium influx; prevents action potential along the neuron	Carbamazepine Phenytoin	200 mg bid–qid 1,000 mg first 24 h, then 300–400 mg/d	Sedation, confusion, nausea, rash, bone marrow depression	Paroxysmal lancinating pains, plexopathies, postherpetic neuralgia
		Valproate Gabapentin	200–500 mg hs 900–2,400 mg/d		
Benzodiazepines	Unknown; does have anticonvulsant effects	Clonazepam	1.5 mg/day, titrate 0.5–1 mg q 3 days, dose should not exceed 20 mg/d	Sedation, dementia, hypotension, dizziness, respiratory depression	Second-/third-line approach, for patients who are refractory to antidepressant/ anticonvulsant therapy, for lancinating or paroxysmal pain
Corticosteroids	Reduce production of prostaglandins by inhibiting phospholipase activity, exact mechanism unknown	Dexamethasone	16–24 mg/d, 40 mg IV stat then 10 mg IV q 6 h for cord compression	Candidiasis, gastritis, fluid retention, insomnia, hypertension, hyperglycemia, psychosis	Refractory neuropathic pain, epidural cord compression, brachial and lumbosacral plexopathies RSD
		Prednisone	40–100 mg/day		
Hormones	Unknown	Calcitonin	100–200 IU/day SC; use skin test to rule out hypersensitivity	Nausea, urinary frequency, hypersensitivity reactions	Sympathetically maintained pain, acute phantom pain

(Continued on next page)

Appendix 10a. Adjuvant Drugs for Neuropathic Cancer Pain *(Continued)*

Category	Mechanism of Action	Specific Drugs	Dose	Side Effects	Indications
Local anesthetics	Block sodium channels at the site of nerve injury to reduce abnormal spontaneous and evoked neural discharges, stabilize nerve membrane	IV lidocaine	5 mg/kg infused over 30–60 minutes (serum levels 1–3 μg/ml)	Dizziness, nausea, tremors, nervousness, headache, paresthesias	Opioid-refractory, antidepressant/anticonvulsant refractory continuous dyesthesias; second-line approach for lancinating and continuous dyesthesias
		Oral mexilitine	150 mg at bedtime x 7 days then 150–250 mg tid if tolerated; can increase to 1,200 mg/d		
	Theoretically inhibits inflammatory response or ectopic impulse generation in cutaneous nerve branches, capsaicin cream thought to deplete substance P	Cutaneous: EMLA® (2.5% lidocaine & 2.5% prilocaine), lidocaine (5%–10%), capsaicin cream (0.025% & 0.075%)	Apply 4–5 times/day, treat for at least 4–6 weeks even if no relief first 2 weeks	Burning with application	Allodynia, hyperesthesia, postherpetic neuralgias, diabetic neuropathy, postsurgical neuropathic pain
Neuroleptics	Exact mechanism of action unknown, haloperidol potentiates morphine sulfate	Methotrimeprazine	5–10 mg IV q 6–8 h	Sedation, confusion, orthostatic hypotension, extrapyramidal symptoms	Trigeminal neuralgia, for patients with excessive opioid side effects
		Fluphenazine	1–5 mg 0.5–5 mg bid-qid		
		Haloperidol pimozide	0.2–0.3 mg/kg/d		
NMDA antagonists (experimental only)	Antagonize the excitatory amino acid (NMDA) involved in pain transmission, reduces the development of the "wind-up" phenomenon, refractory neuropathic pain	Dextromethorphan	40–60 mg·1 g/day short-term	Excessive salivation, purposeless movements, behavioral and cognitive changes	Postherpetic neuralgia, phantom pain, stump pain, postsurgical pain, allodynia
		Ketamine	Oral: 50 mg qid SC/IV: 0.2 mg/kg/h Epidural: usually combined with morphine		

(Continued on next page)

Appendix 10a. Adjuvant Drugs for Neuropathic Cancer Pain (Continued)

Category	Mechanism of Action	Specific Drugs	Dose	Side Effects	Indications
Beta$_2$ antagonist	Inhibits response to adrenergic stimuli	Propranolol	40 mg/d	Bradycardia, hypotension, rash	Trigeminal neuralgia, phantom pain, diabetic neuropathy
Alpha$_2$ agonist	Inhibits the release of endogenous norepinephrine from presynaptic adrenergic fibers, increases GABA activity (an inhibitory neurotransmitter)	Clonidine	Transcutaneous patch: 0.1 µg q 7 days Epidural: 30 µg/h	Sedation, dry mouth, orthostatic effects, weight gain, decreased libido, withdrawal	Opioid refractory pain, generalized neuropathic pain, sympathetically mediated pain
NSAIDs	Blocks conversion of arachadonic acid to prostaglandin E2 in the periphery	Ketorolac (experimental for neuropathic pain)	Continuous SC infusion: 120 mg/24 h	Gastropathy, renal failure, platelet dysfunction	Trigeminal neuralgia, reflex sympathetic dystrophy refractory to other treatment modalities

Abbreviations: bid—twice per day; EMLA—eutectic mixture of lidocaine and prilocaine; GABA—Gamma-aminobutyric acid; IU—International Units; RSD—reflex sympathetic dystrophy; po—oral; qid—four times per day; SC—subcutaneous; tid—three times per day

Doses are oral unless otherwise indicated.

Note. From "Cancer-Related Neuropathic Pain," by J. Brant, 1998, Nurse Practitioner Forum, 9(3), pp. 159–160. Copyright 1998 by W.B. Saunders Co. Reprinted with permission.

Appendix 10b. Cancer-Related Postoperative Pain Syndromes

Pain Syndrome	Associated Signs and Symptoms	Affected Nerves
Postradical neck dissection	A tight, burning sensation in the area of sensory loss Dyesthesias and shocklike pain may be present. Second type of pain may occur, mimicking a drooped shoulder syndrome.	Cervical plexus
Postmastectomy pain	Tight, constricting, burning pain in the posterior arm, axilla, and anterior chest wall. Pain exacerbated by arm movement	Intercostobrachial
Postthoracotomy pain	Aching sensation in the distribution of the incision with sensory loss with or without autonomic changes Often exquisite point tenderness at the most medial and apical points of the scar with a specific trigger point Secondary reflex sympathetic dystrophy may develop.	Intercostal
Postnephrectomy pain	Numbness, fullness, or heaviness in the flank, anterior abdomen, and groin Dyesthesias are common.	Superficial flank
Postlimb amputation	Phantom limb pain usually occurs after pain in the same site before amputation. Stump pain occurs at the site of the surgical scar several months to years after surgery and is characterized by a burning dyesthetic sensation that is exacerbated by movement.	Peripheral endings and their central projections

Note. From "Cancer-Related Neuropathic Pain," by J. Brant, 1998, *Nurse Practitioner Forum, 9*(3), p. 157. Copyright 1998 by W.B. Saunders Co. Reprinted with permission.

Appendix 11. Nonsteroidal Anti-Inflammatory Drugs

Drug	Usual Dose	Maximum Dose
Acetaminophen	650 mg q 4 h	975 mg q 6 h
Aspirin	650 mg q 4 h	6,500 mg in 24 hrs
Carprofen	100 mg tid	100 mg tid
Choline magnesium trisalicylate	1,000 mg tid	1,500 mg tid
Diflunisal	500 mg bid	500 mg tid
Etodolac	200 mg q 4–6 h	400 mg q 4–6 h
Fenoprofen calcium	300 mg q 6 h	600 mg q 6 h
Ibuprofen	400 mg q 6 h	600 mg q 6 h
Ketoprofen	25 mg q 6–8 h	60 mg q 6–8 h
Magnesium salicylate	650 mg q 4 h	650 mg q 4 h
Meclofenamate sodium	50 mg q 6 h	100 mg q 6 h
Mefenamic acid	250 mg q 6 h	Use for one week
Naproxen	250 mg q 6–8 h	1.25 g qd
Naproxen sodium	275 mg q 8 h	1.375 g qd
Sodium salicylate	325 mg q 3–4 h	650 mg q 3–4 h

Appendix 12. Paraneoplastic Syndromes

Disorder	Finding	Associated Malignancy
Cutaneous		
Sweet's syndrome (acute febrile neutrophilic dermatosis)	Tender erythematous plaques	Acute myelogenous leukemia, lymphoma, genitourinary (GU) cancers, breast cancer, stomach cancer
Acanthosis nigricans	Hyperpigmentation and velvety hyperkeratosis on flexural surfaces	Gastrointestinal (GI) adenocarcinoma
Paraneoplastic pemphigus	Generalized mucocutaneous blistering	Lymphoma, thymoma, chronic lymphocytic leukemia, sarcoma, bronchogenic squamous cell carcinoma
Amyloidosis	Pink or yellow elevated nodules, translucent papules, waxy appearance	Multiple myeloma, macroglobulinemia
Acquired ichthyosis	Generalized dry scaling of the skin with accentuation over the shins	Hodgkin's disease
Gardner's syndrome	Multiple epidermoid cysts, desmoid tumors, fibroma, and lipoma. Hallmark is intestinal polyposis of the colon and rectum.	Colon adenocarcinoma
Neurofibromatosis	Neurofibroma, axillary freckling	Neurofibrosarcoma, pheochromocytoma, leukemia
Endocrine		
Syndrome of inappropriate antidiuretic hormone (SIADH)	Hyponatremia from excessive urine output	Small cell lung cancer, carcinoid, esophageal cancer, duodenal cancer, colon cancer, pancreatic cancer, prostate cancer, thymoma, lymphoma
Cushing's syndrome	Excessive production of ectopic adrenocorticotrophic hormone; increased pigmentation, hypokalemia	Small cell lung cancer, thymoma, pancreatic cancer, carcinoid, pheochromocytoma, thyroid cancer
Hypocalcemia	Decrease serum calcium, parathyroid hormone-related protein	Bone metastasis from cancer of the lung, prostate, breast, ovary, head and neck, bladder, or kidney
Hypophosphatemia	Decrease serum phosphorus	Mesenchymal tumors (arising from connective or fibrous tissue)
Hyperthyroidism	Decrease thyroid-stimulating hormone, increase T_3 and T_4	Lung cancer

(Continued on next page)

Appendix 12. Paraneoplastic Syndromes *(Continued)*

Disorder	Finding	Associated Malignancy
Gynecomastia	Increase in breast tissue	Lung cancer, adrenal cancer, testicular cancer, hepatoma, breast cancer in men
Acromegaly	Overproduction of growth hormone	Carcinoid, pheochromocytoma, pancreatic cancer
Carcinoid syndrome	Flushing, diarrhea, bronchospasm	GI cancers, cancer of the larynx, lung, breast, ovary, or testicle
Hypoglycemia	Decrease serum glucose	Fibrosarcoma, mesothelioma, hepatoma, GI adenocarcinoma, cancer of the breast, lung, kidney, or ovary
Hypercalcemia	Increase serum calcium	Cancer of the breast, lung, kidney, or ovary
Hyperpyrexia and fever	Increased in temperature, release of pyrogens from the tumor, inability to detoxify endogenous endotoxin	Hepatic metastasis, Hodgkin's disease, lymphoma, sarcoma
Nephrotic syndrome	Massive edema with proteinuria hypoalbuminemia	Hodgkin's disease
Hematologic		
Disseminated intravascular coagulation	Thromboplastin-like agent fibrinolytic system activation, increased fibrin degradation products	Acute promyelocytic leukemia, prostate cancer
Trousseau's syndrome	Deep venous thrombosis	Cancer of lung, colon, pancreas, breast, ovary, or prostate
Hypercoagulability	Disruption of clotting factors such as protein C, protein S, tissue plasminogen factor, antithrombin III	Adenocarcinoma, multiple myeloma
Musculoskeletal		
Hypertrophic osteoarthropathy	Digital clubbing and tenderness along the distal long bones	Non-small cell lung cancer, lung metastasis
Neurologic		
Lambert-Eaton myasthenic syndrome	Mediator of voltage-gated calcium channel antibodies, proximal muscle weakness of limbs	Cancer of bladder, kidney, breast, stomach, colon, prostate, or gallbladder, small cell lung cancer, lymphoma, sarcoma, thymoma
Sensory neuronopathy	Affects the cell bodies of sensory neurons in dorsal root ganglion	Carcinomas

(Continued on next page)

Appendix 12. Paraneoplastic Syndromes *(Continued)*

Disorder	Finding	Associated Malignancy
Motor neuronopathy	Disorder of anterior horn cells	Lymphoma
Paraneoplastic cortical cerebellar degeneration	Injury to the Purkinje cells of the cerebellum, ataxia, dysarthria, dysphagia, dementia	Small cell lung cancer, breast cancer, ovarian cancer, GU cancers, colon cancer, prostate cancer, sarcoma, neuroblastoma, Hodgkin's disease, lymphoma

Paraneoplastic syndromes can affect a variety of body systems, including endocrine, hematological, epithelial, nervous, renal, gastrointestinal, immunologic, and musculoskeletal. They most commonly are associated with cancer of lung, breast and stomach. Diagnosis is difficult because signs and symptoms represent other clinical abnormalities. Treatment is based on removing the underlying cancer with cancer treatment or suppressing the mediator causing the syndrome.

Barnett, M.L. (1999). Hypercalcemia. *Seminars in Oncology Nursing, 15,* 190–201.
Cohen, P.R., & Kurzrock, R. (1997). Mucocutaneous paraneoplastic syndromes. *Seminars in Oncology, 24,* 334–359.
Gobel, B.H. (1999). Disseminated intravascular coagulation. *Seminars in Oncology Nursing, 15,* 174–182.
Hall, T.C. (1997). Paraneoplastic syndromes. *Hospital Practice, 22,* 105–124.
Haylock, P.J. (1998). Metastatic disease: Nursing implications. *Seminars in Oncology Nursing, 14,* 171–246.
Keenan, A.M.M. (1999). Syndrome of inappropriate secretion of antidiuretic hormone in malignancy. *Seminars in Oncology Nursing, 15,* 160–167.
Keffer, J.H. (1996). Endocrinopathy and ectopic hormones in malignancy. *Hematology/Oncology Clinics of North America, 10,* 811–824.

Appendix 13. Physical Exam Techniques

• **Chvostek's sign:** Used to evaluate hypocalcemia
Technique: Tap the facial nerve.
Positive sign: Twitching of muscles around the mouth, nose, or eyes

• **Fluid wave:** To evaluate for ascites
Technique: Procedure requires three hands; consequently, assistance from the patient or another examiner is needed. Ask patient to lie supine. Ask patient or another examiner to press the edge of the hand and forearm firmly along the vertical midline of the abdomen. This position helps to stop the transmission of a wave through the adipose tissue. Place your hands on each side of the abdomen and strike one side sharply with your fingers. Feel for the wave impulse with the fingers of the other hand.
Positive sign: Feeling a fluid wave may indicate ascites; however, this test is not conclusive because a fluid wave can be detected in patients without ascites or not detected in patients with ascites.

• **Homans' sign:** Evaluative test for deep venous thrombosis
Technique: Flex the patient's knee slightly with one hand, and dorsiflex the foot with the other hand.
Positive sign: Complaint of calf pain, indicating thrombosis

• **Iliopsoas muscle test:** Evaluative test for appendicitis
Technique: Ask the patient to lie supine and place your hand over the lower thigh. Ask the patient to raise the leg, flexing at the hip, while you push downward against the leg.
Positive sign: Lower quadrant pain is experienced.

• **Jugular vein measurement:** Indicates volume and pressure in the right side of the heart
Technique: Ask the patient to slowly lean back into a supine position. Using a ruler, measure the vertical distance between the angle of Louis (manubriosternal joint) and the highest level of jugular vein pulsation on both sides. Record the measurement. Note symmetry of right and left jugular veins.
Positive sign: Measurement greater than 2 cm. Distention on one side suggests localized abnormality. Bilateral distention indicates cardiac etiology.

• **Murphy's sign:** Evaluation of gallbladder disease
Technique: Palpate liver
Positive sign: Pain on inspiration during palpation of liver or gallbladder that causes the patient to stop breathing

• **Neurologic-specific tests:** Evaluation for accuracy of movements and coordination
1. Finger-to-finger test: Ask patient to use the index finger and alternately touch his or her nose and your index finger. Position your index finger about 18 inches from the patient and change location of your finger several times.
2. Finger-to-nose test: Ask the patient to close their eyes and touch his or her nose with the index finger of each hand.
3. Heel-to-shin test: Can be performed with patient standing, sitting, or supine. Ask the patient to run their heel of one foot up and down the shin of the opposite leg. Repeat with other leg.
Positive sign: Abnormal movement or incoordination of movement
4. Rapid rhythmic alternating movements: To evaluate fine motor skills and coordination. Ask the seated patient to pat his or her knees with both hands, alternately turning up the palm and the back of the hands or have the patient touch the thumb to each finger on the same hand, sequentially from the index finger to the little finger and back.

(Continued on next page)

Appendix 13. Physical Exam Techniques *(Continued)*

• **Obturator muscle test:** To evaluate for a ruptured appendix or a pelvic abscess
  Technique: Ask patient to lie supine and flex the right leg at the hip and knee to 90 degrees. Hold the leg just above the knee, grasp the ankle and rotate the leg laterally and medially.
  Positive sign: Pain in the hypogastric region indicates irritation of the obturator muscle.

• **Pulse paradoxus:** To evaluate for cardiac tamponade, constrictive pericarditis, or chronic pulmonary obstructive disease
  Technique:
  1. Ask patient to breathe easily and as normal as possible.
  2. Apply sphygmomanometer and inflate until no sounds are audible.
  3. Deflate cuff gradually until sounds are audible only during expiration and note the pressure.
  4. Deflate cuff further until sounds are audible during inspiration and note the pressure.
  Positive sign: A difference greater than 10 mm Hg, the paradoxical pulse is exaggerated. Associated findings include low blood pressure and a weak rapid pulse.

• **Rinne test:** To evaluate hearing for air and bone conduction
  Technique: Place the base of the vibrating tuning fork against the patient's mastoid bone. Time the interval and ask the patient to tell you when the sound is no longer heard, noting the time in seconds. Quickly position the vibrating tuning fork 1–2 cm from the auditory canal and ask the patient to tell you when the sound is no longer heard. Continue to time the interval to determine the length of time the sound is heard by air conduction. Compare the number of seconds the sound is heard by bone conduction versus air conduction.
  Negative sign: Bone conduction is heard longer than air conduction in affected ear, indicating conductive hearing loss. Positive Rinne or equal to the air conduction heard longer than bone conduction in affected ear, indicating sensorineural hearing loss.

• **Scratch test:** To evaluate for hepatomegaly
  Technique: With stethoscope over the liver, lightly scratch the abdominal surface moving toward the liver. The sound will be magnified over the liver.
  Positive sign: A liver size greater than 4–8 cm in the midsternal line and liver span greater than 8 cm

• **Trousseau's sign:** To evaluate for hypocalcemia
  Technique: Apply sphygmomanometer and inflate midway between systolic and diastolic pressures.
  Positive sign: Spasm of the hand during three to four minutes of exercise while the cuff is inflated

• **Weber test:** To evaluate lateralization of sound
  Technique: Place the base of the vibrating tuning fork on the midline vertex of the patient's head. Ask patient if the sound is heard equally in both ears or is better in one ear.
  Positive sign: Lateralization to affected ear indicates hearing loss. Lateralization to better ear, unless conductive loss, indicates sensorineural hearing loss.

Appendix 14. Topical Corticosteroid Preparations*

Group 1. Highest Potency
Betamethasone dipropionate in optimized vehicle 0.05% cream, ointment, solution (Diprolene®a)
Clobetasol propionate 0.05% cream, ointment, solution (Temovate®b)
Halobetasol propionate 0.05% cream, ointment (Ultravate®c)
Diflorasone diacetate 0.05% cream, ointment (Psorcon®d)

Group 2. High Potency
Amcinonide 0.1% ointment (Cyclocort ®e)
Betamethasone dipropionate 0.05% ointment (Diprolene®a)
Desoximetasone 0.25% cream and ointment (Topicort®f)
Fluocinonide 0.05% cream, gel, ointment, solution (Lidex®g)
Halcinonide 0.1% cream, ointment (Halog®c)

Group 3. Medium-High Potency
Amcinonide 0.1% cream (Cyclocort)
Betamethasone dipropionate 0.05% cream (Diprolene)
Diflorasone diacetate 0.05% cream, ointment (Florone®h, Maxiflor®i)

Group 4. Medium Potency
Desoximetasone 0.05% cream (Topicort LP®f)
Flurandrenolide 0.05% ointment (Cordran® i)
Hydrocortisone butyrate 0.1% ointment (Locoid®k)
Hydrocortisone valerate 0.2% ointment (Westcort®c)
Mometasone furoate 0.1% cream, ointment (Elocon®a)
Triamcinolone acetonide 0.1% ointment (Aristocort®e, Kenalog®c)

Group 5. Low Potency
Alclometasone dipropionate 0.05% cream (Aclovate®b)
Betamethasone valerate 0.1% cream (Valisone®a)
Flurandrenolide 0.05% cream (Cordran®l)
Fluocinolone acetonide 0.025% cream (Synalar®m, Synemol®m, Fluonid®i)
Hydrocortisone butyrate 0.1% cream (Locoid®k)
Hydrocortisone valerate 0.2% cream (Westcort)
Triamcinolone acetonide 0.1% cream or lotion (Aristocort, Kenalog)

Group 6. Mild Potency
Desonide 0.05% cream (Tridesilon®n)
Fluocinolone acetonide 0.01% solution (Fluonid®i, Synalar®m)

Group 7. Lowest Potency
Dexamethasone 0.1% gel, ointment (Decadron®υ)
Hydrocortisone 0.5%, 1%, and 2.5% cream, ointment, lotion (Hytone®d, Synacort®m, Nutracort®p)

---

* It is recommended that one become familiar with and use one agent from each category, making the selection on the basis of cost, cosmetic acceptability, and efficacy.

a Schering Corp., Kenilworth, NJ ; b Glaxo Wellcome Inc., Research Triangle Park, NC; c Westwood-Squibb, Princeton, NJ; dDermik Laboratories, Inc., Collegeville, PA; e Fujisawa Healthcare, Inc., Deerfield, IL; f Hoechst Marion Roussel, Kansas City, MO; g Syntex Laboratories, inc., Palo Alto, CA; h The Upjohn Co., Kalamazoo, MI; i Allergan, Inc., Irvine, CA; i Oclassen Pharmaceuticals, Inc., Corona, CA; k Ferndale Laboratories, Inc., Ferndale, MI; l Eli Lilly & Co., Indianapolis, IN; m Medicis, Phoenix, AZ; n Bayer Corp., West Haven, CT; o Merck & Co., West Point, PA; p Alcon Laboratories, Inc., Fort Worth, TX

Note. From Primary Care Medicine (p. 907), by A.H. Goroll, L.A. May, and A.G. Mulley, 1995, Philadelphia: J.B. Lippincott Co. Copyright 1995 by J.B. Lippincott Co. Reprinted with permission.

Appendix 15. Topical Nasal Steroids

Action: Aerosol preparations deliver corticosteroids to the airways with minimal systemic absorption.
Indications: For relief of nasal congestion from environmental allergens causing allergic rhinitis.

Contraindications: Hypersensitivity to the product.

Special considerations: The development of localized infections of the nose and pharynx with *Candida albicans* has been reported. The incidence may increase when the patient is immunocompromised.

Generic	Brand Name	Adult Dosage
Azelastine	Astelin®[a]	2 sprays per nostril bid
Beclomethasone	Vancenase®[b], Beconase®[c]	1 spray per nostril bid–qid
Budesonide	Rhinocort®[d]	2 sprays per nostril bid or 4 sprays qd
Dexamethasone	Decadron®[e]	2 sprays per nostril bid–tid
Flunisolide	Nasalide®[f], Nasarel®[f]	2 sprays per nostril bid–qid
Triamcinolone	Nasacort®[g]	2 sprays per nostril qd–bid

[a] Carter-Wallace, Inc., New York, NY; [b] Schering Corp. Kenilworth, NJ; [c] Glaxo Wellcome Inc., Research Triangle Park, NC; [d] Astra Pharmaceuticals, LP, Wayne, PA; e Merck & Co., Inc., Whitehouse Station, NJ; [f] Dura Pharmaceuticals, San Diego, CA; [g] Rhône-Poulenc Rorer Pharmaceuticals, Inc., Collegeville, PA

Appendix 16. Tumor Markers

Tumor Marker	Reference Value	Application in Cancer	Comments
Antigens			
Alpha-fetoprotein (AFP)	< 8.5 ng/ml	Testicular cancer, choriocarcinoma, cancer of the pancreas, colon, lung, stomach, biliary system and liver	Also elevated in cirrhosis, hepatitis, and liver injury
Carcinoembryonic antigen (CEA)	0–5.0 ng/ml	Cancers of the breast, lung, prostate, pancreas, stomach, colon, and rectum	Elevated in smokers, COPD, pancreatitis, hepatitis and inflammatory bowel disease
CA- 19-9	< 37 U/ml	Cancers of the pancreas, colon, and stomach	–
CA-125	< 35 U/ml	Cancers of the ovary, pancreas, breast, and colon	–
CA-27-29	0–38 U/ml	Breast cancer	–
Prostate-specific antigen (PSA)	0–4.0 ng/ml	Prostate cancer	Often used as a screening tool for prostate cancer
Enzymes			
Lactic dehydrogenase (LDH)	100–215 U/l	Lymphoma, seminoma, acute leukemia, and metastatic cancer	Also elevated in hepatitis and myocardial infarction
Prostatic acid phosphatase (PAP)	0–3.2 ng/ml	Metastatic cancer of the prostate, myeloma, lung cancer and osteogenic sarcoma	–
Hormones			
Parathyroid hormone	11–54 pg/ml * depends upon the type of method used	Etopic hyperparathyroidism from cancers of the kidney, lung (squamous cell), pancreas, and ovary and myeloma	Also elevated in primary hyperparathyroidism
Estrogen receptors	Greater than 10% nuclear reactivity is considered positive	Breast cancer	Used to evaluate prognosis and base treatment
Progesterone receptors	Greater than 10% nuclear reactivity is considered positive	Breast cancer	Used to evaluate prognosis and base treatment
Calcitonin	M < 40 pg/ml F < 20 pg/ml	Medullary thyroid, small-cell lung cancer, breast cancer and carcinoid	–
Antidiuretic hormone	< 285 mOsm/kg	Small-cell lung cancer and adenocarcinomas	Also elevated in SIADH in pneumonia and porhyria

(Continued on next page)

Appendix 16. Tumor Markers *(Continued)*

Tumor Marker	Reference Value	Application in Cancer	Comments
Adrenocorticotropic hormone (ACTH)	Up to 70 pg/ml	Cancers of the lung, prostate, gastrointestinal tract, and neuroendrocrine system	Also elevated in Cushing's disease
Human chorionic gonadotrophin	< 25 mg/ml	Choriocarcinoma, germ cell testicular cancer, etopic production in cancer of stomach, pancreas, lung, colon, and liver	Also elevated in pregnancy
Proteins			
Serum immunoglobulins		Myeloma, lymphoma	Also elevated in connective tissue disease, benign monoclonal gammopathy, chronic renal failure
IgG	800–1700 mg/dl	IgG myeloma	
IgA	85–490 mg/dl	IgA myeloma	
IgM	50–370 mg/dl	Waldenstrom's	
IgE	0–120 IU/ml	IgE myeloma	
Beta-2 microglobulin	0–1.8/l	Myeloma and lymphoma	–

Tumor markers are cellular products that are abnormally elevated by malignancies. These markers may be useful in diagnosis and prognosis of cancer and in monitoring of cancer treatments. Special considerations need to be given tot he sensitivity and specificity of each marker.

Normal values will differ according to the laboratory.

Appendix 17. Dermatomes and Areas of Sensory Innervation by Certain Peripheral Nerves

Dermatomes, Anterior View

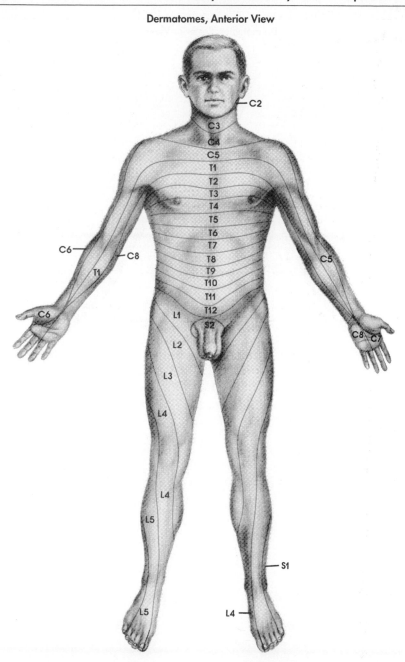

(Continued on next page)

Appendix 17. Dermatomes and Areas of Sensory Innervation by Certain Peripheral Nerves (Continued)

Dermatomes, Posterior View

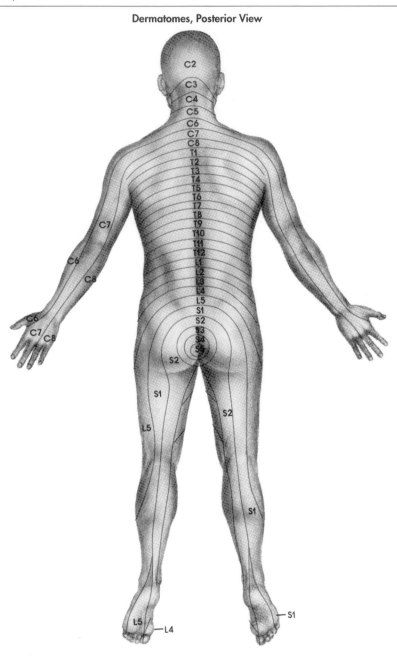

(Continued on next page)

Appendix 17. Dermatomes and Areas of Sensory Innervation by Certain Peripheral Nerves (Continued)

Areas of Sensory Innervation, Anterior View

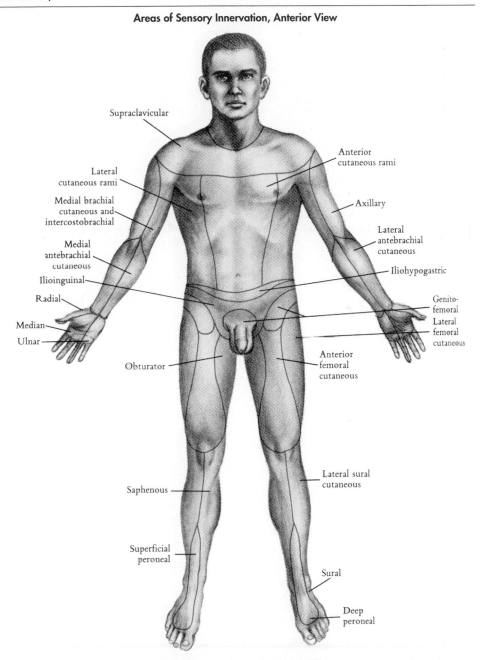

(Continued on next page)

Appendix 17. Dermatomes and Areas of Sensory Innervation by Certain Peripheral Nerves (Continued)

Areas of Sensory Innervation , Posterior View

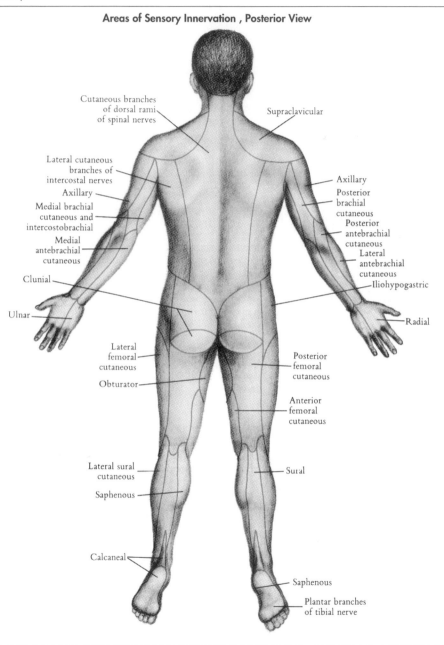

Cutaneous branches of dorsal rami of spinal nerves

Supraclavicular

Lateral cutaneous branches of intercostal nerves

Axillary

Medial brachial cutaneous and intercostobrachial

Medial antebrachial cutaneous

Clunial

Ulnar

Axillary

Posterior brachial cutaneous

Posterior antebrachial cutaneous

Lateral antebrachial cutaneous

Iliohypogastric

Radial

Lateral femoral cutaneous

Obturator

Posterior femoral cutaneous

Anterior femoral cutaneous

Lateral sural cutaneous

Saphenous

Sural

Calcaneal

Saphenous

Plantar branches of tibial nerve

Note. From *Mosby's Guide to Physical Examination* (2nd ed.) (pp. 628–631), by H.M. Seidel, J.W. Ball, J.E. Dains, and G.W. Benedict (Eds.), 1991, St. Louis: Mosby. Copyright 1991 by Mosby. Reprinted with permission.

Appendix 18. Additional Resources

Bates, B. (1995). *A guide to physical examination* (6th ed.). St. Louis: Mosby.

Berger, A., Portenoy, R.K., & Weissman, D.E. (1998). *Principles and practice of supportive oncology.* Philadelphia: Lippincott-Raven.

Carey, C.F., Lee, H.H., & Woeltje, K.F. (1998). *The Washington manual of medical therapeutics* (29th ed.). Philadelphia: Lippincott-Raven.

Casciato, D.A., & Lowitz, B.B. (1995). *Manual of clinical oncology* (3rd ed.). Boston: Little, Brown & Co.

Cutler, P. (1998). *Problem solving in clinical medicine: From data to diagnosis* (3rd ed.). Baltimore: Williams & Wilkins.

DeVita, V.T., Hellman, S., & Rosenberg, S.A. (Eds.). (2000). *Cancer: Principles and practice of oncology* (6th ed.). Philadelphia: Lippincott-Raven.

DiGregorio, G.J., & Barbier, E.J. (1998). *Handbook of commonly prescribed drugs* (13th ed.). West Chester, PA: Medical Surveillance.

Fauci, A.S., Braunwald, E., Isselbacher, K.J., Wilson, J.D., Martin, J.B., Dasper, D.L., Hauser, S.L., & Longo, D.L. (1998). *Harrison's principles of internal medicine* (14th ed.). New York: McGraw-Hill.

Goodheart, H.P. (1999). *A photoguide to common skin disorders: Diagnosis and management.* Baltimore: Williams & Wilkins.

Goroll, A.H., May, L.A., & Mulley, A.G. (1995). *Primary care medicine* (3rd ed.). Philadelphia: Lippincott-Raven.

Katzung, B.G. (1998). Basic and clinical pharmacology (7th ed.). Norwalk, CT: Appleton & Lange.

Medical Economics Company. (1999). *Physicians desk reference* (53rd ed.). Montvale, NJ: Author.

Medical Economics Company. (1999). *Physicians desk reference for herbal medicine.* Montvale, NJ: Author.

Moss, K., & Arbogat, S.L. (1997). *Nurse's manual of infectious diseases.* Boston: Little, Brown & Co.

Seidel, H.M., Ball, J.W., Benedict, G.W. & Dains, J.F. (1999). *Mosby's guide to physical examination* (4th ed.). St. Louis: Mosby.

Uphold, C.R., & Graham, M.V. (1999). *Clinical guideline in adult health* (2nd ed.). Gainsville: Barmarrâe Books.

Wallach, J. (1998). *Handbook of interpretation of diagnostic tests* (6th ed.). Philadelphia: Lippincott-Raven.

Yarbro, C.H., Frogge. M.H., Goodman, M., & Groenwald, S.L. (Eds.). (1997). *Cancer nursing: Principles and practice* (4th ed.). Boston: Jones & Bartlett.

Index

Index

Page references in **boldface** indicate a chapter on the topic.
A letter *f* after the page number indicates a figure or figures; the letter *t* indicates a table.
Drug names are given in the generic form, followed by the trade names (when available).

A

B

F

I

N

Q

R

S